Clinical Problems in

ACUTE CARE MEDICINE

James J. Heffernan, M.D.

Associate Visiting Physician, Department of Medicine
Boston City Hospital

Associate Professor of Medicine, Department of Medicine
Boston University School of Medicine, Boston, Massachusetts

Robert A. Witzburg, M.D.

Associate Director, Department of Medicine
Boston City Hospital

Associate Professor of Medicine, Department of Medicine
Boston University School of Medicine, Boston, Massachusetts

Alan S. Cohen, M.D.

Chief of Medicine, Boston City Hospital
Director, Thorndike Memorial Laboratory

Conrad Wesselhoeft Professor of Medicine
Boston University School of Medicine, Boston, Massachusetts

1989
W. B. SAUNDERS COMPANY
Harcourt Brace Jovanovich, Inc.
Philadelphia   London   Toronto
Montreal   Sydney   Tokyo

W.B. SAUNDERS COMPANY
Harcourt Brace Jovanovich, Inc.

The Curtis Center
Independence Square West
Philadelphia, PA 19106

Library of Congress Cataloging-in-Publication Data

Clinical problems in acute care medicine / [edited by] James J.
Heffernan, Robert A. Witzburg, Alan S. Cohen.
    p. cm.
    1. Critical care medicine. 2. Medical emergencies.
I. Heffernan, James J. II. Witzburg, Robert A. III. Cohen, Alan S.
    [DNLM: 1. Acute Disease. 2. Critical Care. WB 105 C6408]
RC86.7.C54 1989
616'.028—dc19
DNLM/DLC
ISBN 0-7216-1155-9   88-11337

Editor: John Dyson
Designer: Joanne Carroll
Production Manager: Bill Preston
Manuscript Editor: Tom Stringer
Cover Designer: Ann O'Donnell
Illustration Coordinator: Lisa Lambert
Indexer: Ellen Murray

Clinical Problems in Acute Care Medicine   ISBN 0-7216-1155-9

Last digit is the print number: 9   8   7   6   5   4   3   2   1 *to Anita, Lorraine, and Joan*

CONTRIBUTORS

Note: An asterisk denotes contributors who are formerly of Boston City Hospital.

EDWARD AGURA, M.D.*
Hematology Fellow, Fred Hutchinson Cancer Research Center, Seattle, Washington
Beta Blocker Overdose

CARL S. APSTEIN, M.D.
Chief of Cardiology, Boston City Hospital; Professor of Medicine, Boston University School of Medicine, Boston, Massachusetts
Acute Myocardial Infarction; Unstable Angina

GARY J. BALADY, M.D.
Staff Cardiologist, University Hospital; Assistant Professor of Medicine, Boston University School of Medicine, Boston, Massachusetts
Ventricular Dysrhythmias and Sudden Death

M. ANITA BARRY, M.D., M.P.H.
Director, Community Infectious Disease Epidemiology Program, Department of Health and Hospitals; Assistant Professor of Medicine, Boston University School of Medicine; Boston City Hospital, Boston, Massachusetts
Toxic Shock Syndrome

DAVID BERNARD, M.D.
Professor of Medicine, Boston University School of Medicine; Staff Physician, University Hospital, Boston, Massachusetts
Acute Renal Failure; Nephrolithiasis

BARBARA BJORNSON, M.D.*
Staff Hematologist/Oncologist, Malden Hospital, Malden, Massachusetts
Hyperleukocytic and Hyperviscosity Syndromes

v

RITA BLANCHARD, M.D.
Assistant Visiting Physician, Boston City Hospital; Assistant Professor of Medicine, Boston University School of Medicine, Boston, Massachusetts
Disseminated Intravascular Coagulation; Thrombocytopenia; The Prolonged Partial Thromboplastin Time: Anticoagulant Overdose and Common Congenital Factor Deficiencies

CHARLES MICHAEL BLISS, M.D.
Visiting Physician, Boston City Hospital; Associate Professor of Medicine, Boston University School of Medicine, Boston, Massachusetts
Acid Peptic Disease

MARK J. BRAUER, M.D.
Associate Visiting Physician, Boston City Hospital; Associate Clinical Professor of Medicine, Boston University School of Medicine, Boston, Massachusetts
Hemolytic Syndromes; Transfusion Reactions

JOHN B. CADIGAN, III, M.D.
Assistant Visiting Physician, Boston City Hospital; Instructor of Medicine, Boston University School of Medicine, Boston, Massachusetts; Staff, The Guild Medical Center, Norwood, Massachusetts
Supraventricular Tachycardia: Diagnosis and Treatment

ALAN S. COHEN, M.D.
Chief of Medicine, Boston City Hospital; Director, Thorndike Memorial Laboratory; Conrad Wesselhoeft Professor of Medicine, Boston University School of Medicine, Boston, Massachusetts

RAVIN DAVIDOFF, M.D.*
Staff Cardiologist, Veterans Administration Medical Center, Albany, New York
Adrenal Insufficiency; Cushing's Syndrome; Pheochromocytoma

CHAD DEAL, M.D.*
Assistant Professor of Medicine, Case Western Reserve University School of Medicine; Staff, University Hospitals of Cleveland, Cleveland, Ohio
Acute Presentations of Common Rheumatic Disorders; Anaphylaxis; Angioedema; Septic Arthritis

ROCHELLE L. EPSTEIN, M.D.*

Director of Biological Sciences, Department of Medicine, University of Chicago, Chicago, Illinois
Acute Sinusitis and Its Complications; Pyelonephritis; Pelvic Inflammatory Disease

ARTHUR H. ESKEW, M.D.

Assistant Visiting Physician, Boston City Hospital; Instructor of Medicine, Boston University School of Medicine, Boston, Massachusetts
Thromboembolic Disease

ROBERTA M. FALKE, M.D.*

Staff Oncologist, Winchester Hospital, Winchester, Massachusetts
Acute Complications of Chemotherapy; Cancer Pain: Acute Management

JAMES FELDMAN, M.D.

Associate Director of Emergency Services, Boston City Hospital, Assistant Professor of Medicine, Boston University School of Medicine, Boston, Massachusetts
Heat Illness

DAVID FELSON, M.D.

Assistant Visiting Physician, Boston City Hospital; Assistant Professor of Medicine, Boston University School of Medicine, Boston, Massachusetts
Approach to the Patient with Acute Rheumatic Disease; Soft Tissue Rheumatism; Acute Low Back Pain; Crystal-Induced Arthritis

EDWARD FISCHER, M.D.

Department of Neurosurgery, University Hospital/Boston City Hospital, Boston, Massachusetts
Management of Acute Head Injury

ELYSE FOSTER, M.D.

Assistant Visiting Physician, Boston City Hospital; Assistant Professor of Medicine, Boston University School of Medicine, Boston, Massachusetts
Diseases of the Cardiac Conduction System

CLAIRE FRITSCHE, M.D.*
Assistant Professor of Medicine, Medical College of Wisconsin, Milwaukee, Wisconsin
Metabolic Acidosis; Metabolic Alkalosis; Respiratory Acid-Base Disorders

GARY R. GARBER, M.D.
Staff Cardiologist, University Hospital; Instructor of Medicine, Boston University School of Medicine, Boston, Massachusetts
Hemoptysis

ROBERT GOLDMAN, M.D.
Private Practice, Neurology, New Haven, Connecticut
Spinal Cord Compression

WILLIAM HALE, M.D.*
Gastroenterology, New Canaan Medical Group, New Canaan, Connecticut
Intestinal Ischemia; Inflammatory Bowel Disease; Acetaminophen Poisoning; Methanol, Ethylene Glycol, and Isopropyl Alcohol

JAMES J. HEFFERNAN, M.D.
Associate Visiting Physician, Department of Medicine, Boston City Hospital; Associate Professor of Medicine, Department of Medicine, Boston University School of Medicine, Boston, Massachusetts
Shock; Syncope/Transient Loss of Consciousness; Spontaneous Bacterial Peritonitis; Tetanus; Aspiration Syndromes; The Ethanol Withdrawal Syndrome

KAREN HENLEY, M.D.
Assistant Visiting Physician, Boston City Hospital; Instructor of Medicine, Boston University School of Medicine, Boston, Massachusetts
Diabetic Ketoacidosis; Hypoglycemia; Nonketotic Hyperosmolar Coma; Alcoholic Ketoacidosis

BELDON A. IDELSON, M.D.
Visiting Physician, University Hospital; Associate Professor of Medicine, Boston University School of Medicine, Boston, Massachusetts
Hematuria; Uremia

MARTIN JOYCE-BRADY, M.D.

Assistant Visiting Physician, Boston City Hospital; Assistant Professor of Medicine, Boston University School of Medicine, Boston, Massachusetts
Adult Respiratory Distress Syndrome; Acute Respiratory Failure in Chronic Obstructive Pulmonary Disease; Diseases of the Pleura; Tuberculosis

RAYMOND S. KOFF, M.D.

Chief of Medicine, Framingham Union Hospital, Framingham, Massachusetts; Professor of Medicine, Boston University School of Medicine, Boston, Massachusetts
Hepatic Failure; Hepatitis

HOWARD LIBMAN, M.D.

Assistant Visiting Physician, Boston City Hospital; Assistant Professor of Medicine, Boston University School of Medicine, Boston, Massachusetts
Endocarditis; Meningitis and Encephalitis; Brain Abscess; Pneumonia; Legionnaires' Disease; Infection in the Immunocompromised Host; Human Immunodeficiency Virus Infection

WILFRED LIEBERTHAL, M.D.

Assistant Visiting Physician, University Hospital; Assistant Professor of Medicine, Boston University School of Medicine, Boston, Massachusetts
Hypernatremia and Hyponatremia; Hyperkalemia and Hypokalemia

CLAUDIA McCLINTOCK, M.D.*

Staff Gastroenterologist, Woodhull Medical Center, Brooklyn, New York
Upper Gastrointestinal Tract Bleeding

BARBARA A. McQUINN, M.D.*

Private Practice, Neurology, Oakland, California
Transient Ischemic Attacks; Stroke

CAROL M. MEILS, M.D.*

Cardiology Fellow, Department of Cardiology, Johns Hopkins Hospital, Baltimore, Maryland
Cocaine Poisoning

JOSEPH MIASKIEWICZ, M.D.*
Pulmonary Medicine, Puritan Medical Center, Salem, Massachusetts
Asthma

FRANK E. MURRAY, M.B., M.R.C.P.I., M.R.C.P.*
Private Practice, Gastroenterology, Dublin, Ireland
Diarrhea; Acute Pancreatitis; Chronic Pancreatitis; Biliary Tract Disease

JONATHAN NEWMARK, M.D.*
Department of Neurology, University of Louisville, Louisville, Kentucky
Myasthenia Gravis

TERESA A. NOLAN, M.D.*
Private Practice, Hematology, Pittsburgh, Pennsylvania
Superior Vena Cava Syndrome

JOE I. ORDIA, M.D.
Department of Neurosurgery, University Hospital, Boston, Massachusetts;
Associate Professor of Neurosurgery, Boston University School of Medicine,
Boston, Massachusetts
Aneurysmal Subarachnoid Hemorrhage

STEVEN W. PASKAL, M.D.*
Internal Medicine, Harvard Community Health Plan, Medford, Massachu-
setts
Adverse Reactions to Iodinated Contrast Media; Salicylate Intoxication

JON PEHRSON, M.D.
Assistant Visiting Physician, Boston City Hospital; Assistant Professor of
Medicine, Boston University School of Medicine, Boston, Massachusetts
*Pituitary Disorders; Thyroid Disorders; Disorders of Mineral Metabolism;
Pheochromocytoma*

JONATHAN F. PLEHN, M.D.*
Staff Cardiologist, Mary Hitchcock Medical Center, Hanover, New Hampshire; Assistant Professor of Medicine, Dartmouth College of Medicine, Hanover, New Hampshire
Supraventricular Tachycardia: Diagnosis and Treatment; Acute Pericarditis and Cardiac Tamponade; Dissecting Aortic Aneurysm; Blunt Cardiac Trauma

WILLIAM ROBINSON, M.D.*
Private Practice, Gastroenterology, Troy, New York
Diverticular Disease

MICHAEL ROSENBAUM, M.D.*
Assistant Clinical Professor of Dermatology, Boston University School of Medicine, Boston, Massachusetts; Staff, Harvard Community Health Plan, Wellesley, Massachusetts
Toxic Epidermal Necrolysis

HAROLD B. SCHIFF, M.D.*
Private Practice, Neurology, Newton, Massachusetts
Coma; Acute Confusional States

JEREMY D. SCHMAHMANN, M.D., Ch.B.
Instructor of Medicine, Boston City Hospital; Assistant Professor of Medicine, Boston University School of Medicine, Boston, Massachusetts
Acute Inflammatory Polyradiculoneuropathy: The Guillain-Barré Syndrome

DAVID SCHWARTZ, M.D.*
Director, Occupational Medicine, Assistant Professor of Medicine, University of Iowa; Department of Medicine, Division of Pulmonary Diseases, University of Iowa, Iowa City, Iowa
Malaria; Smoke Inhalation and Carbon Monoxide Poisoning; Tricyclic Antidepressants

FEREYDOUN SHAHROKHI, M.D.
Private Practice, Neurology, Medford, Massachusetts
Transient Ischemic Attacks; Stroke; Spinal Cord Compression; Epilepsy

RUTH H. STRAUSS, M.D.
Cardiology Fellow, St. Vincent's Medical Center, Los Angeles, California
Hypertensive Emergencies

DON L. STROMQUIST, M.D.*
Rheumatology, The Hitchcock Clinic, Bedford, New Hampshire
Theophylline

THOMAS L. TREADWELL, M.D.*
Director of Microbiology, Framingham Union Hospital, Framingham, Massachusetts; Assistant Professor of Medicine, Boston University School of Medicine, Boston, Massachusetts
Sepsis

NAGAGOPAL VENNA, M.D.
Associate Director of Neurology, Boston City Hospital; Associate Professor of Neurology, Boston University School of Medicine, Boston, Massachusetts
Headache, Part I: A Clinical Approach; Headache, Part II: Management of Common Headache Syndrome; Myasthenia Gravis; Dizziness and Vertigo: Parts I and II; Acute Inflammatory Polyradiculoneuropathy: The Guillain-Barré Syndrome

JUAN CARLOS VERA, M.D.*
Assistant Visiting Physician, Boston City Hospital; Staff, Veterans Administration Medical Center, Boston, Massachusetts
Acute Complications of Hemoglobinopathies and Thalassemias

BRANT L. VINER, M.D.
Assistant Visiting Physician, Boston City Hospital; Assistant Professor of Medicine, Boston University School of Medicine, Boston, Massachusetts
Malaria

PANTEL S. VOKONAS, M.D.*
Director, Veterans Administration Normative Aging Study, VA Outpatient Clinic, Associate Professor of Medicine and Public Health, Boston University School of Medicine, Boston, Massachusetts
Acute Pulmonary Edema

JOSEPH M. WEINSTEIN, M.D.*
Cardiology, Park Medical Associates, Stoughton, Massachusetts
Sudden Cardiac Death; Cardiopulmonary Resuscitation

LAURA F. WEXLER, M.D.*
Chief of Cardiology Section, Veterans Administration Medical Center; Associate Professor of Medicine, University of Cincinnati Medical Center, Cincinnati, Ohio
Sudden Cardiac Death; Cardiopulmonary Resuscitation

JAMES R. WILENTZ, M.D.*
Private Practice, Cardiology, New York, New York
Shock

ROBERT A. WITZBURG, M.D.
Associate Director, Department of Medicine, Boston City Hospital; Associate Professor of Medicine, Department of Medicine, Boston University School of Medicine, Boston, Massachusetts
Transient Ischemic Attacks; Stroke; Beta Blocker Overdose; Hypothermia

PREFACE

Clinical Problems in Acute Care Medicine is a compilation of selected and focused clinical reviews grounded in the clinical problem mix encountered on the Medical Service of the Boston City Hospital. It has its roots in the long tradition of case discussions and reviews of the medical literature that form the core of Residents' Report. This book is a product of the clinical faculty of the Boston City Hospital and the Boston University School of Medicine. Included among the 59 contributors are 38 former Boston City Hospital house officers and fellows, nine of whom served as Chief Resident in Medicine.

In each article, epidemiology and pathophysiology are explored concisely; the major emphasis, however, is on the clinical features, diagnostic approach, and treatment of acute problems, tied closely in each instance to landmark and recent articles in the medical literature. The accompanying references are critically selected and annotated to demonstrate both the consensus and controversies around a given topic. It is our hope that *Clinical Problems in Acute Care Medicine* will be of value to internists, family practitioners, and emergency physicians, whether they are in practice or in teaching roles; to house officers in training in each of the disciplines; and to medical students.

This book was inspired and sustained by the skill, commitment, and hard work of the house officers and faculty of the Department of Medicine at the Boston City Hospital. In addition, we thank Gretchen Meyers and Leslie Cohen in our departmental office as well as the production and editorial staff at Saunders for their forbearance in this endeavor.

JAMES J. HEFFERNAN
ROBERT A. WITZBURG
ALAN S. COHEN

CONTENTS

SECTION 2
ENDOCRINOLOGY AND METABOLISM

SECTION 3   ·
GASTROINTESTINAL DISEASE

SECTION 4
HEMATOLOGY AND ONCOLOGY

SECTION 5
INFECTIOUS DISEASES

SECTION 6
NEPHROLOGY

SECTION 7
NEUROLOGY

SECTION 8
PULMONARY DISEASE

SECTION 9
RHEUMATOLOGY AND IMMUNOLOGY

SECTION 10
SELECTED TOXICOLOGIC EMERGENCIES

SECTION 11
MISCELLANEOUS DISORDERS

SECTION 1

CARDIOVASCULAR DISEASE

Acute Myocardial Infarction

Carl S. Apstein, M.D.

Acute myocardial infarction (MI) is a common cardiac emergency in the United States, with approximately one million acute MIs occurring per year. The term acute MI refers to myocyte necrosis resulting from myocardial ischemia. The development and size of an MI depend on the severity and duration of the ischemic state. Immediate medical attention and emergency treatment are necessary because 50% of the deaths that are due to acute MI occur within the first hour of its onset. The mechanism of these early deaths is usually ventricular tachycardia or fibrillation. Because the arrhythmias are readily recognizable and potentially reversible, rapid diagnosis and treatment of an acute MI can significantly reduce the death rate. Also, if thrombolytic therapy is given early in the course of acute MI, reperfusion of ischemic myocardium can be accomplished, preventing necrosis and substantially reducing the mortality and morbidity associated with a coronary occlusion.

If the diagnosis is in question, it is better to err on the side of over-diagnosis, treating the patient as a "presumptive MI" or "rule-out MI" until a subsequent evaluation either confirms the diagnosis or fails to do so. The history, physical examination, electrocardiogram (ECG), and serum cardiac enzyme levels provide the most important information for establishing the diagnosis of acute MI.

DIAGNOSIS

History

Most patients with an acute MI complain of chest or upper abdominal pain. The pain is of relatively steady intensity and is usually severe, although there is great variation in pain quality and intensity among patients. The duration of the pain is usually between 30 minutes and several hours. Patients

1

who complain of chest pain of very brief (several minutes) or of long-standing duration (all day or for several days) have rarely sustained an acute MI. The character of the pain is most frequently described as crushing, constricting, or squeezing. Many patients describe the feeling of a heavy weight pressing on their chest, e.g., an "elephant standing on my chest." The location of the pain or chest discomfort is usually in the mid-chest or upper abdomen. The most intense discomfort is usually felt in the sternal or parasternal region, with radiation into the lateral chest unilaterally (usually to the left); bilaterally; or occasionally into the neck, shoulders, arms, lower jaw, and "classically" into the left arm, radiating down the ulnar aspect as far as the elbow or fingers. Pain radiating to the back may occur with an MI, but this should also raise the suspicion of aortic dissection. The radiation of the chest or abdominal pain is highly variable among patients, and occasionally the most intense site of the pain may be one of the usual places of radiation, e.g., the shoulder, neck, jaw, or left arm. In such cases, an acute MI may be misdiagnosed as a toothache, sore throat, bursitis, or arthritic condition.

It is important to watch a patient's hands and face as he describes his chest discomfort. A patient who can point to a small area with one finger to localize the chest pain rarely suffers from an acute MI. Rather, the patient who is having an MI describes a large area (usually the sternal and parasternal region or the epigastrium) and gestures to this entire area to indicate that the area of discomfort is widespread and its limits are hard to define. Very often the patient presses an open hand against the chest to convey a sense of constriction. Commonly, a patient with an acute MI (or angina) will make a tight fist and press it to his chest to describe the squeezing, constrictive nature of the chest discomfort. (This closed fist sign was originally described by the great American cardiologist Dr. Samuel Levine, and it is often referred to as Levine's sign.) The pain of an acute MI has also been described as burning; a dull ache; stabbing; or indigestion, especially if localized in the epigastric region. When a patient with pre-existing angina develops an MI, the character of the chest pain associated with the MI is often similar to that of the pre-existing angina, but the patient usually describes the MI pain as being more intense and of longer duration, commonly saying that the pain is "like my angina, but worse." The face of the patient with an acute MI generally appears anxious and distressed, and such patients often express a feeling of apprehension and fear, a sense of impending doom. The patient who presents a happy demeanor, while complaining of chest pain, is extremely unlikely to have an acute MI.

Occasionally, a patient with an acute MI may present without a significant history of chest or abdominal pain or discomfort. This can occur in patients who are confused or demented, or who have been under anesthesia when their MI occurred. Diabetics may be more prone to "silent" MIs. In other cases, an associated symptom or condition such as nausea and vomiting, congestive heart failure, or a stroke may distract attention from, or diminish the apparent significance of, a history of chest or epigastric pain. The astute clinician should suspect an underlying MI in patients who present with a picture of increased left ventricular congestive failure (dyspnea, orthopnea, paroxysmal noctural dyspnea), especially if the increased congestive heart failure occurred in a patient who is largely at bed rest. (In general, cardiac function is stable or improves and does not deteriorate in a stable patient at bed rest. Thus, deterioration of cardiac function in such a patient implies an active cardiac pathologic process.) In some patients with acute MI, the most significant presenting symptom may be a sense of overwhelming weakness, diaphoresis, nausea and vomiting (especially in inferior MI), decreased mentation (secondary to cerebral hypoperfusion), stroke as a result of cerebral embolism, or evidence of a peripheral arterial embolism. These types of presentations should raise the suspicion of underlying MI.

Other conditions that may present in a fashion similar to an acute MI include musculoskeletal pain, rib fractures, esophagitis, peptic ulcer disease, pericarditis, pleuritis, aortic dissection, a severe anginal episode, pulmonary embolism, increased congestive heart failure that is due to some other condition, and respiratory failure that must be distinguished from congestive heart failure.

Often the history may identify precipitating factors that increase the suspicion of an acute MI. However, this is usually not the case, as most patients are resting or sleeping at the onset of acute MI. About one third of acute MIs occur during physical exertion, but often this is at a usual and not excessive level of activity. Snow shoveling is an activity that occasionally is associated with acute MI. A precipitating factor reported to be associated with an acute MI is increased emotional stress, particularly stress associated with a major life change, such as a change in job or marital relationship. Heavy cigarette smoking, particularly "binge" cigarette smoking, may precipitate an acute MI, and the combination of oral contraceptives and cigarette smoking substantially increases the risk of an MI. Many patients with an acute MI give a good history of an increase in their antecedent anginal symptomatology or the development of frank, unstable angina, which then culminated in the symptoms of an acute MI. As with unstable angina, most cases of acute MI result from a pathologic process in the coronary arteries, i.e., a thrombotic coronary artery occlusion (see later discussion). In a few cases, however, an MI can be precipitated by concomitant conditions that worsen the myocardial oxygen supply-demand imbalance. Therefore, it is important to consider potential contributing conditions such as anemia, poorly controlled hypertension, and aortic stenosis (valvular and muscular subaortic stenosis) in the diagnosis of an acute MI. Similarly, the patient with a history of diabetes and/or an elevated serum cholesterol level is also at increased risk for an acute MI.

Physical Examination

The patient with an acute MI is usually anxious and distressed. Often he spontaneously motions with his hands to indicate a sense of chest pressure or constriction. The patient may have tachypnea or orthopnea secondary to left ventricular failure. Increased sympathetic tone leads to skin pallor, often with cold perspiration. If profound failure and cardiogenic shock are present, the skin is cool and clammy, appearing mottled with peripheral cyanosis. Poor cerebral perfusion can result in confusion and disorientation.

The *vital signs* may be normal or abnormal, but the abnormalities are not diagnostic. Bradycardia or tachycardia may be present, or the heart rate may be normal. Premature beats, especially ventricular premature beats, are common. The blood pressure is usually within the normal range, but if significant left ventricular pump failure is present the systolic pressure may be decreased and diastolic pressure increased. On the other hand, an increased blood pressure may be present if there is a large increase in intrinsic sympathetic tone as a result of the pain and anxiety associated with the acute MI. Hypotension can be precipitated by a large MI with loss of significant cardiac output, but it can also result from treatment with morphine or nitroglycerin.

It is important to recognize that arterial hypotension is not synonymous with cardiogenic shock. Hypotension can result from functional hypovolemia, i.e., inadequate left ventricular filling as a result of intravascular volume depletion or maldistribution of the intravascular volume. Intravenous pooling secondary to systemic venodilation as a result of drug therapy (morphine, nitrates) can cause hypotension. Venodilation can occur as an "autonomic reflex," especially with inferior MI. The inferior and posterior walls of the left ventricle contain afferent vagal fibers that activate the parasympathetic system, causing bradycardia and venodilation (the Bezold-Jarisch reflex). Significant hypotension can result from such a sequence of events and does not necessarily imply large-scale loss of left ventricular muscle.

Blood pressure measurements should be made and peripheral pulses palpated in all four extremities to look for asymmetry, which may indicate the presence of an underlying aortic dissection.

The *temperature* may be slightly elevated, i.e., 101–102° F pr. The fever is the result of myocardial tissue necrosis and may be present from day 1 to day 7 or 8 post-MI.

The *respiratory rate* may be increased, owing to pain, agitation, or increased pulmonary congestion as the result of left ventricular failure.

The ocular fundi may have hypertensive, diabetic, or atherosclerotic changes.

The jugular venous pulse wave, which reflects right atrial and right ventricular diastolic pressure, is usually normal with an uncomplicated acute

MI that affects only the left ventricle. However, a right ventricular infarct may cause significant elevation of the mean jugular venous pressure and an increased A wave. If tricuspid insufficiency occurs, a prominent V wave may be present. With severe left ventricular failure, there may be a secondary increase in right ventricular end-diastolic pressure and a subsequent increased jugular venous A wave. If intravascular hypovolemia is present, the jugular venous pressure is diminished.

The carotid pulse volume is often decreased to palpation if left ventricular stroke volume is diminished. Pulsus alternans may be detected in the presence of severe left ventricular failure. The right and left carotid pulses should be compared, since an aortic root dissection, whose presentation can mimic that of an acute MI, may result in unequal carotid pulses.

Auscultation of the lungs is a critical part of the physical examination for a patient with MI because the presence and extent of rales provide a rough index of prognosis (see Table 1, Killip's Classification of Patients with Acute MI). If the pulmonary congestion is limited to the lung interstitial space, as it may be in the early stages of pulmonary congestion, rales may be absent. However, the chest radiograph shows an interstitial pulmonary edema pattern. High-pitched wheezing, scattered or diffuse, can occur as a result of bronchiolar edema (cardiac asthma).

Examination of the heart itself may be unremarkable in a patient with acute MI, but frequently, important physical signs can be detected. Palpation of the chest often reveals a detectable S_4 gallop or "atrial kick" at the apex. This is usually best appreciated with the patient in the left lateral decubitus position. With an infarct involving the anterior wall or apical region, with the patient in the supine position, a sustained systolic lift reflecting underlying dyskinetic myocardium may be palpated in the left parasternal region or at the apex. (The duration of a systolic lift should be assessed with the patient supine, because normal individuals in the left lateral decubitus po-

TABLE 1. KILLIP'S CLASSIFICATION OF PATIENTS WITH ACUTE MI[1,8]

Class	Definition	% of Patients Admitted to CCU with Acute MI in this Category	Approximate Mortality (%)*
I	No rales; no S_3 gallop	30–40	8
II	Rales limited to <50% of lung fields or an S_3	30–50	30
III	Rales >50% of lung fields (often pulmonary edema)	5–10	44
IV	Shock	10	80–100

Adapted from Killip T, Kimball JT: Treatment of myocardial infarction in a coronary care unit. A two year experience with 250 patients. Am J Cardiol 20:457, 1967.

*Estimated mortality rate in the 1960s. Mortality still rises with increased class, although the values in each class are lower today than in the 1960s.

sition may appear to have a sustained outward apical movement.) A systolic thrill may be palpated between the apical impulse and the left lower sternal border in the case of a ruptured ventricular septum. In the case of a ruptured papillary muscle or severe papillary muscle dysfunction, a systolic thrill may be palpated over the apical impulse with the patient in the left lateral decubitus position.

Auscultation of the heart is a critical part of the physical examination and must be performed in a quiet environment. Although this may be difficult to achieve in an emergency room or CCU, it is imperative to make every effort to do so. The first heart sound is often decreased in intensity as a result of a decrease in left venticular contractile function or an increase in the P-R interval. The second heart sound may be paradoxically split if complete left bundle branch block is present or if left venticular ejection time is prolonged. An S_4 gallop is almost always present in a patient with an acute MI who is in normal sinus rhythm. It indicates the presence of a decrease in left ventricular diastolic compliance (increase in chamber stiffness) and an abrupt increase in left ventricular end-diastolic pressure as atrial contraction is superimposed on a stiff and full left ventricle at end-diastole. The presence of an S_3 gallop indicates extensive left ventricular dysfunction and implies a large amount of infarcted myocardium, which may be a mixture of old and acute infarction. The presence of an S_3 gallop in an acute MI is associated with a 40% mortality rate, compared with a 15% mortality rate if an S_3 gallop is absent. An S_3 gallop is often heard *only* with the patient in the left lateral decubitus position with careful auscultation at the apical impulse. An S_4 gallop is best heard either at the left lower sternal border or at the apical impulse in the left lateral decubitus position.

Systolic murmurs are relatively common in an acute MI. The murmur of papillary muscle dysfunction is best heard at the apical impulse with the patient in the left lateral decubitus position. This murmur may be transient; it depends on the extent of papillary muscle ischemia or infarction, left ventricular size, and left ventricular systolic pressures. Unlike the murmur of rheumatic mitral regurgitation, the murmur of papillary muscle dysfunction is usually not holosystolic nor constant in pitch and intensity. However, it may be diamond shaped and midsystolic, or it may occur in late systole, mimicking the murmur of mitral valve prolapse. Papillary muscle infarction or rupture may cause a murmur of severe mitral insufficiency and is sometimes associated with an apical thrill; these conditions are usually associated with marked pulmonary congestion and pulmonary edema. With rupture of the ventricular septum, a rough holosystolic murmur is present and is usually loudest at the left lower sternal border. The murmur of a ruptured septum or papillary muscle is usually loud, but such patients may be in profound congestive heart failure and have a low-output state; in such cases, the diagnostic murmur may be very soft and difficult to hear. In the presence of a basal systolic murmur, it is important to consider the presence of aortic stenosis (either valvular or muscular subaortic stenosis), which may contribute to the ischemic myocardial state.

It is imperative that all patients be examined sitting upright, leaning forward, holding breath after expiration with careful stethoscopic exploration of the left and right sternal borders in search of a murmur of aortic insufficiency. The presence of aortic insufficiency should raise the suspicion of underlying aortic root dissection as the cause of a patient's chest pain.

Pericardial friction rubs are common in the setting of an acute MI, but they may be transient and not heard unless frequent auscultation is performed with the patient sitting up, leaning forward, and examined during held expiration. They are most common in the first 3 days of an acute MI.

Examination of the abdomen may reveal hepatomegaly and positive hepatojugular reflux in the presence of right ventricular infarction.

Peripheral edema indicates the presence of right ventricular failure and does not occur with uncomplicated left ventricular infarction. The occurrence of a peripheral arterial embolus or an embolic stroke in the setting of an acute MI usually indicates a relatively large anterior or apical MI with a severe wall motion abnormality. A large percentage of such patients develop mural thrombosis in the acute MI setting, but fortunately, only a relatively small number of such mural thrombi embolize.

Although none of the physical findings just described are 100% specific for an acute MI, their presence can aid considerably in making the diagnosis, though their absence does not rule MI out. When the ECG or cardiac enzyme results are not specific, the physical examination may provide the diagnostic information for an acute MI or for a condition that mimics it. Thus, asymmetric pulses, the presence of a murmur of aortic insufficiency, or radiation of the pain to the back raises the suspicion of an aortic dissection. In the patient who presents with chest pain, a pericardial friction rub, and widespread ST segment and T wave abnormalities (or a complete bundle branch block whose secondary ST and T wave abnormalities can mask underlying ischemia), it may be difficult to make the distinction between acute viral pericarditis and acute infarction. In such a case, palpation of a dyskinetic systolic precordial lift may be an extremely valuable sign to suggest the diagnosis of an acute MI.

Laboratory Studies

The laboratory studies important for making the diagnosis of an acute MI include the electrocardiogram and the serum cardiac enzyme levels. Echocardiography, chest radiograph, and radionuclide imaging of the heart may provide corroboratory evidence and are helpful in subsequent patient management.

The Electrocardiogram (ECG)

Almost all patient who have an acute MI will have an abnormal ECG, but the abnormalities may be nondiagnostic and their appearance may be delayed for up to 24 hours after the onset of symptoms. Although it is unusual, a patient can present with classic symptoms of an acute MI and initially have a perfectly normal ECG that does not exhibit ST or T wave abnormalities, or the development of Q waves, until 24 hours have elapsed. Thus, in the initial assessment of a patient with a possible MI, a normal ECG does not rule out this diagnosis.

The typical patient with an acute MI has characteristic ischemic ST segment and T wave abnormalities, which may evolve into a Q wave infarct pattern, depending on the size and transmural extent of the infarct. Development of a Q wave implies either a transmural infarct or a relatively large subendocardial infarct. Conversely, an infarction that is manifested only by ischemic ST segment or T wave abnormalities is due to either a subendocardial infarct or a relatively small transmural infarct. The ECG is often useful in distinguishing between a patient with unstable angina and one with acute MI. Ischemic ST–T wave changes are common during an anginal attack, but development of Q waves or persistence of ischemic ST–T wave changes for longer than 24 hours suggests MI and not simple reversible ischemia, as occurs with unstable angina. Most patients with an acute MI will have some degree of ventricular ectopic activity during the initial 24 hours. (Patients with an acute MI can also develop a variety of arrhythmias and atrioventricular conduction blocks, whose management is discussed in more detail in a later section.) The ECG finding of ventricular ectopy or new conduction disturbance is nonspecific but is contributory diagnostic information for an acute MI.

Cardiac Serum Enzyme Levels

The appearance in the serum of enzymes that are normally contained within myocardial cells is considered to be diagnostic of myocyte necrosis. In general, the extent of the increase in serum enzyme levels is a rough measure of the amount of myocardial necrosis. However, this correlation is not precise, especially if spontaneous or therapeutic reperfusion occurs, since reperfusion has the effect of increasing enzyme washout for a given amount of necrosis. The most important cardiac enzyme for diagnostic purposes is creatine kinase (CK). Characteristically, the serum CK level increases at 6–8 hours post-MI, peaks at about 24 hours post-MI, and declines over 2–4 days post-MI. Reperfusion accelerates and abbreviates this time course and produces a higher peak serum level for a given infarct size. The serum CK level can also increase as result of leakage of this enzyme from skeletal muscle, e.g., after trauma, vigorous exercise, intramuscular injections, seizures, or alcohol intoxication. CK can also be released from brain and kidney with injury to those tissues. Use of the CK *isozyme* levels permits distinction among organ sources. The MB isozyme (CK-MB) is relatively specific for cardiac muscle, but it is also found in intestine, tongue, diaphragm, uterus, and prostate. The CK-MM isozyme is found in skeletal muscle and also, to some extent, in cardiac muscle. The CK-BB isozyme is found in brain and kidney. Thus, it is common practice to use the CK-MB isozyme level to confirm that an elevation of total CK activity in the serum is of cardiac origin.

The serum glutamic oxaloacetic transaminase enzyme (SGOT) is also a useful marker of myocyte necrosis. This enzyme increases at 8–12 hours post-MI, peaks at 18–36 hours post-MI, and declines by 3–4 days post-MI. An increased level of SGOT also occurs with liver injury or skeletal muscle injury.

The enzyme lactate dehydrogenase (LDH) is the last enzyme to manifest an increased serum level post-infarction. It characteristically increases at 24–48 hours post-MI, peaks at 3–6 days post-MI, and declines by 8–14 days post-MI. LDH can also be released from red blood cells, liver, kidney, and skeletal muscle, and after a pulmonary embolism. As with CK, the isozymes of LDH are useful in distinguishing the tissue source of an elevated serum level. The heart is rich in LDH-1, which is also found in red blood cells, kidney, brain, and gastric mucosa. Liver and skeletal muscle have primarily LDH isozymes 4 and 5. The ratio of LDH-1 to LDH-2 yielding a value greater than 1 is suggestive of MI. The value of the serum LDH level is primarily in making a "late diagnosis," i.e., when a patient is seen 1 to 6 days after he or she has experienced symptoms of an acute MI. When a patient is seen immediately after the onset of acute MI, the serum CK and SGOT levels are more helpful in rapidly making the diagnosis of an acute MI.

Chest Radiograph

The chest radiograph is useful in assessing the degree of pulmonary congestion. Careful examination of the mediastinum and aorta is important in assessing the possibility of an aortic dissection. The radiograph may provide other valuable information regarding the origin of chest pain that is non-MI in origin, e.g., rib fractures, pleuritis, and so forth. In correlating the degree of pulmonary congestion on the chest film with a patient's clinical status, it is important to recognize that interstitial pulmonary edema, which can be readily detected on the chest radiograph, may produce no auscultatory findings on physical examination, although such patients are usually dyspneic and tachypneic. Furthermore, the chest film usually "lags" several hours behind the patient's clinical status. Thus, it is a common experience to treat a patient for acute pulmonary congestion appropriately, with gratifying relief of dyspnea and rales and reduction of an elevated pulmonary capilllary wedge pressure, only to find that an immediate chest radiograph shows little change from the pretreatment picture of pulmonary congestion. However, after several hours, the chest film characteristically "catches up" with the improved clinical picture.

Echocardiography

Two-dimensional echocardiography has rapidly become an important laboratory technique for the care of patients with MI. Although no precise diagnostic criteria have been formulated, a careful two-dimensional echocardiographic examination can be diagnostic of MI by identifying regions of impaired contractile function. The echocardiogram is critical in identifying patients with acute MI who have a severe anterior wall or apical wall motion abnormality (i.e., dyskinesis or severe hypokinesis). Such patients are at high risk for mural thrombus formation and subsequent systemic embolization early in the course of an acute MI. Echocardiography can identify such patients before or after mural thrombus formation; in general, these individuals are candidates for anticoagulation (see later discussion). The two-dimensional echocardiogram is also useful for assessing overall left ventricular function.

Radionuclide Cardiac Imaging

Three general types of radionuclide imaging are useful in assessing the patient with a possible acute MI. Technetium pyrophosphate scanning can be helpful in making the diagnosis of an acute infarct. This radiopharmaceutical is an "infarct avid" agent because the pyrophosphate part of the molecule binds to tissue calcium, which is characteristically increased in an infarct region. Thus, this imaging agent accumulates in the infarct area and a positive technetium pyrophosphate scan "lights up" an acute infarct. This technique may also give an estimate of infarct size. The best time for technetium pyrophosphate imaging is 48–72 hours post-MI. The best diagnostic results are obtained with a transmural MI; with a small infarct or a nontransmural infarct, this test is of limited value.

A thallium-201 perfusion imaging scan provides information about the coronary circulation. In general, an acute MI that has not been reperfused appears as an imaging "defect" on a thallium perfusion scan, i.e., the infarct region has fewer counts than the surrounding well-perfused myocardium. Thallium perfusion imaging may also be used to distinguish ischemia from infarction by combined stress testing and thallium scanning. A thallium perfusion defect that is transiently present during exercise stress, but resolves on repeat scanning several hours later, implies reversible myocardial ischemia. In contrast, a thallium perfusion defect that is present acutely during stress testing and is persistent several hours later implies a permanent loss of regional perfusion, consistent with an MI. In general, thallium perfusion imaging is not necessary during the acute assessment of a patient with suspected MI, but it may prove useful later to assess the extent of coronary artery disease when the patient is ready for discharge from the hospital.

Gated blood pool scans are useful for assessing overall cardiac function and defining regions of wall motion abnormality that, if severe, may predispose to thrombus formation. Thus, this type of radionuclide scanning provides much the same information as two-dimensional echocardiography (see previous discussion).

PATHOPHYSIOLOGY

Accurate diagnosis and good clinical management of patients with acute MI require an understanding of the underlying pathophysiologic processes. Infarction occurs because of prolonged, severe myocardial ischemia or oxygen supply-demand imbalance. In over 90% of cases, the problem is one of a decrease in oxygen supply as a result of an abnormality in the coronary arterial circulation; this leads to ischemia and subsequent infarction of the region of myocardium served by the diseased coronary vessel.

In 85–90% of cases, an infarction is triggered by an acute thrombotic occlusion of a coronary artery. In most cases the thrombosis occurs at the site of an atherosclerotic lesion where the plaque has ruptured or become fissured, thereby exposing a thrombogenic surface. The atherosclerotic lesion itself often forms a significant stenosis. In some cases, the atherosclerotic stenosis is relatively mild but serves as a nidus for thrombus formation. In the rare case, a thrombus may form in a coronary artery that appears normal on coronary angiography. In other cases, coronary arterial spasm has appeared to precipitate a coronary thrombosis. The spasm usually occurs in an atherosclerotic vessel but occasionally has been reported to occur in a normal vessel. The initiating step in coronary thrombus formation appears to be platelet aggregation, usually at the site of an atherosclerotic lesion. Thus, this mechanism of thrombus initiation and subsequent myocardial infarction is very similar to the pathophysiology of unstable angina (see Unstable Angina).

Not all infarctions result from a coronary thrombosis. Rarely, a coronary occlusion can result from a coronary embolus from the left atrium or ventricle, or from a piece of vegetation from healed or active endocarditis. A coronary contusion can result in an infarction after cardiac trauma. Other rare forms of coronary occlusive disease include inflammatory diseases of the arterial wall such as the vasculitis associated with systemic lupus erythematosus or polyarteritis nodosa. Occasionally, diffuse infarction can occur from an event that globally reduces oxygen delivery to the myocardium, such as a prolonged period of hypotension or hypoxia, as can occur with significant hemorrhage and severe anemia. Occasionally, a prolonged increase in myocardial oxygen demand, such as occurs with sustained heavy exercise, delirium tremens, or thyrotoxicosis in a patient with limited coronary blood flow, may cause MI. However, the fact that over 90% of acute MIs result from an acute thrombosis of the coronary circulation has resulted in an aggressive attempt to reperfuse the ischemic region by attempted thrombolysis of the occluded artery (see later discussion).

After the development of sustained severe ischemia, an infarct develops in a characteristic way. The myocardium can withstand severe ischemia for approximately 20 minutes before cell necrosis occurs; during these initial 20 minutes the myocytes undergo ischemic injury, but such injury is reversible. If significant collateral flow is present in the region of an occluded artery, this phase of reversible ischemic injury may be present for several hours, during which time reperfusion may completely salvage the ischemic region and prevent necrosis. In the absence of adequate collateral flow, myocyte necrosis begins to occur after approximately 20 minutes of severe ischemia. The subendocardial region undergoes necrosis first, with a progressive "wavefront of necrosis" spreading from subendocardium to epicardium over a course of approximately 3–4 hours, depending on the degree of collateral flow. Thus, interruption of this process by spontaneous or therapeutic reperfusion may transform a potentially transmural infarct into a subendocardial one. Also, if there is good collateral circulation to the subepicardial region, the wavefront of necrosis may spontaneously stop its progression from endocardium to epicardium, resulting in a subendocardial infarction. In such a case, the patient is left with a subendocardial infarct and a viable, but jeopardized, subepicardial region.

The distinction between a transmural and a subendocardial (non-transmural) infarct is clinically important, although it is difficult to distinguish with certainty between these two types of infarcts on clinical grounds. Development of a Q wave on ECG, or of a severe wall motion abnormality on echocardiogram, implies transmural necrosis (or extensive subendocardial necrosis). Although there is not a good correlation between the extent of transmurality of necrosis and the development of Q waves, Q wave infarcts and non–Q wave infarcts (i.e., ST–T wave abnormalities without Q waves) have a different prognosis and natural history. Q wave infarcts have an initial in-hospital mortality rate of approximately 15%, compared with an initial in-hospital mortality rate of 7–8% for non–Q wave infarcts. Thus, the acute mortality rate is approximately 50% lower for a non–Q wave infarct. However, patients followed after an initial non–Q wave infarct had a higher rate of reinfarction and death in the 2 years after hospital discharge than those who had an initial Q wave infarct.[7]

Thus, patients who present initially with a non–Q wave infarct appear to leave the hospital with a viable but jeopardized region of subepicardial myocardium serviced by a diseased coronary vessel. This myocardial region is at risk for subsequent acute infarction. Recent studies have attempted to identify such patients with residual, jeopardized myocardial regions so that aggressive interventions, such as angioplasty or bypass graft surgery, may be considered to improve the coronary circulation to such regions.

The diagnosis of acute MI should include information regarding the region of the left ventricle that is infarcted (anterior, septal, lateral, inferior, or posterior wall) and the occurrence of any evidence of right ventricular infarction (most common in association with an inferior or posterior left ventricular infarction). Assessment as to whether the infarction is transmural or non-transmural (i.e., subendocardial) in distribution, and whether the event represents a first or a recurrent infarction, should also be made. These diagnostic considerations are important in planning appropriate management and follow-up of patients with acute MI (see following discussion).

MANAGEMENT OF ACUTE MYOCARDIAL INFARCTION

Management of acute MI includes the following:
1. General measures
2. Thrombolytic therapy of acute MI
3. Treatment of abnormal hemodynamics
4. Management of arrhythmias and conduction defects
5. Post-myocardial infarction management

General Measures

Patients with a suspected MI should be admitted to hospital and placed in a coronary or intensive care unit setting where arrhythmia monitoring and rapid treatment can be provided. Since the development of the coronary care units (CCU) in the 1960s, there has been approximately a 50% decrease in the mortality rate associated with acute MI. This decrease in mortality rate is probably due to the rapid arrhythmia detection and treatment that is provided by the CCU environment. Additionally, the CCU provides a setting for better hemodynamic monitoring and a specialized staff, experienced in dealing with acute MI patients. A patient with uncomplicated MI should remain in a CCU for 3–5 days. The patient may then be transferred to a less intensive care facility in the hospital where arrhythmia monitoring can continue and he or she can receive instruction about further post-infarction care.

The patient with acute MI requires a quiet, restful environment with medical and nursing reassurance. Light sedation is often useful. Continuous ECG monitoring should be performed, and intravenous lines should be placed in case rapid drug administration becomes necessary. In addition, the IV line facilitates the drawing of blood samples and administration of medications that cannot be taken orally. In general, intramuscular injections should be avoided, since they elevate the serum CK level.

Oxygen by nasal prongs or face mask should be provided to keep the arterial pO_2 greater than 70–80 mmHg.

Initial treatment of chest pain depends on whether the patient is considered to be having a severe anginal episode or an acute MI; this distinction may be difficult or impossible to make. If the duration of chest pain has been relatively short (i.e., less than 20 minutes), it is likely that the ischemic region of the myocardium is still in the phase of reversible injury, in which case myocytes might be salvaged by restoration of a more normal oxygen supply-demand balance. Thus, it is reasonable to treat such patients initially with sublingual *nitroglycerin* or sublingual *nifedipine* and to proceed as outlined in Unstable Angina. Some clinicians argue that even with chest pain of several hours' duration, potentially salvageable regions of ischemic myocardium may exist, and agents such as nitroglycerin or nifedipine may be beneficial. In some cases, use of these agents will promptly relieve the patient's chest pain, suggesting a significant reversible ischemic component. However, in most cases of well-established infarcts, no effect on chest pain is observed.

Both nitroglycerin and nifedipine induce systemic venodilation and may cause hypotension, especially in the patient with a right ventricular infarction, in which right ventricular output is critically dependent on systemic venous return. Should hypotension occur, the patient should have his legs elevated and receive intravenous saline to reverse the hypotension.

Morphine is the agent of choice for analgesia and should be given intravenously, 1–4 mg periodically as needed, to relieve persistent chest discomfort.

An adrenergic beta blocking agent should be considered in the early phase of an acute MI, if there is no evidence of left ventricular failure or atrioventricular nodal block, and especially if the patient has evidence of increased sympathetic tone and adrenergic stimulation. By reducing heart rate and intrinsic contractility, beta blockers can reduce myocardial oxygen demand and thereby reduce the severity of ischemia, potential infarct size, and ischemic-induced ventricular ectopy. They may also reduce the deleterious effects of locally released catecholamines from the ischemic myocardial region; such tissue accumulation of catecholamines may cause necrosis and arrhythmias in the absence of a recognizable increase in sympathetic tone. Use of beta blockers in patients with acute MI without left ventricular failure or other contraindications has been associated with a significant reduction in mortality rate.

If their MI follows an uncomplicated course, many patients will require no additional drug therapy. They should be kept at bed rest for 1–2 days and then be allowed to move between the bed and a bedside chair. Initially, the diet should be liquid and provided in small feedings. In the presence of left ventricular failure, a low-salt diet should be provided. The patient should receive a stool softener to avoid constipation and subsequent straining at stool. No caffeine-containing beverages should be drunk during the early post-MI period because of their potential arrhythmogenic effects as well as their action to increase myocardial contractility and oxygen demand. Most patients should be placed on a low-cholesterol, low–saturated fat diet in the post-MI period, since there is now evidence that such a diet can have a significant effect in reducing the serum cholesterol level, which in turn can reduce the risk of subsequent infarction.

Thrombolytic Therapy of Acute Myocardial Infarction

The modern treatment of acute MI includes the use of thrombolytic agents such as streptokinase (SK) or tissue plasminogen activator (TPA) if such drugs can be given within 4–6 hours of the onset of symptoms. The rationale for such therapy is based on the following four facts:

1. Myocyte necrosis does not occur instantly after a coronary occlusion. Depending on the degree of collateral flow, irreversible injury requires 20 minutes to several hours of ischemia.
2. Reperfusion of ischemic myocardium can prevent progression to irreversible injury.
3. An acute MI is caused by coronary arterial thrombus formation in 85–90% of cases.
4. Intravenous thrombolytic agents can rapidly dissolve such coronary thrombi and permit reperfusion.

In a 12,000-patient randomized trial (GISSI Study[14]), intravenous SK resulted in an overall 20% reduction in acute MI mortality when given within 3–6 hours of symptoms, and a 50% decrease in mortality if given within 1 hour. TPA is likely to be more effective in reducing MI mortality than SK, because TPA is twice as successful as SK in causing coronary thrombolysis when given intravenously during acute MI (36% vs. 66% reperfusion rates for intravenous SK vs. intravenous TPA; TIMI Study).[13]

When the diagnosis of acute MI is made, intravenous TPA should be given if there are no contraindications (detailed guidelines for the use of intravenous SK and intravenous TPA are provided in Table 2) and if it can be administered within 4–6 hours of the onset of symptoms of myocardial ischemia. A patient initially diagnosed as having a severe anginal episode should receive TPA if the "angina" does not respond to the usual therapy and myocardial ischemic symptoms persist for more than 20–30 minutes, indicating likely progression to acute infarction. A patient who has the char-

TABLE 2. BOSTON CITY HOSPITAL GUIDELINES FOR THROMBOLYTIC THERAPY OF ACUTE MI

A. *Indications*
1. Thrombolysis in acute MI less than 4–6 hours old
   a. Presence of acute MI determined by symptoms plus ST segment elevation greater than or equal to 2 mm
   b. Indicated in inferior wall as well as anterior wall acute MI
   c. No age restriction

B. *Contraindications*
1. Thrombocytopenia
2. Acute or recent (within last 10 days) internal bleeding
3. Recent (within 10 days) surgery or major trauma (including CPR)
4. Diabetic hemorrhagic retinopathy
5. CVA or intracranial or intraspinal surgery within last 2 months
6. Atrial fibrillation with underlying valvular disease
7. Subacute bacterial endocarditis
8. Uncontrolled hypertension (diastolic pressure greater than 120)
9. Prior treatment with streptokinase (SK) is contraindication for repeat SK use

C. *Dosage, Preparation, and Administration*
1. Draw baseline TT, PT, PTT, CBC with platelets (do not need to wait for results of coagulation studies before administering tissue plasminogen activator [TPA] or SK). Send blood for type and hold

D. *Use of Streptokinase*
1. Administer 100 mg hydrocortisone IV
2. Give 1.5 million U SK
   a. Reconstitute vials with 5 cc normal saline
   b. Prepare SK in 100 cc normal saline
   c. Administer 100 cc over 30–60 minutes
3. Administer 5000 U heparin IV bolus
4. Monitor vital signs q 15 minutes
5. Notify Cardiology Fellow

E. *Use of TPA*
1. Reconstitute 100 mg TPA with 100 cc of sterile water
2. Give 6 mg TPA IV bolus over first minute
3. Administer 54 mg IV TPA first hour
4. Give 20 mg IV TPA second hour and 20 mg IV over third hour
5. Administer heparin in standard dose, starting 1 hour post-TPA
6. For patients weighing less than 65 kg, use total dose of TPA of 1.25 mg/kg (initial bolus the same; remainder proportionally reduced)

F. *Precautions*
1. No arterial punctures
2. No central lines
3. Watch for reperfusion arrhythmias and conduction defects
4. Venipuncture sites may require prolonged manual compression

acteristic features of acute MI should receive intravenous TPA as promptly as possible; the amount of myocardial salvage is directly proportional to the speed with which reperfusion is accomplished.

Anticoagulation with intravenous heparin for 3–5 days should be initiated immediately after giving intravenous SK or TPA to prevent reocclusion of the coronary vessel. An antiplatelet agent such as aspirin (325 mg qd) should be given on a long-term basis to reduce the risk of coronary restenosis or occlusion. Patients who undergo thrombolytic therapy should be considered for coronary angiography, to be followed by coronary angioplasty or bypass graft surgery in selected cases.

Treatment of Abnormal Hemodynamics

Hemodynamic abnormalities are recognized by an abnormal heart rate (sinus tachycardia or bradycardia), hypotension or shock, and pulmonary congestion or pulmonary edema.

Increased Heart Rate from Sinus Tachycardia

A sinus tachycardia may arise from any of several causes in the setting of acute MI, and each cause requires a different management approach. If the tachycardia is the result of persistent pain, the patient should receive more analgesia. If it is the result of persistent ischemia, appropriate therapies might include nitrates, a calcium channel blocker, or a beta blocker. If it is due to pericarditis, aspirin or another nonsteroidal anti-inflammatory medication is indicated. If it is due to early congestive heart failure, the patient should receive diuretics and possibly nitrates. If the sinus tachycardia is the result of a "hyperdynamic state" as a result of anxiety and increased circulating levels of catecholamines (which can also cause modest hypertension), sedation and beta blockade are the therapy of choice.

Hypertension

Hypertensive patients should have their blood pressure lowered to within the normal range to reduce the work of the heart. Often a tranquil environment and light sedation are all that are required to achieve this in the patient with mild hypertension. If more aggressive therapy is required, a beta blocking agent, a diuretic, or sublingual nitrates or nifedipine may be helpful in reversing the hypertension. Resistant, significant hypertension should be treated with more aggressive antihypertensive agents, such as intravenous nitroglycerin, intravenous nitroprusside, or methyldopa.

Hypotension

The appropriate management of a low blood pressure depends on its underlying cause and the accuracy with which it is measured. It is critical to recognize that significant arterial vasoconstriction can result in a falsely low blood pressure measurement when recorded by the cuff method; in such a case, arterial cannulation is necessary to record the blood pressure accurately.

An increase in vagal tone can cause hypotension. This situation should be suspected in the setting of bradycardia, especially in the presence of an acute inferior or posterior MI, or if significant nausea or vomiting is present. In such cases, the hypotension usually responds to atropine.

Hypotension may also be secondary to hypovolemia. In the absence of significant rales, a hypotensive patient can be put in a modified Trendelenburg's position (legs raised with head dependent to increase venous return) and intravenous crystalloid solutions can be administered. One or two hundred milliliters of saline can be given relatively rapidly with careful auscultation to assess the presence of pulmonary congestion. Monitoring of the respiratory rate and questioning the patient for dyspnea are also important during intravenous fluid loading as a guide to incipient left heart failure, since patients may have significant pulmonary congestion without rales when the pulmonary edema fluid is limited to the interstitial space. If hypotension persists after IV fluid loading, a Swan-Ganz catheter should be placed to assess left ventricular filling pressures more precisely. Measurement of a central venous pressure does not provide reliable information regarding the adequacy of the left ventricular filling pressure; this can only be accurately judged by measurement of the pulmonary capillary wedge pressure.

In the absence of facilities for placement and monitoring of pulmonary capillary wedge pressure catheters, the effects of intravenous fluid loading must be assessed by clinical parameters such as urine output and the presence or absence of rales, and other signs of pulmonary congestion (dyspnea, tachypnea).

In general, if hypotension can be reversed to maintain systolic pressure above 90 mmHg by fluid administration, addition of inotropic agents is usually not necessary. Tables 3 and 4 provide hemodynamic classification and therapy.

Persistent Hypotension Despite Adequate Fluid Replacement. The patient with persistent hypotension should be assessed for the following possibilities:

1. Is the blood pressure measurement accurate? An arterial line should be placed, the cannula flushed, and a high fidelity pressure tracing seen on the monitor before a definite conclusion about significant hypotension is accepted.

TABLE 3.   HEMODYNAMIC SUBSETS IN ACUTE MI

Clinical Subset	Cardiac Index (L/min/m^2)	Pulmonary Capillary Wedge Pressure (mmHg)	Mortality Rate (%)
I. No pulmonary congestion No peripheral hypoperfusion	2.7 ± 0.5	12 ± 7	2.2
II. Isolated pulmonary congestion	2.3 ± 0.4	23 ± 5	10.1
III. Isolated peripheral hypoperfusion	1.9 ± 0.4	12 ± 5	22.4
IV. Both pulmonary congestion and peripheral hypoperfusion	1.6 ± 0.6	27 ± 8	55.5

Modified from Forrester JS, Diamond G, Chatterjie K, Swan JHC: Medical therapy of acute myocardial infarction by application of hemodynamic subsets. N Engl J Med 295:1356, 1404, 1976.

2. What is the patient's usual blood pressure? A systolic BP of 80 mmHg may not have the same significance in a patient whose usual BP is 90 mmHg as it does in one whose usual BP is 140 mmHg. In a patient with a low-preinfarction BP, the adequacy of peripheral perfusion as judged by skin color and warmth, urine output, and mentation may be a better guide to the presence of physiologically significant hypotension than the BP measurement itself.

3. Are any medications being given that could account for the hypotension, e.g., morphine, nitrates, excessive diuretics, negative inotropic agents, or vasodilators?

4. Is severe hypoxia present?

5. Could the hypotension be due to an arrhythmia, such as the development of atrial fibrillation, atrial flutter, or high-degree atrioventricular block?

6. Could the hypotension be due to an underlying mechanical problem, such as pericardial tamponade, right ventricular infarction and failure, ventricular septal defect, mitral insufficiency, or the presence of a large pulmonary embolism? These conditions require specific therapy.

7. Has adequate fluid replacement been administered? The pulmonary capillary wedge pressure (PCWP) is the best guide to the adequacy of fluid replacement. It should be increased to 14–18 mmHg with saline. If hypotension persists with a PCWP of 18, the PCWP should be increased gradually into the low 20s, with careful auscultation of the lungs. Some patients require a relatively high left ventricular filling pressure after an acute MI because of an increase in left ventricular diastolic stiffness. Thus, a greater distending force, as represented by the left ventricular filling pressure or PCWP, is required to maintain adequate preload or sarcomere stretch on the noninfarcted fibers and to maintain adequate diastolic left ventricular filling for an adequate stroke volume.

TABLE 4.   HEMODYNAMIC CLASSIFICATION AND THERAPY

Hemodynamic Category	PCWP*	CI†	Suggested Therapy	Comment
Normal	≤12	2.7–3.5	None	Beta blockade may be beneficial
Hyperdynamic	≤12	≥3.0	Beta blockade Light sedation Reassurance	Tachycardia usually present. Mild hypertension may be present. Rule out underlying cause (persistent pain, ischemia, pericarditis, fever)
Hypotension or shock (from hypovolemia)	≤9	≤2.7	Increase vascular volume	Reassess after PCWP c 18 mmHg. PCWP of 20–25 mmHg may be needed in some cases
Left ventricular failure (mild)	18–22	≤2.5	Diuretics Nitrates Digitalis if congestive heart failure persists	Mild pulmonary congestion; dyspnea, hypoxemia
Left ventricular failure (severe)	≥22	≤1.8	Diuretics Vasodilators Positive inotropic agents (dobutamine, dopamine, digitalis)	Pulmonary congestion and pulmonary edema. Mechanical (positive pressure) ventilation may be helpful
Hypotension or shock from left ventricular pump failure	≥18	≤1.8	Positive inotropic agents Circulatory assist	Rule out surgically correctable lesion (ventricular septal defect, papillary muscle rupture)

*Pulmonary capillary wedge pressure (mmHg).
†Cardiac index (L/min/m²).
Modified from Pasternak RC, Braunwald E, Sobel BE: Acute myocardial infarction. *In* Braunwald E (ed): Heart Disease: A Textbook of Cardiovascular Medicine, 3rd ed. Philadelphia, WB Saunders Co, 1988, p 1273.

8. Should inotropic support be given? If no other cause of the hypotension can be found, and the PCWP has been "cranked up" to the 18–25 mmHg range yet hypotension persists, a positive inotropic agent should be added. Dobutamine and dopamine are particularly useful agents in such circumstances.

Persistent hypotension with an elevated PCWP implies a relatively large infarct and poor prognosis. However, many patients respond favorably to inotropic support and after several hours to days can be weaned from their inotropic agent, or switched to an oral inotropic drug, such as digoxin, and make an acceptable hemodynamic recovery.

Pulmonary Congestion

Pulmonary congestion is recognized by the presence of rales on physical examination or by interstitial pulmonary edema on chest radiograph. Pulmonary congestion occurs because of an elevation of the PCWP in excess of colloid osmotic pressure, which is approximately 25–28 mmHg if the serum albumin concentration is normal. The PCWP represents the hydrostatic force tending to move water from the capillary lumen to the interstitial space; the colloid osmotic pressure is the force retaining fluid within the capillary.

The PCWP reflects left ventricular diastolic pressure. It can become increased as a result of left ventricular *systolic* failure, which results in a higher diastolic volume in the left ventricle because of a decrease in stroke volume. The higher left ventricular diastolic volume causes a higher left ventricular diastolic pressure, which leads to an increase in left atrial, pulmonary venous, and pulmonary capillary pressures. The PCWP can also increase as a result of an increase in stiffness of the left ventricular chamber resulting from the ischemia, edema, and cellular infiltration associated with an MI. This increase in ventricular diastolic stiffness has the effect of increasing the PCWP at even normal diastolic volumes. Thus, systolic failure and an increase in diastolic stiffness are additive in their action to increase the PCWP and cause pulmonary congestion or pulmonary edema.

Acute mitral insufficiency secondary to papillary muscle ischemia or infarction can also cause pulmonary congestion by increasing left atrial pressure and thus PCWP.

Mild Pulmonary Congestion. Mild pulmonary congestion is present if rales are limited to the lower third of the lung field. The chest radiograph shows a pattern of mild pulmonary congestion without gross pulmonary edema. The patient feels slightly short of breath and is modestly tachypneic. The degree of arterial hypoxemia is also mild. As just discussed, the cause of the pulmonary vascular congestion is an elevation of the intracapillary pressure (PCWP) and the goal of therapy is to reduce this pressure.

Diuretics, particularly intravenous furosemide, are usually effective in partially or completely correcting the pulmonary congestion in such circumstances; intravenous furosemide acts initially as a systemic venodilator and subsequently as a diuretic. Nitroglycerin, by virtue of its systemic venodilating effect, also decreases pulmonary congestion. It is important to monitor the arterial blood pressure carefully when these agents are given, because cardiac output can decrease rapidly as the PCWP and left ventricular filling pressure decrease, particularly in the acute MI setting in which the left ventricle is relatively stiff. In such cases, a small decrease in the left ventricular filling pressure can have a marked effect on left ventricular filling volume, stroke volume, and cardiac output.

Pulmonary congestion secondary to mitral insufficiency as a result of papillary muscle ischemia or infarction may also respond to diuretic or nitrate therapy. The severity of the mitral insufficiency often depends on left ventricular size and left ventricular systolic pressures. Nitrates, by their venodilator action, usually decrease left ventricular size, and they may also decrease systolic left ventricular pressure. Both of these actions can significantly decrease the amount of mitral insufficiency. Intravenous nitroprusside can have the same effects. Diuretics, by reducing left ventricular size, can also decrease the amount of mitral insufficiency.

Pulmonary congestion may also represent the consequences of continued myocardial ischemia causing loss of contractility and increased myocardial stiffness in a region that has not become completely infarcted. If such ischemia involves the papillary muscle or underlying LV wall, mitral insufficiency may also result. By relieving the degree of ischemia, nitrates or calcium channel blockers may improve left ventricular function, decrease left ventricular stiffness, or decrease any mitral insufficiency related to a reversible ischemia component.

Severe Pulmonary Congestion. Severe pulmonary congestion or pulmonary edema requires rapid aggressive therapy to reduce the PCWP and avoid severe arterial hypoxemia and respiratory acidosis. Therapy should consist of intravenous diuretics (furosemide), intravenous nitroglycerin or nitroprusside (nitroglycerin is probably preferred, unless there is severe arterial hypertension), and positive pressure mechanical ventilation. If there is concomitant arterial hypotension or a low cardiac output, positive inotropic agents, such as dobutamine or dopamine, should be added and consideration should be given to a circulatory assist device, such as intra-aortic balloon counterpulsation. Rotating tourniquets, intravenous morphine, positioning of the patient upright in bed, and phlebotomy (if the hematocrit is adequate) may all be beneficial or necessary to reverse severe pulmonary congestion or pulmonary edema.

The combination of pulmonary congestion and a low cardiac output has an ominous prognosis because it indicates that stroke volume is low despite an elevated left ventricular filling pressure. The therapeutic goal is to maintain the PCWP at a relatively high level to maintain left ventricular filling and cardiac output, but to keep the PCWP below the level that causes pulmonary congestion. Often a PCWP between 14 and 18 mmHg is adequate, but some patients will require a capillary pressure in the 20–25 mmHg range. In such cases, hemodynamic monitoring with an arterial cannula and a balloon-tipped pulmonary catheter (Swan-Ganz) is often desirable in order to manipulate the PCWP optimally to maintain adequate cardiac output. Cardiac output can be measured by the thermodilution technique with an appropriate pulmonary artery catheter.

Cardiogenic Shock

Cardiogenic shock is characterized by persistent, severe hypotension despite an adequate intravascular volume, i.e., an elevated PCWP. In addition to hypotension, there are signs of peripheral hypoperfusion such as cyanotic extremities with cool, mottled skin; decreased urine output; and a confused, disoriented mental status secondary to cerebral hypoperfusion. The systolic arterial pressure is less than 80 mmHg, and the cardiac index is markedly reduced (< 1.8 L/min/M^2) despite adequate left ventricular filling pressures as indicated by PCWP > 18 mmHg. The systemic vascular resistance is usually elevated, indicating peripheral vascular constriction.

Although most cases of cardiogenic shock result from extensive MI, it is important to rule out other causes, such as drugs with a myocardial depressant effect; respiratory hypoxemia or acidosis; sepsis; hemorrhage; impairment of cardiac output as a result of mechanical ventilation; or a correctable cardiac lesion such as pericardial tamponade, papillary muscle rupture, or rupture of the ventricular septum. If such lesions are thought to be responsible for cardiogenic shock, emergency angiography should be done to confirm the diagnosis, and then emergency surgery performed.

The presence of cardiogenic shock as just defined carries with it an extremely poor prognosis, with mortality rates of 80–90% in most series. Therapy consists of inotropic support with sympathomimetic agents such as dobutamine or dopamine. In some centers, mechanical circulatory assist is performed utilizing devices such as intra-aortic balloon counterpulsation.

Indications for Invasive Monitoring[2]

From the preceding discussion, it is evident that quantitative assessment of arterial pressure, PCWP, and urine output is often necessary for optimal care of the acute MI patient. These data can be obtained by use of intra-arterial cannulation; a pulmonary artery balloon-tipped catheter, which can also measure cardiac output by the thermodilution technique; and an indwelling Foley catheter to assess urine output. In general, indications for invasive monitoring include the following:

1. Persistent hypotension despite reversed Trendelenburg's position and intravenous infusion of several hundred ml of crystalloid solution.
2. Moderate or severe left ventricular failure and pulmonary congestion.
3. Refractory or unexplained sinus tachycardia or other tachyarrhythmias.
4. Unexplained deterioration as manifested by cyanosis, hypoxemia, tachypnea, diaphoresis, or acidosis.
5. Suspected severe mitral regurgitation, ventricular septal defect, or pericardial tamponade.

From these considerations it is evident that the uncomplicated acute MI does not warrant invasive monitoring. This monitoring should not be performed on a routine basis, because these invasive techniques all have a significant risk of morbidity, and because this issue has become more complex as a result of the use of thrombolytic therapy early in the course of acute MI.

Anticoagulant Therapy

As discussed previously, if thrombolytic therapy is given, immediate anticoagulation with intravenous heparin is indicated for 3–5 days, to be followed by long-term antiplatelet therapy with daily aspirin (325 mg qd).

In patients who do not receive thrombolytic therapy and who have no contraindications to anticoagulation, the following approach is recommended:

Indications for Anticoagulation. The use of anticoagulants in the patient with acute MI has been a controversial topic for decades. At this time, the following recommendations seem appropriate for patients who have no contraindication to anticoagulants:

1. Mini-dose heparin (5000 U SQ q8–12 h) is recommended for all patients hospitalized for acute MI, if there is no significant contraindication. This dosage appears to reduce the incidence of deep venous thrombosis significantly, and thereby reduce the incidence of severe pulmonary embolism in patients who are at bed rest. The heparin can be discontinued as patients become ambulatory during the post-MI convalescence phase.

2. Full-dose anticoagulation with heparin (10,000–15,000 U IV, followed by approximately 1000 U/hour to maintain the partial thromboplastin time [PTT] at 1.5–2.5 times normal) is recommended for patients with a high risk of venous thrombosis and pulmonary embolism. Such patients include those with marked obesity, significant left ventricular failure with a low output state, and a past history of venous thrombosis or pulmonary embolism. Patients who show severe motion abnormalities (akinesis or dyskinesis) of the anterior wall or apical regions should also be fully anticoagulated, as they have a significant risk of mural thrombosis and subsequent embolism. The duration of anticoagulation for such patients has not been precisely defined. Anticoagulation should probably continue for 6 months post-infarction, with the patient switched from heparin to sodium warfarin (Coumadin) prior to the time of hospital discharge.

Management of Arrhythmias and Conduction Defects

Most patients with acute MI will develop some form of cardiac arrhythmia, usually ventricular premature beats. Before drug therapy is used, it is important to assess underlying factors that may be responsible for the arrhythmia and attempt to alleviate them, such as the following:
1. Increased catecholamine levels as a result of chest pain and anxiety
2. Congestive heart failure
3. Electrolyte abnormalities, especially hypokalemia
4. Abnormal blood gases (pH, pO_2)
5. Anemia
6. Fever
7. Pericarditis
8. Pulmonary emboli
9. Drug toxicity, especially from caffeine; bronchodilators; digitalis; and antiarrhythmic agents, which themselves can cause sinus bradycardias, conduction defects, and ventricular ectopy

Management of specific arrhythmias is discussed in the following sections.

Sinus Bradycardia

Sinus bradycardia may reflect an increased vagal tone or sinus node ischemia. In the former case, the prognosis is usually good and no treatment is necessary if adequate blood pressure is maintained, there are no associated ventricular premature beats, and the heart rate is above 45. If the bradycardia is associated with hypotension or with a significant frequency of ventricular premature beats, the heart rate should be increased. Ventricular ectopy that appears in the setting of sinus bradycardia is often suppressed with an increase in heart rate. Intravenous atropine can be given in 0.5 mg aliquots and repeated three or four times to increase the heart rate to the range of 60. Atropine is usually most effective in the first 6–8 hours post-MI. Sinus bradycardia that occurs later in the course of an acute MI often represents intrinsic sinus node dysfunction. Atropine should be tried as first therapy. If the bradycardia is not responsive, a temporary pacemaker should be inserted if therapy is required.

Sinus Tachycardia

Sinus tachycardia is discussed under the heading Treatment of Abnormal Hemodynamics.

Atrial Fibrillation, Flutter, and Supraventricular Tachycardia

In the treatment of these arrhythmias, it is important to assess the underlying cause and the hemodynamic consequences of the arrhythmia. If the arrhythmia is associated with an acceptable ventricular rate and is well tolerated hemodynamically in terms of blood pressure, absence of ischemia, or left ventricular failure, specific therapy may not be required. On the other hand, if the arrhythmia is associated with hemodynamic deterioration or causes increased ischemia, treatment is indicated on an emergent basis. The potential therapeutic modalities include direct current cardioversion or pharmacologic therapy with verapamil, a digitalis glycoside, or a beta blocker to control the ventricular rate. The choice of specific therapy should be tailored to the individual situation.

If the rhythm is converted to a sinus mechanism, it is important to try to prevent a recurrence. The usual harbinger of these rhythms is atrial premature contractions; an underlying cause of the atrial ectopy (e.g., incipient congestive heart failure or pericarditis) should be assessed and treated appropriately. Drugs that can reduce atrial ectopy include the digitalis glycosides, beta blockers, quinidine, and procainamide. Maintenance of a high-normal serum potassium level may also be helpful in suppressing atrial ectopy.

Ventricular Ectopic Activity

Almost all patients with acute MI will have some degree of ventricular ectopy. Ventricular ectopy should be suppressed during the first 24–48 hours of an acute MI, when the risk of progression to ventricular tachycardia or ventricular fibrillation (VT/VF) is highest. However, persistent ventricular premature beats (VPBs) beyond the first 48 hours do not always require drug treatment. Generally accepted indications for treatment of ventricular premature contractions during the later course of an acute MI include the following criteria:

1. Frequency > 5–6/minute.
2. The occurrence of repetitive VPBs (two or more sequential VPBs).
3. The occurrence of multi-form VPBs.
4. Occurrence of the "R on T" phenomenon, in which the VPBs occur near the apex of the T wave; such VPBs have a higher than usual propensity to induce ventricular fibrillation.

Treatment initially consists of identifying an underlying cause and reversing it if possible, as discussed previously. If drug therapy is required, intravenous lidocaine is the agent of choice. This medication should be given as a 100 mg bolus, which may be repeated one to three times, depending on patient size and hemodynamic response, and should be followed by an intravenous infusion at 1–4 mg/minute. The dose should be decreased in elderly patients, in the presence of congestive failure or liver disease, and in patients taking propranolol.

Additional useful agents include procainamide, which should be given intravenously in 100 mg aliquots every 6 minutes for seven to ten doses, depending upon the hemodynamic and VPB response. The initial loading dose should be followed by an infusion of 2–6 mg/minute as a maintenance dose. The dose should be decreased in the presence of renal disease.

Adrenergic beta blocking agents may be particularly useful in suppressing VPBs in the early hours of the post-MI period, when sympathetic tone may be increased.

Maintenance of a high serum potassium level may also be helpful in suppressing ventricular ectopy and in decreasing the likelihood of progression to VT/VF.

After ventricular ectopy is suppressed with one of these pharmacologic agents, it is reasonable to reassess the need for such therapy at 24 hours after the initiation of treatment by progressively titrating down the maintenance infusions and observing whether there is any recurrence of the ventricular ectopy. As a general rule, ventricular ectopy is more frequent in the early phase of acute MI; most patients who require early suppression of ventricular premature contractions can be successfully weaned from their antiarrhythmic therapy later in the course of the MI.

The question of "prophylactic therapy," in the absence of VPBs, to prevent serious ventricular arrhythmias such as VT/VF remains controversial. It is probably reasonable to give lidocaine as "prophylaxis" in a patient with an acute MI who is at low risk for lidocaine toxicity. Prophylactic lidocaine may also be useful in a setting in which arrhythmia monitoring is not possible and in which the incidence of ventricular ectopy is high. Thus, in a relatively young patient (< 50 years old), having a first MI, who is in the initial 24 hours of the onset of symptoms, in whom there is no congestive failure or liver disease, prophylactic lidocaine may be beneficial. On the other hand, in older patients or those with left ventricular failure or liver disase, or those who present relatively late after the onset of their MI (> 24 hours), the risk of prophylactic lidocaine therapy probably outweighs the benefits.

Ventricular Tachycardia

Two types of ventricular tachycardia need to be distinguished: slow ventricular tachycardia and rapid ventricular tachycardia.

Slow ventricular tachycardia, also called "accelerated idioventricular rhythm," occurs at rates of approximately 60–110 and often represents an escape rhythm in response to an underlying sinus bradycardia or high-degree atrioventricular block. The potential of this rhythm to deteriorate into rapid ventricular tachycardia or ventricular fibrillation is controversial; slow ventricular tachycardia is certainly not an innocuous rhythm, but it can also be well tolerated in many cases and often does not deteriorate into more serious arrhythmias.

A reasonable therapeutic approach is to monitor such patients carefully if an adequate blood pressure is maintained during the slow ventricular tachycardia. This rhythm can often be abolished by increasing the sinus rate with atropine or a temporary pacemaker. Alternatively, the rhythm can be suppressed with lidocaine. However, before suppressing a slow ventricular tachycardia, one must be certain that there is adequate underlying sinus node activity. If the slow ventricular tachycardia represents an escape rhythm from sinus arrest or severe sinus bradycardia, abolition of the ventricular tachycardia may leave the patient with severe sinus bradycardia or asystole as the post-treatment rhythm.

Rapid ventricular tachycardia is characterized by a rate that is usually greater than 150. Emergency treatment is required because blood pressure and cardiac output are usually markedly decreased and because this rhythm often rapidly deteriorates into ventricular fibrillation. The treatment of choice is direct current countershock, which should be synchronized if possible. Usually, relatively low energies can be utilized; 25 watt-seconds is a reasonable starting level. It is important to assess any underlying causes of ventricular ectopy to try to prevent a recurrence. In general, lidocaine or procainamide should be administered post-cardioversion (doses discussed previously). Often the initiating event of ventricular tachycardia is a VPB. Thus, it is appropriate to treat the patient who has had an episode of rapid ventricular tachycardia with lidocaine or procainamide to attempt to prevent a recurrence by suppressing any VPBs.

Bretylium may also be employed in an attempt to convert ventricular tachycardia and may be used to prevent its recurrence.

Ventricular Fibrillation

Although classic teaching has been that ventricular fibrillation is usually preceded by a "warning" arrhythmia such as ventricular tachycardia or ventricular premature contractions, recent studies have shown that 50% of episodes of ventricular fibrillation have no such warning arrhythmias.[2] The term "primary ventricular fibrillation" refers to an event that is primarily electrical, i.e., is not the result of severe congestive heart failure or cardiogenic shock. Such primary ventricular fibrillation is most common in the first few hours of an MI, but it can occur with a decreasing incidence throughout the acute infarct course. "Secondary" ventricular fibrillation occurs in the setting of severe hemodynamic deterioration and is usually a terminal event.

The treatment of ventricular fibrillation is immediate direct current countershock at relatively high energies, e.g., 400 watt-seconds. Post-defibrillation therapy should be addressed at reversal of underlying causes and suppressive therapy with lidocaine, procainamide, or bretylium.

Atrioventricular Block and Conduction Defects

First-degree atrioventricular block generally requires no specific treatment but should be monitored carefully for progression to higher degrees of atrioventricular block.

Second-degree atrioventricular block is of two types: Mobitz I (Wencke-bach's) or Mobitz II. Mobitz I atrioventricular block usually occurs in the setting of an inferior or posterior wall MI, is generally of a benign prognosis, and is often self-limited. The presence of Mobitz I block implies that the block is at the level of the atrioventricular node and not at the lower His bundle or Purkinje's fibers. In general, no specific therapy is needed if the ventricular rate is maintained above 60 and there is adequate blood pressure and no concomitant bundle branch blocks. If the ventricular rate is too slow, atropine may be tried as therapy. If atropine is not successful, a temporary pacemaker should be inserted. If second-degree atrioventricular block that appears to be Mobitz I is associated with complete right bundle branch block or left bundle branch block, a pacemaker should be inserted because such patients are at relatively high risk for high-grade atrioventricular block (see later discussion).

Mobitz II second-degree atrioventricular block (i.e., nonconducted P waves without progressive lengthening of the P-R interval) should be treated with a temporary pacemaker. Mobitz II block implies block at the level of the bundle of His or lower conducting system; such patients are at significant risk for progression to higher degrees of atrioventricular block.

Third-degree atrioventricular block (complete heart block) generally requires a temporary pacemaker. An exception can be made for Mobitz I block that progresses to third-degree atrioventricular block with a good escape rhythm, usually in the setting of an inferior wall MI. An escape rhythm is adequate if the heart rate is above 50, blood pressure is maintained, and there is a narrow QRS complex indicating an escape focus relatively high in the His-Purkinje system. If a temporary pacemaker is initially withheld because the escape rhythm is adequate but the patient develops ventricular premature beats that warrant therapy, a pacemaker should be inserted before administering antiarrhythmic drugs, since such drugs may abolish the escape rhythm.

In assessing the patient with atrioventricular block, it is important to rule out underlying contributing conditions such as digitalis toxicity, hyperkalemia, quinidine or procainamide toxicity, and effects that are due to beta blockers or calcium channel blockers.

If left ventricular failure is present, an atrioventricular sequential pacemaker may be desirable to maintain the atrial contribution to left ventricular filling.

Prophylactic Temporary Pacemaker Insertion for Bundle Branch Blocks

Certain bundle branch block patterns are associated with a relatively high risk of developing high-degree atrioventricular block in a patient with acute MI. In such cases, insertion of a temporary pacemaker as a prophylactic measure is warranted. The pacemaker protects the patient should high-degree atrioventricular block develop.

For example, a patient with complete left bundle branch block who is a candidate for Swan-Ganz catheter placement should have a temporary pacemaker inserted prior to placement of the catheter, since the Swan-Ganz catheter often produces transient right bundle branch block; in a patient with pre-existing left bundle branch block, the result is complete heart block.

Other high- and low-risk categories for developing high-grade atrioventricular block depend on involvement of both the right and the left bundle branch systems and consideration of whether a bundle branch block is "new" with the acute infarct or has been present chronically.[12]

The following combinations are associated with a relatively low risk (10–13%) of developing high-grade atrioventricular block during the course of an acute MI, and prophylactic temporary pacemaker insertion is generally not indicated for these situations:

1. First-degree atrioventricular block
2. "New" unilateral bundle branch block
3. Old bilateral bundle branch block, i.e., right bundle branch block with left anterior or posterior fascicular block

The following combinations represent an intermediate risk of developing high-grade atrioventricular block (19–20%):

1. First degree atrioventricular block plus "new" unilateral bundle branch block
2. First-degree atrioventricular block plus old bilateral bundle branch block

The following combinations are at relatively high risk (31–38%) of developing high-grade atrioventricular block during the course of acute MI:

1. Bilateral bundle branch block of which one or both components are "new" carries a 31% risk of developing high-grade atrioventricular block.
2. In the setting of additional first degree atrioventricular block, this combination has a 38% risk of developing high-grade atrioventricular block.

It is reasonable to place a prophylactic temporary pacemaker in situations in which the patient is at a 20% or greater risk of developing high-grade atrioventricular block during the course of acute MI.

Post–Myocardial Infarction Care

A detailed discussion of post-MI care is beyond the scope of this book. However, the general considerations that need to be addressed before the patient is discharged are as follows:

1. Post-MI workup: Holter's monitoring, stress testing, and echocardiography
2. Need for chronic antiarrhythmic therapy
3. Need for chronic anticoagulation
4. Need for permanent pacemaker implantation
5. Need for chronic beta blocker therapy
6. Need for cardiac rehabilitation program

KEY FEATURES

I. Diagnosis
  A. History may include one or more of the following:
    1. Prolonged (greater than 20 minutes) characteristic chest or upper abdominal pain (often with radiation to shoulders, arms, neck, jaw, or back), often squeezing or constrictive (positive Levine's sign)
    2. Increased congestive heart failure manifesting as dyspnea
    3. Weakness, diaphoresis, nausea, and vomiting
    4. Stroke
  B. Physical findings depend on the severity of hemodynamic compromise and range from a normal hemodynamic state with a small myocardial infarct to congestive heart failure and profound shock with large infarcts. Characteristic features include the following:
    1. Patient is usually anxious and distressed.
    2. Blood pressure and pulse may be normal, increased, or decreased.
    3. Ventricular ectopy is common.
    4. An S_4 gallop, murmur of papillary muscle dysfunction, and transient pericardial friction rub are common.

      5. Signs of pulmonary congestion may be present, depending on the degree of heart failure.

      6. A sustained apical lift may be present, representing a dyskinetic ventricular bulge.

   C. Laboratory tests

      1. The ECG usually shows ischemic ST–T abnormalities; Q waves may develop; ventricular ectopy is common; and conduction defects may be present. ECG changes may not evolve for 24 hours after the onset of an MI. A normal ECG does not rule out an acute MI.

      2. Serum levels of creatine kinase, SGOT, and LDH are increased.

      3. The chest radiograph may show pulmonary congestion, depending on the degree of heart failure.

      4. The echocardiogram may demonstrate left ventricular wall motion abnormalities or apical thrombus.

      5. Radionuclide studies

         a. Technetium pyrophosphate scan "lights up" acute infarct regions.

         b. Thallium perfusion scan shows a nonreversible defect.

         c. Gated blood pool scan may reveal wall motion abnormalities.

  II. Pathophysiology

An acute thrombotic occlusion of an epicardial coronary artery is the cause of acute MI in 85–90% of cases. After such an occlusion, the rate of myocardial necrosis depends upon the extent of collateral flow. Necrosis starts in the subendocardial layer of the ischemic region after approximately 20 minutes of severe ischemia, and a "wavefront" of necrosis progresses from subendocardium to subepicardium over 4–6 hours. Infarct size is an important determinant of prognosis. The larger the infarct, the greater the likelihood of congestive heart failure, malignant ventricular ectopy, conduction defects, cardiogenic shock, and death.

  III. Treatment

   A. General measures include CCU admission, sedation, analgesia, and appropriate diet.

   B. Immediate thrombolytic therapy with tissue plasminogen activator (TPA) or another effective agent should be given if it can be administered within 6 hours of the onset of symptoms.

   C. Hemodynamic abnormalities require specific precise therapy (see Tables 3 and 4).

   D. Arrhythmias and conduction defects require individualized specific therapy (see text).

   E. Post-MI care includes risk stratification; consideration of coronary angiography and percutaneous transluminal coronary angioplasty (PTCA) or coronary bypass graft surgery; and chronic beta adrenergic blockade therapy, unless contraindicated.

BIBLIOGRAPHY

1. Alpert JS, Braunwald E: Acute myocardial infarction: Pathological, pathophysiological and clinical manifestations. *In* Braunwald E (ed): Heart Disease: A Textbook of Cardiovascular Medicine, 2nd ed. Philadelphia, WB Saunders Co, 1984, pp 1262–1300.

2. Sobel BE, Braunwald E: The management of acute myocardial infarction. *In* Braunwald E (ed): Heart Disease: A Textbook of Cardiovascular Medicine, 2nd ed. Philadelphia, WB Saunders Co, 1984, pp 1301–1333.

2a. Pasternak RC, Braunwald E, Sobel BE: Acute myocardial infarction. *In* Braunwald E (ed): Heart Disease: A Textbook of Cardiovascular Medicine, 3rd ed. Philadelphia, WB Saunders Co, 1988, pp 1222–1313.
    These three chapters from Braunwald's text provide an excellent foundation for the care of patients with MI. There is little else that one needs to read on this subject.

3. Uretsky BF, Farquhar DS, Borezin A, Hood WB: Symptomatic myocardial infarction without chest pain: Prevalence and clinical course. Am J Cardiol 40:498, 1977.
    In a series of 102 consecutive patients with acute MI at the Boston City Hospital, 26% had no chest pain, pressure, or heaviness, but presented with atypical symptoms such as dyspnea, abdominal pain, fatigue, left arm pain, cough, nausea and vomiting, or syncope. Such an atypical presentation occurred more frequently in older patients and was associated with a longer delay between the onset of symptoms and arrival at the hospital, examination by a physician in the emergency room, diagnosis of a possible MI, and transfer from the emergency room to an intensive care unit. Mortality in the atypical presentation group was 50%, compared with 18% in the group who presented with typical chest pain or pressure. This article should alert physicians to consider the diagnosis of acute MI in patients who present with atypical symptoms.

4. DeWood MA, Spores J, Notske R: Prevalence of total coronary occlusion during the early hours of transmural myocardial infarction. N Engl J Med 303:897, 1980.
    This important article documents that coronary arterial thrombus formation is responsible for the coronary arterial occlusion that precipitates acute MI in 85% of cases.

5. Laffel LG, Braunwald E: Thrombolytic therapy. A new strategy for the treatment of acute myocardial infarction. N Engl J Med 311:710, 770, 1984.
    An excellent review of the current status of thrombolytic therapy for acute MI.

6. Reimer KA, Lowe JE, Ramussen MM, Jennings RB: The wavefront phenomenon of ischemic cell death. I. Myocardial infarct size vs. duration of coronary occlusion in dogs. Circulation 56:786, 1977.
    After a coronary artery occlusion, myocardial necrosis occurs first in the subendocardium, where cell death was noted after 40 minutes. With longer periods of occlusion, a "wavefront" of necrosis spread along a transmural axis from endocardium to epicardium. Approximately 4–6 hours was required to produce a completed transmural infarct.

7. Hutter AM, DeSanctis RW, Flynn J, Yeatman LA: Nontransmural myocardial infarction: A comparison of hospital and late clinical course of patients with that of matched patients with transmural anterior and transmural inferior myocardial infarction. Am J Cardiol 48:595, 1981.
    Patients admitted with nontransmural infarction had a significantly lower CCU mortality rate (9%) than patients with a transmural infarct (20%). However, over the subsequent 9 months, recurrent MI was greater in those patients originally admitted for a nontransmural infarction (21% reinfarction rate, compared with only a 3% reinfarction rate following an initial transmural infarction). The overall late mortality rates of the two types of infarcts were comparable.

8. Killip T, Kimball JT: Treatment of myocardial infarction in a coronary care unit. A two year experience with 250 patients. Am J Cardiol 20:457, 1967.
    During the 1960s, coronary care units became accepted as the best environment for the modern treatment of acute MI. This early paper from Killip and Kimball provides a great deal of clinical guidance and a classification of patients with acute MI that has remained highly useful for two decades.

9. Forrester JS, Diamond G, Chatterjie K, Swan JHC: Medical therapy of acute myocardial infarction by application of hemodynamic subsets. N Engl J Med 295:1356, 1404, 1976.
Interpretation of pulmonary capillary wedge pressure and cardiac output measurements, and their relation to prognosis, clinical course, and therapy are the subjects of these classic articles.

10. Nordrehaug JE, Johannessen KA, Von Der Lippe G: Usefulness of high-dose anticoagulants in preventing left ventricular thrombus in acute myocardial infarction. Am J Cardiol 55:1491, 1985.
Fifty-three patients with acute anterior MI were randomized to anticoagulants or placebo. In the placebo group, seven patients (33%) developed left ventricular thrombus compared with none in the anticoagulant group.

11. Visser CA, Kan G, Meltzer RS, Dunning AJ, Roelandt J: Embolic potential of left ventricular thrombus after myocardial infarction: A two-dimensional echocardiographic study of 119 patients. J Am Coll Cardiol 5:1276, 1985.
Left ventricular mural thrombus complicating an MI occurred after an anterior MI ten times more commonly than after an inferior MI. A systemic embolus occurred in 20% of cases. Anticoagulants reduced, but did not completely prevent, embolization.

12. Hindman MC, Wagner GS, Ja Ro M, Atkins JM, Scheinman MM, Rubin M, Morris JJ: The clinical significance of bundle branch block complicating acute myocardial infarction. 2. Indications for temporary and permanent pacemaker insertion. Circulation 58:689, 1978.
This article reviews the clinical course of over 400 patients with acute MI who had some degree of atrioventricular nodal block or bundle branch block. Depending on their specific type and combinations of atrioventricular and bundle branch block, and the acuteness, such patients can be categorized according to their relative risk for developing high-grade atrioventricular block. This classification provides a useful framework for deciding which patients should receive "prophylactic" temporary pacemaker insertion.

13. TIMI Study Group. N Engl J Med 312:932, 1985.
Patients with impending acute MI were randomized into intravenous TPA or intravenous SK treatment groups, and coronary angiography was performed before and after thrombolytic therapy to document the presence of coronary arterial clot and thrombolysis. The intravenous TPA was twice as effective as SK in recanalizing the occluded coronary arteries (66% vs. 36% recanalization rate, respectively).

14. Gruppo Italiano per lo Studio Della Streptochinasi Nell'infarcto Miocardio (GISSI). Lancet 1:397, 1986.
The GISSI Trial provides definitive evidence of the benefits of early intravenous thrombolytic therapy in acute MI. Approximately 12,000 patients with acute MI were prospectively randomized to a "no thrombolytic treatment" control group or an intravenous SK group. Hospital mortality rate was reduced in direct proportion to the speed with which the intravenous SK was given. In patients who received SK within 1 hour of symptoms, the mortality rate was 50% less than that of controls. If SK was given within 3 hours of symptoms, mortality was reduced by 25%. The decrease in mortality rate was 20% in patients who received SK within 3–6 hours of the start of symptoms.

15. Simoons ML, et al: Improved survival after early thrombolysis in acute myocardial infarction. Lancet 2:578, 1985.
This Dutch multi-center trial of thrombolytic therapy for acute MI reports results consistent with the GISSI Trial. Five hundred thirty-three patients with acute MI were randomized to "conventional" or "early thrombolytic" therapy; the mortality rate was 50% lower in the early thrombolytic group (10% vs. 5% mortality rates at 14 days post-MI, respectively). The average time from onset of symptoms to arterial recanalization was 3.3 hours. Recanalization was achieved by a variety of methods, including intravenous and/or intracoronary SK, mechanical perforation of persistent thrombus, and angioplasty in

some cases in which severe residual stenoses persisted after thrombolysis in the infarct-related artery. The results indicate that considerable benefit can be gained by thrombolysis early in the course of acute MI.

Unstable Angina

Carl S. Apstein, M.D.

Unstable angina is a serious condition that warrants immediate hospitalization of the patient for monitoring and treatment in a coronary care unit setting, because the natural history is uncertain and because these patients are at high risk for potentially lethal ventricular arrhythmias and/or progression to myocardial infarction.

HISTORY

Unstable angina can occur in a patient with pre-existing, chronic, stable angina, or it can occur *de novo* in a patient with no previous history of angina. In the patient with pre-existing stable angina, the diagnosis of unstable angina is made when a "crescendo" pattern of chest pain occurs, characterized by more frequent episodes of angina, episodes that are more prolonged than usual, easier to provoke, and more resistant to relief by nitroglycerin or rest. Often, angina will occur spontaneously at rest whereas previously it had only occurred with exertion. Angina of new onset (less than 2 months) is also considered to be unstable because its future course is unknown; although such patients may develop a chronic stable anginal pattern, some will rapidly develop a crescendo pattern or progress to a myocardial infarction. Angina may present not only as the characteristic dull, squeezing chest pain, but also as chest "tightness," which can be similar to a sensation of dyspnea. Therefore, in the patient who complains of progressive inability to "catch his breath" with exertion, unstable angina should be considered as part of the differential diagnosis.[1]

Although most cases of unstable angina result from a pathophysiologic process in the coronary arteries (see later discussion), others are precipitated by concomitant conditions that alter the myocardial oxygen supply-demand balance.[2] Therefore, it is important to consider contributing conditions such as anemia, fever, congestive heart failure, hypertension, arrhythmias, thyrotoxicosis, aortic stenosis, emotional stress, or a recent history of heavy cigarette smoking. In the presence of such factors, a major element of therapy must be treatment of the contributing factors themselves.

PHYSICAL EXAMINATION

During a pain-free interval the patient may have no characteristic physical finding of unstable angina, although other evidence of coronary artery disease may be present as a result of pre-existing myocardial infarction. During and immediately after an anginal episode, there is usually an alteration in heart rate and blood pressure, although these may be masked by beta blocker or calcium channel blocker therapy, and the cardiac examination may provide evidence of ischemic myocardial dysfunction such as the presence of a gallop rhythm (usually an S_4 gallop); a murmur of mitral insufficiency that is due to ischemic papillary muscle dysfunction; a sustained apical lift as a resut of dyskinetic bulging of the ischemic region; and pulmonary congestion, which may cause tachypnea, rales, or wheezing. During an episode of angina, the patient is often anxious and frightened and may be diaphoretic or nauseated. With resolution of the myocardial ischemia, the physical findings may disappear and the cardiac examination can return to normal. The rapidly changing nature of the cardiac examination supports the diagnosis of angina.

LABORATORY STUDIES

The electrocardiogram is the most important laboratory test in the acute evaluation of the patient with unstable angina. It usually shows transient ischemic ST segment elevation or depression; T wave inversion or peaking; or, rarely, acute changes in axis or R wave amplitude. Increased atrioventricular nodal block, bundle branch blocks, and/or ventricular ectopy may also occur.

UNSTABLE ANGINA VERSUS ACUTE MYOCARDIAL INFARCTION

The differentiation of angina from myocardial infarction is initially based on the duration of the chest pain, serial ECG changes, and the appearance of cardiac enzymes in the blood. In general, chest pain or tightness of longer than 30 minutes' continuous duration should be considered to represent myocardial infarction until proved otherwise. Likewise, development of Q waves or persistence of ST–T wave changes for longer than 12–24 hours also suggests myocardial infarction. An increased blood level of cardiac enzymes (creatine kinase or lactate dehydrogenase [LDH]) also implies myocyte necrosis and myocardial infarction rather than uncomplicated angina. In many cases, it is not possible to distinguish a severe episode of angina from a myocardial infarction until 24–48 hours have elapsed so that serial ECGs and blood enzyme levels can be assessed.

PATHOPHYSIOLOGY

The pathophysiology of unstable angina is not completely understood, and it may not be the same in all patients. Mechanisms of unstable angina may include the following:
  1. Progression of the atherosclerotic process itself with stenosis of the major epicardial coronary arteries as a result of growth of atheroma
  2. Coronary arterial spasm
  3. Platelet aggregate formation in the coronary circulation
  4. Thrombus (blood clot) formation, which can partially or completely occlude a coronary artery (myocardial infarction may not occur despite a complete occlusion if there is adequate collateral coronary circulation)
  5. A primary increase in myocardial oxygen demand induced by an increase in heart rate or blood pressure
  6. A decrease in oxygen delivery related to severe anemia or hypoxia[3,4]

Several mechanisms may be present in the same patient, and these can reinforce one another. For example, the process of platelet aggregation results in the release of thromboxane from the platelets, causing coronary spasm. The spasm and consequent reduction in local blood flow may enhance further platelet aggregation and thrombus formation.

TREATMENT

The management of unstable angina varies, depending on whether the patient presents during an episode of angina or during a pain-free interval. In both cases, the patient should be admitted to the hospital, ideally to the coronary care unit with close ECG and hemodynamic monitoring. In the patient who presents during a pain-free interval, it is reasonable to defer medication and to monitor the patient closely in order to establish the diagnosis definitively. If an episode of angina occurs, a physical examination and ECG should be performed rapidly and medication given (to be described). Alternatively, if the patient remains pain-free after admission, he or she can be evaluated subsequently on a more elective basis.

The evaluation of a patient who presents *during* an episode of angina should include a very brief history, an efficient physical examination of the cardiovascular system, and a full 12-lead ECG. Conditions that can exacerbate angina (see preceding discussion) should be assessed and treated appropriately. Antianginal medication should then be rapidly administered. As noted previously, different pathophysiologic mechanisms may be responsible in different patients; accordingly, the sequence of medication administration described in the following should not be considered absolute. These guidelines, adapted from Epstein and Palmeri,[2] provide a reasonable overall approach.

1. If the patient is not hypotensive, sublingual nitroglycerin should be administered even if the patient has taken it prior to the arrival at the hospital. It is not uncommon for a patient's supply of nitroglycerin to have become inactive; therefore, the patient's history of having failed to get relief from sublingual nitroglycerin at home should not be taken as definitive evidence against its potential efficacy. If the angina is relieved by sublingual nitroglycerin, long-acting nitrates, either oral or transcutaneous, should be started. Aspirin therapy and a beta blocker or calcium channel blocker should be added subsequently.

2. If sublingual nitroglycerin is not effective in relieving the patient's angina, intravenous nitroglycerin should be promptly started. The use of intravenous nitroglycerin requires close hemodynamic monitoring to avoid hypotension. Adequate arterial blood pressure during intravenous nitroglycerin therapy requires an adequate left ventricular filling (pulmonary capillary wedge) pressure. If maintenance of an adequate arterial blood pressure becomes problematic, a Swan-Ganz catheter should be inserted and left ventricular filling pressure maintained at an adequate level with intravenous saline; a good range is usually 15–18 mmHg. Inadequate filling pressure, even in the absence of overt hypotension, can be deleterious by reducing stroke volume and cardiac output. The resulting reflex sympathetic stimulation may induce sinus tachycardia with increased myocardial oxygen demand and worsen ischemia. If the angina is controlled with intravenous nitroglycerin, the drug should be slowly tapered over 6–12 hours as the patient is switched to long-acting nitrates, a beta blocker or calcium channel blocker, and daily aspirin therapy.

3. If intravenous nitroglycerin fails to control the angina, a calcium channel blocking agent should be started; sublingual nifedipine is a particularly useful agent to give under these circumstances if there is no hypotension and heart rate is not excessively high.[6–8] A persistent sinus tachycardia, with or without overt hypotension, requires prompt investigation because it may be indicative of either inadequate filling pressures or incipient congestive heart failure. Swan-Ganz monitoring is the most definitive means of differentiating these two diagnoses. If tachycardia is present, diltiazem may be preferable to nifedipine as a calcium channel blocker.[5]

4. Mild sedation; a quiet, tranquil environment; and nasal oxygen may also contribute to the relief of angina.

5. If there is no contraindication, the patient should be anticoagulated with heparin,[9] an antiplatelet agent such as low-dose aspirin or dipyridamole (Persantine) can also be given with the heparin. The addition of an antiplatelet agent to the heparin increases the risk of bleeding complications, but it is usually well tolerated for a short period of time.[6,7]

6. Low-dose aspirin therapy (80–325 mg/day) should be given long-term after an episode of unstable angina.[6-8]

7. Long-term beta blocking therapy should also be considered at this time.

8. Most patients respond to the medical regimen outlined here, and their unstable angina is relieved or "cools down." In such cases, urgent cardiac catheterization is not necessary. In general, elective cardiac catheterization and coronary angiography are recommended to define the coronary pathology and permit consideration of coronary angioplasty or coronary artery bypass graft surgery, depending on the individual patient's circumstances and coronary anatomy.[10]

9. If the patient continues to have angina despite the medical regimen described, more aggressive therapy should be considered. Emergency coronary arteriography should be performed.[10] If the patient is hemodynamically unstable during episodes of angina, intra-aortic balloon counterpulsation may be effective in relieving angina and reducing complications during coronary arteriography. After coronary arteriography is performed, the patient may be considered for intracoronary thrombolytic therapy and/or coronary angioplasty or coronary artery bypass graft surgery.

KEY FEATURES

I. *Diagnosis*
   A. History may include one or more of the following:
      1. "Crescendo" angina (more frequent, prolonged, easier to provoke, harder to relieve)
      2. New onset or increased frequency of angina at rest in addition to angina with minimal exertion
      3. New onset angina (present for less than 1–2 months)
   B. Assess possible contributing conditions, such as aortic stenosis, anemia, hypoxia, fever, thyrotoxicosis, poorly controlled hypertension, arrhythmias, congestive heart failure, heavy cigarette smoking, increased emotional stress
   C. Physical examination may show:
      1. S_3 or S_4 gallop
      2. Murmur of mitral insufficiency (papillary muscle dysfunction)

    3. Sustained apical lift (dyskinetic bulge)

    4. Pulmonary congestion

    5. Findings 1–4 may occur transiently during or after an anginal episode

  D. ECG usually shows transient ST segment depression or elevation and/or T wave abnormalities. Development of Q waves or persistence of ST–T changes for longer than 12–24 hours suggests myocardial infarction.

  E. Cardiac enzymes are not elevated with uncomplicated unstable angina; an increase in cardiac enzyme level implies myocyte necrosis, i.e., myocardial infarction.

II. *Pathophysiology*

  A. One or more of the following mechanisms may be involved:

    1. Progression of atherosclerosis

    2. Coronary arterial spasm

    3. Platelet aggregation at the site of a stenosis or ulcerated atheromatous plaque

    4. Thrombus formation that can partially or completely occlude a coronary vessel

    5. Increased myocardial oxygen demand

    6. Reduced oxygen delivery (anemia, hypoxia)

III. *Management*

  A. The general approach is *initial medical therapy,* which, if successful, is followed by *elective coronary arteriography;* consideration is then given to *coronary artery bypass grafting surgery* (CABG) or *percutaneous transluminal coronary angioplasty* (PTCA).

  B. Medical therapy may consist of one or more of the following:

    1. Sublingual nitroglycerin

    2. Intravenous nitroglycerin

    3. A calcium channel blocker

    4. An antiplatelet and/or anticoagulant agent

    5. Beta blocker therapy

    6. Fibrinolytic therapy

  C. If medical therapy is unsuccessful in relieving angina, emergency coronary arteriography (which may be performed in concert with intra-aortic balloon counterpulsation) and subsequent CABG surgery or PTCA should be considered.

REFERENCES

1. Rutherford JD, Braunwald E, Cohn PF: Chronic ischemic heart disease (Chap. 39). *In* Braunwald E (ed): Heart Disease: A Textbook of Cardiovascular Medicine, 3rd ed. Philadelphia, WB Saunders Co, 1988, pp 1314–1378.

2. Epstein SE, Palmeri ST: Mechanisms contributing to precipitation of unstable angina and acute myocardial infarction: Implications regarding therapy. Am J Cardiol 54:1245–1252, 1984.

    An excellent review of current concepts of the pathophysiology and management of unstable angina.

3. Folts JD, et al: Blood flow reductions in stenosed canine coronary arteries: Vasospasm or

platelet aggregation? Circulation 65:248–254; The effects of cigarette smoke and nicotine on platelet thrombus formation in stenosed dog coronary arteries: Inhibition with phentolamine. Circulation 65:465–469, 1982.

These workers describe an elegant experimental model of "spontaneous" angina. Dogs underwent a 60–80% coronary arterial stenosis by means of an external constricting plastic ring. Blood flow through the stenosed artery showed intermittent spontaneous reductions as a result of platelet aggregates that were eliminated with antiplatelet drugs such as aspirin; coronary vasodilators such as nitroglycerin did not decrease these flow reductions. Cigarette smoke and intravenous nicotine increased the frequency and severity of the coronary flow reductions.

4. Mandelkorn JB, et al: Intracoronary thrombus in nontransmural myocardial infarction and in unstable angina pectoris. Am J Cardiol 52:1, 1983.

   Nine patients with unstable angina underwent coronary angiography; five had evidence of partially or completely obstructive coronary arterial clot, which could be lysed with intracoronary streptokinase.

5. Muller JE, et al: Nifedipine and conventional therapy for unstable angina pectoris: A randomized, double-blind comparison. Circulation 69:728, 1984.

   Nifedipine and "conventional" therapy (isosorbide dinitrate and propranolol) were equally efficacious as the initial treatment of unstable angina; the combination of nifedipine plus conventional therapy appeared to be better than either used alone.

6. Lewis HD, et al: Protective effects of aspirin against acute myocardial infarction and death in men with unstable angina. N Engl J Med 309:396, 1983.

   Twelve hundred male patients with unstable angina were randomized to daily treatment with 325 mg aspirin or placebo for 3 months. At 3 months' follow-up, the aspirin group had a 50% reduction in the rate of death or acute myocardial infarction relative to the placebo group (5% vs. 10%). At 1 year follow-up, the aspirin group had a 43% reduction in mortality rate.

7. Cairns JA, et al: Aspirin, sulfinpyrazone, or both in unstable angina: Results of a Canadian multicenter trial. N Engl J Med 313:1369, 1985.

   Randomized, double-blind, placebo-controlled trial with end-points of nonfatal MI and cardiac death. Aspirin therapy produced a 51% risk reduction, with no additional benefit from sulfinpyrazone.

8. Fitzgerald DJ, et al: Platelet activation in unstable coronary disease. N Engl J Med 315:983, 1986.

   Physicochemical analysis suggesting that platelet activation occurs during spontaneous ischemia in patients with unstable angina. Biochemically selective inhibition of the synthesis or activation of thromboxane A_2 may be effective in such patients.

9. Telford A, Wilson C: Trial of heparin versus atenolol in prevention of myocardial infarction in intermediate coronary syndrome. Lancet 1:1125, 1981.

   In patients who presented with unstable angina or a nontransmural myocardial infarction, early heparin therapy reduced the frequency of progression to a transmural MI from 15% in the non-heparin group to 3% in the heparin treatment group.

10. Unstable Angina Pectoris: National Cooperative Study Group to Compare Surgical and Medical Therapy. II. In-Hospital Experience and Initial Follow-up Results in Patients with One, Two, and Three Vessel Disease. Am J Cardiol 42:839–848, 1978.

    This prospective randomized study compared intensive medical therapy with urgent coronary artery bypass graft surgery in 288 patients with unstable angina. The hospital mortality rate was 5% in the surgical group, vs. 3% in the medical group (p = ns). The surgical group had a higher in-hospital rate of myocardial infarction than the medically treated group (17 vs. 8%, p < 0.05). During a 30-month follow-up period, 36% of the *medically treated patients required coronary artery surgery to relieve unacceptable angina. Late mortality was comparable in the two groups. The results indicated that patients with unstable angina can be managed acutely with intensive medical therapy; most patients had adequate relief of pain, and there was no increase in mortality or infarction rate. Later, elective coronary surgery (or PTCA) can be performed with a low risk and good clinical results if anginal symptomatology or coronary anatomy warrants such an intervention.*

Acute Pulmonary Edema

Pantel S. Vokonas, M.D.

Acute pulmonary edema may be the consequence of any disease process that enhances pulmonary capillary pressure, alters alveolar-capillary membrane permeability, or limits lymphatic drainage of the lungs.[1] The most common mechanism in cardiogenic pulmonary edema is elevated end-diastolic pressure as a result of underlying left ventricular systolic and/or diastolic dysfunction, usually in the setting of underlying ischemic or hypertensive cardiac disease, resulting in increased pulmonary capillary hydrostatic forces. This produces a net flux of fluid first into the interstitium and then into the alveolar spaces. This process can be aggravated by the presence of low colloid osmotic pressure as a result of hypoalbuminemia from any cause.[1,2] The presence of large amounts of edema fluid in the alveoli, in turn, leads to serious ventilation-perfusion disparities with regional arteriovenous shunting of blood through the lungs, resulting in hypoxia (reduced arterial oxygen tension: PaO_2) with a wide alveolar-arterial (A-a) oxygen gradient. Hypoxia may induce regional vasoconstriction, further enhancing the disparity of ventilation to perfusion that already exists. Mitral stenosis is a less common cause of cardiogenic pulmonary edema. Noncardiac causes of pulmonary edema—adult respiratory distress syndrome, pneumonia, smoke inhalation, uremia, near-drowning, and narcotic overdose—are characterized by either low or normal pulmonary capillary pressures.[1,2] Therefore, direct measurement of pulmonary capillary wedge pressure using a Swan-Ganz balloon-tipped catheter is a useful approach in differentiating between cardiogenic and noncardiogenic pulmonary edema.

CLINICAL FEATURES

The clinical picture is characterized by extreme breathlessness, tachypnea, agitation, and expectoration of pink, frothy sputum. Tachycardia, elevated systolic and diastolic blood pressures, diaphoresis, cold, ashen skin, and peripheral cyanosis may also be present, reflecting both low cardiac output and enhanced activity of the sympathetic nervous system. Moist inspiratory rales are heard, first over the bases of both lungs but then extending upward toward the apices as the condition progresses. A third heart sound (S_3) or a summation gallop (S_3 and S_4) is frequently present. A chest roentgenogram may reveal varying degrees of interstitial and alveolar edema as well as pleural effusion. The electrocardiogram (ECG) should be evaluated for cardiac arrhythmias or evidence of acute myocardial infarction.

TREATMENT

Specific measures that are often effective in the treatment of acute pulmonary edema include the following:
1. The patient is placed in an *upright, sitting position.*[1,3]
2. *Oxygen* is administered by means of a well-fitted face mask (Venturi mask or reservoir bag).[3] Inspired oxygen concentrations and flow rates are adjusted to achieve an arterial oxygen tension (PaO_2) of at least 60–70 mmHg.
3. *Morphine sulfate* is given intravenously (3–5 mg), and the dose is repeated in approximately 15 minutes, if necessary. A critical effect of morphine is venodilation resulting in decreased venous return and preload.[1,3] A specific morphine antagonist such as naloxone hydrochloride should be immediately available if respiratory depression occurs.
4. A *rapidly acting diuretic* such as furosemide 20–40 mg is given intravenously.[4]
5. *Vasodilators* may be of additional benefit if arterial blood pressure is either normal or elevated.[5] Nitroglycerin (a venodilator) may be administered sublingually, topically, or intravenously, using a low-flow constant infusion pump, at an initial rate of 5 μg/minute; the dosage is then increased by increments of 5 μg/minute every five minutes. Sodium nitroprusside (a balanced arteriolar dilator and venodilator) is given intravenously at an initial rate of 10–20 μg/minute, and the dose is adjusted upward by increments of 5 μg/min every five to ten minutes until pulmonary edema is relieved or arterial systolic blood pressure falls below 100 mmHg. Intravenous vasodilators should only be administered under conditions of continuous hemodynamic monitoring.
6. In a patient with bronchospasm, *aminophylline* 250–500 mg may be given intravenously.[6] Aminophylline relieves bronchoconstriction; in addition, it has a direct vasodilating effect, promotes diuresis, and may improve cardiac contractility.[1,3]
7. Venous return to the heart may be further reduced by the application of *tourniquets* to three extremities.[1,3] Tourniquets are rotated every 15 minutes and removed sequentially when no longer needed. If reduction

in venous return using this method is inadequate, particularly in the presence of marked venous distention, *phlebotomy* with the removal of 300–500 cc of blood should be considered.

8. *Digitalis,* given intravenously, may be of benefit, particularly in patients with atrial flutter or fibrillation associated with rapid ventricular rates.[3,7] However, in the treatment of acute cardiac failure, digitalis should, in general, be considered an ancillary measure to improve cardiac contractility compared with rapid effectiveness of measures already outlined.

9. When a critically ill patient with acute pulmonary edema fails to respond to the preceding measures, particularly when arterial blood gases suggest rapidly progressive deterioration (severe hypoxia and hypercapnia), *endotracheal intubation* should be performed and continuous positive pressure ventilation applied.[1,3] Further improvement in arterial oxygenation can be achieved, if necessary, by the application of *positive end-expiratory pressure (PEEP).*[8]

Common factors that may precipitate pulmonary edema include arrhythmias, hypertension, myocardial infarction, infection, hypoalbuminemia, excessive intake of salt, and discontinuation of cardiac medications. These should be identified and, whenever possible, corrected. Noninvasive studies such as echocardiography, radionuclide cardiography, ambulatory ECG monitoring, and, if indicated, cardiac catheterization and angiographic studies may be performed at a later time to assess the specific cardiac disease involved.

KEY FEATURES

The hallmark of cardiogenic pulmonary edema is elevated pulmonary capillary hydrostatic pressure. This usually results from elevated left ventricular end-diastolic pressure in the setting of ischemic or hypertensive cardiac disease. Ventricular dysfunction may be systolic, diastolic, or both. Mitral stenosis is a less common cause of elevated pulmonary hydrostatic pressure.

Noncardiogenic pulmonary edema generally results from a failure of pulmonary capillary integrity and usually arises in the setting of toxic inhalation, aspiration, systemic infection, or major metabolic/immunologic disturbance.

Low colloid osmotic pressure may exacerbate either form of pulmonary edema.

Direct measurement of pulmonary capillary wedge pressure is the most reliable means of differentiating between cardiogenic and noncardiogenic pulmonary edema when the clinical picture is uncertain.

Major clinical features of cardiogenic pulmonary edema include extreme dyspnea, tachypnea, agitation, and tachycardia. Hypertension is usually noted; chest pain suggestive of ischemia, diaphoresis, cool extremities, and cyanosis are not uncommon. An S_3 or summation gallop is usually present, and in severe cases the patient produces copious amounts of pink, frothy sputum.

There are no specific ECG features. Chest roentgenograms reveal varying degrees of interstitial or alveolar edema with or without pleural effusion.

Treatment measures include postural maneuvers, oxygen administration, and pharmacologic intervention (see text). The patient should be monitored acutely with strong consideration given to the possibility of myocardial infarction.

REFERENCES

1. Robin ED, Cross EC, Zelis RM: Pulmonary edema. N Engl J Med 288:239–304, 1973.
    Definitive review of pulmonary edema, including pathophysiologic mechanisms, multiple etiologies, functional disturbances, and therapeutic considerations; an outstanding source of information.

2. Sprung CL, Rackow EC, Fein IA, et al: The spectrum of pulmonary edema. Differentiation of cardiogenic, intermediate and noncardiogenic forms of pulmonary edema. Am Rev Respir Dis 124:718, 1981.
    Clinical study of 20 patients evaluating the utility of protein determinations in pulmonary edema fluid and serum, in addition to clinical and hemodynamic data, in differentiating between cardiac and noncardiac forms of pulmonary edema. Edema fluid to serum protein ratios <0.5 were consistent with cardiac and ratios >0.7 with noncardiac forms of pulmonary edema. A mixed or "intermediate" form of pulmonary edema identified in six patients is also discussed.

3. Ramirez A, Abelman WH: Cardiac decompensation: Current concepts. N Engl J Med 290:499, 1974.
    Excellent outline of specific treatment modalities and rationale for their use in acute cardiac failure.

4. Dikshit K, Vyden JK, Forrester JS, et al: Renal and extrarenal hemodynamic effects of furosemide in congestive heart failure after myocardial infarction. N Engl J Med 288:1087, 1973.
    Acute clinical study involving 20 patients with myocardial infarction demonstrated that critical relief of symptoms of acute pulmonary congestion frequently preceded apparent diuresis following administration of furosemide. These effects were probably related to a rapid increase in peripheral venous capacitance (venodilation resulting in diminution of cardiac preload) occurring before a rise in renal plasma flow.

5. Miller RR, Fennell WH, Young JB, et al: Differential systemic arterial and venous actions and consequent cardiac effects of vasodilator drugs. Prog Cardiovasc Dis 24:353, 1982.
    Review discussing the clinical use and differential hemodynamic effects of various vasodilator agents commonly employed in the management of severe heart failure.

6. Mitenko PA, Ogilvie RI: Rational intravenous doses of theophylline. N Engl J Med 289:600, 1973.
    Pharmacokinetic data from studies using intravenous theophylline (aminophylline) in patients with acute bronchial asthma suggest that plasma drug concentrations of 10 mg/ L (μg/ml), corresponding to optimal bronchodilation, can be achieved safely by giving a

loading dose of 4.5 mg/kg IV over 15–30 minutes, followed by a continuous infusion of
0.72 mg/kg/hour. Toxic side effects include hypotension and cardiac arrhythmias.

7. Smith TW, Braunwald E, Kelly RA: The management of heart failure. *In* Braunwald E
    (ed): Heart Disease: A Textbook of Cardiovascular Medicine, 3rd ed. Philadelphia, WB
    Saunders Co, 1988, pp 485–543.
    Comprehensive resource on the use of digitalis glycosides and other inotropic agents
    in the treatment of congestive heart failure.

8. Rizk NW, Murray PF: PEEP and pulmonary edema. Am J Med 72:381, 1982.
    Emphasizes the effect of PEEP in increasing arterial PaO₂ and lung compliance by
    opening distal airways; recruiting alveoli; and possibly redistributing excess lung water to
    sites where it interferes less with gas exchange, thereby partially reducing ventilation-
    perfusion disparities. PEEP does not decrease the net flux of fluid into alveoli or the quantity
    of extravascular lung water.

Sudden Cardiac Death

Joseph M. Weinstein, M.D.
Laura F. Wexler, M.D.

Sudden cardiac death is defined as a witnessed unexpected death occurring outside the hospital within 1 hour of the onset of symptoms. The
exact incidence is unknown, but it is estimated that 500,000 people in the
United States die suddenly each year.[4]

The vast majority of sudden cardiac deaths are secondary to coronary
artery disease; it is estimated that two thirds of patients dying from atherosclerotic coronary artery disease die suddenly before reaching a hospital.
Other less common diseases associated with sudden death include (1) valvular
heart disease, primarly aortic stenosis; (2) primary myocardial disease, including both hypertrophic and dilated congestive cardiomyopathies; (3) the
prolonged QT syndrome: (4) ruptured aortic aneurysm; (5) massive pulmonary embolism; (6) intracerebral hemorrhage; (7) pulmonary hypertension;
(8) cardiac tumors; and (9) a variety of congenital disorders associated with
arrhythmias, including right ventricular dysplasia, hereditary prolonged QT
syndrome, and pre-excitation syndromes (Wolff-Parkinson-White syndrome). Reports suggest two other important causes of sudden death: anorexia nervosa and vigorous exercise.[3,9] As was found in instances of sudden
death in patients on liquid protein diets, the mechanism of sudden death
in patients with anorexia nervosa appears to be ventricular tachyarrhythmias,
probably related to QT prolongation. Exercise has long been thought to
reduce the risk of coronary artery disease, but recent findings suggest that

the risk of sudden death may be transiently increased during vigorous exercise.

Despite the high prevalence of diffuse, severe coronary artery disease among victims of sudden death, evidence of a new acute myocardial infarction (MI) is found in less than 50% of successfully resuscitated patients.[1,2,7,8] In such patients, the cause of death is almost always ventricular tachycardia and/or fibrillation. Ventricular tachycardia is not instantly fatal but results in hemodynamic compromise from decreased diastolic filling, loss of effective atrial contraction, and an altered sequence of ventricular contraction. The hemodynamic compromise produces further myocardial ischemia, which leads to an increased propensity to ventricular fibrillation. Other lethal arrhythmias may also occur, including severe bradyarrhythmias and asystole.

The identification of patients at risk for sudden death is the first important step in decreasing the magnitude of the problem. The major risk factors for sudden death are similar to those for coronary disease—hypertension, left ventricular hypertrophy, diabetes mellitus, elevated serum cholesterol, cigarette smoking, male sex, and age greater than 50. Most victims of sudden death have a previous history of heart disease, and certain features have been shown to identify the patient at highest risk. Survivors of an MI are at increased risk of sudden death, particularly within the first 6 months. The presence of high-grade ventricular ectopy, especially repetitive forms (pairs, triplets, or ventricular tachycardia), on pre-discharge continuous ambulatory ECG monitoring correlates with risk of subsequent sudden death.[5,6] Even more ominous is the combination of high-grade ventricular ectopy and a depressed left ventricular ejection fraction.[5] These patients seem to be at especially high risk for lethal ventricular arrhythmias and deserve special attention from the physician.

Once a patient has had an episode of sudden death and has been resuscitated, the key issue becomes how to prevent a recurrence. The risk of recurrent sudden death is actually highest (approximately 25%) in patients who do not show evidence of a new acute transmural MI. Patients who are resuscitated from ventricular fibrillation in the setting of an acute MI have an overall recurrence rate of 2%. Most investigators have found that the occurrence of ventricular fibrillation during the acute phase of an acute MI does not affect overall late mortality.

Many centers recommend that the majority of post-infarction patients with or without a history of ventricular fibrillation during the acute event should undergo a series of noninvasive tests following recovery from their MI, including ambulatory monitoring; some examination of left ventricular function, such as radionuclide scanning or two-dimensional echocardiography; and exercise testing. The objective is to select out patients at high risk for sudden death as well as recurrent ischemia who might be candidates for more aggressive medical or surgical therapy. The approach to the sudden death patient who has *not* shown evidence of an acute MI should be even more aggressive in terms of trying to identify the mechanism of the initial event and establishing adequate therapy to reduce the risk of recurrence. There are two approaches to the evaluation of such patients. The first, continuous ECG monitoring usually with exercise stress testing, is based on the observations (1) that risk of recurrence of lethal ventricular arrhythmias is markedly enhanced in patients having complex ventricular ectopy (pairs, triplets, ventricular tachycardia) on ambulatory monitoring; and (2) that in the coronary artery disease population, elimination or substantial reduction of complex ectopy after oral administration of antiarrhythmic drugs can reduce the risk of subsequent sudden death.[2,6] The long-term value of this type of antiarrhythmic therapy in noncoronary artery disease patients at high risk for recurrent sudden death, e.g., idiopathic cardiomyopathy patients, has not been proved. This approach is time consuming, often requiring multiple 24-hour monitor recordings before and after serial oral administration of several drugs.[2] A more critical limitation of this approach is that in order to prove that a drug effectively reduces the frequency of complex ventricular ectopy, the patient must have substantial and reproducible baseline complex ectopy with which to compare post-drug recordings. Many patients resuscitated from sudden death have little, if any, ventricular ectopy on ambulatory monitoring.

The second approach to evaluation of sudden death patients is electrophysiologic (EP) testing.[8] In this technique, catheters introduced into the right, and sometimes left, ventricle deliver timed electrical stimuli to the endocardium. Nonsustained or sustained ventricular tachycardia will be precipitated in a large proportion of susceptible patients, i.e., those resuscitated from sudden death. In cases in which the arrhythmia causing the original sudden death attack was documented, the catheter-induced arrhythmia will often have the same morphologic appearance as the spontaneous arrhythmia. Catheter stimulation is repeated after serial intravenous drug testing; abolition of the catheter-induced arrhythmia appears to correlate with a reduced risk of recurrent sudden death in the future. In patients who have serious arrhythmias that are unresponsive to drug therapy, EP testing can also be used to "map" the endocardium in search of a specific initiating focus on the endocardium that can be surgically resected. EP testing is not available in all centers, and it is an invasive test with some morbidity. It is clearly indicated for survivors of sudden death who do not have significant arrhythmias on ambulatory monitoring.

One randomized prospective clinical trial of the invasive and noninvasive approaches to therapy in patients with symptomatic ventricular tachyarrhythmias has been reported. This study suggests that therapy selected by the invasive approach is superior to the noninvasive approach in terms of preventing recurrences of symptomatic ventricular tachycardia or ventricular fibrillation. This study was limited in size, and further long-term trials are required to establish whether or not EP testing is superior to ambulatory monitoring in specific patient populations.[11]

It has been clearly shown that patients who remain refractory to medical treatment are at high risk for a recurrence of suddent death.[12] With the advent of the automatic implantable cardioverter-defibrillator, patients who are intolerant or resistant to medications can now be provided with an effective form of therapy. The implantable defibrillator, or AICD, is a self-contained device that can diagnose and treat hemodynamically significant ventricular tachyarrhythmias. Early clinical experience demonstrates a significantly improved survival in this high-risk group of patients.[13]

KEY FEATURES

  I. Etiologic factors
   1. Most common predisposing factor is severe diffuse coronary artery disease.
   2. A new acute myocardial infarction (MI) is not seen in the majority of victims of sudden death who are resuscitated.
   3. Ventricular fibrillation is the arrhythmia responsible for the majority of cases of sudden death.
 II. Identification of the patient at risk
   1. Risk factors for sudden death are similar to those for coronary disease
     a. Hypertension
     b. Left ventricular hypertrophy
     c. Cigarette smoking
     d. Diabetes mellitus
     e. Male sex
     f. Age greater than 50
   2. Most patients who have sudden death have an antecedent history of heart disease.
     a. History of MI in the last 6 months
     b. History of high-grade (complex) ventricular ectopy
     c. Depressed left ventricular ejection fraction
III. For victims of sudden cardiac death who are successfully resuscitated:
   1. Treatment with antiarrhythmic agents is indicated, with documentation of suppression of high-grade ectopy.
   2. Two modalities exist:
     a. Electrophysiologic testing
     b. Serial 24-hour continuous ECG monitoring
IV. Community-wide instruction in cardiopulmonary resuscitation is essential to reduce the excessive mortality rate from out-of-hospital cardiac arrest.

REFERENCES

1. Eisenberg MS, Hallstrom A, et al: Long term survival after out-of-hospital cardiac arrest. N Engl J Med 306:1340–1344, 1982.
   Patients who survive an out-of-hospital cardiac arrest and are treated for their ventricular ectopy have a good prognosis for long-term survival.

2. Graboys TB, Lown B, Podrid PS, DeSilva RA: Long-term survival of patients with malignant ventricular arrhythmias treated with antiarrhythmic drugs. Am J Cardiol 50437–443, 1982.
   Successful treatment of malignant ventricular ectopy can be accomplished with continuous electrocardiographic monitoring and trials of antiarrhythmics. When high-grade ectopy is abolished, the recurrence of sudden death is significantly decreased and the need for invasive procedures is abolished.

3. Isner JM, Roberts WC, Heymsfield JB, Yager J: Anorexia nervosa and sudden death. Ann Intern Med 102:49–52, 1985.
   Sudden death in patients with anorexia nervosa may result from ventricular tachyarrhythmias, related to a prolonged QT interval.

4. Lown B: Sudden cardiac death: The major challenge confronting contemporary cardiology. Am J Cardiol 43:313–321, 1979.
   A review of the problem of sudden death, and approaches to ventricular ectopy.

5. Mukhari J, Rude RE, Poole K, et al: Risk factors for sudden death after acute myocardial infarction: Two year follow-up. Am J Cardiol 54:31–36, 1984.
   The presence of ventricular ectopy and left ventricular dysfunction early after MI identifies the patient at highest risk for sudden death.

6. Olson PC, Lyons KP, Troop P, Burman SM, Piters KM: Prognostic implications of complicated ventricular arrhythmias early after hospital discharge in acute myocardial infarction: A serial ambulatory electrocardiography study. Am Heart J 108:1221–1228, 1984.
   Patients with complicated ventricular ectopic activity at discharge from the hospital after an MI were significantly more likely to suffer sudden death compared with those without complicated ventricular ectopy.

7. Ruskin JN, McGovern B, Garan H, DiMarco JP, Kelley E: Antiarrhythmic drugs: A possible cause of out-of-hospital cardiac arrest. N Engl J Med 309:1302–1305, 1983.
   Antiarrhythmic drugs may exacerbate ventricular ectopy in some cases.

8. Ruskin JN, DiMarco JP, Garan H: Out-of-hospital cardiac arrest: Electrophysiologic observations and selection of long-term antiarrhythmic therapy. N Engl J Med 303:607–613, 1980.
   The role of electrophysiologic testing in survivors of sudden death.

9. Sislovick DS, Weiss NS, Fletcher RH, Lasky T: The incidence of primary cardiac arrest during vigorous exercise. N Engl J Med 311:874–877, 1984.
   The risk of cardiac arrest is transiently increased during vigorous exercise. However, habitual exercise is associated with a decreased risk of sudden death.

10. Velebit V, Podrid P, Lown B, Cohen BH, Graboys TB: Aggravation and provocation of ventricular arrhythmias by antiarrhythmic drugs. Circulation 65:886–894, 1982.
    Antiarrhythmic agents may paradoxically increase high-grade ventricular ectopy rather than controlling these arrhythmias. As this is not a predictable occurrence, continuous electrocardiographic monitoring is needed to document an antiarrhythmic effort before long-term therapy is begun.

11. Mitchell LB, Duff HJ, Manyari DE, Wyse DG: A randomized clinical trial of the noninvasive and invasive approaches to drug therapy of ventricular tachycardia. N Engl J Med
317:1681, 1987.
    *Antiarrhythmic therapy selected by electrophysiologic testing appears to be superior
in preventing recurrences of symptomatic ventricular tachyarrhythmias than therapy selected by the noninvasive approach.*

12. Wilber DJ, Garan H, et al: Out-of-hospital cardiac arrest: Use of electrophysiologic testing
in the prediction of long-term outcome. N Engl J Med *318*:19, 1988.
    *The persistence of inducible ventricular tachyarrhythmias on electrophysiologic test-
ing despite medical therapy is a significant risk factor for recurrence of sudden death.*

13. Fogoros RN, Fiedler SB, Elson JJ: The automatic implantable cardioverter-defibrillator in
drug-refractory ventricular tachyarrhythmias. Ann Intern Med *107*:635, 1987.
    *The automatic implantable cardioverter-defibrillator is extremely effective in detecting
and correcting malignant ventricular tachyarrhythmias. In patients who are resistant to
medical therapy, the defibrillator significantly improves survival.*

Cardiopulmonary Resuscitation

Joseph M. Weinstein, M.D.
Laura F. Wexler, M.D.

The patient who suffers an episode of out-of-hospital sudden death is dependent on the community's ability to provide both basic and advanced cardiac life support. Some cerebral perfusion must be restored within approximately 4 minutes, or the patient runs a high risk of permanent neurologic sequelae. Recognition of cardiac arrest by a bystander and institution of effective cardiopulmonary resuscitation (CPR) are the cornerstones of a successful outcome.[10,11] It has been on this premise that widespread instruction in basic life support has been provided to some communities. The presence of an advanced life support system is also crucial, as CPR alone is incapable of terminating most lethal arrhythmias. Paramedics are now capable of performing defibrillation and drug administration in the field and have increased the survival of patients suffering from sudden cardiac death. In one study, 43% of patients with out-of-hospital ventricular fibrillation were successfully resuscitated with bystander-administered CPR followed by advanced cardiac life support.

BASIC LIFE SUPPORT

The principles of CPR remain assisted ventilation and maintenance of circulation via chest compression. Two techniques are recommended by the

American Heart Association (AHA), based on how many rescuers are present: In one-rescuer CPR, 15 consecutive chest compressions are followed by 2 ventilations and the compressions are delivered at a rate of 80 beats per minute. With two-rescuer life support, 5 chest compressions are delivered followed by 1 ventilation. This is done at a rate of 60 compressions and 12 ventilations per minute. Chest compressions are performed with the heel of one hand over the other at the mid-sternum and the hands interlocked. The shoulders should be directly over the sternum with elbows locked and with the downward thrust coming from the shoulders. The sternum should be compressed 1½–2 inches with each compression.

The mechanism of blood flow in CPR has been a topic of renewed interest.[1,6,9] It was previously assumed that forward blood flow was generated during closed chest massage by compression of the heart between the vertebrae and the sternum. However, studies have demonstrated the importance of the generalized increase in intrathoracic pressure during chest compressions in producing forward blood flow rather than direct cardiac compression. Based on observations in both animals and humans, it is known that the heart behaves as a conduit during CPR: pressure within all cardiac chambers and great vessels increases during chest compression and blood is propelled forward because the major veins collapse at the thoracic inlet while the great arteries remain patent because of their muscular framework. There are two practical correlates of these observations. First, the duration of chest compression should be at least 50% of the pumping cycle in order to exert a sustained increase in pressure on all cardiac chambers and intrathoracic great vessels. There is ample clinical evidence that this pattern improves forward blood flow compared with rapid brief compressions. Second, maneuvers that further increase intrathoracic pressure, such as abdominal binding, intermittent abdominal compressions, and simultaneous ventilation and chest compression, may enhance blood flow during closed chest compressions. These latter techniques remain experimental, and although they appear promising, they are unproved and are not yet recommended for routine CPR.

Mouth-to-mouth breathing remains an accepted method for initial ventilation, but the necessity of controlling the airway with an endotracheal tube as soon as possible should not be overlooked. The advantages of improved ventilation with supplemental oxygen are obvious, but the prevention of aspiration is also vital. Furthermore, there is a substantial body of data that support the use of endotracheal administration of certain medications: epinephrine, atropine, and lidocaine can all be given by the endotracheal tube if peripheral or central venous access cannot be quickly established. Medications that *cannot* be given via the respiratory tract include sodium bicarbonate, norepinephrine, calcium chloride, and bretylium. Thus, it is essential that intravenous access be established as soon as possible. The question of whether peripheral or central access is optimal remains debated: some authors feel that there is more rapid onset of action with centrally administered medications, but other studies show no significant differences. Finally, there appears to be no indication for intracardiac injections of medications. The complications associated with this technique make it a poor route for administration of drugs, and it offers no advantages over central venous access.

ADVANCED LIFE SUPPORT

Although CPR is essential to a good outcome in cardiac arrest, closed chest massage and artificial respirations alone will rarely reverse the underlying mechanism that led to the cardiac arrest. Access to medications and defibrillation equipment is essential. If ventricular fibrillation is documented, defibrillation should be attempted and repeated once if unsuccessful before further drug therapy is instituted. Defibrillation produces simultaneous depolarization of all cardiac cells, which may allow a stable cardiac rhythm to emerge. Electrical defibrillation is most effective early after the onset of ventricular tachycardia/fibrillation and in the presence of a normal pH and PO_2. The energy levels to be used initially remain debated; current AHA guidelines recommend 200–300 joules for the first defibrillation.[10] Studies have suggested that maximum energy levels should be used from the start, i.e., 360 joules.[7] Repetitive defibrillation may be effective, in that thoracic resistance is decreased with subsequent countershocks.[5] Finally, it has been shown that fibrillation amplitude is a good predictor of outcome, with coarse fibrillation responding better to therapy than fine fibrillation.[3,12]

DRUG THERAPY FOR RESISTANT OR RECURRENT VENTRICULAR TACHYCARDIA/FIBRILLATION

CPR will not prevent the development of both metabolic and respiratory acidosis, which in turn can markedly diminish the likelihood of successful defibrillation and a return of effective cardiac contraction. One of the most controversial areas in resuscitation physiology concerns the acid-base abnormalities that develop. It is now known that arterial blood gases may not adequately reflect the state of acid-base abnormalities in the tissues. Arterial PCO_2 is frequently normal or low, reflecting hyperventilation, whereas venous blood usually reveals hypercarbia and acidemia. This gap in arterial and venous carbon dioxide content is most likely a manifestation of the poor perfusion that is present in states of cardiac arrest.

In its most recent revision of advanced cardiac life support guidelines, the American Heart Association no longer recommends the automatic administration of sodium bicarbonate. Complications of bicarbonate administration include metabolic alkalosis, hypernatremia, and hyperosmolarity. It has also been recently shown that when bicarbonate is given, carbon dioxide is generated, and this may worsen the venous respiratory acidemia. There is also data suggesting that carbon dioxide may diffuse intracellularly and into the central nervous system, causing a deterioration of intracellular and central nervous functions. However, bicarbonate should be used if severe pre-existing metabolic acidosis or hyperkalemia is known to have contributed to the patient's deterioration. After 10 minutes of CPR, the physician must weigh the risks and benefits of bicarbonate administration and treat on this basis.[10]

Epinephrine is also a useful drug when initial attempts at defibrillation are unsuccessful. It is a powerful chronotropic and inotropic agent and also increases peripheral vascular resistance, which may promote coronary and cerebral perfusion during CPR. Furthermore, epinephrine may convert fine fibrillation into a coarse pattern, increasing the likelihood of a successful defibrillation. Doses of 1 mg are given initially and are repeated every 5–10 minutes as needed.

Antiarrhythmics are of key importance to a resuscitation effort, both to facilitate defibrillation and to prevent recurrent ventricular tachycardia. Lidocaine continues to be the initial agent of choice. It acts both by suppressing ventricular ectopic foci and by decreasing conduction throughout the reentry pathways. It is given in serial intravenous bolus injections of 1 mg/kg and then 0.5 mg/kg, followed by continuous infusion of 1–4 mg/minute. The danger of lidocaine toxicity must be considered in the elderly and in patients with liver disease and severe congestive heart failure. A second choice for ventricular fibrillation and ventricular tachycardia is bretylium.[4] Bretylium acts by raising the ventricular fibrillation threshold as well as increasing the effective refractory period. It is given as a loading dose of 5 mg/kg, followed by an infusion of 1–4 mg/minute. Bretylium may be particularly effective in cases of refractory ventricular fibrillation. Acute administration of bretylium is associated with a transient period (approximately 10 minutes) of increased sympathetic stimulation, which may result in a brief period of enhanced ventricular ectopy. Following this phase, hypotension is the major unwanted side effect. Procainamide is also an effective antiarrhythmic and may work when both lidocaine and bretylium have failed. An initial dose of 500–1000 mg is administered slowly over 5–10 minutes, followed by an infusion of 1–4 mg/minute. The major side effect of procainamide is hypotension; conduction system depression leading to heart block may also occur.

The use of intravenous calcium for asystole and electromechanical dissociation has been revised. There is no evidence to suggest that it improves the likelihood of resuscitation or survival. When administered in the previously recommended dosages, blood concentrations would remain significantly elevated for 10–15 minutes. This is most likely because of the small volume of distribution in these patients. Therefore, calcium administration is now recommended only if patients are suspected of having hypocalcemia or hyperkalemia, having received a toxic amount of calcium channel blockers, or if cardiac arrest is associated with recovery from cardiopulmonary bypass.[10]

There are two situations encountered during CPR that deserve special mention. Electromechanical dissociation (EMD) refers to the presence of sustained cardiac electrical activity in the absence of pulse, blood pressure, or heart sounds. The differential diagnosis includes exsanguinating hemorrhage, acute cardiac tamponade (usually secondary to cardiac rupture), massive pulmonary embolus, and profound myocardial depression from massive infarction or severe cardiomyopathy. Accordingly, a trial of volume infusion, pericardiocentesis, and vasopressors is indicated and rarely may lead to a successful outcome. The second situation is that of asystole, which occurs infrequently as an initial cause of cardiac arrest. Epinephrine, atropine, and isoproterenol remain the initial therapies of choice, followed by transvenous pacing. The prognosis of cardiac arrest associated with asystole is exceedingly poor.[8]

Although studies have led to advances in cardiopulmonary resuscitation, the majority of patients suffering a cardiac arrest still do not survive. Patients who suffer cardiac arrest and require CPR within the hospital setting have a 5–15% chance of leaving the hospital; those who suffer from a concurrent chronic illness, i.e., pneumonia, renal failure, cancer, etc., have a much worse prognosis.[2] Patients who suffer sudden death outside the hospital either from primary ventricular fibrillation or from ventricular fibrillation associated with an acute myocardial infarction have a somewhat better prognosis, depending on access to a mobile resuscitation unit.[11] Research continues not only in techniques to improve coronary perfusion pressures and myocardial salvage but also in terms of effective cerebral resuscitation. Maneuvers to increase blood flow to the brain and to prevent neurologic compromise are essential to a good outcome from CPR. Although increasing our resuscitative armamentarium will help, the prevention of sudden death seems the area with more promise.

KEY FEATURES

I. *Basic cardiopulmonary resuscitation* (CPR)
   1. Onset of CPR should be within 4 minutes of cardiac arrest to keep neurologic sequelae to a minimum.
   2. Compression/ventilation ratio:

      a. With one-rescuer CPR, 15 compressions followed by 2 ventilations, at a rate of 80 beats per minute.

      b. With two-rescuer CPR, 5 compressions followed by 1 ventilation, at a rate of 60 beats per minute.

    3. Compressions should last for 50% of the pumping cycle.

  II. *Advanced life support*

    1. The airway should be controlled with an endotracheal tube and supplemental O_2 provided.

    2. Defibrillation should be attempted as soon as ventricular tachyarrhythmia is documented.

      a. Initiate defibrillation with 200–300 joules.

      b. Multiple defibrillations may be required.

      c. Defibrillations are most successful with normal metabolic parameters.

    3. Intravenous access is essential.

    4. Medications should be administered if initial defibrillation is unsuccessful.

      a. Epinephrine for inotropic and chronotropic support.

      b. Lidocaine and/or bretylium to control ventricular tachyarrhythmias; procainamide if these are ineffective.

      c. Volume repletion and vasopressors as needed for reversal of hypotension.

    5. Treatment of asystole includes:

      a. Epinephrine

      b. Atropine

      c. Isoproterenol

      d. Transvenous pacing

REFERENCES

1. Babbs CF, et al: Knowledge gaps in CPR: Synopsis of a panel discussion. Crit Care Med 8:181–187, 1980.
   Review of major controversies in CPR.

2. Bedell SE, Delbanco TI, Cook EF, Epstein FH: Survival after cardiopulmonary resuscitation in the hospital. N Engl J Med 309:569–576, 1983.
   Identification of prognostic indicators affecting outcome in in-hospital CPR.

3. Gascho JA, Crampton RS, Cherwek ML: Determinants of ventricular fibrillation in adults. Circulation 60:231–237, 1979.

4. Haynes RE, Chinn TL, Copass MK, Cobb LA: Comparison of bretylium tosylate and lidocaine in management of out of hospital ventricular fibrillation: A randomized clinical trial. Am J Cardiol 48:353–356, 1981.
   Bretylium and lidocaine are equally effective in the first line management of ventricular fibrillation.

5. Kerber RE, Grayzel J, Hoyt R, Marcus M, Kennedy J: Transthoracic resistance in human defibrillation. Circulation 63:676–682, 1981.
   Human transthoracic resistance is directly proportional to chest size. Resistance declines with subsequent shocks, as well as with large paddles and firm pressure.

6. McIntyre KM, Parisi AF, Benfari R, Goldberg AH, Dealin JE: Pathophysiologic syndromes of cardiopulmonary resuscitation. Arch Intern Med 138:1130–1133, 1978.
   Review of major complications of CPR, both properly and improperly performed.

7. Morgan JP, Hearne SF, Raizes GS, White RD, Giuliani ER: High-energy versus low-energy defibrillation: Experience in patients (excluding those in the intensive care unit) at Mayo Clinic–affiliated hospitals. Mayo Clinic Proc 59:829–834, 1984.
   High levels of delivered energy are more effective in initial defibrillation attempts, as compared with low levels.

8. Myerburg RJ, Estes D, Zaman L, Luceri RM, Kessler KM, Throbman RG, Castellanes A: Outcome of resuscitation from bradyarrhythmic or asystolic cardiac arrest. J Am Coll Cardiol 4:1118–1122, 1984.
   Outcome for victims of pre-hospital cardiac arrest from bradyarrhythmias or asystole has improved slightly, but these groups still have a very high mortality rate.

9. Sanders AB, Meislen HW, Ewy GA: The physiology of cardiopulmonary resuscitation: An update. JAMA 252:3283–3286, 1984.
   A review of the physiology of CPR, including the latest theories on closed chest massage, mechanisms of blood flow, and utility of open chest massage.

10. Textbook of Advanced Cardiac Life Support. Dallas, American Heart Association, 1987.
    Classic reference source used in the Advanced Cardiac Life Support course—extremely well written and referenced.

11. Thompson RG, Hallstrom AP, Cobb LA: Bystander initiated cardiopulmonary resuscitation in the management of ventricular fibrillation. Ann Intern Med 90:737–740, 1979.
    Patients whose CPR was initiated by bystanders had a much better prognosis, as opposed to those patients whose CPR was first performed by paramedical personnel.

12. Weaver WD, Cobb LA, Dennis D, Ray R, Hallstrom AD, Copass MK: Amplitude of ventricular fibrillation waveform and outcome after cardiac arrest. Ann Intern Med 102:53–55, 1985.
    Outcome with coarse ventricular fibrillation is much better than with fine ventricular fibrillation. This is in part a result of delay in initiation of therapy.

Diseases of the Cardiac Conduction System

Elyse Foster, M.D.

Diseases of the cardiac conduction system are diverse in etiology and may affect any site along its anatomic course. The clinical manifestations, the prognosis of the disorder, and the need for treatment are dependent on both the cause and the site affected. The most common causes include infiltrative (or degenerative) disease, coronary artery disease, drug toxicity, autonomic dysfunction (carotid sinus hypersensitivity), and endocarditis. Infiltrative disease and carotid sinus hypersensitivity are more likely to present with chronic symptoms, whereas ischemic disease, drug effects, and endocarditis often have an acute presentation.

Normal conduction begins in the sinus node and travels along intraatrial pathways to the atrioventricular (AV) node. The AV node is composed of two distinct anatomic regions: the compact portion and the penetrating portion (also known as the bundle of His). The bundle of His divides into the right bundle branch; and the left bundle branch, which again divides into the left anterior and left posterior fascicles. Each of these anatomic sites is discussed separately in the following text.

SINUS NODE DYSFUNCTION

Sinus node dysfunction may be manifested as sinus bradycardia, sinus arrest, or sinoatrial block with or without associated tachyarrhythmias. When it occurs on the basis of degenerative disease, it is termed sick sinus syndrome or bradycardia-tachycardia syndrome and usually presents with chronic or recurrent cerebral symptoms.[1,2] Elective insertion of a permanent pacemaker is the treatment of choice, with the addition of pharmacologic therapy to control tachyarrhythmias. Acute management with isoproterenol, atropine, or temporary pacemaker are occasionally necessary if altered mentation, angina, or hemodynamic impairment is present. The need for antiarrhythmic drugs or cardioversion in the management of tachyarrhythmias may also necessitate a temporary pacemaker. Antiarrhythmic drugs may suppress sinus node activity, and cardioversion of a tachyarrhythmia may result in absent atrial activity in patients with sick sinus syndrome.

Ischemic sinus node dysfunction is uncommon. Sinus bradycardia, sinus arrest, and sinoatrial block occur in only about 5% of acute myocardial infarctions (MI).[3] Ischemic sinus node dysfunction is most often associated with an inferoposterior or lateral wall MI.[3] Atropine is the treatment of choice for symptomatic and hemodynamically significant sinus bradycardia or sinoatrial block. Temporary pacemaker insertion is the second-line treatment if the arrhythmia is unresponsive to or recurs following atropine. Isoproterenol should be avoided because of its pro-arrhythmic and positive inotropic effects.

Sinus node function is also influenced by many commonly used cardiac drugs, including beta blockers and calcium channel blockers. Patients with underlying sinus node disease may be very sensitive to these agents and may present with symptomatic bradycardia. Isoproterenol is the treatment of choice for cases of excessive beta blockade, although this should be used with caution in patients with coronary artery disease, and temporary pacemaker insertion may be required.

ATRIOVENTRICULAR NODAL DISEASE

AV block may be intranodal (within the compact portion of the AV node) or infranodal (within the His bundle or the bundle branches). Although the precise level of the block can be determined only by invasive electrophysiologic studies, important clues are available from the surface ECG. The type of AV block and rate of the escape rhythm provide these clues and have important prognostic value.

First-degree AV block (prolongation of the P-R interval) is usually intranodal but may be infranodal when accompanied by a bundle branch block. It is commonly seen in clinical situations associated with increased vagal tone (e.g., inferior MI) or during therapy with digitalis or calcium channel blockers (diltiazem and verapamil). First-degree AV block does not require specific treatment or withdrawal of the offending drug. Patients with first-degree AV block complicating an acute MI require very close observation, because the progression to second- or third-degree AV block may be as high as 60%, depending on the associated conduction abnormalities.[4]

Second-degree AV block may be associated with a Mobitz I (Wenckebach's) or Mobitz II pattern. Mobitz I block (progressive P-R prolongation preceding the nonconducted P wave) is almost always intranodal in location and is often seen in the presence of an acute inferior MI or digitalis excess. In the setting of an acute inferior MI (when no bundle branch block is present), atropine should be administered if the heart rate is less than 45 or if there is hemodynamic compromise. If the slow rate does not respond to atropine or recurs after the initial dose, a temporary pacemaker should be inserted. Mobitz I block in the setting of digitalis excess can usually be managed by withdrawing digoxin under observation.

Mobitz II second-degree AV block (constant P-R interval preceding the nonconducted P wave) is usually infranodal in origin and almost always associated with a bundle branch block. It signifies more extensive damage to the conduction system and is rarely responsive to atropine therapy. It more often occurs in the setting of an acute anterior MI and is more likely to progress to complete heart block. Therefore, temporary pacemaker insertion is indicated, although a large number of these patients with MI succumb to pump failure.[5] When Mobitz II AV block occurs as a result of progressive degenerative disease, elective permanent pacemaker insertion is usually indicated.

Second-degree AV block occurring with a 2:1 conduction ratio may be a manifestation of type I or type II AV block. The level of block cannot be discerned from the surface ECG unless (1) higher conduction ratios are present in the same patient; or (2) a bundle branch block is present, which makes Mobitz II block more likely. The treatment depends on the clinical setting.

Complete heart block (CHB), or third-degree AV block (no P waves are conducted, and the atrial rate is greater than the ventricular rate), may be intranodal or infranodal in location. Intranodal block is accompanied by a junctional escape rhythm with a narrow complex at a rate of 40–60 beats/ minute. There are three exceptions. Intranodal block may be associated with a wide complex escape focus if a concomitant bundle branch block is present, and, rarely, intranodal block is associated with a ventricular escape mechanism. Infranodal block within the His bundle is often associated with a narrow complex junctional escape focus. In general, the clinical setting, the treatment, and the prognosis of intranodal CHB are similar to that of Mobitz I second-degree AV block. It usually responds to atropine or isoproterenol with an increase in the rate of the junctional pacemaker or return of AV conduction. Although there is some disagreement, most cardiologists believe that a temporary pacemaker should be placed in patients with acute inferior MI and CHB, especially for a rate less than 45 or if ventricular ectopy requiring treatment is present.[4]

Infranodal CHB is associated with an idioventricular escape rhythm characterized by a wide QRS complex at a rate of 30–40. Because of the slower escape rate, it is more likely to be symptomatic. Pharmacologic therapy is less likely to be effective in accelerating the rate; therefore, temporary pacemaker insertion is nearly always indicated. In the setting of a chronic degenerative process, elective insertion of a permanent pacemaker should be performed expeditiously because the complications of an indwelling temporary pacing wire increase with time. However, in the setting of an acute MI, a delay of 2–3 weeks is advisable because of changes in pacing threshold that may occur in the healing myocardium and because of the increased risk of perforation in recently infarcted myocardium.

BUNDLE BRANCH BLOCK

Disease confined to the bundle branches requires acute management only in the setting of an acute MI. Although cardiovascular mortality, including sudden death, is increased in patients with chronic bundle branch block, death usually results from the underlying disease or from ventricular arrhythmias.[6,7] Progression to CHB does occur, but it is usually heralded by syncope or other symptoms and rarely presents as sudden death.[6,7]

On the other hand, when a bundle branch block complicates an acute MI, the risk of progression to higher-degree AV block (Mobitz II second-degree AV block or CHB) is increased. In the following situations, the risk exceeds 20% and prophylactic temporary pacemaker insertion is indicated to avoid the possibly disastrous occurrence of these rhythm disturbances in a patient with acute MI. These situations include:

1. First-degree AV block and bifascicular bundle branch block, whether

recent or old (i.e., right bundle branch block and left anterior hemiblock or left posterior hemiblock; alternating right bundle branch block; and left bundle branch block)
2. New bundle branch block and first-degree AV block
3. New bifascicular bundle branch block in the absence of first-degree AV block[4,5,8]

In certain instances during acute myocardial infarction, extensive hemodynamic impairment exists in addition to bradyarrhythmias. Ventricular pacing alone may not restore the blood pressure in these cases. Temporary AV sequential pacing may be required, because these patients are dependent on atrial contraction for maintenance of cardiac output.[9]

Swan-Ganz catheter insertion has been associated with an approximately 5% incidence of right bundle branch block secondary to trauma as the catheter passes the septum.[10] In the presence of a pre-existing LBBB, this could potentially result in CHB; therefore, temporary pacemaker insertion is generally recommended when Swan-Ganz catheterization is indicated in a patient with LBBB.

External temporary pacing has been shown to be both safe and effective.[11] If an external pacemaker is available, it may provide sufficient prophylaxis in this group of patients deemed at high risk so that insertion of a temporary transvenous pacemaker may be avoided. The disadvantages of this technique are that it may be very uncomfortable and requires sedation. If prophylactic use is intended, the pacing threshold should be determined and capture with adequate perfusion should be documented.

KEY FEATURES

The most common causes of cardiac conduction abnormalities are degenerative or infiltrative disease, coronary artery disease, and drug toxicity.

Sinus node dysfunction is usually termed "sick sinus syndrome" and may be associated with tachyarrhythmias. Emergency temporary pacemaker insertion is rarely necessary.

The level of AV block may be intranodal or infranodal. Infranodal block is associated with a Mobitz II second-degree AV block or third-degree AV block with idioventricular escape rhythm. It is usually symptomatic and requires temporary pacer insertion. Intranodal block usually responds to vagolytic therapy (atropine).

Indications for temporary pacemaker insertion in the absence of an acute myocardial infarction (MI) include the following:
1. Symptomatic sinus bradycardia unresponsive to atropine
2. Prolonged episodes of sinoatrial block or sinus arrest without escape rhythm

3. Second-degree AV block with symptomatic bradycardia unresponsive to atropine
4. Complete heart block with junctional escape rhythm and symptoms
5. Infranodal complete heart block with idioventricular escape rhythm
6. Cardioversion or antiarrhythmic drug therapy in patient with tachyarrhythmia and known sick sinus syndrome
7. Permanent pacemaker failure in pacemaker dependent patient
   Indications for temporary pacemaker insertion in the presence of
acute MI include the following:
1. Complete heart block
2. Mobitz I second-degree AV block with symptomatic bradycardia or when recurrent after dose of atropine
3. Mobitz II second-degree AV block
4. Symptomatic sinus bradycardia
5. Sinus arrest or sinoatrial block
6. High-risk bundle branch block (see text)
7. Swan-Ganz catheter insertion in the presence of a left bundle branch block

REFERENCES

1. Mond H: The bradyarrhythmias: Current indications for pacing (Part II). PACE 4:438, 1981.
   A good review of this subject, which includes indications and results of permanent pacemaker insertion in patients with high-degree AV block during acute MI, sick sinus syndrome, and other bradyarrhythmias.

2. Kulberthuis HH: Experience with permanent pacing in the sick sinus syndrome. Cardiovasc Clin North Am 14:189–194, 1983.
   Brief review of sick sinus syndrome, which usually presents with chronic neurologic symptoms. Permanent pacemaker insertion provides symptomatic relief but does not improve long-term survival, which is usually reduced as a result of underlying cardiac disease.

3. Parameswaran R, Ohe T, Goldberg H: Sinus node dysfunction in acute myocardial infarction. Br Heart J 38:93–96, 1976.
   A retrospective chart review of 431 patients with acute MI, excluding patients with cardiogenic shock or congestive failure, revealed 20 (4.6%) patients with sinus node dysfunction. Of 13 patients with sinus bradycardia, only 2 required temporary pacemaker insertion and none required permanent pacing. Of 7 patients with brady-tachy syndrome, 5 required temporary pacemaker insertion and 4 required permanent pacing.

4. DeGuzman M, Rhahimtoola SH: What is the role of pacemakers in patients with coronary artery disease and conduction abnormalities? Cardiovasc Clin North Am 13:191–207, 1982.
   An excellent review of the vascular supply to the conduction system and the effects of ischemia and infarction on cardiac conduction. In a series of 684 patients with acute MI, AV block without associated bundle branch block occurred in 12% of patients and was associated with a mortality of 29%. The overall incidence of bundle branch block in patients with acute MI was 9%, and it was more frequent with anterior MI. Twenty-nine per cent of those patients developed AV block, and the overall mortality rate was 20%. High-risk bundle branch block is defined, and indications for temporary pacemaker insertion are discussed.

5. Hindman MC, Wagner GS, JaRo M, Atkins JM, Scheinman MM, DeSanctis RW, Hutter AH Jr, Yeatman L, Rubenfire M, Pujura C, Rubin M, Morris JJ: The clinical significance

of bundle branch block complicating acute myocardial infarction. 1. Clinical characteristics, hospital mortality, and one-year follow-up. Circulation 58:679–688, 1978.

Four hundred ninety-four patients with bundle branch block and acute MI were identified in a retrospective chart review. Thirteen per cent were in cardiogenic shock prior to the development of bundle branch block and had an 84% in-hospital mortality rate. The remainder of the patients had an in-hospital mortality and 1-year mortality rate of 28% and 28%, respectively. Sixty-seven per cent of deaths were attributable to severe congestive heart failure, but the other 15 patients (9%) died as a result of AV block, and 9 of these 15 died when temporary pacemaker could not be inserted successfully.

6. McNaulty JH, Rhahimtoola SH, Murphy E, DeMots H, Ritzmann L, Kanarek PE, Kauffman S: Natural history of "high risk" bundle branch block. N Engl J Med 307:137–143, 1982.

   Five hundred fifty-four patients with chronic bifascicular and trifascicular block were followed for an average of 42 months. The 5-year mortality rate that could have been due to a bradyarrhythmia was 6%, including patients with sudden death of undocumented cause. Heart block occurred in 19 patients, and temporary pacemaker insertion was unsuccessful in only 2 patients. Although patients with syncope had a higher incidence of heart block than those without (17% vs. 2%), this study shows that permanent pacemaker insertion is not indicated unless a bradyarrhythmia can be documented.

7. Fisch GR, Zipes DB, Fisch C: Bundle branch block and sudden death. Progr Cardiovasc Dis 23:187–224, 1980.

   An extensive literature review on the association of bundle branch block and sudden death.

8. Hindman MC, et al: The clinical significance of bundle branch block complicating acute myocardial infarction. 2. Indications for temporary and permanent pacemaker insertion. Circulation 58:689–699, 1978.

   The patients at most risk for developing high-degree AV block (31–38%) were those with bilateral bundle branch block (right bundle branch block and left anterior hemiblock, right bundle branch block and left posterior hemiblock, or alternating bundle branch block) of new or indeterminate onset. Patients with a new unilateral bundle branch block and first-degree AV block or with first-degree AV block and old bilateral bundle branch block were at intermediate risk (19–20%). Prophylactic temporary pacing is recommended for these patients. Patients who progressed to high-degree AV block had a risk of sudden death or recurrent high-degree AV block (28%), and the mortality rate was decreased in those with permanent pacemakers (60% vs. 10%).

9. Haffajee CI: Temporary cardiac pacing: Modes, evaluation of function, equipment, and trouble shooting. 3:515, 1985.

   A good review of temporary cardiac pacing with a discussion of temporary AV sequential pacing.

10. Stein PD, Mathur VS, Herman MV, Levine HD: Complete heart block induced during cardiac catheterization of patients with pre-existent bundle branch block. The hazard of bilateral bundle branch block. Circulation 34:783–791, 1974.

    A report of five cases and a review of the literature. The incidence of right bundle branch block complicating right heart catheterization ranged between 0.5% and 12%. The incidence might be expected to be higher with the stiffer catheters used during cardiac catheterization than with Swan-Ganz catheters.

11. Falk RH, Zoll PM, Zoll RH: Safety and efficacy of noninvasive cardiac pacing. N Engl J Med 309:1166–1168, 1983.

    Sixteen normal volunteers and fifteen patients underwent testing of an external cardiac pacemaker. In ten patients, the pacemaker was tested prophylactically because these individuals were considered at high risk for bradyarrhythmias during cardioversion; in five patients, the pacemaker was used therapeutically. Failure to pace occurred in only one patient with a severe dilated cardiomyopathy, and only one patient was unable to tolerate the discomfort of the procedure.

Ventricular Dysrhythmias and Sudden Death

Gary J. Balady, M.D.

Approximately 500,000 Americans die each year from sudden cardiac death. Major efforts continue in an attempt to establish an effective means of identifying and treating patients at risk for this entity, which claims one life per minute in the United States alone. Individuals who are at the greatest risk of sudden death include:

1. *Survivors of out-of-hospital cardiac arrest.* These patients have a 12–34% recurrence rate in one year.[1] However, if the cardiac arrest was associated with a myocardial infarction (MI), the recurrence rate is only 2% in one year.[2]

2. *Patients who demonstrate recurrent sustained accelerating ventricular tachycardia.* Most members of this group have underlying coronary artery disease or cardiomyopathy. These patients are at a 40% risk of mortality within one year. Sustained ventricular tachycardia can be defined as a ventricular tachycardia that persists for more than 30 seconds or produces loss of consciousness.

3. *Patients who demonstrate a prolonged QT interval and have had an episode of ventricular tachycardia or syncope.* The prolonged QT syndrome, which may lead to a polymorphic ventricular tachycardia known as "torsades de pointes,"[3] can be either acquired or congenital. The acquired form is most often drug induced, e.g., from group IA antiarrhythmics, phenothiazines, or tricyclic antidepressants. It also is found to occur in patients with hypokalemia, myocarditis, and increased intracranial pressure. The congenital form is the result of an autonomic nervous system imbalance and, unlike the acquired form, is treated with beta adrenergic blocking agents.

4. *Subgroups of patients who have suffered a myocardial infarction.* Frequent or repetitive ventricular premature beats (VPBs) demonstrated on a 24-hour Holter's monitor recording imply a higher mortality rate, especially when associated with a reduced left ventricular ejection fraction. A precise definition of "frequent VPBs" remains controversial, and includes greater than five VPBs per hour, multifocal VPBs, and repetitive forms.[4] Post-MI

patients in whom electrophysiologic testing yields repetitive ventricular ectopy may be at higher risk of sudden death, although this finding is as yet inconclusive.[5]

Individuals who demonstrate VPBs in the absence of cardiac disease are *not* felt to be at greater risk of sudden death.[1]

Therefore, risk analysis of a given individual with ventricular dysrhythmias depends on the patient's mode of initial clinical presentation and on the demonstration of underlying cardiac disease.

Holter's monitoring is a useful tool in qualifying and quantitating ventricular dysrhythmias. Patients should be physically active during Holter's monitoring and should maintain a log of daily activities and symptoms in order to yield maximum information. Of note, the inherent variability in the occurrence of ventricular ectopy has been reported to be about 25% in 24 hours.[4] Thus, in the assessment of the therapeutic effectiveness of a particular drug, 80% reduction in isolated VPB frequency and elimination of repetitive ventricular beats must be observed to evaluate drug effect.[6]

Exercise testing can be employed as an adjunctive measure to provoke ventricular dysrhythmias, in addition to Holter's monitoring. Invasive electrophysiologic (EP) testing is a very useful method of studying ventricular dysrhythmias in a given patient. However, its availability is often limited to specialized tertiary care centers, limiting the practicality of this method for broad application. Patients who should be considered for EP testing are those who are at high risk for sudden death, and also those in whom a dysrhythmic cause of palpitations, dizziness, or syncope is suspected but not documented by noninvasive methods.[5,7]

The ultimate goal in identifying patients with ventricular dysrhythmias and assessing their risk of sudden cardiac death is to establish an effective treatment that would reduce their subsequent cardiac morbidity and mortality. Patients with no underlying cardiac disease do not require treatment for ventricular dysrhythmias unless they are symptomatic. A careful history and physical examination, as well as an ECG, exercise testing, and echocardiogram should be performed to assess the presence of heart disease. Cardiac catheterization should be performed in those patients whose history suggests coronary artery disease, when the noninvasive workup is otherwise unrevealing. However, therapy in high-risk patients can be instituted, keeping in mind that there are no conclusive data stating that such therapy is effective in reducing cardiac mortality. There is, however, evidence confirming that EP test–guided therapy reduces the incidence of sudden death in patients with a documented history of sudden death. Therefore, a carefully designed treatment plan with specific goals in mind, rather than empiric therapy, is recommended.

Currently available antiarrhythmic drugs and their dosages are outlined in Table 1.

TABLE 1. ANTIARRHYTHMIC DRUGS

Drug	Dosage	Side Effects
Group I		
A. Quinidine	200–600 mg q6h po	GI; CNS; thrombocytopenia; prolonged QT
Procainamide	100 mg q 5 minutes to total of 1 gm IV, then 2–4 mg/minute drip	Lupus-like syndrome; prolonged QT; hypotension
	250–1000 mg q4h po	
Disopyramide	100–200 mg q6h po	Urinary hesitancy; constipation; prolonged QT; congestive heart failure
B. Lidocaine	1 mg/kg IV bolus, then repeat dose of ½ initial bolus in 20 minutes, then 1–4 mg/minute	CNS: dizziness, slurred speech, altered mental status, seizures
Tocainide	400 mg q8h po (1200–1800 mg/day)	CNS (as above); nausea, vomiting, anorexia
Mexiletine	200–400 mg q8h po	CNS; GI: nausea, dyspepsia
C. Encainide	25–50 mg q8h po	Proarrhythmia; CNS: dizziness, blurred vision; GI: nausea
Flecainide	50–200 mg bid po	CNS: dizziness, tremors, blurred vision; GI: nausea; congestive heart failure
Lorcainide*		
Propafenone*		
Group II: Beta Adrenergic Blocking Agents		
Propranolol	10–80 mg qid po	Drowsiness; impotence; bradycardia; congestive heart failure
	80–120 mg bid po†	
Group III		
Bretylium	5 mg/kg initially, with additional doses of 10 mg/kg to maximum of 30 mg/kg	Hypotension, nausea; vomiting, parotid pain
Amiodarone	800–1600 mg qid for 1–3 weeks, then 600–800 mg qid for 1 month, then 200–400 mg qid	Hypothyroidism; hyperthyroidism; pulmonary toxicity; congestive heart failure; corneal microdeposits; elevated liver function tests; GI; CNS
Group IV: Calcium Channel Blocking Agents		
Verapamil	80–120 mg qid po	Hypotension; bradycardia; constipation

*Investigational use only.
†Recommended post-MI dose.[10]

Survivors of sudden death without coincident MI, as well as patients with recurrent sustained ventricular tachycardia, should be considered for treatment guided by EP testing. Such testing is performed in a well-controlled environment in which the ventricle is directly stimulated to induce ventricular tachycardia, while varied drug regimens are assessed for their ability to prevent the recurrence of inducible ventricular dysrhythmias.

Patients with prolonged QT syndrome and demonstrable ventricular tachycardia should be evaluated to identify a cause and to correct inciting factors (e.g., discontinuation of group IA antiarrhythmic therapy). An intravenous bolus of magnesium sulfate has been shown to be effective in terminating torsade de pointes rhythm.[8] Electric cardioversion, lidocaine, and isoproterenol have also led to the successful return of sinus rhythm. Temporary atrial or ventricular pacemaker insertion may be needed in cases in which the long QT interval is due to a marked bradycardia, such as that seen in intracranial hemorrhage.

Treatment of ventricular dysrhythmias in post-MI patients in the absence of sustained recurrent ventricular tachycardia remains far from clear. If therapy is instituted, it must be given with an understanding of the benefits and risks of treatment. Antiarrhythmic drugs, notably group IA, may actually induce ventricular tachycardia and fibrillation.[9] They should be administered with close observation for the development of a prolonged QT interval. Initial empiric use of lidocaine in post-infarction patients has been shown to be effective in reducing the incidence of sudden death in one controlled study; however, the authors reported a 15% incidence of unwarranted side effects as a result of therapy.[10] One could argue that the infrequent occurrence of ventricular fibrillation in the early acute MI patient (about 2%) and the high rate of successful cardioversion in the coronary care unit (CCU) setting make careful observation without empiric lidocaine a reasonable option, especially in the elderly, who have a higher incidence of side effects to lidocaine. Institution of beta adrenergic blocking drugs, timolol or propranolol hydrochloride (Inderal), within 7–10 days after an MI has been demonstrated to reduce cardiovascular morbidity and mortality in these patients.[11] This is a recommended course of therapy in post-MI patients in whom there is no contraindication of beta blockade, e.g., congestive heart failure or obstructive lung disease.

Several new modes of therapy are being evaluated for use in patients who do not respond to conventional forms of treatment. These include investigational drugs; endocardial electrosurgery, antitachycardia pacemakers, and implantable defibrillators.

KEY FEATURES

Patients who are at highest risk for sudden death include survivors of ventricular fibrillatory arrest; patients with prolonged QT syndrome and ventricular tachycardia or syncope; patients with recurrent sustained accelerating ventricular tachycardia; and post-MI patients with ventricular ectopy and a reduced ejection fraction.

Patients without cardiac disease who demonstrate asymptomatic ventricular dysrhythmias are *not* at great risk and do not warrant therapy.

Evaluation of patients with ventricular dysrhythmias includes mode of initial clinical presentation, 24-hour Holter's monitoring, exercise stress testing, and electrophysiologic testing.

Use of antiarrhythmic drugs should not be empiric, but rather guided by careful evaluation via Holter's monitor recording or electrophysiologic testing. Both of these methods are limited in their usefulness.

Multiple antiarrhythmic drugs are available for use, though the potential benefits of their use must be weighed against their inherent risk of inducing ventricular dysrhythmias.

REFERENCES

1. Surawicz B: Prognosis of ventricular arrhythmias in relation to sudden cardiac death: Therapeutic implications. J Am Coll Cardiol 10:435, 1987.
    A review of studies regarding ventricular dysrhythmias. This article defines the high-risk patient and outlines the strategy for treatment.

2. Cobb LA, Werner JA, Trobaugh GB: Sudden cardiac death. Mod Concepts Cardiovasc Dis 49:37–42, 1980.
    A very good review on management of the post-resuscitation patient, with special attention to the treatment of ventricular dysrhythmias in this group.

3. Smith WM, Gallagher JJ: "Les Torsades de Pointes": An unusual ventricular arrhythmia. Ann Intern Med 93:578–584, 1980.
    An early but comprehensive article that defines torsades de pointes in terms of etiology, recognition, and management.

4. Rosenthal ME, Oseran DS, Gange E, Peter T: Sudden cardiac death following acute myocardial infarction. Am Heart J 109:865–876, 1985.
    A superb review that discusses the approach to risk stratification and post-MI patients, with pertinent information regarding sudden death, ventricular dysrhythmias, and methods of assessment and treatment.

5. Rahimtoola SH, Zipes DP, Akhtar M, Burchell H, Mason J, Myerburg R, O'Rourke R, Ruskin J, Schlant R, Surawicz B: Consensus statement of the conference on the state of the art of electrophysiologic testing in the diagnosis and treatment of patients with cardiac arrhythmia—Part 2. Mod Concepts Cardiovasc Dis 56:61, 1987.
    Important summary of the indications for intracardiac electrophysiologic testing.

6. Morganroth J, Michaelson EL, Horowitz LN, et al: Limitations of routine long-term electrocardiographic monitoring to assess ventricular ectopic frequency. Circulation 58:408–414, 1978.
    This article discusses the variability in ventricular premature beat frequency during 24-hour Holter's monitoring. The limitations of routine 24-hour ambulatory monitoring are presented.

7. Brugada P, Wellens HJJ: Programmed electrical stimulation of the human heart. *In* Josephson ME, Wellens HJJ (eds): Tachycardias: Mechanisms, Diagnosis, Treatment. Philadelphia, Lea and Febiger, 1984.

An excellent overview of the present role of electrophysiologic testing in cardiology.

8. Tzivoni D, Keren A, Cohen A, et al: Magnesium therapy for "Torsades de Pointes." Am J Cardiol 53:528–530, 1984.
    A landmark report on the use of intravenous magnesium sulfate as emergent and effective therapy for torsades de pointes.

9. Ruskin JN, McGovern B, Garan H, et al: Anti-arrhythmic drugs: A possible cause of out-of-hospital cardiac arrests. N Engl J Med 309:1302–1306, 1983.
    Presents evidence that antiarrhythmic drugs can cause increases in life-threatening ventricular arrhythmias. This study effectively provokes thought on the benefit-risk ratio of antiarrhythmic drug therapy.

10. Lie KI, Wellens HJJ, Van Copelle FJ, Durrer D: Lidocaine in the prevention of primary ventricular fibrillation. N Engl J Med 29:1324–1326, 1974.
    A frequently quoted study (actually the only controlled data) that found a statistically significant reduction of primary ventricular fibrillation using prophylactic lidocaine in all patients admitted to the coronary care unit with a diagnosis of myocardial infarction. The incidence of primary ventricular fibrillation was 9% in the control group, with no ventricular fibrillation occurring in the lidocaine-treated group. There was a 15% incidence of unwarranted side effects in the lidocaine-treated group.

11. Frishman WH, Furberg CD, Friedwald WT: Beta-adrenergic blockade for survivors of acute myocardial infarction. N Engl J Med 310:830–837, 1984.
    An excellent comprehensive review discussing the pros and cons of the use of beta adrenergic blocking drugs in post-MI patients as a prophylaxis against sudden death.

Supraventricular Tachycardia: Diagnosis and Treatment

John B. Cadigan, M.D.
Jonathan F. Plehn, M.D.

Supraventricular tachycardia (SVT) is a generic term for those tachyarrhythmias sustained by electrical impulses originating in or cycling through the atria and/or the atrioventricular (AV) node. Specific types of SVT include sinus tachycardia, sinoatrial re-entrant tachycardia, intra-atrial re-entrant tachycardia, AV nodal re-entrant tachycardia, automatic atrial and junctional tachycardia, atrial flutter, atrial fibrillation, and multifocal atrial tachycardia. Strictly speaking, SVT implies supraventricular impulse formation at rates greater than 100 beats per minute, but it typically occurs at rates greater than 150.

Although SVT is usually not life threatening, in patients with impaired systolic or diastolic cardiac function these tachyarrhythmias may lead to diastrous consequences. Tachycardias may exacerbate ischemic conditions by increasing the myocardial oxygen demand, and patients whose cardiac output is compromised at baseline may develop hypotension or congestive heart failure because the relative time for diastolic filling decreases with an increase in heart rate. In those types of SVT causing loss of the "atrial kick" (e.g., atrial fibrillation or re-entrant AV nodal tachycardias), up to 30% of ventricular filling is lost, resulting in an increase in atrial pressure, a decline in myocardial contractility as a result of the Frank-Starling mechanism, and a reduction in cardiac output.[1] The loss of normal sequential AV contraction (as in AV nodal re-entrant tachycardia) may also exacerbate congestive heart failure if the atrium contracts against a closed mitral valve leading to an increase in left atrial pressure and subsequent pulmonic congestion.

The vast majority of SVTs are caused by one of two physiologic mechanisms: re-entry or automaticity (Table 1).[2] Re-entry requires the existence of two separate pathways with different refractory periods and conductivities. The pathways must be electrically connected both proximally and distally. Pathologic environments such as ongoing ischemia or electrolyte abnormalities are thought to set the stage for the establishment of such conditions by creating a variety or "dispersion" of refractory periods in neighboring cardiac tissue. SVT is often initially established with the occurrence of a supraventricular premature beat. This is then conducted down the pathway with the shorter refractory period (and usually the longer conduction time), being blocked in the adjoining conduction tissue with the longer refractory period. The former pathway is known as the alpha pathway and the latter, the beta pathway. Once the impulse reaches the distal connection of the two pathways, the one that was originally refractory to conduction (beta) may now be able to conduct in a retrograde direction back to the proximal junction. If the first pathway is no longer refractory, the impulse may "re-enter" at

---

TABLE 1.   MECHANISMS OF SUPRAVENTRICULAR TACHYCARDIA

Re-entry
Sinoatrial re-entrant tachycardia
Intra-atrial re-entrant tachycardia
Atrioventricular *nodal* re-entrant tachycardia (AVNRT)
Atrioventricular re-entrant tachycardia
    Wide QRS complex: antidromic type (i.e., WPW syndrome)
    Narrow QRS complex: orthodromic type
Atrial flutter (intra-atrial re-entry)
Atrial fibrillation (chaotic widespread atrial re-entry)

Increased Automaticity
Sinus tachycardia
Automatic atrial tachycardia
Automatic nodal tachycardia
Multifocal atrial tachycardia

the proximal connection and establish re-entry tachycardia by repetitive cycling through this re-entry loop.

Although most re-entry mechanisms leading to SVT occur within sinoatrial, atrial, or AV nodal tissue, the presence of accessory AV nodal bypass tracts, which usually have increased rates of conduction but also increased refractory periods, may also predispose the patient toward SVT. Re-entry by way of these accessory pathways is known as atrioventricular re-entrant tachycardia (AVRT). In these cases, the impulse may propagate in the antegrade direction over the normal AV conduction system (alpha pathway) but return by way of the bypass tract (beta pathway), setting up a re-entrant tachycardia with a normal sequence of ventricular activation and hence a "narrow complex SVT." Occasionally, however, antegrade conduction may occur over the bypass tract with retrograde conduction through the normal pathway, thus causing abnormal ventricular activation and a "wide complex SVT." The presence of these AV nodal bypass tracts may be revealed in the surface ECG, as in the Wolff-Parkinson-White syndrome, or they may be concealed and detected only during intracardiac electrophysiologic testing.

Increased automaticity is the second major mechanism for generating SVT. In this case, an ectopic pacemaker cell extrudes potassium rapidly during phase 4 of its action potential, causing an early return to its electrical threshold and thus depolarization. This ectopic cell may have a faster rate of spontaneous discharge than the heart's intrinsic pacemaker and may take over control of the heart rate. Unlike re-entry SVT, which usually begins suddenly, often precipitated by a premature atrial depolarization, automatic tachycardias often demonstrate a warm-up period in which the rate gradually increases initially and slows down prior to termination. It should be noted that although this warm-up phenomenon strongly supports an etiology of automaticity, it sometimes occurs with re-entry mechanisms as well. Conditions leading to increased automaticity include ischemia, hypoxia, electrolyte imbalance, acidosis, and conditions causing catecholamine excess (e.g., congestive heart failure).

DIAGNOSIS

The type of SVT is generally distinguished by use of an ECG, but the physical examination may also suggest its mechanism. For example, an AV nodal re-entrant SVT may depolarize the ventricle before the atrium, causing the right atrium to contract against a closed tricuspid valve, and thereby generating "cannon A waves" in the jugular veins. Fine flutter waves may be seen in the neck veins during periods of atrial flutter. An irregularly irregular rhythm with varying intensities of the first heart sound may be observed in atrial fibrillation.

In the examination of the surface ECG of any tachycardia, the first question to ask is whether it is ventricular or supraventricular in origin. The presence of narrow QRS complexes (under 120 msec) virtually rules out a ventricular origin; however, the differentiation of wide complex tachycardias may be more difficult.

SVT producing wide QRS complexes may result from pre-existing bundle branch block; rate-dependent bundle branch block; or accessory atrioventricular bypass tracts, as in the Wolff-Parkinson-White syndrome. Underlying bundle branch block may be permanent, as is seen in fibrosis of the conduction system; or temporary, as may be observed in electrolyte or metabolic abnormalities. Tachycardia-dependent ventricular aberrancy occurs as a result of differences in the refractory periods of the bundle branches, the right usually being longer than the left. If impulses are conducted to the ventricles rapidly, they may find the right bundle refractory but may conduct down the left bundle, causing a right bundle branch block pattern of aberrancy. This phenomenon may be seen in any cardiac conduction tissue, and left bundle branch block morphologies may also be seen. It is often difficult to distinguish between the wide, often bizarre, QRS tachycardia of SVT with ventricular aberrancy and that of ventricular tachycardia. The following are helpful points for distinguishing between these two arrhythmias:

1. The presence of AV dissociation strongly suggests ventricular tachycardia.
2. When compared with prior ECGs at nontachycardic rates, aberrancy is suggested if the initial deflection (intrinsicoid deflection) of the QRS complex is in the same direction.
3. A QRS complex of ventricular origin is often greater than 140 msec with a leftward axis. Aberrant QRS complexes often have a normal axis with a QRS not exceeding 120 msec.
4. Aberrant conduction may be intermittent and rate related.
5. Aberrant complexes often have a typical right bundle branch block pattern with a triphasic QRS complex (RSR') in lead V1 and an R' wave of greater amplitude than the R wave. Leads I and V6 maintain small narrow Q waves, consistent with normal early septal activation.
6. With ventricular tachycardia, the QRS complex in V1 is often biphasic and the normal septal Q waves in I and V6 are often missing. If the QRS complex is triphasic, the R wave amplitude is greater than that of the R' wave.[4]
7. In patients with underlying bundle branch block who develop SVT, the initial deflections of the QRS complexes are often in the same direction as in the pre-existing complexes and the width of the SVT QRS does not exceed the underlying QRS by more than 80 msec.
8. Wide complex SVT as a result of conduction down an accessory AV

pathway is extremely difficult to differentiate from ventricular tachycardia unless one notes delta waves on a prior tracing during normal sinus rhythm.

Once it has been determined that a tachycardia is supraventricular in origin, one must further characterize the mechanism so that proper treatment may be pursued. One should first determine if the rhythm is regular or irregular. Regular SVT includes sinus tachycardia, automatic atrial and junctional tachycardia, sinus and AV nodal re-entrant SVT, re-entrant SVT with a bypass tract (AVRT), and atrial flutter.

Regular Rhythm SVT

Sinus Tachycardia

Sinus tachycardia is an acceleration of normal sinus rhythm at rates greater than 100 beats per minute and usually no greater than 180. Causes include exertion, anxiety, fever, sepsis, hypovolemia, anemia, thyrotoxicosis, ischemia, congestive heart failure, pulmonary emboli, or drug effect (e.g., caffeine, aminophylline, or alcohol). Treatment is aimed at the underlying clinical process.

Sinus Node Re-entrant Tachycardia

Only about 10% of SVT is accounted for by this mechanism. It characteristically occurs at a slower rate than AV nodal re-entrant tachycardia (AVNRT), averaging rates less than 130 beats per minute. P waves are usually indistinguishable from those appearing during normal sinus rhythm, and the only way to differentiate sinus node re-entrant tachycardia from sinus tachycardia is observation of its abrupt onset and termination.

AV Nodal Re-entrant Tachycardia (AVNRT)

Impulse re-entry within the AV node is due to the presence of dual intranodal pathways. A characteristically extremely regular tachycardia is the clinical expression of AVNRT. P waves are formed by retrograde conduction into the atria almost simultaneously with that to the ventricles. As a result, the P waves may be invisible on the surface ECG tracing because they are "buried" in the QRS complex, or they may precede or follow the QRS in 5% of cases. This type of SVT was previously known as "paroxysmal atrial tachycardia" (PAT) and represents about 60% of regular SVT, excluding sinus tachycardia and atrial flutter.[5] Although usually occurring at rates of 140–160 beats per minute, AVNRT may reach rates of 220 beats per minute.

Atrioventricular Re-entrant Tachycardia (AVRT): AV Re-entrant Tachycardia With a Bypass Tract

AVRT may manifest as either a narrow or a wide QRS complex rhythm. Narrow QRS complex AVRT is the second most common cause of paroxysmal regular SVT and accounts for about 30% of such cases according to some investigators. This is an orthodromic tachycardia with initial conduction down the alpha pathway (AV node), and re-entry is through an anomalous beta pathway that bypasses the AV node. In the less common, antidromic forms of this tachycardia, there is antegrade conduction down the beta accessory pathway and re-entry via the alpha (normal AV nodal) pathway.[6] In the antidromic form, a wide complex SVT results; this may be seen in patients with Wolff-Parkinson-White syndrome. The beta pathway in this syndrome is called a Kent bundle, and it connects the atrium to the ventricle. One often cannot differentiate an AVNRT from an orthodromic AVRT without the aid of sophisticated electrophysiologic testing. Fortunately, this is not usually a problem because the precipitating causes and standard treatments are the same.[7]

It should be noted that both AVNRT and AVRT can be found in otherwise normal individuals. In addition, these tachycardias are frequently observed in patients having recently ingested nicotine, caffeine, or alcohol; having high levels of circulating catecholamines; having metabolic derangements; or with high atrial pressures causing increased atrial stretch.

Atrial Flutter

Intra-atrial re-entry probably accounts for most forms of atrial flutter. Atrial rates vary from 250 to 350 beats per minute but occur most commonly at 300 beats per minute. The ECG often demonstrates the classic sawtooth atrial flutter waves in lead V1 and the inferior leads. Because the AV node is incapable of conducting impulses at such rapid rates, there is block at this level, usually at a ratio of 2:1. Thus, atrial flutter should be suspected in any patient presenting with a regular ventricular rate of 150 beats per minute. Although the AV nodal block seen with flutter is usually regular and constant, it may be intermittent, making it difficult to distinguish this arrhythmia from the irregular rhythm of atrial fibrillation. If the flutter waves are not initially apparent, carotid sinus massage may increase AV nodal block, thus lowering the ventricular response and making atrial activity more obvious. The placement of a standard transvenous temporary pacemaker electrode in the esophagus behind the left atrium may also enhance diagnosis of the supraventricular rhythm. Paroxysmal atrial flutter may occur in patients without cardiac pathology, but in general it is associated with organic heart disease such as rheumatic or ischemic cardiomyopathies.

Automatic Atrial Tachycardia

Typically, automatic atrial tachycardia occurs in the face of conditions known to cause increases in intracellular (phase 4) depolarization, such as excess digitalis administration, hypokalemia, hypoxemia, or ischemia. It differs from sinus tachycardia in that the pacemaker impulse emanates from an area of the atrium outside of the sinus node; therefore, the P wave morphology and the PR segment length may be appreciably different. Inverted P waves may be encountered in lead I and the inferior leads. Usually the tachycardia develops gradually after a warm-up period and may decelerate gradually as well.

Automatic Junctional Tachycardia

As we have mentioned, most forms of paroxysmal SVT involve re-entry through the AV node. Uncommonly, spontaneous depolarization in the lower portion of the AV node (the junction) may accelerate and become the predominant pacemaker. An important clinical situation in which this occurs is that of digitalis toxicity, noted most commonly in patients requiring digitalis for control for chronic atrial fibrillation. Digitalis may block the upper AV node but increase the rate of depolarization of the junctional pacemaker cells, resulting in a junctional tachycardia. In this case, one may fail to see a P wave on the surface ECG or it may appear after the QRS complex, often deforming the T wave, or just before the QRS complex. As these P waves are manifestations of retrograde atrial depolarization, their axis is usually superior and they are inverted in the inferior leads, particularly in the ECG lead. The point to remember is that in any patient with atrial fibrillation on digitalis, regularization of the ventricular rate suggests a junctional rhythm and digitalis toxicity should be suspected.

Irregular SVT

The presence of an irregular SVT (varying R-R intervals) suggests either an irregular ectopic pacemaker (as in atrial fibrillation of multifocal atrial tachycardia) or irregular conduction through the AV node (as is sometimes seen with atrial flutter, particularly when the patient is digitalized).

Atrial Fibrillation

Atrial fibrillation results from chaotic atrial impulses reaching the ventricle by random conduction through the AV node. The rate of conduction is dependent on the refractoriness of the AV node and may be slowed by increases in vagal tone. The ventricular response in atrial fibrillation varies widely and is irregular. The height of the fibrillatory waves may be quite small or even indiscernible. However, in cases of "coarse fibrillation" occurring at slower rates, it may be difficult to distinguish from a rapid atrial flutter with variable AV nodal block. Atrial fibrillation usually implies the presence of underlying cardiac or systemic disease and is seen commonly with mitral and tricuspid valvular disase, cardiomyopathies, hypertension, pericarditis, coronary artery disase, pulmonary emboli, alcohol abuse, and thyrotoxicosis.

Multifocal Atrial Tachycardia

Multifocal atrial tachycardia (MAT) is diagnosed by the presence of at least three P wave morphologies with varying PR intervals and heart rates greater than 100 beats per minute. This rhythm is seen in conditions causing increased automaticity and results form the firing of multiple atrial ectopic foci. It is usually seen in the presence of severe chronic lung disease and may be exacerbated by the use of bronchodilator preparations such as aminophylline. Other causes include diabetes, ischemia, and severe congestive heart failure. As with any automatic arrhythmia, MAT is extremely resistant to treatment. In general, the rhythm is treated by eliminating or improving the predisposing conditions.

TREATMENT

On first encountering a patient with SVT, one must determine if the arrhythmia is causing significant hemodynamic compromise requiring emergent therapy. The presence of moderate or severe hypotension, severe congestive heart failure, or angina suggests the use of an aggressive approach, specifically electrical cardioversion, if the arrhythmia is considered susceptible to this treatment modality. If the patient displays no symptoms or is mildly symptomatic, a more conservative approach, dependent upon the underlying cause of the arrhythmia, is warranted. The management of some of the more commonly encountered types of SVT is discussed in the following sections.

AVNRT and AVRT

In these situations, one attempts to manipulate the requisite conditions for re-entry by altering the refractory periods or the conduction times of the pathways involved in the circuit. This may be effected by performing maneuvers known to enhance vagal tone, such as the application of carotid sinus pressure, coughing or Valsalva's maneuver, or elicitation of the diving reflex. In the first case, one should first auscultate the carotid arteries and avoid manipulating any arteries in which bruits are noted. Firm pressure is applied in a circular motion to the area just beneath the mandible over the carotid sinus for no longer than 5 seconds. This may be repeated and, if the tachycardia persists, attempted on the opposite side. Only one carotid should be massaged at any one time. Concurrent use of Valsalva's maneuver may enhance the response. Abrupt termination of the arrhythmia suggests a re-entry mechanism as its basis. Slowing of the arrhythmia bespeaks an automatic or intra-atrial mechanism such as sinus tachycardia or atrial flutter. If carotid sinus massage is ineffective, verapamil may be given by slow intravenous bolus administration utilizing an initial dose of .0375–.075 mg/kg, repeating (or doubling) every 5 minutes until 15 mg has been administered. Over 90% of AVNRT is converted in this manner.

It should be noted that verapamil must be used cautiously, as it may cause hypotension and is contraindicated in patients with more than mild hypotension. In the latter case, the use of a vasopressor agent such as norepinephrine bitartrate (Levophed) or metaramine may increase peripheral vascular resistance and, therefore, blood pressure, causing a reflex vagal response that may ablate the AVNRT or AVRT. In patients with hypertension or known coronary artery disease, this regimen should be avoided. Other medications that are less frequently used in these cases today are intravenous digitalis, propranolol, and edrophonium chloride (Tensilon). Observation and simple sedation are also often effective.

In the case of patients with suspected or manifested AV bypass tracts, one must be cautious with the use of digitalis or verapamil. In SVT generated by AVNRT or by AVRT, conversion to sinus rhythm may be aided with these medications. However, these medications are known to decrease the refractoriness of the fast pathway and decrease conduction through the AV node. If the SVT involves a purely atrial mechanism, such as with atrial fibrillation or flutter, use of these two drugs may cause preferential conduction down the accessory pathway and a consequently rapid ventricular response. This may lead to induction of ventricular fibrillation. When a wide complex SVT is detected and suspected to be a result of AVRT or when an atrial-based SVT such as atrial fibrillation or flutter occurs in a patient with a history of Wolff-Parkinson-White syndrome manifested by delta waves, medications that specifically prolong the accessory pathway's refractory period should be used. These include the type IA antiarrhythmics (quinidine, procainamide, and disopyramide), and beta blockers. Amiodarone (which at the time of this writing is not approved for this indication by the FDA) has been shown to be particularly useful in the conversion of SVT in patients with AV bypass tracts.[8] Finally, patients with wide complex tachycardias that are due to anomalous AV conduction should undergo intracardiac electrophysiologic testing to define the reaction of the accessory pathway's refractory period to various medications.

Atrial Fibrillation and Flutter

Assuming the patient is hemodynamically stable or no more than mildly symptomatic from these arrhythmias, one concentrates on controlling what may be a very rapid ventricular response. This is performed by increasing AV nodal block through the administration of verapamil or digitalis. Both arrhythmias may be managed with intravenous verapamil if rapid ventricular rate control is desired. Administration of 2.5 mg every three minutes up to 10–15 mg is usually effective. In about 8% of cases, there is an associated conversion of atrial flutter to normal sinus rhythm with verapamil therapy, though this would not be expected, owing to the intra-atrial generation of the tachycardia. Digitalis in the form of digoxin has historically been the drug of choice in controlling ventricular rates in these disorders. However, recent work has strongly suggested that digitalis does not actually convert atrial fibrillation to sinus rhythm.[9] Digoxin (0.25–0.5 mg) may be given as a loading dose intravenously. Titration to ventricular response may be accomplished with sequential 0.25 mg doses intravenously or orally every 3–4 hours up to a total of 1.5 mg. Larger loading doses than this often result in toxicity. In the case of atrial flutter, a type IA antiarrhythmic may be started in hope of chemical cardioversion after an adequate blocking effect of the AV node has been attained with digoxin or verapamil. Early conversion of atrial fibrillation should not be attempted unless the patient is hemodynamically unstable, as preliminary anticoagulation may be required to prevent thromboembolization from the left atrium.

Multifocal Atrial Tachycardia

The most effective therapy for MAT is reversal of the underlying pulmonary problem and correction of any acidemia, electrolyte imbalances, or hypoxemia. If these measures fail, rate control may be attempted with verapamil or with the cautious use of selective beta blockers. The efficacy of metoprolol has been reported, but its use exacerbates pre-existing pulmonary problems. Digitalis and type IA antiarrhythmics are usually unsuccessful in this condition.[10,11]

Electrical Cardioversion and Overdrive Pacing

In the setting of significant hypotension, angina, or severe congestive heart failure as a result of rapid ventricular rate, emergency electrical cardioversion of SVT must be considered. In any but the most critical of situations, parenteral sedative-muscle relaxants should be administered prior to cardioversion. Digitalis toxicity markedly increases the risk of dysrhythmic sequelae resulting from electrical cardioversion. If digitalis use is known or suspected, test administration of synchronized cardioversion at extremely low power settings should be considered. Overdrive pacing of regular re-entrant supraventricular tachydysrhythmias is often effective as an alternative treatment modality.

CONCLUSIONS

This article discusses the diagnosis, mechanisms, and treatment of supraventricular tachyarrhythmias. They form a diverse group of arrhythmias with varying underlying mechanisms, causes, and treatments. They are, in general, benign tachyarrhythmias, but at times constitute life-threatening emergencies. Although they are often easily corrected, problematic SVTs can be the most challenging, frustrating, and difficult arrhythmias encountered by the clinician.

KEY FEATURES

The supraventricular tachycardias (SVT) have in common a mechanism of impulse generation, propagation, and sustained action arising in the atrial or atrioventricular nodal tissues.

The two primary physiologic mechanisms resulting in SVT are (1) re-entry circuit and (2) increased automaticity.

Approximately 60% of cases of regular SVT result from AV nodal re-entry; 30% involve concealed accessory bypass tracts.

Both narrow and wide complex SVTs exist. The presence of a narrow complex (0.12 msec) virtually rules out ventricular tachycardia.

Wide complex SVT may be observed with AVRT conducted ante-gradely down a bypass tract or in the settings of underlying or rate-related bundle branch block. SVT with aberrant conduction is suggested if the initial QRS deflection is identical to that of the native rhythm, if there is a right bundle branch block configuration that is triphasic in V1 with R' greater than R, and if small Q waves are noted in leads I and V6.

Ventricular tachycardia is suggested if the wide complex QRS has a left axis deviation but the native rhythm does not, if there is a biphasic QRS or triphasic QRS with R greater than R' in V1, or if the QRS is wider than 140 msec with no underlying bundle branch block.

Synchronized electrical cardioversion must be considered whenever SVT results in hemodynamic compromise manifested in angina, hypotension, or congestive heart failure.

AV nodal re-entrant tachyarrhythmias respond well to vagotonic maneuvers (e.g., carotid sinus massage, coughing or Valsalva's maneuver, or elicitation of the diving reflex) or to medications that slow conduction in the AV node (e.g., verapamil or digitalis).

Automatic SVTs, atrial flutter, and atrial fibrillation initially require control of the ventricular rate and correction of predisposing conditions.

REFERENCES

1. Naito M, et al: Am J Cardiol 46:625, 1980.
   The role of atrial systole and the hemodynamic results of abnormal atrioventricular activation.

2. Gilman RF, Zipes DP: Basic electrophysiologic mechanisms of the development of arrhythmias: Clinical application. Med Clin North Am 68:795, 1984.
   A comprehensive overview of SVT.

3. Josephson ME, Wellens HJ: Tachycardias: Mechanisms, Diagnosis, Treatment. Philadelphia, Lea and Febiger, 1984.
   A comprehensive text of SVT, their diagnosis, electrophysiology, and treatment.

4. Wellens H, et al: Am J Med 64:27, 1978.
   A "classic" paper reviewing the ECG differential diagnosis of tachycardia with widened QRS complexes.

5. Wu D, et al: Am J Cardiol 41:1045, 1978.
   Reviews the clinical electrocardiographic and electrophysiologic features of 79 patients with paroxysmal SVT, excluding those secondary to ventricular pre-excitation.

6. Baylor College of Medicine Cardiology Series 7:(11), 1984. Dreifus LS, Michelson EL. Supraventricular tachycardia: Its pathophysiology, diagnosis and treatment. McIntosh, HD.
   An excellent review of SVT for the internist. Not as detailed or sophisticated as Josephson's text.

7. Berold SS, et al: Am J Cardiol 39:97, 1977.
   Discusses the mechanisms of AV nodal re-entry tachycardias and tachycardias secondary to conduction via accessory bypass tracts.

8. Rosenbaum MB, et al: Am J Cardiol 38:934, 1976.
   The clinical efficacy of amiodarone as an antiarrhythmic agent.

9. Falk RH, Knowlton AA, Bernard SA, Gotlieb NE, Battinelli NJ: Digoxin for converting recent-onset atrial fibrillation to sinus rhythm. A randomized, double-blinded study. Ann Intern Med 106:503, 1987.

10. Levine J, et al: N Engl J Med 312:21, 1985.
    The treatment of MAT with verapamil.

11. Grayboys T (editorial): N Engl J Med 312:43, 1985.
    A good, concise overview of SVT, including MAT, with pertinent references.

Acute Pericarditis and Cardiac Tamponade

Jonathan F. Plehn, M.D.

Acute pericarditis is a condition that is frequently diagnosed in the emergency room. Although its presentation is usually benign, its course may rapidly deteriorate into cardiac tamponade and the physician must be aware of the disease in all of its manifestations.

ANATOMY AND PATHOPHYSIOLOGY

The pericardium is a double-layered sac that surrounds the heart, supports its position in the thorax, and serves to prevent the spread of infection from contiguous organs to the heart itself. The visceral pericardium is immediately adherent to the epicardial fat layer surrounding the heart and is separated from the parietal pericardium by a potential space that normally contains up to 50 cc of fluid secreted by the epithelial cells of the surrounding pericardial layers.

When a disease process leads to inflammation or irritation of the pericardium, the common reaction is transudation or exudation of fluid. Although a pericardial effusion is often seen in cases of acute pericarditis, other conditions, such as congestive heart failure, hypothyroidism, or trauma, can also cause effusion without actual pericardial inflammation.[1]

The most common cause of acute pericarditis is viral, usually a Coxsackie B or an Echo virus. This type of pericarditis is often seen in the spring or fall, when enteroviral infections are most prevalent. Bacterial pericarditis is less frequently seen on an emergent basis but should be suspected in children and in those adults presenting with pre-existing or coexisting bacterial infections, a recent history of thoracic surgery, or a history of immunosuppression. Other relatively common causes of pericarditis include connective tissue disease, uremia, radiation therapy, post–myocardial infarction (Dressler's) syndrome, and post-cardiotomy syndrome.[1-3]

Pericardial inflammation usually, but not always, leads to the accumulation of a pericardial effusion. This fluid may cause hemodynamic compromise of the heart by compression and resultant restriction to cardiac filling, which, in turn, may lead to diminished cardiac output and occasionally frank shock.[4] Although cardiac tamponade is usually associated with large effusions, this is not always the case. Small effusions that have rapidly accumulated may also cause tamponade and are usually the result of bleeding from either surgery or some other form of trauma.

PRESENTATION

The most common symptom of acute pericarditis is sharp pleuritic chest pain that may radiate to the shoulders and is classically worse in the supine position. The pain may, however, masquerade as a myocardial infarction (MI) or as an abdominal disorder. MI or ischemic pain is usually of a duller type and is often described as a pressure sensation. In addition, ischemic pain often radiates down the arm to the hand, may be relieved with sublingual nitroglycerin, is not exaggerated with inspiration or coughing, and is not relieved by sitting up. Both conditions may be accompanied by a slight fever, but myocardial ischemia is much more commonly associated with nausea and diaphoresis. Congestive heart failure is more frequently seen in cases of MI but may be seen when pericarditis accompanies acute myocarditis.

PHYSICAL EXAMINATION

The pericardial friction rub is usually a three component scratchy sound, which, in this form, is virtually pathognomonic of pericardial inflammation. The first component is caused by ventricular ejection in systole, and the other two parts are due to the early rapid ventricular filling phase and the later diastolic filling phase caused by atrial contraction. Less frequently, two or only one of these components will be evident. The rub is frequently evanescent, which often leads to debate regarding its presence by examining physicians. A key point to remember about the pericardial rub is that its presence does not exclude a large effusion, since the rub may be due to a pleural-pericardial interaction instead of friction between the visceral and parietal pericardium.

As pericardial fluid accumulation leads to impairment of cardiac filling, neck vein distention appears and is often noted up to the angle of the jaw. The two venous pulsations that are normally observed (A and V waves) appear as a single wave, owing to impediment to right ventricular filling and consequent loss of the Y descent. The sign of pulsus paradoxicus occurs when arterial pressure drops more than 10 mmHg with normal inspiration. Although this sign is almost always seen in cardiac tamponade, it may be masked by associated left ventricular hypertrophy, aortic insufficiency, or congestive heart failure. In addition, it may also be demonstrated in other conditions, most notably acute asthma. Kussmaul's sign, a rise or failure of the neck veins to collapse with normal inspiration, is seen in only about a third of patients with tamponade and is much more common in constrictive pericarditis.[4]

DIAGNOSTIC STUDIES

An electrocardiogram is the first test to order in cases of suspected acute pericarditis. This may demonstrate diffuse, upsloping ST segment elevation and P-R segment depression in the early stages of the disease. With time, there is return to baseline of the ST segment, T wave inversion, and finally reversion to normal. Any of these stages may be bypassed in the progression of the pericarditic ECG.[5] The ECG findings of pericarditis classically differ from those of acute MI in that the ST segment elevation of ischemia or injury has a concave rather than a convex shape facing upward, and the distribution of involved leads is usually limited to those reflecting affected cardiac segments. Pericarditic changes are frequently diffuse, with ST segment elevation seen in all leads except AVR and V1, where ST segment depression is noted. Early repolarization abnormalities, which are most commonly seen in young black males, may confound the picture but are usually limited to the right precordial leads.

The chest film may be useful in identifying a pericardial effusion but suffers from a low sensitivity for fluid and a lack of specificity. The "water flask heart" sign, although often indicative of a large pericardial effusion, may also represent a dilated cardiomyopathy with four chamber enlargement.

Echocardiography provides the best screening test for pericardial effusion.[6] Using a two-dimensional sector scanner, as little as 10 cc of pericardial fluid may be detected. Thus, the technique is exquisitely sensitive but may not be specific because the normal heart may be surrounded by as much as 50 cc of fluid, thus raising the possibility of a false positive diagnosis. In addition, the failure to detect pericardial fluid does not exclude a diagnosis of noneffusive pericarditis.

Until recently, there was no reliable means to diagnose cardiac tamponade noninvasively. The echocardiographic finding of diastolic right atrial indentation has now been shown to correlate very highly with the hemodynamic definition of tamponade.[7] Marked respiratory variation of flow across left-sided valves is a useful pulsed Doppler manifestation of tamponade and pulsus paradoxicus.[8]

The hemodynamic hallmark of cardiac tamponade is the finding of diastolic equalization of cardiac chamber pressures. A Swan-Ganz flow-directed right heart catheterization is performed, and the pulmonary capillary wedge pressure in end-diastole is usually found to be within 6 mmHg of the right atrial, right ventricular, and pulmonary capillary wedge pressures.[4]

Once the diagnosis of pericarditis is firmly established, a cause must be sought. If the patient has no history of predisposing disease processes and has no other symptoms suggestive of a specific cause, blood tests must be obtained. A CBC and renal profile should be taken, and if fever is present or a leukocytosis exists, blood should be drawn for cultures. In addition, a tuberculin skin test should be administered and serum screening for collagen vascular diseases should be considered. If the work-up fails to reveal a cause, the pericarditis is usually assumed to be virally induced.

The necessity and timing of an elective pericardiocentesis are controversial. Some physicians prefer to obtain samples of pericardial fluid in all patients; if the picture is highly suggestive of a viral cause and there is no hemodynamic compromise, other physicians prefer to follow the patient clinically and with echocardiography, without obtaining fluid. If an infectious cause other than viral is suspected, and if the echocardiogram has demonstrated at least a moderate-sized effusion that might be safely aspirated with a needle, pericardiocentesis should be undertaken by an experienced cardiologist. This is a procedure fraught with a great number of complications, and many physicians will consult a thoracic surgeon to drain the effusion and biopsy the pericardium under direct visualization in the operating room.[8]

TREATMENT

The specific treatment of acute pericarditis will, of course, depend on its cause. Hospital admission is required for all patients other than those with probable viral pericarditis exhibiting small or nonexistent effusions.

Infectious endocarditis may be life-threatening and must be rapidly and aggressively managed with intravenous antibiotics and drainage. Uremic pericarditis usually responds to dialysis but may require the addition of anti-inflammatory agents, including steroids. Viral pericarditis, the most common form, is usually self-limited but requires the administration of analgesics and anti-inflammatory agents. Aspirin 650 mg qid or indomethacin 25 mg tid is a reasonable initial therapy. In patients with extreme discomfort, a drug such as oxycodone hydrochloride (Percodan), which combines a potent analgesic and an anti-inflammatory agent (aspirin), should be prescribed.

Many cardiologists do not routinely admit all younger patients with viral pericarditis to the hospital. Bed rest for at least a week is suggested, and serial echocardiograms should be obtained to ensure that the effusion is not increasing. Post-MI (Dressler's) syndrome has become a relatively rare condition for unexplained reasons. It may appear from 2 weeks to 2 years after an MI and is treated in the same manner as viral pericarditis. Post-pericardiotomy syndrome, which is seen after cardiac surgery, is, like Dressler's syndrome, probably an autoimmune phenomenon and is treated similarly with analgesics and anti-inflammatory agents. In some cases, corticosteroids may be required because these latter two conditions are often refractory to initial medical therapy.

The only effective treatment for cardiac tamponade is pericardial drainage. This condition may develop quite abruptly and may lead to a patient's rapid demise. Although fluid loading and the use of intravenous sympathomimetic amines and afterload reducers may provide temporary support for the patient with tamponade and shock, the usefulness of these agents in this setting is debatable.[9] The rapid removal of even small amounts of pericardial fluid by pericardiocentesis often results in dramatic improvement in blood pressure and can be life-saving. Echocardiography should first be used to confirm the presence of a sizable effusion that can be safely tapped. Once the effusion is successfully located by a percutaneous needle placement, a Teflon catheter with side holes may help to assist drainage. This may be left in place for several days to prevent reaccumulation of fluid. If fluid reaccumulation becomes a problem, a surgeon should be consulted to perform a pericardiotomy (window) or a stripping.

KEY FEATURES

Acute pericarditis is a condition commonly seen in the emergency room.

The classic presentation is of sharp pleuritic chest pain radiating to the shoulders and exacerbated by assumption of the supine position; the pain may, however, mimic other conditions such as myocardial infarction (MI) or acute gastrointestinal syndromes.

The key to diagnosis of acute pericarditis is a compatible history, a pericardial friction rub on auscultation, and characteristic electrocardiographic changes.

Echocardiography is extremely valuable in detecting associated pericardial effusion and in grossly estimating the size of effusion. The echocardiogram may be oversensitive for effusion, however, and failure to visualize an effusion does not exclude the diagnosis of pericarditis.

A cause of the pericarditis must be aggressively sought. Bacterial pericarditis requires prompt drainage of effusion and administration of intravenous antibiotics.

In patients with an unexplained cause of their pericarditis after a thorough work-up, a viral cause should be suspected. These patients should be followed closely both clinically and with serial echocardiography. Acute hospitalization may not be absolutely required.

Treatment of noninfectious endocarditis and viral endocarditis requires bed rest; analgesia; and the use of anti-inflammatory agents, including aspirin or indomethacin.

Cardiac tamponade can develop very quickly and can cause life-threatening hypotension. It may be seen in acute or chronic pericarditis or in noninflammatory causes of effusion.

Although fluid loading and institution of pressors and vasodilators may temporarily maintain blood pressure in cardiac tamponade, reports question the efficacy of medical therapy. Pericardiocentesis or intra-operative pericardiotomy and drainage should be pursued as soon as possible.

REFERENCES

1. Roberts WC, Spray TL: Pericardial heart disease: A study of its causes, consequences and morphologic features. *In* Spodick DH (ed): Pericardial Disease. Philadelphia, FA Davis, 1976, pp 11–65.
   A well-organized review of the pathophysiology of pericardial disease, with good illustrative material.

2. Lorell BH, Braunwald E: Pericardial disease. *In* Braunwald E (ed): Heart Disease: A Textbook of Cardiovascular Medicine, 3rd ed. Philadelphia, WB Saunders Co, 1988, pp 1484–1534.
   An extensive review of pathophysiology, diagnosis, and treatment. A good discussion of the various causes of pericarditis is included.

3. Spodick DA: The normal and diseased pericardium: Current concepts of pericardial physiology, diagnosis and treatment. J Am College Cardiol 1:240, 1983.
   A brief overview of pericardial disease by one of the most prolific writers in this area. This article is a good introduction to the subject.

4. Shabetai R: Tamponade. *In* Shabetai R: The Pericardium. New York, Grune and Stratton, 1981, pp 224–278.
   A careful and detailed discussion of the mechanisms of cardiac tamponade by an author who has devoted much of his time to the investigation of this subject.

5. Spodick DA: Electrocardiogram in acute pericarditis. Distribution of morphologic and axial changes by stages. Am J Cardiol 33:470, 1974.
   A description of the classic evolutionary pattern of the electrocardiogram in acute pericarditis.

6. Shah PM: Echocardiography in pericardial diseases. *In* Reddy PS, Leon DE, Shaver JA (eds): Pericardial Disease. New York, Raven Press, 1982.
   Reviews the extremely important application of echocardiography to the diagnosis of this disease and how this technique has contributed to our understanding of the physiology of some of the disease manifestations.

7. Miller SW, Feldman L, Palacios I, et al: Compression of the superior vena cava and right atrium in cardiac tamponade. Am J Cardiol 50:1287, 1982.
   A comparison of the echocardiographic and angiographic findings in cardiac tamponade.

8. Callaham M: Pericardiocentesis in traumatic and nontraumatic cardiac tamponade. Ann Emerg Med 13:924, 1984.
   A good review of the clinical and emergent management of pericardial disease.

9. Kerber RE, Jascho JA, Litchfield R, Wolfson P, Ott D, Pandian NJ: Hemodynamic effects of volume expansion and nitroprusside compared with the pericardiocentesis in patients with acute cardiac tamponade. N Engl J Med 307:929, 1982.
   A critique of the current medical management of tamponade.

Dissecting Aortic Aneurysm

Jonathan F. Plehn, M.D.

Dissecting aortic aneurysm is an acute, life-threatening condition that demands rapid diagnosis and early intervention. The mortality rate of this condition in untreated patients is quite high, ranging from 13% in the first twelve hours to approximately 74% in the first two weeks.[1] Thus, rapid detection and aggressive treatment are extremely important in attempting to modify the natural history of the disease.

PATHOGENESIS

Aortic dissection occurs when a rupture in the medial layer of the aortic wall opens up a tissue plane that expands either proximally or distally as a result of the shearing force of systemic blood pressure. The division of the aortic medial wall creates an "intimal flap," which is pushed into the aortic lumen by the dissecting hematoma. As the dissection progresses, it may occlude branch arteries of the aorta by dissecting into them or by occluding their lumens with the intimal flap.

The initial event precipitating the dissection is still in question,[2,3] but in most cases, a tear in the intimal layer of the aorta can be documented in contiguity with the medial dissection. In addition, there is some evidence that degeneration of the medial layer of the aortic wall may predispose the patient to progression of the dissection once the tear has occurred. Certain conditions associated with an increased frequency of medial degeneration are also associated with aortic dissection, such as Marfan's syndrome and hypertension.

The site of the intimal tear and subsequent area of dissection extension bear a direct relationship to the clinical presentation, prognosis, and management of this condition. DeBakey has developed the most popular classification system,[4] in which tears occurring in the ascending or transverse aortic arch before the left subclavian artery are called type I or II and those occurring beyond the subclavian are termed type III. Type I dissections involve both the proximal aorta and the area lying distal to the subclavian. Type II dissections involve only the proximal aorta. Aortic dissections most commonly begin in the ascending aorta and rarely initiate in the abdominal aorta.

Over two thirds of the cases of aortic dissection occur in the 40–70-year-old age group and afflict males two to three times as frequently as females. Conditions commonly associated with aortic dissection include hypertension (more commonly seen with descending aortic dissections), Marfan's syndrome, bicuspid or unicommissural aortic valve, coarctation of the aorta, and pregnancy.[5] Trauma and atherosclerosis bear only a mild or non-existent relationship to dissection.[2,3] Iatrogenic causes, such as retrograde aortic catheterization or cardiac surgical procedures, are well documented.

CLINICAL PRESENTATION

The clinical presentation of dissection is related to the involved areas of the aorta.[6] The sudden onset of sharp chest pain, often of excruciating intensity, is the most common symptom seen in this condition and is usually associated with a type I or II dissection. The pain often radiates to the back and may be migratory. The sharp quality and migratory nature help to distinguish the presentation from that of myocardial infarction (MI). Type III dissections usually cause back pain, which is also frequently of a migratory nature. It should be emphasized that location of the pain is not absolutely diagnostic of the extent or location of the dissection. In addition, there is a small subgroup of patients who experience painless dissection.

The most dramatic presentations of aortic dissection occur in patients with ascending arch disease. The abrupt onset of congestive heart failure is almost always due to acute aortic insufficiency precipitated by retrograde dissection into the annular area. The development of hypotension often results from cardiac tamponade caused by rupture of the dissecting hematoma into the pericardial sac. Other rupture sites include the pleural cavity, usually on the left side, and the gastrointestinal tract.

Many of the manifestations of aortic dissection are caused by luminal compromise of the aortic branch arteries. Although coronary artery dissection is rarely reported, innominate, carotid, and subclavian artery obstruction is frequently observed. The patient may present with a pulseless extremity, a pulse inequality, or, in the case of carotid occlusion, a cerebrovascular accident. Obstruction of more distal arteries can cause acute renal failure, gastrointestinal hemorrhage as a result of mesenteric bowel infarction, and spinal artery ischemia.

Additional complications may arise from compression of extrinsic structures. Horner's syndrome may occur with superior sympathetic ganglion involvement. Tracheal deviation and superior vena caval syndrome may also result from compression.

Finally, aortic rupture may lead to aortocardiac fistulae (usually into right-sided chambers) and esophageal and pulmonary hemorrhage.

PHYSICAL EXAMINATION

Probably the most important clue to diagnosis of aortic dissection is the loss or diminution of peripheral pulses as a result of luminal obstruction. Therefore, all pulses should be carefully checked for strength and symmetry. Manometric measurements should be taken in both arms and legs in suspicious situations. The new auscultation of a decrescendo, blowing diastolic heart murmur suggests aortic root involvement and acute aortic regurgitation and is observed in over two thirds of patients with ascending aorta involvement.[6] This may be overlooked when it results in the more impressive picture of acute congestive heart failure and therefore should be considered as a possible cause in any case in which the etiology of acute congestive failure is not immediately apparent. Other findings on physical examination include the presence of new bruits over areas of luminal narrowing and either central or peripheral neurologic deficits. A pulsatile sternoclavicular joint is rarely seen in this condition.

LABORATORY TESTS

A chest roentgenogram is an important early screening test. A widened mediastinum should raise the question of dissection immediately, though a lack of widening does not exclude the diagnosis. Observation of a calcified aortic knob with extension of the aortic wall 4 or 5 cm beyond the calcification is pathognomonic of this condition.[7]

Electrocardiography is another study to pursue that is particularly useful if no ischemic changes are noted, as it may help to rule out a diagnosis of myocardial ischemia or infarction. Unfortunately, if ischemia is noted, the diagnosis will remain in question because coronary artery dissection may rarely occur, causing a similar picture.

Cardiac and abdominal ultrasound have been shown to be effective screening tests for dissection. Ultrasonography can be performed rapidly in the emergency room, under monitored conditions, and has the added advantage of being able to visualize the entire aorta when performed by a skilled technician.[8] Recent reports have also documented the utility and accuracy of transesophageal echocardiography. Color flow Doppler mapping may define the entry point of the dissection.[9]

If there continues to be a strong suspicion of dissection after the ultrasound examination has been performed, aortography is the next diagnostic step.[10] The abdominal aortogram may more clearly delineate the extent of aortic involvement and pinpoint the site of the intimal tear. It should be noted that retrograde aortography has been shown to be an extremely safe procedure in this condition but may be time consuming in a period when time is of the essence. Digital subtraction angiography has also been reported to diagnose and demonstrate the extent of dissection successfully.

The sensitivity of aortography has been called into question,[11] and many authorities now believe that contrast-enhanced, computed tomographic (CT) body scanning may provide a more accurate method to detect the presence and extent of dissection.[12] Magnetic resonance imaging (MRI) may also provide useful diagnostic information.

TREATMENT

In general, treatment is based on the location of dissection. In all cases, aggressive medical therapy must be pursued initially to prevent extension of the dissection. Two factors that are largely responsible for progression of the dissecting hematoma are systemic blood pressure and the rate of rise of systolic pressure (dP/dT), which is also known as the "shearing force." Control of these parameters, at least in the very early stages, is important for a successful outcome. Ideally, then, medical management of acute aortic dissection would both lower systemic blood pressure and reduce the shearing force caused by cardiac ejection.[7]

Trimethaphan (Arfonad) is an intravenous drug that rapidly reduces blood pressure while causing a decrease in dP/dT. It is given at a rate of 1–2 mg/minute. Unfortunately, tachyphylaxis rapidly develops with this drug and its antisympathetic side effects restrict its usefulness. Sodium nitroprusside (Nipride) is an alternative drug of choice in this condition. It is better tolerated and can be easily titrated to lower blood pressure without causing severe hypotention. It should be started at 0.5 µg/minute and titrated to the point at which systolic pressure is lowered by 20–40 mmHg in the normotensive patient or to a level of 100–120 mmHg total. Because nitroprusside has the deleterious additional effect of increasing dP/dT, a negative inotropic agent, preferably intravenous propranolol, should be administered concomitantly. This is given as an initial 0.5 mg intravenous bolus, which is then followed approximately every five minutes by repeated 0.5 mg boluses to the point at which a bradycardiac rate response is attained. If neither sodium nitroprusside nor trimethaphan can be effectively used in a patient, intramuscular reserpine at a rate of 1–2 mg every four to six hours can be administered. Cimetidine and antacids should be given simultaneously to reduce reserpine's ulcerogenic potential.

Surgery has been shown to reduce mortality significantly in patients with ascending aortic dissection and should be undertaken promptly in these individuals.[13,15] The previously described tests should be performed to determine the extent of dissection, and many surgeons require aortography with tomograms to identify the site of the intimal tear. Modern day surgical techniques include resection of the aneurysm at the site of the intimal tear, oversewing the two free ends of the aorta, and then reconnecting these with a Dacron graft or by direct anastomosis. If aortic insufficiency is found, either valvular resuspension or valve replacement is performed.

Most evidence in the literature suggests that type III dissections should be managed medically unless the dissection is noted in progress, the pain is intractable, there is unremitting systemic hypertension, or there is evidence of circulatory compromise of a major organ. However, some authorities prefer to repair all acute aortic dissections no matter where they are found.[14]

PROGNOSIS

Modern therapeutic techniques have clearly influenced the history of this disease. Mortality rates are greatly affected by major associated complications, with the possible exception of acute aortic insufficiency.[15] Overall in-hospital survival rates of 60–80% are reported for patients with acute ascending dissections treated surgically, and an 80% survival rate is reported for those with descending dissections treated medically.[13,15] Because dissection is known to recur, careful long-term management of blood pressure with oral drugs that reduce dP/dT (such as beta blockers) and noninvasive follow-up of aortic anatomy with echocardiography or CT scan are mandatory.

KEY FEATURES

Aortic dissection is a life-threatening condition that has a high mortality rate in its early stages.

Predisposing conditions include Marfan's syndrome, bicuspid or unicommissural aortic valve, pregnancy, recent aortic surgery or catheterization, and hypertension.

Dissection may involve the ascending and/or the descending aorta, and its location affects presentation, treatment, and prognosis.

The most common presentation is severe, migratory chest or back pain with pulse deficits. The finding of a new aortic insufficiency murmur with accompanying chest pain is highly suggestive of an ascending aorta dissection.

Initial diagnostic tests include chest film and ECG. Echocardiography provides an excellent screening test, and angiography, CT scan and MRI are highly diagnostic in this condition.

All patients should be stabilized initially with medication to lower the systemic blood pressure and shearing forces (dP/dT), which may extend the dissection. This usually includes intravenous sodium nitroprusside and propranolol.

Early surgical intervention is suggested for patients with acute or chronic dissection involving the ascending aorta. Medical treatment is preferred in dissection confined to the descending aorta, unless there is unremitting pain, hypertension, aneurysm expansion, or vascular compromise of a major organ.

Although appropriate therapy will lead to an in-hospital survival rate of up to 80% overall, post-discharge care must include tight blood pressure control, preferably with a beta blocker, and follow-up of aortic anatomy with noninvasive imaging techniques such as echocardiography or CT scanning.

REFERENCES

1. Hirst AE, Varner VJ, Hohns VJ Jr, Kime SW Jr: Dissecting aneurysm of the aorta: A review of 505 cases. Medicine (Baltimore) 37:217–279, 1959.
   An exhaustive review of prior studies providing good natural history data.

2. Larson EW, Edwards WD: Risk factors for aortic dissection: A necropsy study of 161 cases. Am J Cardiol 53:849–855, 1984.
   Examines the pathologic associations of aortic dissection in a large-scale retrospective study.

3. Roberts WC: Aortic dissection: Anatomy, consequences, and causes. Am Heart J 101:195–214, 1981.
   A good pictorial demonstration of the anatomy of aortic dissection, with a review of pathologic studies.

4. DeBakey ME, Henly WS, Cooley DA, et al: Surgical management of dissecting aneurysms of the aorta. J Thorac Cardiovasc Surg 49:130–149, 1965.
   The classic surgical article outlining the DeBakey classification and surgical protocol.

5. Hirst AE, Gore IG: The etiology and pathology of aortic dissection. In Doroghazi RM, Slater EE (eds): Aortic Dissection. New York, McGraw-Hill, 1983.
   A good description of pathology and possible risk factors for this condition.

6. Slater EE, DeSanctis RW: The clinical recognition of dissecting aortic aneurysm. Am J Med 60:625–633, 1976.
   An overview of the presenting signs and symptoms in 124 cases of aortic dissection.

7. Wheat MW Jr: Acute dissecting aneurysms of the aorta: Diagnosis and treatment—1979. Am Heart J 99:373–387, 1979.
   One of the major contributors to the literature describes the pathophysiologic approach of medical and surgical therapy.

8. Victor MF, Mintz GS, Kotler M, Wilson AR, Segal BL: Two dimensional echocardiograpic diagnosis of aortic dissection. Am J Cardiol 48:155–159, 1981.
   Documents the accuracy of two-dimensional echocardiography as compared with angiography and describes the typical ultrasound findings.

9. Takamofo S, Omoto R: Visualization of thoracic dissecting aortic aneurysm by transesophageal Doppler color flow mapping. Herz 12:187, 1987.

10. Smith DC, Jang GC: Radiological diagnosis of aortic dissection. In Doroghazi RM, Slater EE (eds): Aortic Dissection. New York, McGraw-Hill, 1983.
    An in-depth presentation of the angiographic findings in this condition, including many excellent illustrative studies.

11. Shuford WH, Sybers RG, Weens HS: Problems in the aortographic diagnosis of dissection aneurysm of the aorta. N Engl J Med 280:225–231, 1969.
12. Thorsen MK, San Dretto MA, Lawson TL, et al: Dissecting aortic aneurysms: Accuracy of computed tomographic diagnosis. Radiology 148:773–777, 1983.
    Documents the accuracy and utility of this technique and compares it with angiography and postmortem examination.
13. Dalen JE, Alpert JE, Cohn LH, Black H, Collins JJ: Dissection of the thoracic aorta: Medical or surgical therapy? Am J Cardiol 24:803–808, 1974.
    A 10-year review of cases at the Peter Bent Brigham Hospital comparing medical and surgical therapies and their benefit on dissections at different locations.
14. Miller DC, Stinson EB, Dyer PE, et al: Operative treatment of aortic dissections: Experience with 125 patients over a sixteen-year period. J Thorac Cardiovasc Surg 78:365–382, 1979.
    An evaluation of an aggressive, uniform surgical approach to aortic dissection, with the inclusion of long-term follow-up data. The authors diverge from standard practice in recommending surgery as the treatment of choice for acute descending aortic dissection.
15. Doroghazi RM, Slater EE, DeSanctis RW, et al: Long-term survival of patients with treated aortic dissection. J Am Coll Cardiol 3:1026–1034, 1984.
    A retrospective review and follow-up of 156 cases. This study relates presenting signs and symptoms to prognosis and compares the relative success of medical and surgical therapy.

Blunt Cardiac Trauma

Jonathan F. Plehn, M.D.

Blunt chest trauma is a common clinical problem in the emergency room setting. Whereas the diagnosis of pulmonary contusion is often easily made with a chest radiograph or lung scan, the reliable detection of cardiac trauma is not as secure. A review of the literature reveals a paucity of definitive data on this subject, and the development of multiple new cardiac imaging techniques has further confused the picture. This article attempts to set forth what little information is well established in this area.

The appropriate approach to the patient with blunt chest trauma is poorly defined. The primary question in the emergency room setting often regards the selection of patients for admission. Which physical findings or objective tests can help to pinpoint a patient who is likely to run into trouble if he is not monitored or treated? If the patient is admitted, what is his prognosis and what are his risks for undergoing the noncardiac surgery that victims of multiple trauma often require? What are the potential late sequelae of blunt cardiac trauma?

Until the work of Bright and Beck in 1934,[1] it appeared that blunt chest trauma with resultant myocardial contusion carried an extremely ominous prognosis. They found that of 168 cases previously described, 157 resulted in death. Realizing that only the most severe cases had probably been reported and that their own experience differed substantially from this picture, they developed a dog model for blunt chest trauma. They concluded that the heart could stand a great deal of blunt injury and that successful recuperation was the rule, not the exception. However, with the advent of the high-speed automobile and the rise in apparent drunken driver–related accidents, the incidence of steering wheel chest injuries has skyrocketed and it has become important to identify the relatively small percentage of patients at risk for serious sequelae.

PATHOLOGY

Blunt cardiac injuries have historically been divided into categories of concussion, laceration, and contusion. Concussion implies that the organ has been subjected to severe jarring but that no detectable damage is found on anatomic examination. Laceration indicates that there has been loss of organ integrity by tearing. Finally, contusion involves myocardial bruising. Blunt myocardial trauma may result in transmural, subepicardial, or subendocardial injury. Initially, there is extravasation of red blood cells into the areas between myocardial fibers with edema of the fibers themselves. With time, there is leukocytic infiltration and macrophage entry into the area. There may be fragmentation or necrosis of the muscle fibers during this period and eventual scar formation. Areas of transmural necrosis are subject to the same wall stresses that occur in myocardial infarction (MI), presenting the possibility of aneurysm formation and even myocardial rupture.[2]

Three situations may produce this pathology. The heart, lying between the sternum and the thoracic vertebral column, may swing against these structures at times of rapid acceleration or deceleration; a steering wheel injury illustrates the latter event and is the most common cause of blunt chest trauma. In addition, the heart may be pinned between the sternum and vertebral column in a crush injury. Finally, extreme increases in either intrathoracic or intra-abdominal pressure may lead to contusion.

Besides the myocardial effects of blunt heart trauma, the valvular structures and supporting structures (i.e., papillary muscles and chordae tendineae) may also be affected. Parmley's classic retrospective analysis of necropsy data from the Armed Forces Institute of Pathology found acute valvular incompetence to be uncommon, but when it did occur, it was most frequently found in the mitral and tricuspid positions.[3] On the other hand, rupture of a cardiac wall was not that uncommon, occurring in over half of the cases, with right ventricular rupture being the most common location. It should be recognized that Parmley's study included only the most severe cases of blunt chest trauma, those resulting in death, which as stated previously is an uncommon situation. Pericardial laceration and hemopericardium are also relatively common findings at autopsy. Interestingly enough, coronary artery rupture is rare and, despite earlier claims to the contrary, acute coronary thrombosis resulting directly from blunt chest trauma has rarely been documented.

Fortunately, the skeletal structures usually serve in more of a protective than a destructive capacity, as evidenced by the surprisingly small percentage of contusions or lacerations observed in the Parmley review. Examining the records of 546 autopsy cases of proven blunt cardiac injury, the authors could find only 105 cases of cardiac contusion or laceration. In the 67 patients who died immediately from trauma, only 12 deaths could be directly ascribed to cardiac injury. In a more recent study,[4] there were 15 deaths out of 100 patients presenting with significant blunt chest trauma; however, only 5 of these patients had evidence of cardiac trauma on necropsy examination. In none of these five could death be considered cardiac-related.

Although it appears that there is a low mortality rate resulting from blunt cardiac injury, it is well known that blunt chest trauma may result in fatal cardiac arrest as a result of ventricular arrhythmias without any obvious anatomic damage observed at autopsy. In addition, because today's emergency rooms are dealing with such a high volume of these injuries, it is important to identify the small percentage of patients requiring inpatient observation and treatment.

CLINICAL PRESENTATION

The description of the clinical presentation of blunt cardiac trauma varies tremendously in the literature. Some authors claim that victims often present with typical anginal pain, whereas others dispute this entirely.[5] The recent consensus favors the view that if chest pain is present, it is most often musculoskeletal in origin. Most patients appear relatively asymptomatic unless they have sustained rib fracture or some other associated form of musculoskeletal injury.

In rare instances, patients may present with new murmurs that are due to valvular incompetence or to a high-output state secondary to increased sympathetic drive. Acute congestive heart failure has been reported but is a very unusual presenting symptom. Of more concern is the state of the pericardium and great vessels. Cardiac tamponade can occur as a result of hemopericardium, ventricular rupture, aortic dissection, or transection. The patient should be checked for jugular venous distention, pulsus paradoxicus, distant heart sounds, or a large cardiac silhouette on chest film. The presence of unequal peripheral pulses suggests the diagnosis of aortic dissection.

After it is clear that the patient's vital signs are stable, it must be decided which further tests should be ordered. It is at this point where the confusion really begins, since a large variety of tests are available at most modern hospitals but there are very few studies demonstrating their utility in risk stratification.

DIAGNOSTIC STUDIES

Electrocardiography. Studies confirm that the electrocardiogram (ECG) is of extremely limited value in the diagnosis and prognosis of cardiac contusion.[4,6] The most common findings are nonspecific ST segment and T wave abnormalities. Because many of the patients in this population are young, early repolarization abnormalities that persist on sequential ECGs are frequently noted. Arrhythmias are common in the setting of blunt chest trauma and were seen in 73% of the subjects in Potkin's series of patients receiving Holter's monitoring within 12 hours of admission.[4] This particular investigation did not include isolated premature supraventricular beats but found that premature ventricular contractions were most common (seen in 70% of patients). Ventricular couplets were seen in 9%, and tachycardia was noted in only 3% of patients. Heart block is also commonly seen, but in the great majority of patients, there is right bundle or left bundle branch block (usually the former), which is transient. Atrioventricular nodal block is rare. Also uncommon is the development of a clear-cut myocardial injury pattern (horizontal ST segment elevation or depression) or new Q wave formation.

Chest Films. Although diagnostic of pulmonary contusion, this modality is of minimal value in searching for signs of cardiac trauma. Its only importance lies in its ability to suggest the presence of significant pericardial effusions.

Cardiac Enzymes. In the emergency room setting, only the measurement of total creatine kinase (CK) is generally possible at most hospitals. This parameter is nonspecific, since most patients have sustained significant skeletal muscle trauma, thus raising the total CK levels. Use of the CK-MB isoenzyme, which is more specific for cardiac muscle, would make more sense because if positive, it would seem very diagnostic of myocardial cell damage with subsequent enzyme extrusion. However, this test usually takes a long period of time to be performed and was not of any obvious prognostic value in two reports.[4,7] In Potkin's study of the five patients with autopsy proved myocardial contusion, only one had a significant elevation in the percentage of CK-MB.

Echocardiography. Two-dimensional echocardiography has the advantage of being extremely portable, rapidly performed, of no known risk to the patient, and relatively inexpensive. Most regions of the heart can be evaluated for myocardial form and function, valvular integrity, pericardial fluid, and aortic dissection. Doppler ultrasound can evaluate intracardiac blood flow and detect small amounts of valvular regurgitation. A study of myocardial contusion in a dog model demonstrated a high sensitivity, specificity, and predictive accuracy of this medium in a blind analysis.[8] Two small series have documented the utility of echocardiography in the clinical situation as well.[9,10]

Radionuclide Studies. Much has been written evaluating nuclear medicine studies in cases of blunt chest trauma. It is generally agreed that technetium-99m pyrophosphate scanning is neither sensitive nor specific in this area. In Potkin's series, only 2 patients out of 100 had positive scans and none of the five contusions diagnosed at autopsy was considered positive using this test.[4] Thallium-201 perfusion scanning seeking to document necrotic or edematous, unperfused areas of myocardium has been equally disappointing. There is some hope that either first-pass or equilibrium gated blood pool scanning will be useful in these patients. Sutherland and colleagues[11] documented a 55% incidence of focal wall motion abnormalities in patients suffering from multisystem trauma and severe blunt chest injury. Of patients demonstrating wall motion abnormalities, 64% were noted to have isolated right ventricular findings, 17% left ventricular, 17% combined, and 2% septal. Eighty-four per cent of these patients reverted back to normal wall motion over time, and only 3 patients of the 42 with wall motion defects died of cardiac causes. Although this technique holds some promise, it has not as yet been shown to be prognostic in terms of in-hospital complications or mortality.

TREATMENT

Thus, the accuracy of prospective diagnosis and prognosis of blunt cardiac trauma is unclear. In light of present knowledge, it is prudent to obtain a 12-lead ECG in the emergency room setting. If there is still some question about admitting the patient, a portable two-dimensional echocardiogram can rule out most significant forms of cardiac dysfunction. If after initial history, physical examination, ECG, and echocardiogram, there is enough concern to admit the patient, continuous telemetry should probably be instituted with bed rest for a 48-hour period. If premature ventricular contractions are noted to occur frequently or repetitively, the patient should be admitted to a coronary care unit setting and an intravenous antiarrhythmic such as lidocaine started.

During the initial period of the patient's hospitalization, cardiac isoenzymes may be measured and echocardiography, first-pass and/or gated equilibrium blood pool scans performed for further evaluation. The patient should be treated symptomatically in the meantime. If there are no further sequelae and all noninvasive imaging tests are normal, it is likely that the patient may be discharged and followed as an outpatient.

CONCLUSION

Because there is no gold standard with which to compare the various noninvasive methods of blunt cardiac trauma evaluation, it is unclear at present how we can facilitate our evaluation of this condition in the acute setting. In addition, most reported studies have failed to indicate the clinical prognostic value of any of these tests. Fortunately, the vast majority of patients sustaining blunt chest trauma do well without intervention. Nevertheless, it is probably wise to err on the side of caution in the evaluation and treatment of this condition until future, in-depth analysis of risk stratification with noninvasive testing is reported.

KEY FEATURES

Blunt chest trauma is a common occurrence and is most often caused by a deceleration event in the form of a steering wheel injury.

Most patients are relatively unaffected by blunt chest trauma and cardiac contusion is rare, owing to the protective effect of the surrounding rib cage.

The challenge facing the emergency room or primary care physician is the question of whom to admit to the hospital for closer monitoring and possibly treatment. The amount of internal injury may be disproportionate to that of external injury, and cardiac contusion, in rare instances, can have disastrous consequences.

The pathology of cardiac contusion includes the extravasation of red blood cells into areas between myocardial fibers, followed by leukocytic and macrophage infiltration. There may be areas of necrosis with eventual scar formation. Myocardial injury may be full-thickness, subendocardial, or subepicardial.

Besides cardiac contusion, valve rupture may occur, usually involving the mitral or tricuspid apparatuses. Myocardial rupture can occur, as well as pericardial laceration and aortic dissection. Blunt chest trauma may also cause cardiac arrest as a result of ventricular fibrillation. This may occur without the postmortem finding of structural cardiac damage.

Although electrocardiography provides the first line of diagnosis, it is insensitive and nonspecific. Common findings include nonspecific ST segment and T wave abnormalities, premature ventricular contractions, and transient right bundle branch and sometimes left bundle branch block.

Creatine kinase MB isoenzymes are difficult to obtain acutely and are not predictive of clinical course.

Two-dimensional echocardiography has been sensitive, specific, and predictive in a controlled laboratory study of blunt cardiac trauma but has not as yet been field-tested in a prospective manner. Doppler ultrasound has the potential to detect mild valvular imcompetence and may also be a worthwhile screening procedure.

Technetium-99m pyrophosphate (hot spot) scans and thallium-201 perfusion scans have been disappointing in this area. First-pass and equilibrium gated blood pool scans have diagnosed wall motion abnormalities in a high percentage of patients and should be considered in the early evaluation of blunt cardiac trauma. The right ventricle and anterior left ventricular walls are the most common areas affected.

Patients with some evidence of cardiac trauma should be monitored with telemetry initially and treated symptomatically. We prefer to observe these patients for at least 48 hours and obtain early follow-up in the post-discharge period.

The field of blunt cardiac trauma remains an ill-defined area that requires future investigation into early risk stratification, treatment, and long-term follow-up.

REFERENCES

1. Bright EF, Beck CS: Nonpenetrating wounds of the heart: A clinical and experimental study. Am Heart J *10*:293, 1934.
   An early pioneering work in this area, this monograph exhaustively reviews the earlier reports of blunt cardiac trauma and summarizes the author's experimental animal studies.

2. Symbas PN: Cardiac trauma. Am Heart J 92:387, 1976.
   This is a short and fairly superficial review of both penetrating and nonpenetrating trauma. Some of the author's suppositions are ill founded, based on earlier, poorly performed investigations.

3. Parmley LF, Manion WC, Mattingly TW: Nonpenetrating traumatic injury of the heart. Circulation *18*:371, 1958.
   In their analysis of 546 autopsy studies, the authors present a detailed account of the pathology of severe blunt cardiac trauma.

4. Potkin RT, Werner JA, Trobaugh GB, et al: Evaluation of noninvasive tests of cardiac damage in suspected cardiac contusion. Circulation 66:627, 1982.
   This is probably the best study available in this area. It analyzes the relative values of serial ECGs, Holter's monitoring, and CK-MB isoenzyme measurement in a prospective fashion. It is a good model for future studies evaluating other cardiac imaging techniques.

5. Harley DP, Mena I, Narahara KA, Miranda R, Nelson RJ: Traumatic myocardial dysfunction. J Thorac Cardiovasc Surg 87:386, 1984.
   The authors examined the use of electrocardiography, creatine kinase isoenzymes, and first-pass and equilibrium gated radionuclide angiography in evaluating this condition. The authors found evidence of segmental wall motion abnormalities in 74% of their patients but, unfortunately, did not correlate this with in-hospital or post-discharge outcome.

6. Pearce W, Blair E: Significance of the electrocardiogram in heart contusion due to blunt trauma. J Trauma 16:136, 1976.
   This study is useful only for its description of ECG abnormalities in the setting of blunt trauma. The ECG findings are compared with only a very rough clinical estimation of the severity of cardiac trauma.

7. Lindsey D, Navin TR, Finley PR: Transient elevation of serum activity of MB isoenzyme of creatine phosphokinase in drivers involved in automobile accidents. Chest 74:15, 1978.

This paper documents the insensitivity of the ECG but also claims the CK-MB iso-enzyme to be a good marker for cardiac contusion based on its frequent elevation in patients experiencing blunt chest trauma. Again, this test is not correlated with clinical outcome and its sensitivity is not based on a good reference standard of contusion (the latter obviously being very difficult to find).

8. Pandian NG, Skorton DJ, Doty DB, Kerber RE: Immediate diagnosis of acute myocardial contusion by two-dimensional echocardiography: Studies in a canine model of blunt chest trauma. JACC 2:488, 1983.

    The authors document the high sensitivity, specificity, and predictive value of two-dimensional echocardiography in a closed-chested dog model using controls. They list the echocardiographic findings of localized cardiac contusion that should be applicable to human studies.

9. Miller FA, Seward JB, Gersh BJ, Tajik AJ, Mucha P Jr: Two-dimensional echocardiographic findings in cardiac trauma. Am J Cardiol 50:1022, 1982.

    This is the only clinical report of the use of two-dimensional echocardiography in the literature. Unfortunately, it only reports findings in seven patients and does not attempt to analyze the predictive value of the test in clinical follow-up.

10. Reid CL, Kawanishi, DT, Rahimtoola SH, Chandraratma PAN: Chest trauma: Evaluation by two-dimensional echocardiography. Am Heart J 113:971, 1987.

    This echocardiography study evaluated 39 patients with blunt chest trauma.

11. Sutherland GR, Driedger AA, Holliday RL, Cheung HW, Sibbald WJ: Frequency of myocardial injury after blunt chest trauma as evaluated by radionuclide angiography. Am J Cardiol 52:1099, 1983.

    This study documents the surprisingly common finding of segmental wall motion abnormalities as detected by radionuclide angiography. The authors reported a 55% incidence of segmental abnormalities in a group of 77 victims of multisystem trauma including blunt chest trauma. In most cases (84%), the findings were transient.

Shock

James R. Wilentz, M.D.
James J. Heffernan, M.D.

The management of shock remains a challenge in the acute care setting, demanding rapid diagnosis and prompt institution of therapy. The patho-physiologic endpoint of the various shock states is inadequate perfusion of critical organs leading to widespread ischemia and cellular damage. The clinical hallmarks are hypotension with systolic arterial pressure <90 mmHg or significantly below a hypertensive patient's norm; and evidence of hy-poperfusion manifested especially in abnormal mental status and skin changes, oliguria, and lactic acidosis.[1] Early recognition and treatment are of the utmost importance, since the mortality rate rises rapidly with duration and irreversible shock may develop as a result of a loss of capillary integrity and irremediable end-organ damage.[1,5,10,11]

CLASSIFICATION

Cardiogenic Shock. Cardiogenic shock is hypoperfusion with or without hypotension as a result of primary failure of cardiac output.[2] This is most commonly due to acute myocardial infarction (MI), occurring in 10–15% of such patients, and carries a mortality rate of 75–90%. Cardiogenic shock in the setting of acute MI generally represents the loss of >40% of left ventricular muscle, acute ventricular septal or free-wall rupture, acute mitral regurgitation, or large saccular aneurysm formation. An important group of patients with a significantly better prognosis are those with right ventricular infarction whose RV failure results in low LV filling pressures as the cause of low cardiac output, which can be easily reversed with volume infusion and increase of venous return.[4] Less common causes of cardiogenic shock are outflow and inflow tract obstructions, as in aortic stenosis, idiopathic hypertrophic subaortic stenosis, mitral stenosis, and rarely atrial myxoma; other tumors and thrombus; acute aortic or mitral regurgitation as a result of endocarditis or disintegration of abnormal collagen; decompensated chronic cardiomyopathy; and prolonged arrhythmia only if the rate is outside that required to generate an adequate output or (uncommonly, in noncompliant hearts) as a result of loss of atrioventricular synchrony. The hemodynamic profile shows (1) elevated PCWP >18 mmHg (or elevated CVP with normal PCWP in RV infarct), (2) decreased CI <2 L/min/M², and (3) elevated SVR ≥2000 dyne-sec/cm⁵.

Maldistributive Shock. Maldistributive shock is defined as hypoperfusion-hypotension that is due to abnormal vascular volume distribution with preserved cardiac function. Causes include *sepsis* with gram-negative bacilli, staphylococci (includes toxic shock syndrome), pneumococci, Neisseria, and others; *endocrinopathies* such as diabetic ketoacidosis, hyperosmolar coma, adrenal crisis, diabetes insipidus, myxedema, and hypoglycemia; *CNS lesions*, especially with intracranial hypertension: *anaphylaxis*; and *microcirculatory sludging*, as in polycythemia vera, hyperviscosity states, and sickle cell crisis. The hemodynamic profile shows (1) normal or *low* PCWP ≤10 mmHg (in absence of coexisting LV dysfunction) and CVP <5 mmHg; (2) elevated or normal CI ≥2 and often >5 L/min/M²; (3) low SVR <950 dyne-sec/cm⁵; (4) in late stages, cardiac failure may supervene, leading to a low CI with elevated SVR and PCWP.

Hypovolemic Shock. Hypovolemic shock is hypoperfusion-hypotension as a result of critical loss of blood volume (either whole blood or plasma filtrate). This is most commonly due to hemorrhage, with loss of either 30% of venous or less of arterial blood producing shock. Other causes include states of plasma or fluid-electrolyte loss such as burns and skin trauma, pancreatitis, ascites, pheochromocytoma, massive vomiting with or without diarrhea, heat, diabetes mellitus or insipidus, salt-losing nephropathy, adrenal insufficiency, and diuretic abuse. The hemodynamic profile shows (1) low PCWP ≤10 mmHg (in absence of coexisting LV dysfunction) and CVP <5 mmHg; (2) usually normal CI ≥2 L/min/M²; and (3) elevated SVR ≥1600 dyne-sec/cm⁵.

Obstructive Shock. This form of shock is defined as hypoperfusion-hypotension that is due to failure of effective cardiac output from factors extrinsic to heart muscle or valves. Causes include (1) pericardial tamponade, with equalized elevated diastolic pressures in all cardiac chambers impeding filling, i.e., PCWP, CVP >10–15 mmHg, PCWP minus CVP <5 mmHg and PA, RV systolic pressues <40 mmHg; (2) pulmonary embolus, with elevated RV diastolic and CVP >10–15 mmHg, normal or low PCWP ≤10 mmHg and PA, RV systolic pressures ≥40 mmHg; and (3) pulmonary hypertension with elevated PA/RV systolic pressure ≥60 mmHg, elevated CVP >10–15 mmHg, and low or normal PCWP ≤10 mmHg. Pulmonary embolus and hypertension cause LV failure by obstructing RV output, thereby impeding LV filling. All these states show a low CI ≤2 L/min/M² and an elevated SVR ≥1600 dyne-sec/cm⁵.

PATHOPHYSIOLOGY

Shock of any type results in inadequate tissue perfusion. Compensatory mechanisms initially serve to maintain core organ perfusion, but ultimately lead to worsening total body ischemia. Elevated sympathetic tone and catecholamine release cause arteriolar and venular constriction, shunting cardiac output from skeletal muscle to core, at the cost of tissue necrosis and acidosis. Renal ischemia causes elevated renin-angiotensin-aldosterone production, at first supporting volume and blood pressure, but then leading to further arteriolar constriction. Splanchnic ischemia shunts blood to heart and brain but causes mucosal damage, with fluid loss and entry of toxins from the gastrointestinal tract.

As acidosis and poor perfusion persist, arteriolar tone fades and the gradient for transcapillary leak increases, generating further intravascular fluid loss and interstitial edema. End-organ damage then ensues.

Shock Lung. Shock lung, a form of the adult respiratory distress syndrome, may occur either while perfusion is still jeopardized or after its return—generally 24–48 hours after the onset of shock. This syndrome results from transcapillary leakage and interstitial and alveolar edema as a result of endothelial ischemic injury, septic and other toxins, and complement and platelet-leukocyte activation. It is exacerbated by a low plasma oncotic pressure and a high PCWP. Shock lung is characterized by low pressure (except in cardiogenic shock) pulmonary edema, decreased lung compliance (with high-peak inspiratory pressures if mechanically ventilated), and intrapulmonary shunting with ventilation-perfusion mismatches leading to hypoxemia and a significant A-a gradient.

Kidney. Prerenal azotemia, with intense sodium retention and a low urine sodium concentration (in the absence of diuretic therapy), progresses to acute renal tubular necrosis with isosthenuria and muddy brown casts.

Heart. Profound acidosis of any cause is a significant myocardial depressant that may play a role even early in noncardiogenic shock. In late stages of shock, a myocardial depressant factor (MDF) may be liberated into the circulation as a result of pancreatic ischemia, leading to profound heart failure.

Blood. Disruption of endothelium may lead to disseminated intravascular coagulation with microthrombosis and widespread tissue destruction.

CLINICAL FEATURES

History. The history is often unobtainable from the patient; nonetheless, a determined search among family and friends may point to the cause of shock and its duration.

Physical Examination. Examination of the patient may be very helpful in determining the type of shock. *General appearance*: agitation, confusion, prostration, hypotension. *Skin*: altered temperature (cold and clammy—cardiogenic; warm—early septic), profound pallor, cyanosis if a significant A-a gradient has already developed, purpura if disseminated intravascular coagulation supervenes. *Lungs*: tachypnea; rales in cardiogenic shock or if adult respiratory distress syndrome (ARDS) has occurred or if pneumonia is the source of sepsis. *Heart*: tachycardia; S_3 gallop if cardiogenic, other specific findings referable to valvular disease, etc., are found. *Abdomen*: the liver may be enlarged if CHF is chronic; ascites may be a clue to fluid loss and a septic site. *Extremities*: thready peripheral pulses.

Laboratory. Blood count may show leukocytosis with immature forms. The hematocrit may be normal if less than a few hours have passed after acute blood loss. Chemistries may show metabolic acidosis, respiratory alkalosis, and respiratory acidosis with hypoxia if ARDS occurs. Lactate levels are elevated, and the level may correlate with prognosis. Cardiac enzymes and ECG may show evidence of infarction. BUN, creatinine, and urinary sodium may aid in assessment of hydration and glomerulotubular function. A guaiac test of stool or gastric aspirate may show the source of blood loss. Coagulation tests and blood smear may show evidence of disseminated intravascular coagulation.

TREATMENT

Monitoring. After recognition of shock and acute stabilizing measures, prompt institution of dependable monitoring is essential for further treatment.[1-3,10,11] A radial (or femoral) *arterial catheter* should be inserted to allow continuous arterial pressure monitoring and assessment of arterial blood gases. A *pulmonary arterial catheter* or CVP line should be inserted. In patients with clear-cut absence of left ventricular dysfunction and pulmonary disease, the CVP may well reflect left-sided filling pressure; however, if either is present or if management of shock requires complex adjustments of hemodynamics, a more direct assessment of LV filling with a pulmonary capillary wedge tracing is mandatory. The PA catheter should be inserted only by personnel trained in and comfortable with the procedure and the interpretation of the data obtained. The flow-directed, balloon-tipped thermodilution catheter can be inserted at the bedside through the internal jugular, subclavian, or median antecubital vein and allows measurement of PCWP, as well as PA, RV, and RA (central venous) pressures, calculation of cardiac output and peripheral resistance, and direct measurement of core body temperature. Risk of PA catheter placement is increased in bacteremia, coagulopathy, and pulmonary hypertension. Technical considerations include the following:

1. *Site*: An internal jugular or antecubital approach in a ventilated patient carries a lower risk of pneumothorax; subclavian placement is the most stable site and most easily protected against respiratory equipment and secretions.

2. *Lung zone*: To reflect the LV diastolic pressure properly, the catheter tip must be in a position where a continuous open conduit of blood exists between the tip and the LV. This exists in lung zone 3, where both arterial and venous pressures are higher than intrapulmonary pressure. In shock with low pulmonary venous pressure, especially with PEEP above 10 cm H_2O, this may not be the case and the tracing will not show the normal PCW waveform. In ventilated patients, the PCWP should be taken in end-expiration to minimize this effect. Pulmonary veno-occlusive disease and mitral stenosis will also introduce a gradient between the PCWP and the LV diastolic pressure.

A urinary catheter should be placed to allow assessment of renal function and fluid therapy.

Volume Manipulation. If the patient is not in clear-cut cardiogenic shock, place him or her in a supine position and rapidly infuse 300–500 ml crystalloid. In hemorrhage, the fluid of choice is obviously *blood*. A controversy has raged regarding the merits of *crystalloid* and *colloid* replacement fluids. Although theoretical considerations suggest that maintenance of plasma colloid oncotic pressure should decrease the tendency for transcapillary leak, recent work shows this to be of little importance, at least in the pulmonary circulation. Available crystalloids include *lactated Ringer's,* which may help maintain alkalinity when hepatic function is intact; and *normal saline.* Available colloids include *salt poor albumin,* with a short half-life in the intravascular space; *dextran,* with an incidence (though low) of anaphylaxis and interference with clotting and blood grouping, and *hydroxyethyl starch,* which is a polysaccharide with less effect on coagulation and less chance of anaphylaxis; (one third may remain in the intravascular space at 24 hours). In cardiogenic shock with pulmonary edema, *furosemide* may be used to decrease LV filling pressure in conjunction with measures to increase cardiac output.

Correction of Acidosis and Hypoxia. This is essential to the maintenance of cardiac function in all forms of shock. *Sodium bicarbonate* may be given in intravenous boluses and by infusion if necessary to maintain pH at 7.1 acutely and at 7.3 over time. (This may also be an adjunct to volume therapy, since each 50 ml bolus contains 44.5 mEq sodium.) Intubation and mechanical ventilation may be required to maintain the PaO_2 $\geqslant 80$ mmHg. PEEP may also minimize transudation of fluid into the alveoli.

Correction of Disseminated Intravascular Coagulation. Disseminated intravascular coagulation with prominent arterial thrombosis requires prompt heparin treatment.

Cardiac Output and Peripheral Resistance. Manipulation of cardiac output and peripheral resistance must be tailored to the specific hemodynamics. An increase in cardiac output must be weighed against the increase in myocardial oxygen consumption.

Sympathomimetic Agents

1. *Dopamine* is an endogenous catecholamine with beta, alpha, and specific dopaminergic effects. At dosages of $\leqslant 5$ μg/kg/min, it has a dilating effect on both the renal and mesenteric circulations with minimal effect on cardiac output; at dosages of 5–8 μg/kg/min, a beta-1 effect linearly increases cardiac output without an increase in SVR and maintains the renal and mesenteric sparing effect; at dosages >8 μg/kg/min, there is a continued increase in cardiac inotropy, but this is offset by the increasing alpha effect, elevating the SVR. This last phenomenon becomes predominant at doses >20 μg/kg/min. At high doses, dopamine has a significant tachycardic and arrhythmogenic effect.
2. *Dobutamine* is a synthetic catecholamine with primarily beta-1 and minimal alpha action; in doses of 2.5–10 μg/kg/min, it increases cardiac output linearly, with decreases in SVR and PCWP and minimal effect on heart rate and renal and hepatic blood flow.
3. *Isoproterenol* in doses of 0.5–4 μg/min is a pure beta agonist with

peripheral and coronary vasodilating effects as well as cardiac inotropism and chronotropism. Tachycardia and/or dysrhythmias are commonly induced and limit isoproterenol's usefulness. It is relatively strongly contraindicated in coronary disease because of its marked increase in myocardial oxygen consumption.

4. *Norepinephrine* is an endogenous catecholamine with primarily alpha and less beta effect in doses of 2–8 μg/min. It is useful to support core blood pressure by increasing SVR; however, high doses are associated with marked increments in SVR and loss of renal, mesenteric, skeletal muscle, and skin perfusion as well as a severe afterload increase that may further compromise cardiac function. It has little effect on heart rate.

5. *Phenylephrine* is a synthetic pure alpha stimulator. Doses of 5–20 μg/min are useful to support blood pressure in patients with a low SVR, but it has the same disadvantages as norepinephrine.

Vasodilators

These agents may be useful in increasing cardiac output in cardiogenic shock, but they are not of proven efficacy in other shock states.

1. *Nitroprusside* is a primary arteriolar, and, to a lesser extent, alpha venular dilator that decreases SVR and afterload, with generally less effect on preload. Doses utilize range from 10 to 500 μg/min. Cyanide toxicity may develop in the setting of renal failure. The drug may have a coronary steal effect and may reflexly increase heart rate and thereby myocardial oxygen consumption.

2. *Nitroglycerin* is primarily a venodilator with limited arteriolar dilating effect except in the coronary circulation. In doses of 10–500 μg/min, it may be extremely helpful in treating ongoing ischemia during cardiogenic shock.

Mechanical Assistance. Intra-aortic balloon counterpulsation (IABP) may result in salvage of 5–10% of patients who would otherwise have died in cardiogenic shock when used in patients who will go on to definitive therapy of ischemia (see later discussion). The military anti-shock trousers (MAST suit) bind the legs and abdomen, causing rapid influx of pooled venous blood to the central circulation (an easily reversible fluid challenge), and increase the portion of cardiac output perfusing core organs in shock and during CPR. Although it is still considered experimental, it is potentially extremely useful in treating hypovolemic and maldistributive shock. It is contraindicated in head trauma or intracranial disease and in cardiogenic shock.

Corticosteroids. Corticosteroids have been used in all forms of shock; however, they have now been shown definitively to be of *no* benefit in reversing shock or prolonging life and should not be used in patients with shock other than when adrenal insufficiency is suspected.[6,7]

Naloxone and Other Agents. Naloxone is a pure opiate antagonist that has been shown to reverse endotoxic, hemorrhagic, and spinal shock in animals presumably by displacing endogenous opioids (endorphins) released in these states. There is no convincing evidence of benefit from naloxone in human shock states, after some initial interest,[8,9] but its use is routine when narcotic overdose is a consideration. Prostaglandin inhibitors, vasodilating prostaglandins, protease inhibitors, angiotensin inhibitors and antagonists, antihistamines, and endotoxin antibodies have shown some promise of efficacy in various shock states.

Specific Strategies. Specific strategies must be developed for specific states of shock. In *cardiogenic shock,* one directs initial therapy at restoring cardiac output and reversing pulmonary edema while preparing definitive therapy. Certain *pressor-vasodilator combinations* may be particularly useful—this therapy has been nicknamed the "medical balloon" because of its increase in cardiac output and decrease in afterload. One scheme is to use dopamine only in renal sparing doses, add dobutamine if a further increase in cardiac output is needed, add nitroprusside if SVR remains elevated (maintaining systolic arterial pressure >80–90 mmHg), and add nitroglycerin or furosemide if PCWP is still elevated. Once a decision is made for aggressive definitive therapy, the IABP should be inserted early (in patients with appropriate arterial anatomy) to stabilize the situation. Definitive therapy for cardiogenic shock is dictated by the causative lesion. *Myocardial revascularization* by thrombolysis with or without percutaneous transluminal coronary angioplasty (PTCA) has been used successfully to reverse shock in acute infarction, as has coronary bypass surgery. A surgical approach may be necessary to correct mechanical defects in acute infarction such as septal or free-wall rupture, aneurysm formation, and mitral regurgitation; or to correct non–infarct-related lesions such as acute aortic or mitral valvular regurgitation or critical aortic stenosis. It should be remembered that cardiogenic shock in the setting of end-stage cardiomyopathy has a grim prognosis with little to be gained from IABP placement except in patients carefully selected for transplantation or mechanical implants.

In *hemorrhagic-maldistributive* shock, rapid aggressive volume replacement is required along with early use of antibiotics and perhaps methylprednisolone in sepsis. One must bear in mind that at least in the early stage, the lesion is *not* a failure of cardiac output. In "warm" shock with a low SVR, an *active agent* such as norepinephrine may be appropriate in doses required to maintain systolic arterial pressure ≥90 mmHg. The dose of dopamine required to accomplish this may well be above that with a renal and mesenteric dilating effect and may cause unacceptable tachycardia and arrhythmia.

KEY FEATURES

All shock states are characterized by relative or absolute hypotension and signs of tissue hypoperfusion.

1. *Cardiogenic shock*: Results from primary failure of cardiac output, usually in the setting of acute myocardial infarction. Treatment of shock with RV infarction is different and prognosis is better than is the case with LV infarction.
2. *Maldistributive shock*: Abnormal vascular volume distribution with or without preserved cardiac function, most commonly seen in sepsis.
3. *Hypovolemic shock*: Results from hemorrhage or loss of fluid/electrolytes (e.g., with massive vomiting).
4. *Obstructive shock*: Failure of effective cardiac output resulting from extracardiac factors. Major subsets include pulmonary embolism, pulmonary hypertension, and pericardial tamponade.

Hemodynamic profile of shock subtypes:

	PCWP (mmHg)	CVP (mmHg)	PAP syst (mmHg)	CI L/min/M²	SVR (dyne-sec/cm⁵)
Cardiogenic	>18	↑ →	↑ →	<2	≥2000
RV infarct		↑ ↑	↓	<2	≥2000
Maldistributive	≤10	<5		≥2	<950
Hypovolemic	≤10	<5		≥2	≥1600
Obstructive					
Tamponade	>10–15	>10–15	<40	<2	≥1600
Pulmonary embolus	≤10	>10–15	>40	<2	≥1600
Pulmonary hypertension	≤10	>10–15	>60	<2	≥1600

Persistent tissue hypoperfusion results in lactic acidosis, ischemic damage, vascular leak, activation and release of toxic mediators, further volume loss, multi-organ damage, and, ultimately, irreversible shock; late stages of various shock subtypes are often indistinguishable.

Salient clinical features include altered mental status (agitation, confusion, obtundation); cutaneous pallor or cyanosis, occasionally purpura, and in early septic shock, warm flushing; tachypnea and hyperventilation with rales in cardiogenic shock or when ARDS supervenes; an S_3 gallop in cardiogenic shock; protean other cardiac findings related to etiology—increased A_2–P_2 split and RV heave and prominent P_2 with pulmonary embolus; diminished heart sounds and/or pericardial rub preceding tamponade, pansystolic murmur with septal or papillary rupture, etc.

Abnormalities in routine laboratory screen vary with causes.

Prompt recognition and rapid institution of stabilizing measures are essential.

Central hemodynamic monitoring is indicated unless hypovolemic shock is the obvious cause and responds promptly to volume resuscitation.

Early management requires volume manipulation (the cornerstone in hypovolemic states), correction of acidemia and hypoxemia, and pharmacologic cardiovascular support with inotropic agents and vasopressors (primarily sympathomimetic infusions) and unloading agents.

Adjunctive treatment may be indicated with mechanical assistance devices—

military anti-shock trousers in hypovolemic situations and intra-aortic balloon counterpulsation in instances of cardiogenic shock in which a remediable underlying lesion is suspected.

Ultimate survival depends on both the aggressive management of the shock state and the rapid identification and treatment of the underlying cause.

REFERENCES

1. Shine KI (moderator): Aspects of the management of shock. Ann Intern Med 93:723, 1980.
    Edited transcription of a conference sponsored by the UCLA School of Medicine. Literature-based discussion focusing primarily on specific interventions for the management of various shock states.

2. Resnekov L: Cardiogenic shock. Chest 83:893, 1983.
    Review of the definition, pathophysiology, diagnosis, and management of cardiogenic shock.

3. Rude RE: Pharmacologic support in cardiogenic shock. Adv Shock Res 10:35, 1983.

4. Cama-Canella I, Lopez-Sendon J, Gamallo C: Low output syndrome in right ventricular infarction. Am Heart J 98:614, 1979.
    Representative series describing the clinical and hemodynamic features of ten patients with right ventricular infarction and low output syndrome. Stresses the finding of disproportionately increased right atrial pressure in relation to left ventricular filling pressure. Right atrial pulse tracings were noted to be similar to those seen in constrictive pericarditis. Mortality rate of 40% was felt in part to reflect concurrent left ventricular damage.

5. Parker MM, Parillo JE: Septic shock: Hemodynamics and pathogenesis. JAMA 250:3324, 1983.

6. Bone RC, Fisher CJ, Clemmer TP, Slotman GJ, Metz CA, Balk RA, and the Methylprednisolone Severe Sepsis Study Group: A controlled clinical trial of high-dose methylprednisolone in the treatment of severe sepsis and septic shock. N Engl J Med 317:653, 1987.

7. The Veterans Administration Systemic Sepsis Cooperative Study Group: Effect of high-dose glucocorticoid therapy on mortality in patients with clinical signs of systemic sepsis. N Engl J Med 317:659, 1987.
    Pair of large, multicenter, randomized, double-blind, placebo-controlled clinical trials of high-dose methylprednisolone in severe sepsis and septic shock that definitively demonstrated no benefit from glucocorticoid administration in prevention or reversal of shock or in mortality at 14 days. Patients treated with methylprednisolone died more often from infection, and a subset of patients with azotemia at enrollment demonstrated a significantly higher mortality rate at 14 days.

8. Peters WP, Johnson MW, Friedman PA, Mitch WE: Pressor effect of naloxone in septic shock. Lancet 1:529, 1981.
    Uncontrolled trial suggesting a pressor response to naloxone in patients with septic shock not receiving corticosteroids.

9. DeMaria A, Craven DE, Heffernan JJ, McIntosh TK, Grindlinger GA, McCabe WR: Naloxone versus placebo in treatment of septic shock. Lancet 1:1363, 1985.
    Prospective, randomized, double-blind, placebo-controlled trial of naloxone at standard dosage as adjunctive therapy in the treatment of septic shock. No significant difference

was noted in mean systolic blood pressure rise between naloxone- and placebo-treated groups. Overall survival rates at 48 hours and 7 days were similar.

10. Billhardt RA, Rosenbush SW: Cardiogenic and hypovolemic shock. Med Clin N Amer 70:853, 1986.
    General review of pathophysiology and management.

11. Karakusis PH: Considerations in the therapy of septic shock. Med Clin N Amer 70:933, 1986.
    General review.

Syncope/Transient Loss of Consciousness

James J. Heffernan, M.D.

Transient loss of consciousness not clearly related to a known overriding medical condition such as major trauma, shock, drug overdose, or acute cardiac disease is a common clinical entity, accounting for 3% of visits to a major urban emergency room in one series.[7] The causes of brief loss of consciousness are legion. Incidence rates of specific phenomena very widely as a function of the clinical setting and the population studied, although most causes fall under a limited number of headings. Plum has estimated incidence rates for these major groups (Table 1).[1]

The evaluation and management of patients with known or presumed seizure disorder, sudden death, or dysrhythmia are discussed elsewhere in this text. This article is directed toward evaluation of the patient with transient loss of consciousness on an unknown basis, with a specific focus on syncope.

TABLE 1.   PRINCIPAL CAUSES AND APPROXIMATE FREQUENCIES OF BRIEF LOSS OF CONSCIOUSNESS

Syncope	
Vasovagal/psychophysiologic	55%
Cardiovascular	10%
Central nervous system	
First seizure	10%
Other	5%
Drug-metabolic	5%
Undiagnosed, including hysteria	15%

From Plum F: Brief loss of consciousness. *In* Wyngaarden JB, Smith LH Jr (eds): Cecil Textbook of Medicine, 17th ed. Philadelphia, WB Saunders Co, 1985, p 1983.

PATHOPHYSIOLOGY

Syncope is defined physiologically as transient loss of consciousness associated with unresponsiveness and inability to maintain postural muscle tone as a result of cerebral hypoperfusion. In most studies of syncope, the operational definition is that of an episode of transient loss of consciousness and postural tone not clearly attributable to seizure, vertigo, dizziness, coma, shock, or other states of altered consciousness.[4,5] Use of the term syncope implies spontaneous recovery, not requiring specific resuscitative measures.[2,6] The specific causes of transient loss of consciousness/syncope are legion; those cited most often include vasodepressor episodes precipitated by psychoemotional stress or pain, cardiovascular reflex mechanisms triggered by physiologic events (e.g., cough, micturition, or defecation syncope), orthostatic hypotension, tachydysrhythmias, cardiac conduction disturbances and bradydysrhythmias, valvular aortic stenosis, hypertrophic cardiomyopathy, mitral valve prolapse, pulmonary hypertension, pulmonary embolism, anaphylaxis, drug reactions, subclavian steal syndrome, carotid sinus hypersensitivity, migraine headache, transient ischemic attack, and psychiatric disorders, especially conversion reactions. In up to 50% of instances, a cause is not established despite careful evaluation.[3–5,7,8] One in four patients is admitted to a hospital on initial presentation after transient loss of consciousness, and half of such admissions are to intensive care units.[4,8] An association between vasodepressor syncope and sudden death exists, substantiated by both epidemiologic and physiologic data.[2]

Clinical reviews of brief loss of consciousness/syncope are not strictly comparable, having been conducted on different patient populations in different settings: emergency room patients;[7] medical inpatients;[3] medical intensive care unit patients;[8] and combined medical inpatients and outpatients.[4,13] Nonetheless, despite differences in study design, a number of findings have recurred consistently.

DIAGNOSIS

In all reviews cited, the history and physical examination have formed the cornerstone of diagnosis. Vasodepressor/psychogenic episodes and seizures account for up to 70% of presentations to an emergency room after transient loss of consciousness. In such a setting, the history and physical examination provide the most important diagnostic information in 85% of patients in whom a diagnosis can be established.[7] In a large prospective study of inpatients and outpatients with syncope, history and physical examination yielded the diagnosis in 49% of those instances in which a diagnosis was ultimately made and a simple 12-lead electrocardiogram (ECG) brought the diagnostic yield to 60%.[5] Of 108 patients with syncope admitted to an intensive care unit, the admission history, physical examination, chest radiograph, routine blood tests, and ECG formed the basis for diagnosis in 72% of instances in which a diagnosis was achieved by any means.[8] In general, routine blood tests have been helpful, if at all, in confirming abnormalities already suspected.[4,5,7]

A variety of more extensive diagnostic procedures have been broadly applied to the evaluation of brief loss of consciousness/syncope. Most of these have shown no independent clinical utility, e.g., skull roentgenograms, lumbar puncture, and radionuclide brain scan. Head computed tomograms have revealed significant lesions in patients with focal neurologic findings, but these lesions have rarely borne any identifiable relationship to the syncopal episode that prompted the study. Electroencephalograms have been performed in as many as half of the patients in the various series and are nonspecifically abnormal in a number of cases but contribute independently to the diagnosis of a cause of syncope only rarely, with confirmation of a seizure disorder in less than 5% of instances.[3,4,7,8]

Prolonged electrocardiographic monitoring, either in an intensive care unit or on a 24-hour Holter monitor tracing, has proved useful in most clinical reviews. One in six such tests performed has demonstrated a cause of syncope and this has accounted for up to 27% of diagnoses made,[3,4,7,8,13] although most patients do not have syncope during monitoring and most symptomatic patient show no rhythm disturbance during symptomatic episodes.[5] Frequent or repetitive premature ventricular complexes (PVCs) and sinus pauses are associated independently with overall mortality and sudden death.[13]

Electrophysiologic study has shown some utility in selected populations; the cause of syncope has generally been identified in 10–36% of such tests performed.[3,4,12] In one report of a highly selected population of 25 patients with recurrent syncope, many with known underlying cardiac disease and/ or ECG abnormalities, a putative cause was found in 68%.[9] The diagnosis of the cause of syncope identified by electrophysiologic study usually rests on the demonstration of inducible sustained ventricular tachycardia/fibrillation with programmed extrasystoles, significant H-V interval prolongation, sinus pauses after pacemaker-induced tachycardia and inducible supraventricular arrhythmias.

Cardiac catheterization, pulmonary angiography, and cerebral angiography have all yielded the cause of syncope in highly selected populations at rates of up to one in four tests performed, although these tests combined contribute less than 10% to the total pool of diagnoses made.[3,4] In light of the high cost and relatively low yield of most of the aforementioned diagnostic procedures, it is not surprising that one group estimated a cost of $23,000 per definitive diagnosis among inpatients admitted for syncope in 1982.[3]

TREATMENT

Syncope may be a marker of life-threatening illness or a benign and self-limited event. The prevention of future episodes obviously depends on the identified cause. With drug-induced syncope, the offending agent should be withdrawn.[11] An appropriate antidysrhythmic can be instituted in situations in which a tachydysrhythmia is clearly implicated; electrophysiologic study or ambulatory electrocardiographic monitoring can be utilized to corroborate efficacy. Serious conduction system disturbances may necessitate pacemaker insertion. Cardiac surgery to correct vascular, valvular, or muscular abnormalities plays a role in a small number of cases, as occasionally does cerebrovascular surgery or systemic anticoagulation. Carotid sinus hypersensitivity may respond to avoidance of precipitating circumstances, to vagolytic medications, to neck surgery (as for a compressing mass lesion), or to a pacemaker, although vasodepressor responses are not always corrected by such interventions.[10] Anticonvulsant therapy is obviously indicated when a seizure disorder is identified as the cause. In 15–50% of cases of syncope, no cause is identified and in the largest single group with an identified cause, i.e., vasodepressor syncope, no specific treatment is indicated.

PROGNOSIS

The prognosis of those under 30 years of age presenting to an emergency room after a syncopal episode is excellent. The prognosis for those between 30 and 70 years of age with a diagnosis of a vasodepressor/psychogenic or unknown cause as the basis for loss of consciousness is also excellent.[7] Identification of a cardiovascular basis for syncope is of prognostic importance, suggesting a substantial 1 year mortality and morbidity rate.[4,7,8] Identification of a noncardiovascular basis for syncope is associated with an intermediate but much lower risk, whereas failure to identify a cause of syncope carries only the risk of co-morbid disease.

KEY FEATURES

Vasodepressor syncope is the most common cause of transient loss of consciousness in nearly all clinical populations studied.

Patients with seizures may account for up to 29% of individuals presenting to an emergency room after transient less of consciousness.

Patients with serious cardiac problems are more heavily represented among hospitalized patients or those with recurrent episodes of transient loss of consciousness.

In 15–50% of instances, no cause is identified.

Clinical history and physical examination are sufficient to identify the cause in 49–85% of cases for which an cause is identified by any means; ECG improves the yield by up to 12%.

Ambulatory ECG monitoring should be considered in any instance in which the cause is not immediately apparent.

Other intensive diagnostic procedures should be limited to selected populations.

Identification of a cardiovascular cause of syncope has been associated with a 1 year mortality rate of 19–30%.

Prognosis is excellent in general for those under 30 years of age, or in those 30–70 years old with vasodepressor/psychogenic syncope or no identified cause.

Treatment is predicated on the identified cause, if any.

REFERENCES

1. Plum F: Brief loss of consciousness. *In* Wyngaarden JB, Smith LH Jr, eds: Cecil Textbook of Medicine. 17th ed. Philadelphia, WB Saunders, 1985, pp 1983–1986.
    Comprehensive and well-organized discussion of the topic of brief loss of consciousness with special emphasis on the various forms of syncope. Pragmatic and clinically useful approach. (See also Plum F, Posner JB: Disturbances of consciousness and arousal in the 18th edition of the Cecil Textbook of Medicine.)

2. Engel GL: Psychologic stress, vasodepressor (vasovagal) syncope and sudden death. Ann Intern Med 89:403, 1978.
    Well-reasoned and heavily referenced discussion of the association between vasodepressor syncope and sudden death with, more fundamentally, an attempt to establish the relationship of psychologic and physiologic factors underlying both entities. Stresses the importance of uncertainty in settings of stress, and actual or threatened injury predisposing to autonomic liability with conflicting activity of "fight-flight" and "conservation-with-drawal" mechanisms.

3. Kapoor WN, Karpf M, Maher Y, Miller RA, Levey GS: Syncope of unknown origin. JAMA 247:2687, 1982.
    Retrospective review of features of the work-up of syncope in an inpatient population of 121 patients of mean age 63.1 years. Extensive diagnostic studies identified a definitive cause of syncope in only 13 patients: ECG monitoring in 7/67 tests; cardiac catheterization in 3/14; electrophysiologic study in 3/13. Glucose tolerance test, head CT scan, radionuclide brain scan, lumbar puncture, and skull roentgenograms did not yield the diagnosis in any case. EEGs were abnormal in 26 of 67 tests performed but not definitively in any instance. Cost per patient evaluation was $2463 and per definitive diagnosis was $23,000.

4. Kapoor WN, Karpf M, Wieand S, Peterson JR, Levey GS: A prospective evaluation of patients with syncope. N Engl J Med 309:197, 1983.
    A cause of syncope was identified in 107 of 204 patients who were prospectively evaluated after presenting with a history compatible with a syncopal event. All patients underwent a standardized basic evaluation; all but some of those with vasodepressor syncope or orthostatic hypotension underwent electrocardiographic monitoring of at least 24 hours' duration (190), while smaller clinical subgroups underwent head CT scan (65), EP studies (23), EEG (100), or angiography (36). History and physical examination revealed the cause of syncope in 52 instances, basic laboratory examination in none, and ECG in

12. *Prolonged ECG monitoring identified the cause in another 29 cases, EP study in 3, cardiac catheterization in 7, cerebral angiography in 2, EEG in 1, and post mortem examination in 1. The mortality rates of patients with an identified cardiovascular cause, an identified noncardiovascular cause, and no identified cause of syncope were 30%, 12%, and 6.4%, respectively. Sudden death rates were 24%, 4%, and 3%.*

5. Kapoor WN, Karpf M, Levey GS: Issues in evaluating patients with syncope (editorial). Ann Intern Med 100:755, 1984.

   General discussion of the difficulties encountered attempting to establish a cause of syncope with a plea to limit the use of intensive, low-yield procedures.

6. Lipsitz LA: Syncope in the elderly. Ann Intern Med 99:92, 1983.

   Excellent general description of the causes of syncope with a special focus on the increased risks of co-morbid disease, multiple medications, and physiologic changes associated with aging.

7. Day SC, Cook EF, Funkenstein H, Goldman L: Evaluation and outcome of emergency room patients with transient loss of consciousness. Am J Med 73:15, 1982.

   Retrospective review of the evaluation and outcome of 198 patients who presented to an emergency room after transient loss of consciousness. A presumptive diagnosis was made in 87% of cases, with a vasovagal/psychogenic cause identified in 40%, seizure disorder in 29%, a cardiac cause in 9%, a toxic/metabolic cause in 6.5%, and other CNS causes in 2.5%. The history and physical examination were sufficient for diagnosis in 85% of cases for which a diagnosis was ultimately obtained. Blood chemistries, ECG, Holter monitoring, and EEG provided definitive information in a limited number of instances. Low, medium, and high prognostic risk groups were defined on the basis of analysis of simple clinical parameters.

8. Silverstein MD, Singer DE, Mulley AG, Thibault GE, Burnett O: Patients with syncope admitted to medical intensive care units. JAMA 248:1185, 1982.

   Retrospective review of 108 patients admitted to a medical intensive care unit for syncope. A cardiovascular cause was identified in 36%, a noncardiovascular cause in 17%, and no cause in 47%. Of all etiologic diagnoses, 72% were made on the basis of information immediately available at the time of patient presentation, 14% on the basis of ICU monitoring, and 14% after further tests. Syncope with an identified cardiovascular cause was associated with a one year mortality of 19%; syncope with a noncardiovascular cause or no identified cause carried a one year mortality of 6%, felt to reflect co-morbid disease.

9. DiMarco JP, Garan H, Harthorne JW, Ruskin JN: Intracardiac electrophysiologic techniques in recurrent syncope of unknown cause. Ann Intern Med 95:542, 1981.

   Retrospective review of 25 patients with recurrent syncope who underwent electrophysiologic (EP) study after extensive noninvasive cardiac and neurologic evaluation failed to demonstrate a specific cause (although most patients were known to have underlying anatomic or electrocardiographic abnormalities). EP study yielded or confirmed a diagnosis in 17 of 25 cases; therapy based on the results of EP testing was associated with resolution of symptoms in 14 and improvement in 1 of 17 treated patients.

10. Sugrue DD, Wood DL, McGoon MD: Carotid sinus hypersensitivity and syncope. Mayo Clin Proc 59:637, 1984.

    Case report and general discussion noting contributions from both cardioinhibitory and vasodepressor components.

11. Swiryn S, Kim SS: Quinidine-induced syncope. Arch Intern Med 143:314, 1983.

    Case report of quinidine-associated syncope and more general discussion of the long QT syndrome.

12. Teichman SL, Felder SD, Matos JA, Kim SG, Waspe LE, Fisher JD: The value of elec-

trophysiologic studies in syncope of undetermined origin: Report of 150 cases. Am Heart J *110*:469, 1985.

Large clinical series of 150 patients who underwent electrophysiologic study after an extensive standard evaluation failed to yield an unequivocal cause of syncope or near-syncope. Concomitant heart disease was noted in 75 of 150 patients and abnormal baseline ECG in 129 cases. Electrophysiologic abnormalities that could explain syncope were detected in 54 of 150 patients (36%). Results compared with other studies in the literature.

13. Kapoor WN, Cha R, Peterson JR, Wieand HS, Karpf M: Prolonged electrocardiographic monitoring in patients with syncope. Am J Med 82:20, 1987.

Follow-up of previous study (see reference 4), focusing on results of prolonged electrocardiographic monitoring in patients with syncope, in whom a cause was not assigned by history, examination, and ECG. Frequent or repetitive ventricular ectopy and sinus pauses were identified as independent ECG predictors of sudden death and mortality.

Hypertensive Emergencies

Ruth H. Strauss, M.D.

Hypertension becomes a medical emergency as a result of the direct effects of extremely high systemic blood pressure manifesting in a number of clinical settings, most notably aortic aneurysm dissection, cerebrovascular accident, encephalopathy, left ventricular decompensation, coronary artery disease, toxemia of pregnancy, and renal failure. Malignant hypertension, defined as a diastolic BP >130 mmHg in association with papilledema (grade IV Keith-Wagener retinopathy), leads to certain death from renal destruction if left untreated; accelerated hypertension, defined as markedly elevated diastolic pressure associated with retinal hemorrhages and exudates (grade III Keith-Wagener retinopathy), may have a more chronic destructive course but will lead to the malignant phase if neglected. Because 1–7% of all hypertensives may develop malignant hypertension and the estimated prevalence of hypertension in the United States is 23 million people, the significance of the problem should not be underestimated.[1]

CLINICAL FEATURES

Malignant hypertension gives rise to a necrotizing arteriolitis, with myointimal proliferation of the arteriolar wall as well as intimal destruction with fibrin deposition, microthrombus formation, and luminal narrowing.[2] In the kidney, this pathology is responsible for uremia and ensuing death in the untreated state; similarly, these pathologic changes result in the microangiopathic hemolytic anemia associated with advanced cases. Cerebral vascular autoregulation becomes abnormal in prolonged and severe hypertension, and altered permeability of the vasculature to protein and other intravascular constituents gives rise to the cerebral edema implicated in encephalopathy. Elevated blood pressure is not solely responsible for these changes, as elegant animal models have demonstrated that humoral factors such as renin, angiotensin II, and vasopressin are also responsible for vasoconstriction, sodium and water depletion, and vascular lesions; repletion of sodium and water, despite persistently elevated blood pressure, healed nephrosclerotic lesions in animals with malignant hypertension.[3,4]

Clinical features of malignant hypertension include the elevated blood pressure and retinal findings mentioned; neurologic symptoms of headache, dizziness, visual disturbance or frank loss, somnolence, stupor, coma, seizures, or focal deficits; and weight loss, anorexia, nausea, or vomiting. Other crises requiring immediate attention, such as aneurysmal dissection, myocardial ischemia or failure, toxemia, intracranial hemorrhage, stroke, and catecholamine excess, have well-known symptoms and features outlined elsewhere in this text and in selected references.[7-9] Laboratory abnormalities in malignant hypertension include schistocytes on peripheral blood smear and anemia if either renal failure or microangiopathy has supervened; and urinary sediment showing hematuria, pyuria, granular or hyaline casts, and nonnephrotic range proteinuria. Electrolytes (serum) may demonstrate low sodium concentration secondary to a pressure natriuresis or low potassium secondary to elevated aldosterone levels. Left atrial enlargement and left ventricular hypertrophy are often evident in the ECG. Azotemia is present in renal failure, a widened cardiac and aortic silhouette on chest radiograph will be noted in proximal aortic dissection, and evidence of pulmonary edema will be seen in left ventricular decompensation. Altered ST–T segments occur in the setting of myocardial ischemia complicated by severe hypertension. Cerebrospinal fluid abnormalities, notably increased pressure and protein content, are seen in encephalopathy.[6]

TREATMENT

Although rapid reduction of blood pressure takes precedence in the management of malignant hypertension and its complications, isolated severe hypertension demands a search for a remediable cause. Although ≤ 5% of all hypertension is secondary (nonessential), the prevalence of secondary forms may be substantially higher in the population with severe disease; this is especially true of renovascular hypertension, as notably documented by Davis and coworkers,[5] who found the incidence of renovascular disease to be 31% in their series of malignant or accelerated hypertensives. Thus, once urgently treated, patients with severe elevations of BP should be strongly considered for radiologic evaluation for renal artery stenosis. Urinary metanephrines, vanillylmandelic acid, and catechols can be collected to rule out pheochromocytoma. Although Cushing's disease and hyperaldosteronism are less likely causes of malignant hypertension, they may also be excluded electively.

It should be noted that severely elevated levels of BP do not always accompany hypertensive emergency; this is particularly true of women with toxemia of pregnancy or children with hypertension in the setting of glomerulonephritis, in whom BPs of 160/110 mmHg can be clinically dangerous. Although the clinical setting may demand *rapid* reduction of pressure, the *level* of reduction must be clinically determined beforehand and agents should be carefully chosen; caution must be exercised to avoid precipitous falls in pressure, particularly in cerebrovascular disease.

Therapy is directed at carefully controlled BP reduction through appropriate agents for the clinical setting. Nitroprusside is the mainstay of therapy in many settings, including malignant hypertension with or without encephalopathy;[1] ventricular decompensation; ischemic heart disease;[7] and, with a beta blocker, in aortic dissection. The last-named condition may be managed with trimethaphan. Administration of nitroprusside requires ICU monitoring but is the most accurate method for controlling rate of fall of blood pressure. Diazoxide is also used in hypertensive emergencies, but experience has dictated that mini-boluses are preferable to the previously utilized 300-mg bolus, to avoid precipitous falls in BP. In aortic dissection, this drug, and other direct vasodilators, is avoided, owing to its induction of a reflex rise in cardiac output and dP/dT. Phentolamine is reserved for emergencies of catechol excess, such as pheochromocytoma or central-agonist cessation-induced rebound. Diuretics should be administered concomitantly with the cited agents, since most other antihypertensive drugs lead to volume expansion, which ultimately interferes with control. Most authors agree that reduction to approximately 160/110 mmHg is adequate lowering to remove a patient from danger without engendering problems of organ hypoperfusion; in the setting of intracerebral hemorrhage, a reduction of only 20–30% is warranted if systolic pressure is ≥200 mmHG, based on studies by the Clinical Management Study Group.[8,9]

Other agents that may be used to sustain treatment once immediate BP lowering has been effected include parenteral or oral methyldopa, beta blocker, or hydralazine; angiotensin-converting enzyme inhibitors; centrally acting sympathetic agonists such as clonidine or guanabenz; or the peripheral alpha receptor antagonist prazosin.

Devising a well-reasoned, simplified antihypertensive regimen after the emergency and employing nursing and/or paramedical assistance in patient education are the best weapons against recurrence of many hypertensive emergencies.

KEY FEATURES

Diastolic BP ≥ 130 mmHg with grade III or IV Keith-Wagener retinopathy demands immediate attention; lower blood pressure elevations are important in pregnant women and in children.

Laboratory abnormalities may provide a clue to etiology of disease, although frequently they merely provide evidence of severity of disease.

Level of BP reduction must be carefully monitored to avoid hypoperfusion of organ systems.

A wide variety of antihypertensive agents exist; usually there is a preferable drug for a particular hypertensive crisis; thorough knowledge of agents and their mechanisms of action helps define appropriate agent for setting.

Simplified oral regimen and patient education are essential to outpatient management after crisis is resolved.

REFERENCES

1. Kaplan N: Hypertensive crisis (Chap. 4). *In* Kaplan N: Clinical Hypertension, 3rd ed. Baltimore, Williams and Wilkins, 1982, pp 193–209.
   Basic summary of definitions, pathophysiology, differential diagnosis, and treatment. Other chapters in book give detailed discussion of agents used in treatment; secondary causes; and special conditions, including childhood hypertension and hypertension in the setting of pregnancy.

2. Kincaid-Smith P: Malignant hypertension: Mechanisms and management. Pharmac Ther 9:245–269, 1980.
   Definitive review of pathology, including vascular lesion production and healing; hormonal factors responsible for transition from benign to malignant phase; and approach to treatment.

3. Woods JW: Malignant hypertension: Clinical recognition and management. Cardiovasc Clin North Am 9:311–328, 1978.
   Short, concise review of disease and treatment.

4. Mohring J, et al: Effects of saline drinking on malignant course of renal hypertension in rats. Am J Physiol 230:849–857, 1976; Vasopressor role of ADH in the pathogenesis of malignant DOC hypertension. Am J Physiol 232:F260–F269, 1977.
   Rat models of malignant hypertension, utilizing unilateral renal artery clipping or deoxycorticosterone administration, demonstrate sodium loss, hyperreninemia, and microangiopathic hemolytic anemia as in humans. Hypertension was corrected by saline administration, which stopped malignant phase lesions, as well as by antiserum to vasopressin.

5. Davis BA, Crook JE, Vestal RE, Oates JA: Prevalence of renovascular hypertension in patients with grade III or IV hypertensive retinopathy. N Engl J Med 301:1273–1276, 1979.
   Important article emphasizing that although renovascular hypertension is seen in a small portion of the total hypertensive population, its distribution in patients with advanced retinopathy is high: 31% of 123 patients with either malignant or accelerated hypertension proved to have the diagnosis (with a higher prevalence in white hypertensives than in blacks).

6. Healton EB, Brust JC, Feinfeld DA, Thomson GE: Hypertensive encephalopathy and the neurologic manifestations of malignant hypertension. Neurology 32:127–132, 1982.
    Prospective study of 41 admissions for malignant hypertension with neurologic evaluation before and after antihypertensive treatment; delineation of problems distinguishing cause, effect, and correlation; symptoms outlined and cerebrospinal fluid laboratory abnormalities given.

7. Keith TA: Hypertension crisis: Recognition and management. JAMA 237:1570–1577, 1977.

8. Ledingham JGG: Management of hypertensive crises. Hypertension (Suppl III) 5 (III):114–119, 1983.
9. Richardson DW, Raper AJ: Management of complicated hypertension including hypertensive emergencies. Cardiovasc Clin North Am 9:227–241, 1978.
10. McRae, RP Jr, Liebson, PR: Hypertensive Crisis. MCNA 70:749, 1986.
    Four references on treatment of all aspects of hypertensive crisis, including cerebrovascular accidents, aortic aneurysm dissection, toxemia of pregnancy, left ventricular failure, and coronary artery disease with ischemia.

SECTION 2
ENDOCRINOLOGY AND METABOLISM

Pituitary Disorders

Jon Pehrson, M.D.

ACUTE VASCULAR DISORDERS

Pituitary Apoplexy

Pituitary apoplexy is the rapid loss of one or more trophic pituitary hormones, usually in association with hemorrhage into a previously existing neoplasm or vascular malformation involving the pituitary-hypothalamic region. Clinically, patients usually present with a severe headache of acute onset. Neurologic manifestations such as stupor, coma, meningismus, and focal neurologic findings depend on the location and extent of hemorrhage and on damage/compression of contiguous brain structures. The endocrine manifestations of pituitary apoplexy depend on the underlying endocrine status of the patient at the time of the apoplectic event and on the severity and extent of acute pituitary hormone deficiencies.[1] For example, a patient with intact pituitary function right up to the time of pituitary apoplexy may only present with acute glucocorticoid deficiency (owing to rapid loss of ACTH) and diabetes insipidus (owing to rapid loss of ADH); a patient with pre-existing panhypopituitarism may present with mixed signs and symptoms of myxedema coma, acute glucocorticoid deficiency, and diabetes insipidus. Obviously, it is most useful if the patient's underlying pituitary status is known prior to the apoplectic event. Acute thyroid-stimulating hormone (TSH) deficiency produces hypothyroidism; however, the onset of clinical and biochemical hypothyroidism may be delayed for days or weeks because depletion of circulating thyroid hormone stores occurs very slowly (the half-life of thyroxine is 6–7 days). Consequently, thyroid function tests should be monitored at weekly intervals in patients with pituitary apoplexy and

121

normal initial thyroid function tests. Treatment with parenteral or oral thyroxine should be initiated if total and free thyroxine levels decrease during this period. Patients with evidence of pre-existing TSH deficiency and hypothyroidism should be treated as if they were in myxedema coma (see section on hypothyroidism in Article II–2). Acute loss of ACTH secretion produces acute adrenal glucocorticoid deficiency manifested by postural hypotension or circulatory collapse and occasionally hypoglycemia; adrenal mineralocorticoid secretion is spared. Acute adrenal glucocorticoid deficiency is a medical emergency and requires rapid intravenous stress doses of glucocorticoids. A bolus of 100–200 mg of hydrocortisone intravenously followed by a continuous intravenous drip at 10 mg/hour is the most desirable regimen. However, the large doses of parenterally administered dexamethasone frequently used by neurosurgeons to combat cerebral edema in apoplectic vascular neurologic events are more than adequate for acute glucocorticoid replacement in these patients. (For details of signs, symptoms, and treatment of acute glucocorticoid deficiency, please refer to Articles II–8 and II–9.) Acute loss of ADH causes acute diabetes insipidus, characterized by large volumes of dilute urine resulting in water loss, dehydration, and hypernatremia. The acute diabetes insipidus may be transient (hours to days) or permanent. Transient diabetes insipidus may be followed by a period of inappropriate ADH secretion (syndrome of inappropriate antidiuretic hormone [SIADH]). This SIADH is thought to be the result of leakage of ADH from damaged hypothalamic neurons. The SIADH usually resolves in a matter of days (rarely a few weeks) and may be followed by partial or complete diabetes insipidus, depending on the extent of loss of ADH-containing hypothalamic neurons. The acute loss of growth hormone and gonadotropins does not produce immediate life-threatening sequelae. Pituitary apoplexy is an endocrinologic *and* neurosurgical emergency. Consequently, patients with presumed pituitary apoplexy should undergo rapid assessment by both a competent endocrinologist and a neurosurgeon. The underlying hypothalamic pituitary neoplasm or vascular malformation resulting in the hemorrhage and neurologic damage may require acute neurosurgical intervention. Thyroid function tests, cortisol levels, electrolytes, and urine osmolality should be obtained at the initial presentation. Parenterally administered stress doses of glucocorticoids should be initiated as rapidly as possible. If the patient appears myxedematous, parenteral replacement with thyroxine should also be initiated. Treatment of acute diabetes insipidus is discussed in the next section. Rapid endocrinologic and neurosurgical evaluation and treatment of patients with pituitary apoplexy are of paramount importance.

Sheehan's Syndrome

Sheehan's syndrome, or postpartum pituitary necrosis, is the result of infarction of the enlarged, vascular pituitary gland of pregnancy in association with significant peripartum uterine hemorrhage. The highly vascular pituitary gland enlarges during pregnancy. This enlargement and the hypercoagulable state of pregnancy are thought to predispose the pituitary to thrombosis and ischemic necrosis when a large peripartum hemorrhage occurs. Clinically, patients may present with acute onset of loss of ACTH (glucocorticoid deficiency) and less commonly, ADH (diabetes insipidus); however, loss of trophic pituitary hormones may occur slowly weeks or months after the peripartum hemorrhage. In spite of teachings to the contrary, there is no predictable pattern of hormone loss and virtually every variation and combination of pituitary hormone deficiency has been described in Sheehan's syndrome. Clinical manifestations of these deficiencies include postural dizziness (ACTH deficiency leading to glucocorticoid deficiency); lethargy, fatigue, and cold intolerance (TSH deficiency leading to hypothyroidism); polyuria (ADH deficiency); postpartum oligomenorrhea or amenorrhea (gonadotropin deficiency); and absent or poor postpartum lactation (prolactin deficiency). CT scans have demonstrated a partially empty sella in patients with Sheehan's syndrome, presumably owing to the shrinkage of the pituitary gland as a result of necrosis. Sheehan's syndrome should be suspected in any woman with a significant peripartum or postpartum hemorrhage who presents with signs and symptoms of pituitary hormone deficiencies. Sheehan's syndrome has occasionally been confused with pituitary hormone deficiencies as a result of enlargement of a prolactinoma during pregnancy or with the recently described entity of postpartum lymphocytic hypophysitis. As such, a careful history and physical examination to elucidate other signs and symptoms of autoimmune endocrinopathies, a CT scan, and a basal prolactin level are probably indicated in any patient in whom the diagnosis of Sheehan's syndrome is entertained. Documentation of pituitary hormone deficiencies with a few brief endocrine tests is simple, and it is imperative because deficiencies of pituitary hormones usually mandate life-long treatment: ACTH deficiency with replacement of glucocorticoids, TSH deficiency with replacement doses of thyroxine, and diabetes insipidus with DDAVP. Gonadotropin deficiency can be treated with sex steroid replacement (estrogens and a progestational agent). Patients with Sheehan's syndrome and gonadotropin deficiency who desire further pregnancy can undergo ovulation induction with exogenous gonadotropins; however, this is quite costly and tedious.

ANTIDIURETIC HORMONE (ADH)

The osmolality of extracellular body fluids is one of the most tightly regulated parameters in humans.[2,3] Although osmolality is largely determined by the serum sodium concentration, osmolality is adjusted by changes in water retention and excretion rather than by changes in sodium retention or excretion. Osmoreceptors in the hypothalamus respond rapidly to changes in extracellular fluid osmolality. These osmoreceptors are located in close proximity to and impinge upon ADH neurons located in the supraoptic and paraventricular nuclei of the hypothalamus. ADH is transported in the axons of these neurons which terminate in the posterior pituitary region and infundibulum. A rise in osmolality results in release of ADH into the systemic circulation. ADH acts on nephron collecting duct cells and allows intraluminal water to be dragged along the osmotic gradient in the hypertonic renal medulla. Consequently, water is retained, a concentrated urine is excreted and extracellular osmolality is restored to normal. Conversely, intake of hypotonic fluids that results in a decrease in osmolality results in inhibition of ADH secretion. In the absence of ADH, the collecting duct cells become impermeable to water, a dilute urine is excreted, and osmolality rises back to normal. This system is extremely sensitive, and as little as a 1% increase in osmolality produces a 2–10-fold increase in ADH secretion, whereas a 1% decrease in osmolality shuts off ADH secretion almost totally. As a result, serum osmolality is usually maintained at a level of approximately 287 ± 5 mOsm/kg, approximately midway between the shutoff threshold of ADH (280 mOsm/kg) and the threshold for thirst (295 mOsm/kg). Thirst probably serves as a backup mechanism for the preservation of osmolality.

Obviously, the preservation of extracellular fluid osmolality requires a normal thirst mechanism, an intact functioning osmoreceptor, normal synthesis and secretion of ADH, normal action of ADH on the renal collecting duct cells, and generation of a hypertonic environment in the interstitium of the renal medulla. Interference at any of these levels compromises the patient's ability to conserve water. Inability to consume enough water to keep pace with urinary or insensible losses will result in dehydration and hypernatremia. Conversely, inability to shut off ADH secretion or action may result in dilutional hyponatremia, especially in patients given a free water load.

There are several other important influences on ADH secretion. Receptors in the cardiac atria and the aortic arch respond to perceived volume deficits. Neuronal pathways from these receptors impinge upon ADH neurons and may override osmolar control of ADH secretion. Consequently, perceived volume deficits may result in ADH secretion and result in dilutional hyponatremia from retention of free water. This can occur with *true* volume deficits (hemorrhage, fluid losses from diarrhea, third-spacing of intravascular fluids) or from *perceived* volume deficits with maldistribution of body fluids (congestive heart failure, cirrhosis, patients on positive end-expiratory pressure [PEEP]). Teleologically, this is the body's way of repairing a volume deficit with any kind of fluid it can retain, even at the expense of extracellular fluid osmolality.

Neurons from the chemoreceptor trigger zone in the brain stem can also stimulate ADH secretion and cause dilutional hyponatremia. Nausea and drugs that stimulate this chemoreceptor trigger zone (morphine, etc.) can lead to a neurogenic dilutional hyponatremia from excess ADH secretion. Occasionally, irritating lesions in the lung or thoracic cavity may stimulate ADH secretion through neuronal pathways and cause dilutional hyponatremia.

Deficient ADH Secretion

Causes of deficient ADH secretion or action can be broken down into the anatomic areas affected as follows:

I. Neurogenic
   A. Destruction of osmoreceptors and/or ADH neurons
      1. Neoplastic diseases (primary or metastatic involving the hypothalamus)
      2. Hypothalamic injury
         a. Anoxic brain damage
         b. Marked hypoglycemic coma
         c. Hemorrhage
         d. Head trauma
         e. Surgery
   B. Inhibition of ADH secretion by drugs
      1. Alcohol (acutely rising levels only)
      2. Some phenothiazines-butyrophenones
      3. Opiates (in low doses)
II. Nephrogenic
   A. Inhibition of ADH renal effects
      1. Lithium
      2. Demeclocycline
      3. Methoxyflurane
      4. Barbiturates
      5. Glyburide
   B. Renal defects (nephrogenic diabetes insipidus)
      1. Hypokalemia
      2. Hypercalcemia
      3. Familial/sporadic nephrogenic diabetes insipidus
      4. Pyelonephritis
      5. Polycystic kidney disease
      6. Postobstruction
      7. Sickle cell trait/disease
      8. Medullary "washout" (solute diuresis, primary polydipsia)

Clinically, patients with inadequate ADH secretion or action present with polyuria, polydipsia, and a dilute urine. Dehydration and hypernatremia are present if patients are unable to compensate for urinary water losses by oral intake of water. Chronic renal disease, especially interstitial renal diseases, is characterized by a reduced ability to produce a hypertonic environment in the renal medullary interstitium. However, these patients usually only have mildly increased urine volumes because they can produce isosthenuric urine (approximately 300 mOsm/kg).

A markedly dilute urine in the presence of mildly decreased plasma osmolality suggests primary polydipsia. Many patients with primary polydipsia have psychiatric disorders or are on medications that lead to a dry mouth that is ameliorated by constant intake of water. Conversely, a dilute urine in the face of plasma hyperosmolality suggests neurogenic (central) or nephrogenic (renal) diabetes insipidus. In most patients, a careful history and physical examination with special attention to diseases or drugs that may affect the central nervous system or kidney will help to elucidate the pathophysiology. The distinction between neurogenic and nephrogenic diabetes insipidus can be established by the urinary response to exogenously administered ADH or by the measurement of the plasma ADH level. Patients with neurogenic diabetes insipidus usually have a rise in urine osmolality in response to exogenous ADH and low plasma ADH levels, whereas patients with nephrogenic diabetes insipidus have a minimal response of urine osmolality to exogenous ADH and high ADH levels. In most circumstances, the urinary osmolality response to ADH readily distinguishes neurogenic from nephrogenic diabetes insipidus and measurement of ADH levels are probably only necessary in equivocal cases.

In an acutely ill patient with an obvious reason for neurogenic diabetes insipidus (surgery, head trauma, etc.), the pathophysiology is usually obvious; detailed testing is unnecessary and treatment should be instituted immediately. For example, the acutely ill patient with head trauma, hypernatremia, and large volumes of dilute urine almost certainly has central diabetes insipidus.[4] The urinary response to exogenously administered ADH (as judged by urine volume and urine specific gravity/osmolality) not only confirms the diagnosis but also initiates the treatment. In less urgent circumstances, a dehydration test can be performed; a careful baseline weight and postural vital signs should be obtained prior to restricting fluids. During fluid restriction, the patient's weight, postural vital signs, urinary volume, and urinary osmolality (or specific gravity) are obtained at hourly intervals. When urine osmolality has plateaued or clinically significant dehydration has occurred (as judged by significant postural hypotension or greater than 3% loss in basal body weight), a blood sample for a serum sodium concentration and osmolality is obtained to assess the adequacy of the dehydration. Five units of aqueous vasopressin is administered subcutaneously. Urine osmolality is measured 1 hour later. A rise in the urinary osmolality after vasopressin of greater than 9% suggests neurogenic diabetes insipidus, whereas a rise of less than 9% suggests nephrogenic diabetes insipidus. If results are equivocal, measurement of the ADH level in the patient's serum obtained just prior to the administration of aqueous vasopressin will distinguish neurogenic from nephrogenic diabetes insipidus.[5]

Treatment of acute neurogenic diabetes insipidus involves replacement of the water deficit and urinary losses (usually parenterally). In cases when diabetes insipidus may be transient (postsurgical, post–head trauma), replacement of the water deficit and hourly urinary losses may be adequate to maintain normal fluid and electrolyte balance. However, this becomes more difficult when urinary volumes are high and/or a significant water deficit already exists. Aqueous (short-acting) vasopressin can be given subcutaneously at a dosage of 2.5–5.0 U every few hours to decrease urinary water losses and allow correction of water deficits. A *short-acting* vasopressin preparation is mandatory, since transient diabetes insipidus seen postsurgically or after head trauma may be followed by SIADH, necessitating rapid alterations in therapy. In situations in which subcutaneous perfusion may be comprised (elderly patients, shock, vacillating blood pressures, treatment with pressors), the absorption of subcutaneous vasopressin may be inadequate or erratic. In these patients, aqueous vasopressin should be administered as a constant intravenous infusion. We have found that doses as low as 0.025–0.05 U/hour will reproducibly control neurogenic diabetes insipidus with no pressor effects.

In patients with permanent, complete neurogenic diabetes insipidus, intranasal administration of 50–100 μg of DDAVP once or twice daily usually controls urine output to manageable levels. Doses may be held during the waking hours until urine output increases; this will avoid water intoxication and hyponatremia.

Partial neurogenic diabetes insipidus can be treated with oral fluid intake in alert, ambulatory patients if the deficit is mild. Some patients require a small dose of DDAVP at bedtime to curtail nocturia. Drugs that enhance secretion or action of ADH, such as chlorpropamide or clofibrate, can also be used in patients with partial neurogenic diabetes insipidus. Hypoglycemia (chlorpropamide) and cholelithiasis (clofibrate) may limit the use of these drugs in patients.

Nephrogenic diabetes insipidus can be treated with withdrawal of the offending drug (lithium, demeclocycline) or with a thiazide diuretic. Thiazides ameliorate nephrogenic diabetes insipidus by volume contraction (allowing increased salt and water resorption to occur in the proximal nephron) and by antagonizing the formation of free water in the ascending limb of the loop of Henle. In psychiatric patients on lithium, the high urinary volumes may be the result of a combination of nephrogenic diabetes insipidus and an acquired primary polydipsic component. Gradual restriction of free water intake with careful monitoring of serum sodium concentration and/or osmolality may reveal that the patient's lithium-induced nephrogenic diabetes insipidus is relatively mild and that the primary cause of the high urine volumes is a coincidental primary polydipsia. Unfortunately, some psychiatric patients cannot be managed without lithium and significant true nephrogenic diabetes insipidus produces intolerable urine volumes. Thiazide diuretics have been used in these patients; however, lithium levels may rise during treatment with thiazides. Amiloride (a potassium-sparing diuretic) has been reported to reduce this nephrogenic diabetes insipidus without significant lithium toxicity occurring.

Excess ADH

Excessive secretion or action of ADH results in water retention and dilutional hyponatremia. ADH secretion can be influenced by many non-osmotic stimuli, such as nicotine, acetylcholine, opiates (high doses), nausea, other drugs (carbamazepine, vincristine, cyclophosphamide), thoracic lesions (pneumonia, lung abscess), and, most importantly, by perceived or true volume deficits. Finally, ADH may be increased when it leaks from hypo-thalamic neurons (post–head trauma, post-surgery) or when it is ectopically produced by certain carcinomas (oat cell carcinoma of the lung, pancreatic carcinoma, thymoma).[6]

In one sense, certain hyponatremic states can be thought of as *"inap-propriate,"* in that the excessive ADH secretion is not a physiologic but rather a pathologic phenomenon. Examples of this are ectopic ADH production from tumors, leakage of ADH from damaged neurons, drug- or nausea-induced ADH secretion, or drugs that simulate or stimulate the action of ADH on the renal tubule. In these states, water retention in excess of normal total body sodium stores occurs and dilutional hyponatremia results. Urinary sodium concentrations are usually greater than 20 mEq/L. Presumably, this enhanced urinary sodium excretion is due to decreased renal tubular resorption of sodium from the mild volume expansion induced by water retention. Hypothyroidism has also been associated with hyponatremia and inability to excrete a free water load and is due to a combination of decreased cardiac output, decreased glomerular filtration rate, and inappropriately elevated levels of ADH. Occasionally, pure glucocorticoid deficiency has been associated with mild hyponatremia, presumably as a result of mild postural hypotension and resetting of the osmostat. For these reasons, the syndrome of inappropriate ADH usually requires the absence of any signs associated with a semiphysiologic stimulus for ADH secretion, such as edema or postural hypotension. In addition, some investigators feel that normal thyroid function tests and glucocorticoid levels should be included as criteria for SIADH.

Conversely, many hyponatremic states can be thought of as an appropriate physiologic response of ADH to perceived volume deficits. ADH hypersecretion in association with increased total body sodium stores is almost always characterized by maldistribution of body fluids and intravascular volume, as in cirrhosis, nephrosis, and congestive heart failure, and in ventilatory patients on PEEP. In contrast, "appropriate" ADH hypersecretion in association with decreased total body sodium is usually characterized by true volume contraction as a result of causes such as blood loss, diarrhea, vomiting, diueretic use, salt-losing nephropathy, or mineralocorticoid deficiency. Urinary sodium concentrations obviously vary in these states and are usually high in patients with salt-losing nephropathy, mineralocorticoid deficiency, and duiuretic use. Urinary sodium values are most helpful if obtained *prior to treatment* with intravenous fluids in interpreting the pathophysiology of hyponatremia.

Signs and symptoms of hyponatremia depend on the underlying pathophysiology, the degree of hyponatremia, and the rate at which hyponatremia has developed. Underlying causes are usually obvious in most patients and many times are multifactorial. Hyponatremia produces variable neurologic signs, which range from mild cognitive dysfunction to frank stupor, coma, and seizures. Although one would think the degree of hyponatremia would correlate with the neurologic manifestations, the rate at which hyponatremia develops has a more profound influence. Rapid drops in the serum sodium concentration produce more neurologic symptoms, whereas slow decreases in the serum sodium concentration may be associated with minimal manifestations. For these reasons, the treatment of the hyponatremic patient involves elucidation and treatment of the underlying or aggravating cause and a careful assessment of the degree of compromise that is attributable to the hyponatremia. Correction of a true volume deficit with intravenous normal saline may be all that is required to restore normal serum sodium levels in a patient with diarrhea, vomiting, diuretic use, or blood loss. Correction of maldistribution of body fluids or vascular volume in patients with nephrosis or congestive heart failure may also correct hyponatremia. Restriction of hypotonic fluids or free water during treatment of any of these cases is usually helpful and depends on the degree of hyponatremia and the symptoms attributable to hyponatremia. In patients with a neoplastic source of ectopic ADH, reduction in tumor mass may be associated with improvement in hyponatremia. In general, in patients with readily apparent and treatable causes of hyponatremia the prognosis is good and hyponatremia resolves. Unfortunately, many causes of hyponatremia are not totally correctable. Restriction of free water and hypotonic fluids may result in reasonable serum sodium values in patients with neoplastic sources of ADH secretion and in patients with cirrhosis and congestive heart failure. If this is unsuccessful, treatment with demeclocycline, a drug that antagonizes the action of ADH at the level of the kidney, has been used in doses of 600–1200 mg/day. A lag phase of several days may be noted before improvement in hyponatremia occurs. Unfortunately, in patients with maldistribution of body fluids such as in cirrhosis or congestive heart failure, worsening of renal function has limited this drug's use. Intravenous normal saline balanced with administration of furosemide is quite effective for management of inpatient hyponatremia but must be individually tailored for each patient. We have found that treatment with hypertonic saline is rarely necessary even in severely hyponatremic cases if underlying and aggravating factors of hyponatremia are aggressively treated and normal saline and furosemide are used. Hypertonic saline should probably be reserved for severely hyponatremic patients with marked neurologic symptoms who have not responded to normal saline and furosemide.

KEY FEATURES

ACUTE VASCULAR DISORDERS

Apoplectic events involving the pituitary gland only occur when there is a pre-existing pituitary/hypothalamic neoplasm or vascular malformation or after a significant postpartum hemorrhage.

The signs and symptoms of pituitary apoplexy depend on the patient's underlying endocrine status, the amount of damage or compromise to contiguous brain structures, and the severity and pattern of hormonal dropout.

The key to successful treatment of acute pituitary insufficiency is suspicion of the disorder and rapid clinical and biochemical assessment; treatment should be initiated rapidly and should be based on the clinical examination and immediately available laboratory results.

Neurosurgical assessment and treatment are just as important as medical assessment and treatment.

Acute ADH insufficiency is usually readily apparent, attributable to an obvious cause, and should be rapidly diagnosed and treated.

ANTIDIURETIC HORMONE

Acute neurogenic diabetes insipidus is usually readily predictable in certain clinical situations. Acute diabetes insipidus may be transient, permanent, or followed by a period of SIADH; treatment regimens must be adapted to rapid changes in free water balance (short-acting drugs, predictable absorption and effect, frequent monitoring of serum and urinary osmolality).

Hypernatremia usually occurs when a defect in water conservation is combined with an inability to keep pace with water losses. The cause of inadequate water conservation is usually readily apparent or easily elucidated.

Hyponatremic states are the result of retention of total body water in excess of total body sodium. Total body sodium may be normal, increased, or decreased.

States of normal total body sodium and excess free water are usually the result of inappropriate secretion or action of ADH as a result of tumors, leakage of ADH, or drug effects.

Hyponatremia with decreased total body sodium is usually due to true volume deficits.

Hyponatremia with increased total body sodium is almost always the result of maldistribution of body fluids/blood volume with a perceived volume deficit stimulating ADH secretion.

REFERENCES

1. Thomas JP, et al: Medical management of pituitary disease. Clin Endo Metab 12:771–788, 1983.
   Discussion of pituitary abnormalities and management; organized into sections on each pituitary hormone.

2. Baylis PH: Posterior pituitary function in health and disease. Clin Endo Metab 12:747–790, 1983.
   Excellent review of ADH and oxytocin with several good tables and figures.

3. Robertson GL, et al: Neurogenic disorders of osmoregulation. Am J Med 72:339–353, 1982.
   Detailed discussion of physiology and pathophysiology of neural osmoregulation, including thirst, osmoreceptor function, and alterations from drugs and diseases.

4. Shucart WA, Jackson I: Management of diabetes insipidus in neurosurgical patients. J Neurosurg 44:65–71, 1976.
   Pragmatic overview of treatment of ADH disorders in neurosurgical patients.

5. Moses AM, Notman DD: Diabetes insipidus and syndrome of inappropriate ADH secretion (SIADH). Adv Intern Med 27:73–100, 1982.
   Comprehensive discussion of pathophysiology and treatment of disorders of water balance.

6. Buckalew VM: Hyponatremia; pathogenesis and management. Hosp Prac 21:49–58, 1986.
   Extremely well-written and organized discussion of hyponatremia.

Thyroid Disorders

Jon Pehrson, M.D.

HYPERTHYROIDISM

Hyperthyroidism is commonly caused by autonomously functioning thyroid tissue (toxic multinodular goiter, toxic nodule), thyroid-stimulating immunoglobulin (Grave's disease), or inflammation of the thyroid gland (thyroiditis). Grave's disease and toxic multinodular goiter account for the large majority of patients who require acute medical care for hyperthyroidism.[1] The profound effect of thyroid hormones on the metabolic rate of tissues and the body's response to this demand account for the common signs and symptoms of hyperparathyroidism. The increased metabolic rate results in increased oxygen and food consumption, heat production and catabolism. Increased number of cardiac beta adrenergic receptors, direct myocardial stimulation by thyroid hormones, and the increased oxygen demand result in markedly increased cardiac output, tachycardia, decreased total peripheral resistance, and shortened circulatory times. The age of the patient, underlying cardiovascular disease, and concomitant medications obviously influence the mode of presentation of hyperthyroidism. Generally, younger patients commonly present with nervousness, tremor, insomnia, voracious appetite, heat intolerance, palpitations, goiter, and weight loss; older patients may present with atrial fibrillation, congestive heart failure, apathy, cachexia, and muscle weakness. Marked hyperthyroidism with fever and agitation characterizes thyroid storm. Thyroid storm usually occurs in a previously hyperthyroid patient and is commonly precipitated by such things as infection, anesthesia, parturition, and medications. The mortality rate in untreated thyroid storm is quite high, and awareness of the condition and prompt treatment substantially reduce the morbidity and mortality. Although treatment of hyperthyroidism is fairly standardized, therapy must be individually tailored to each patient, especially in elderly patients with coexistent cardiovascular disease who present with atrial fibrillation and congestive heart failure.[2] In patients whose congestive heart failure and atrial fibrillation are due mainly to the effects of hyperthyroidism, therapy with antithyroid drugs (propylthiouracil, iodides) and beta adrenergic blockers results in marked improvement. However, patients with previously compromised cardiac function may have their condition worsened by overzealous use of fluids and beta adrenergic blockers and congestive heart failure may worsen during treatment.[3] Many times this becomes apparent only after therapy has been initiated; therefore, patients require frequent examination during treatment and continued adjustment of dosages of beta adrenergic blockers and fluids. Digitalis may only be useful in patients with coexistent digitalis responsive cardiac disorders, and exclusive use of digitalis to control the ventricular response in atrial fibrillation is limited by the large doses of digitalis required to control the rate; toxicity is frequently observed. Many patients with atrial fibrillation and hyperthyroidism revert to normal sinus rhythm when their hyperthyroidism is controlled. Chemical or electrocardioversion of patients who are still hyperthyroid is probably useless, since most of these patients revert to atrial fibrillation unless their hyperthyroidism is controlled. Persistence of atrial fibrillation after 3–4 months of euthyroidism usually indicates that an underlying cardiac disease is responsible for the atrial fibrillation. Systemic emboli occur in a significant (8–15%) percentage of patients with atrial fibrillation and hyperthyroidism, usually in individuals with congestive heart failure or underlying valvular disease—anticoagulation is probably prudent in this subset of patients. Rough guidelines for the treatment of thyroid storm or severe hyperthyroidism are as follows:

- Propylthiouracil (po or via nasogastric tube 300–400 mg q6h)
- Iodides (only after propylthiouracil has been absorbed)
- SSKI* 1–3 drops po q6–8h or sodium iodide 1–2 gm IV/day
- Propranolol 20–80 mg po q6h (must be carefully individualized)
- Intravenous fluid supplementation (must be carefully individualized)
- Glucocorticoids (hydrocortisone 10 mg/hour or dexamethasone 8 mg/24 hours)

Aggressive multi-drug treatment significantly lowers thyroid hormone levels in a matter of only a few days, and treatment can be reduced to lower doses of propylthiouracil (450–600 mg/day). Iodides and glucocorticoids can be rapidly discontinued and propranolol doses tapered down to allow more accurate physical assessment of the patient's underlying status. In patients who present in thyroid storm, elucidation and treatment of a possible precipitating cause should take place as rapidly as possible. Prognosis in properly treated young patients is excellent, whereas elderly patients with coexistent disease obviously fare less well and require more meticulous care.

HYPOTHYROIDISM

Hypothyroidism in adults results from destruction (autoimmune, post-^{131}I treatment, large local doses of external ionizing radiation) or surgical removal of the thyroid gland. Rarely (5%), hypothyroidism is due to hypothalamic-pituitary dysfunction. Hypothyroidism is usually a slowly progressive process that takes place over years or decades, resulting in insidiously progressive symptoms and signs. Unfortunately, these symptoms and signs are frequently erroneously attributed to the normal aging process, dementia, or coexistent medical problems. It is useful to think of hypothyroidism as a disease characterized by generalized slowing of the bodily processes (such as slow elimination of lipids, drugs, and free water; slowed skeletal and cardiac muscle action; slowed nervous system function; slowed gastrointestinal function; etc.).[4] Signs and symptoms of hypothyroidism include the following:

---

*SSKI = saturated solution of potassium iodide.

- Cold intolerance
- Irritability
- Delayed relaxation phase of deep tendon reflexes
- Coarse hair
- Weight gain (modest)
- Weakness
- Thick, dry, scaly skin
- Diminished cognitive function, dementia
- Constipation
- Low-output congestive heart failure (dilated cardiomyopathy with pericardial and pleural effusions, decreased ECG voltage)
- Hypothermia
- Lethargy, lassitude
- Hoarse voice
- Bradycardia
- Decreased sensation, hearing, taste, smell

Common laboratory abnormalities observed in hypothyroidism include a mild normochromic, normocytic anemia; mild hyponatremia; hypercholesterolemia; and mildly elevated creatine kinase values. Ninety-five per cent of cases of hypothyroidism are due to primary hypothyroidism and are characterized by low thyroxine (T_4) levels and elevated thyroid-stimulating hormone (TSH) levels. Hypothalamic pituitary diseases are characterized by low TSH levels and usually deficiencies in other anterior pituitary hormones. It is important to determine the extent of anterior pituitary hormone deficiency before treating these patients with thyroid hormones, since treatment may precipitate an adrenal crisis in a patient who has decreased ACTH reserve.

Treatment of mild to moderate hypothyroidism is not an emergency and should take place slowly over a period of weeks, especially in older patients and patients with underlying cardiovascular disease. Initial dosage of thyroxine is usually 0.025 mg orally, increased by 0.025-mg increments every one to three weeks until T_4 and T_3 are normal. Suppression of TSH may take many months in patients who have been hypothyroid for prolonged periods of time. The worsening or onset of angina pectoris during thyroid replacement may indicate underlying coronary vascular disease, and replacement should be slowed or stopped until assessment of the patient's cardiovascular status is completed. In selected patients, revascularization of the coronary arterial system prior to obtaining euthyroidism has been accomplished without significant morbidity and mortality. Younger patients with recent onset of hypothyroidism usually can be treated more rapidly. Usual replacement doses average 1.8–2.0 μg/kg of oral thyroxine daily; however, older patients may require as little as one half this amount.[5]

Myxedema Coma

The end of the spectrum of hypothyroidism is myxedema coma. This occurs in previously hypothyroid patients and is frequently precipitated by an event such as an infection, cold exposure, administration of drugs, or general anesthesia. Patients are almost always obviously mxyedematous, with hypothermia, low cardiac output, and slowed relaxation phase of deep tendon reflexes. Mild hyponatremia is commonly present, especially if the patient has received a recent load of hypotonic fluids. Myxedema coma is a medical emergency, and immediate treatment is required. Precipitating causes obviously should be actively investigated and treated. Supportive measures include parenteral D5NS* or plasma expanders to treat shock, passive warming (severe hypothermia may require warmed parenteral fluids), and maintenance of adequate ventilation. Required drugs should be administered intravenously, since gastrointestinal, subcutaneous, or intramuscular absorption is slow and unreliable in myxedema. Intravenous administration of thyroxine in doses sufficient to saturate empty intracelluar and extracellular binding sites requires 400–500 μg of L-thyroxine. Thereafter, 50–100 μg intravenously daily should be continued until oral replacement is possible. Stress doses of glucocorticoids should be administered, since (1) occasionally hypothyroidism may be due to hypothalamic pituitary dysfunction, and (2) autoimmune adrenal dysfunction may coexist with autoimmune thyroid disease. The common belief that hypothyroidism per se causes inadequate adrenal responses to stress is not supported by adequate studies. However, treatment with stress doses of glucocorticoids is probably harmless and may be life-saving in patients with inadequate endogenous glucocorticoids.

KEY FEATURES

Hyperthyroidism in young patients presents with nervousness, palpitations, voracious appetite, heat intolerance, and goiter; older patients may be atypical and present with atrial fibrillation, weakness, or weight loss.

Treatment of severe hyperthyroidism involves treatment of precipitating factors as well as treatment of the hyperthyroidism. Young patients usually recover; older patients require meticulous individual care and dosage adjustment.

Myxedema coma occurs in previously hypothyroid patients, usually with obvious signs and symptoms and a precipitating cause. Treatment

*D5NS = 5% dextrose in normal saline.

involves aggressive supportive measures, intravenous thyroxine, and treatment of precipitating factors.

REFERENCES

1. Chopra IJ, et al: Pathogenesis of hyperthyroidism. Ann Rev Med 34:267–281, 1983.
   The current thinking on the pathogenesis of Grave's disease is nicely summarized.

2. Hartzband PI, et al: The treatment of hyperthyroidism. Disease-a-Month 27:1–74, 1983.
   A detailed, complete discussion of all treatment modalities (acute and chronic) for hyperthyroidism, with a good section on thyroid storm.

3. Feely J, et al: Use of beta-adrenoreceptor blocking drugs in hyperthyroidism. Drugs 27:425–436, 1984.
   Excellent current review of all published literature concerning beta adrenergic blockers in the management of hyperthyroidism.

4. Hall R, et al: Hypothyroidism: Clinical features and complications. Clin Endo Metab 8:29–38, 1979.
   System by system review of clinical manifestations with succinct explanations.

5. Robuschi G, et al: Hypothyroidism in the elderly. Endo Rev 8(2):142–153, 1987.
   Comprehensive discussion of diagnosis and treatment of hypothyroidism in the elderly.

Disorders of Mineral Metabolism

Jon Pehrson, M.D.

CALCIUM

Hypercalcemia

Approximately one half of circulating calcium is bound (albumin, globulins) such that calcium levels must be interpreted with respect to levels of endogenous binders.[1] The normal total serum calcium level is 8.5–10.5 mg/dl in a patient with normal levels of calcium binders. Total serum calcium is lowered in hypoproteinemic patients by a factor of 0.8 mg/dl of calcium per 1 gm/dl of albumin. The unbound, or ionized, calcium level is physiologically the most important determinant of (1) feedback on parathyroid hormone (PTH) and (2) signs and symptoms of hypercalcemia. Consequently, determinations of levels of calcium binders (albumin, globulin) are important in the assessment of a patient's calcium status. Alkalosis produces enhanced binding of calcium onto protein binders; conversely, acidosis is associated with decreased binding of calcium to protein binders.

Hypercalcemia produces a constellation of signs and symptoms that are profoundly influenced by the rate of calcium increase.[2] Generally, rapidly progressive hypercalcemia produces more marked symptoms than slowly progressive hypercalcemia.

Hypercalcemia causes several reproducible abnormalities, including the following:
- Paresthesias
- Lethargy, stupor, coma
- Shortened QT interval
- "Coving" of ST segments
- Widened T waves (extreme hypercalcemia)
- Constipation
- Abdominal pain
- Pruritus
- Muscle weakness, fatigue
- Arrhythmias (ventricular tachycardia, ventricular fibrillation at high levels)
- Polyuria, polydipsia (nephrogenic diabetes insipidus)

Severity of symptoms is related to absolute calcium levels and to the rate of rise. Symptoms and signs resolve with treatment, but delays are commonly observed, especially in older patients. Dehydration will exacerbate hypercalcemia of any cause, and the correction of dehydration is the most important initial step in treatment.[3]

The causes of hypercalcemia are many; the major causes are listed in Table 1. Generally, outpatient hypercalcemia is most commonly due to primary hyperparathyroidism, while inpatient hypercalcemia is usually due to cancer.

A careful history, physical, and laboratory evaluation usually elucidate

TABLE 1. MAJOR CAUSES OF HYPERCALCEMIA

Factitious (prolonged tourniquet time)	Primary hyperparathyroidism
Vitamin D intoxication	Cancers
Vitamin A intoxication	Bone metastases (lung, breast,
Adrenal insufficiency	prostate, lymphoproliferative/
Hyperthyroidism	hematogenous)
Granulomatous disease (tuberculosis, sarcoidosis, berylliosis)	Humorally mediated (squamous cell of lung, head/neck, esopha-
Tertiary hyperparathyroidism (post–renal transplant, etc.)	gus; renal cell, transitional cell bladder carcinoma, ovary)
Familial hypocalciuric hypercalcemia	Coexistent primary hyperparathyroidism
Lithium	
Immobilization of adolescents or patients with Paget's disease of the bone	Rhabdomyolysis (recovery phase of acute tubular necrosis)

the cause of hypercalcemia in most patients. Asymptomatic hypercalcemia is found in many elderly patients and is usually due to primary hyperparathyroidism. Marked hypercalcemia is almost always due to malignancy or dehydration in a previously hypercalcemic patient.

Treatment

Mild hypercalcemia (serum calcium 10.5–12.0 mg/dl) usually requires only a careful diagnostic work-up and is rarely associated with systemic symptoms unless co-existent hypoproteinemia is present. Significant hypercalcemia (greater than 13.0 mg/dl) generally requires aggressive treatment, especially if significant neurologic or cardiovascular complications are present. Initial treatment consists of administration of normal saline at 200–500 ml/hour, depending on the patient's fluid status. Hypercalcemia commonly results in a nephrogenic diabetes insipidus that causes fluid losses prior to the patient's presentation. Administration of normal saline is recommended in most hypercalcemic patients because (1) they are usually volume depleted and (2) infusion of normal saline usually results in prompt lowering of calcium levels. This process may require a Foley catheter to monitor urine outputs and/or a central venous line to monitor volume status. Aggressive fluid administration should be followed by administration of a diuretic such as furosemide in doses of 10–80 mg intravenously to induce a sodium and calcium diuresis only after intravascular volume has been adequately replaced and expanded. This "flushout" procedure is remarkably effective in the majority of cases and will restore calcium to a safe level. Replacement and monitoring of potassium and magnesium levels are quite important, especially in patients undergoing large saline diuresis. Further treatment is quite controversial, is variable, and is influenced by the underlying cause of the hypercalcemia.[4]

Calcitonin. Dosage is 200–800 MRC units intramuscularly in divided doses two to three times daily. This treatment is very effective in primary hyperparathyroidism and in hypercalcemia associated with immobilization states. Effect in hypercalcemia of malignancy is much more variable and may be quite transient.

Oral Phosphates. Oral phosphates can be given 1.5–2.0 gm orally per day in divided doses three to four times per day. The predominant indication arises in patients with hypophosphatemia in association with hypercalcemia; phosphate therapy should never be used in hyperphosphatemic patients (vitamin D intoxication, immobilization).

Glucocorticoids. Glucocorticoids are most effective in vitamin D intoxication and hypercalcemia in malignancies known to be steroid responsive (lymphoma, leukemia, multiple myeloma). Dosage of prednisone is 40–80 mg per day. Glucocorticoids in combination with calcitonin prolongs the effectiveness of calcitonin.

Mithramycin. Dosage is 25 µg/kg intravenously every 2–5 days. Therapy is simple and very effective in hyperparathyroidism and hypercalcemia of malignancy associated with increased osteoclast activity (squamous cell carcinoma of the head, neck, lung; renal cell carcinoma; etc.). Effect may not take place for several days but may last for days or even weeks. Mithramycin can be given in an outpatient oncology clinic setting. The drug may cause problems with marrow toxicity and thrombocytopenia in cancer patients previously treated with chemotherapy. Increased toxicity is seen with renal failure or hepatic failure.

Prostaglandin Inhibitors. Indomethacine dosage is 100–150 mg per day. These drugs have unpredictable, variable responses. They may interfere with preservation of intrarenal hemodynamics in patients with volume contraction, congestive heart failure, and dehydration.

Intravenous Phosphates. These agents should only be used as a last resort in hypercalcemic patients refractory to other treatments in association with hypophosphatemia. Dosage should never exceed 50 mmol per day. Danger of ectopic calcification exists.

Dialysis. Dialysis against a low-calcium bath is effective but is usually only used as a last resort in refraction hypercalcemia.

Generally, removal or ablation (chemotherapy, radiation) of tumors associated with humorally related hypercalcemia may result in dramatic improvement in the hypercalcemia. Frequently, patients are treated with multiple drugs and improvement in the hypercalcemia is probably multifactorial. In patients in whom hypercalcemia is a significant complication of malignancy, control of the hypercalcemia may be an important determinant of patient well-being. Unfortunately, hypercalcemia frequently accounts for readmission of oncology patients to the hospital and difficulties in controlling the hypercalcemia prolong their hospital course.

Hypocalcemia

Hypocalcemia must also be interpreted with respect to endogenous calcium binders (mainly albumin: 0.8 mg/dl calcium per 1 gm/dl albumin), since the unbound (ionized) calcium levels determine the signs, symptoms, and severity of hypocalcemia. This is an important point, because abnormalities in ionized calcium levels may be present in patients with abnormalities of binding proteins. True (ionized) hypocalcemia is almost always caused by deficient production or action of parathyroid hormone (PTH) and/or vitamin D. Occasionally, precipitation of calcium by phosphate (rhabdomyolysis, exogenous parenteral phosphate therapy, renal failure with retention of phosphate) or chelating agents (large volumes of blood products) produces hypocalcemia. Hypocalcemia is frequently present in patients with multi-organ failure and sepsis; the etiology is multifactorial, and hypocalcemic patients have a poorer prognosis. Rapid decreases in ionized calcium produce more marked symptoms and signs than gradual hypocalcemia. Signs and symptoms of hypocalcemia include the following:

- Tetany
- Laryngospasm, seizures, muscle weakness, paresthesias (circumoral, acral)
- Chvostek's and Trousseau's signs
- Carpopedal spasm
- Hypotension
- Prolonged QT interval

Usually, a careful history and physical examination and a few simple biochemical tests reveal the cause of hypocalcemia. Common causes of hypocalcemia include the following:

- Hypoparathyroidism (surgery, autoimmune, infiltrative)
- Hypomagnesemia (decreased PTH and decreased PTH action)
- Renal failure (acute and chronic)
- Hypoalbuminemia (factitious)
- Vitamin D deficiency or resistance
- Phosphate overload (renal failure, iatrogenic, rhabdomyolysis)
- Acute pancreatitis (especially hemorrhagic, worsened by hypomagnesemia)
- "Hungry bones" after parathyroidectomy
- Chelating agents

Treatment

Treatment is obviously influenced by severity of the hypocalcemic signs and symptoms. Hypomagnesemia is a commonly overlooked cause that is easily treated with magnesium repletion (see section on hypomagnesemia) and is refractory to even parenteral calcium treatment. Treatment of frank hypocalcemic tetany involves parenteral calcium replacement with 200–300 mg of elemental calcium until tetany resolves. This can be given as either calcium gluconate (93 mg of calcium/10 ml) or calcium chloride (360 mg of calcium/10 ml). If tetany recurs, 15 mg/kg of calcium should be administered intravenously over 4–6 hours. After acute hypocalcemic tetany is treated, futher therapy is dictated by the patient's clinical status, follow-up calcium values, and the underlying cause. Permanent hypoparathyroidism (surgery, infiltration, etc.) usually requires large doses of vitamin D (50,000 U/day) with supplemental calcium. Correction of hyperphosphatemia (antacid phosphate binders, dialysis) is frequently necessary in renal failure patients. In hypomagnesemic patients, magnesium repletion is commonly associated with resolution of hypocalcemia.

MAGNESIUM

Hypomagnesemia

One third of extracellular magnesium circulates bound to proteins, and the remaining two thirds is free or unbound. Normal magnesium levels range from 1.6 to 2.1 mEq/L. Because only 1–2% of body stores of magnesium are extracellular, magnesium levels may not always accurately reflect total body stores. However, clinically significant magnesium deficiency is usually associated with low serum magnesium levels. One third to two thirds of dietary magnesium is absorbed in the ileum, and this absorption is partially influenced by vitamin D. Unbound magnesium is filtered by the glomerulus, 10–20% is resorbed in the proximal convoluted renal tubule, and 60–70% is absorbed in the thick ascending limb of Henle. The remainder is poorly absorbed in sites distal to these. Unlike ionized calcium levels, ionized magnesium levels are not under tight homeostatic hormonal control. As such, hypomagnesemia occurs when intake, GI absorption, or renal resorption is decreased. Conversely, hypermagnesemia almost never occurs with intact renal function.

Hypomagnesemia produces signs and symptoms of neuromuscular excitability that include tremor, fasciculations, tetany, dysphagia, carpopedal spasm, nystagmus, muscle weakness, paresthesias, supraventricular tachyarrhythmias, ventricular arrhythmias, and seizures. In addition, severe hypomagnesemia causes hypocalcemia (as a result of deficient PTH production and action) and is frequently associated with hypokalemia. Potassium depletion may be due to other factors in critically ill patients, but repletion of body stores of potassium is difficult unless hypomagnesemia is also corrected. This is presumably a result of suboptimal function of the sodium/potassium ATPase in the hypomagnesemic patient. Although the causes of hypomagnesemia can be thought of as due to decreased intake, decreased gastrointestinal absorption, increased renal losses, or shifts into intracellular compartments, hypomagnesemic patients frequently have a combination of these factors. Causes of hypomagnesemia include those listed in Table 2.

Treatment. Mild or incidentally discovered hypomagnesemia may be treated with oral replacement with magnesium oxide tablets or magnesium-containing antacids. Unfortunately, the cathartic effects of oral magnesium preparations limit their use and significant magnesium deficiency usually requires parenteral replacement. Hypomagnesemic patients usually need 1.0–2.0 mEq/kg of parenteral magnesium (1 gm of magnesium sulfate con-

TABLE 2.   CAUSES OF HYPOMAGNESEMIA

Renal losses
   Solute diuresis (glucose, mannitol, urea, sodium)
   Diuretics
   Renal tubular resorption defects (renal tubular acidosis, postobstructive
      diuresis, diuretic phase of acute tubular necrosis)
   Aminoglycosides
   Cisplatin
   Hyperaldosteronism
   Acute alcohol ingestion
Decreased gastrointestinal absorption (small bowel resection or irradia-
      tion, malabsorption, steatorrhea)
   Chronic diarrhea
   Decreased intake
   Starvation
Postoperative patients (multifactorial)
Intracellular shifts
   Insulin therapy (especially treated diabetic ketoacidosis)
   Respiratory alkalosis
   Alcohol withdrawal
Sequestration
   Healing bones
   Pancreatitis

tains 8.1 mEq of magnesium) over several days. One third to two thirds of parenterally administered magnesium is lost in the urine, and patients with normal renal function can excrete up to 40–60 gm of magnesium sulfate in 24 hours. Repletion can be given intravenously or intramuscularly; intravenous supplementation may be simpler and certainly less painful. However, large rapid intravenous doses are *quite dangerous* and IV flow rates must be monitored if large amounts of magnesium sulfate are added to the IV solution. A rough guide for intravenous repletion is 8–12 gm of magnesium sulfate intravenously on day one and 5–6 gm per day on days 2–5 for severely depleted patients. Extreme caution and much lower doses must be used in conjunction with frequent monitoring of serum magnesium levels in patients with poor renal function or reduced urine flow rates. In severely hypomagnesemic patients wth arrhythmias or seizures, intravenous administration of 2–4 gm of magnesium sulfate as a 10–20% solution over five to ten minutes may be used, followed by intravenous repletion over several days.[5]

Hypermagnesmia

Hypermagnesemia is fairly rare and is almost always caused by exogenous magnesium loads (magnesium sulfate IV solutions, enemas, antacids) in a patient with impaired renal function (acute or chronic renal failure, urinary obstruction, toxemia, severe volume contraction).[6] Levels in excess of 4–5 mEq/L are usually required before signs and symptoms become apparent. Levels of 5–10 mEq/L are usually associated with loss of deep tendon reflexes and ECG changes (P-R interval and QRS prolongation, bradycardia). Levels in excess of 10–15 mEq/L may result in muscle paralysis, complete heart block, and asystole. Treatment of hypermagnesemia includes removal of the exogenous magnesium load and correction of reversible causes of renal insufficiency. Dialysis to remove magnesium may be necessary if levels remain dangerously elevated. Intravenous calcium (100–200 mg), which may antagonize some of the effects of hypermagnesemia, can be given in the interim.

HYPOPHOSPHATEMIA

Phosphorus is found throughout the body in many forms that play important roles in the maintenance of cellular structure and function. Body stores are 700–800 gm; 85% of this is in the bone, and the remaining 15% is in the soft tissue (muscle, liver). Only 1% of the total body phosphorus is in the extracellular compartment and is in the form of phosphates. Serum phosphorus levels range from 2.5 to 4.5 mg/dl and may vary as much as 2 mg/dl during the course of a day. This is predominantly due to intracellular shifts of phosphorus when carbohydrates are ingested. Intracellular phosphorus is present in many forms of obvious structural and functional importance, such as ATP, ADP, 2,3-DPG, phospholipids, NAD/NADH, RNA, DNA, and glycolytic pathway intermediates. As with other predominantly intracellular elements (potassium, magnesium), depletion of total body phosphorus may occur in spite of normal extracellular levels. Common clinical examples of this situation are catabolic patients at initial presentation (burns, starvation, diabetic ketoacidosis, alcoholic ketoacidosis). When these patients are treated and "nutritional recovery" is initiated by administration of calories and/or insulin, phosphates are rapidly shifted intracellularly as glycolysis takes place, marked hypophosphatemia becomes apparent, and tissues (such as formed elements of the blood, central nervous system, etc.) may manifest dysfunction as a result of hypophosphatemia.[7] Hypophosphatemia that is due to rapid intracellular shifts can also occur in spite of normal total body phosphorus. This occurs in marked respiratory alkalosis, presumably owing to the intracellular alkalosis stimulating glycolysis. Antacids that bind dietary phosphates and phosphates in intestinal secretions can lead to marked phosphorus depletion. Finally, there are several conditions associated with decreased gastrointestinal absorption of phosphates (vitamin D deficiency, malabsorption) or enhanced renal losses of phosphates (primary or secondary hyperparathyroidism, diuretics, renal tubular defects, solute diuresis, volume expansion). In practice, most patients who display clinically significant hypophosphatemia or phosphorus depletion have a combination of several of the cited causes.[8] Not uncommonly, hypophosphatemia becomes apparent 1 to 2 days after admission of an ill patient, owing to medical treatment that does not take phosphorus depletion and intracellular shifts into account. For example, consider the chronically malnourished alcoholic patient suffering from chronic pancreatitis (with malabsorption and vitamin D deficiency) and gastritis (treated with phosphate-binding antacids) who enters the hospital dehydrated in moderate alcoholic ketoacidosis and alcohol withdrawal (respiratory alkalosis) and is treated with intravenous glucose and saline (intracellular shift of phosphates).

Severe phosphorus deficiency (<1 mg/dl) is usually seen in the following situations:
- Alcoholic ketoacidosis with withdrawal
- Treated diabetic ketoacidosis
- Burns
- Nutritional recovery syndrome
- Hyperalimentation with inadequate phosphorus repletion
- Respiratory alkalosis

Clinical manifestations of phosphorus depletion or hypophosphatemia vary from mild to severe and are obviously influenced by coexisting metabolic derangements and underlying diseases. Frequently, abnormalities of potassium, magnesium, and calcium may coexist in the hypophosphatemic patients and clinical manifestations such as muscle weakness may be due to a combination of these abnormalities. Unfortunately, there are almost no highly specific, classic manifestations that can be solely attributed to phosphorus abnormalities and repaired completely by phosphorus repletion alone. The main areas of clinical expression of phosphorus depletion include those listed in Table 3.

Treatment. Phosphorus levels of <1 mg/dl are considered severe and usually require treatment, especially if there is evidence of tissue hypoxia, significant respiratory or skeletal muscle weakness, hemolysis, bleeding,

TABLE 3.   CLINICAL EXPRESSION OF PHOSPHORUS DEPLETION

Central nervous system
  Altered cognitive function
  Delirium/confusion
  Obtundation/coma
  Seizures
Muscle
  Weakness/myopathy
  Increased creatine kinase
  Frank rhabdomyolysis
Hematologic
  Decreased 2,3-DPG (impaired oxygen release from hemoglobin)
  Hemolysis/spherocytosis
  Platelet dysfunction
  WBC dysfunction
Skeletal
  Bone pain and osteomalacia

infection, or altered central nervous system function. Phosphorus levels of 1.0–2.5 mg/dl are considered moderately decreased and probably should be treated if clinical signs and symptoms consistent with phosphorus depletion are present. If patients are able to take fluids or medications orally, replacement can be given as potassium phosphate tablets or capsules (1 gm of phosphorus per day), or more simply as a quart of skim milk per day (1 gm of phosphorus per quart). Phosphasoda contains 1.5 gm of phosphorus/ml, but it is quite hyperosmotic and may produce diarrhea. In hypophosphatemic patients who cannot take oral medications or food or in severely hypophosphatemic patients with clinical signs of phosphorus deficiency, parenteral therapy can be used. Initial dosage should be 0.08–0.16 mmol of phosphorus/kg* given over 6–8 hours and should never exceed 0.24 mmol of phosphorus/kg in one 6–8 hour infusion.[9] Phosphorus levels should be monitored to avoid hyperphosphatemia, which may cause dangerous hypocalcemia.

KEY FEATURES

- Calcium levels must be interpreted in the light of the levels of binders, since free calcium levels are the most physiologically important.
- Markedly elevated calcium levels are treated with large amounts of fluid replacement (normal saline), followed by a program of saline diuresis with careful replacement of potassium and magnesium losses.
- Therapy of acute hypercalcemia is governed by the severity of the hypercalcemia and the underlying cause. Treatments may vary markedly from patient to patient and must be individually tailored to the patient's cardiovascular and renal status and underlining cause of the hypercalcemia.
- Interpret calcium levels with respect to level of calcium binders and signs of symptoms of hypocalcemia.
- Search for underlying cause.
- Correct secondary factors (hyperphosphatemia, hypomagnesemia).
- Examine the patient carefully during treatment for signs and symptoms of neuromuscular excitability.
- Magnesium is a predominantly intracellular cation important in many enzymatic reactions throughout the body.
- Magnesium is not under tight homeostatic control, and as such decreased intake, decreased gastrointestinal absorption, or enhanced renal losses readily result in hypomagnesemia.
- Hypomagnesemia produces signs and symptoms of neuromuscular excitability.

---

*Concentrated parenteral potassium phosphate usually contains 4 mEq potassium and 3 mmol phosphorus/ml.

- Significant magnesium depletion almost always requires parenteral replacement.
- Hypermagnesemia is rare unless renal function is impaired.
- Severe hypophosphatemia and clinical phosphorus deficiency occur in several very predictable clinical settings.
- Watch for hypophosphatemia during treatment in patients at high risk (respiratory alkalosis, refeeding, alcohol withdrawal, alcoholic and diabetic ketoacidosis).
- Severe hypophosphatemia is often accompanied by other metabolic abnormalities (hypokalemia, hypocalcemia, hypomagnesemia).
- Hypophosphatemia should be treated with oral supplementations if possible. Many patients go through a hypophosphatemic phase during hospitalization and recovery; not all of these patients require treatment. Remember: don't treat yesterday's lab value, treat today's patient.

REFERENCES

1. Agus ZA, et al: Disorders of calcium and magnesium homeostasis. Am J Med 72:473–488, 1982.
    Scholarly discussion of divalent cation homeostatic mechanisms and common abnormalities.

2. Heath DA: The emergency management of disorders of calcium and magnesium. Clin Endocrinol Metab 9:487–502, 1980.
    Very brief but complete discussion of treatment aspects of acutely ill patients.

3. Lee DR, et al: The pathophysiology and clinical aspects of hypercalcemic disorders. West J Med 129:278–320, 1978.
    The best review of hypercalcemia to date; understandable explanations and clinical applications.

4. Mundy GR: The hypercalcemia of malignancy: Pathogenesis and management. Metab 31:1247–1277, 1982.
    Well-organized, complete overview of the hypercalcemia of cancer with excellent section on treatment aspects.

5. Geiderman JM, et al: Magnesium—the forgotten electrolyte. JACEP 8:204–208, 1979.
    Excellent discussion of hypomagnesemia. Packed with valuable information and superbly referenced.

6. Mordes JP, Wacker WE: Excess magnesium. Pharmacol Rev 29:273–293, 1978.
    Lengthy article on hypermagnesemia and its effects on tissues.

7. Knochel JP: The pathophysiology and clinical characteristics of severe hypophosphatemia. Arch Intern Med 137:203, 1977.
    A classic article that covers every aspect of phosphorus, including basic science investigations. Essential background reading for an understanding of phosphorus abnormalities.

8. Kreisberg RA: Phosphorus deficiency and hypophosphatemia. Hosp Pract 12:121–128, 1977.
    Clinically oriented review of phosphorus abnormalities frequently encountered in practice; good table of treatment modalities.

9. Lentz RD, et al: Treatment of severe hypophosphatemia. Ann Intern Med 89:941–944, 1978.
    Superb article on treatment with dosage guidelines and an excellent table of contents of commonly used phosphorus preparations.

Diabetic Ketoacidosis

Karen Henley, M.D.

Diabetes mellitus (DM) is a complex disorder that has its basis in insulin deficiency. The pathogenesis of diabetes mellitus is unknown, but it is most likely multifactorial in orgin. These factors include genetic predisposition; gene transformation; and exposure to specific viruses, toxins, and antibodies. Thus, the current division of diabetes mellitus into specific subtypes is, at best, crude and, possibly, inaccurate. Those patients who have an absolute insulin deficiency and, therefore, are at increased risk to develop ketosis are termed type I (or IDDM or ketosis-prone). Patients who have type II DM have a *relative* insulin deficiency (in relationship to their elevated serum glucose). The insulin these individuals secrete protects them from developing ketosis because much less insulin is needed to inhibit free fatty acid metabolism and ketone production than to normalize blood glucose.[1] It should be understood that under certain conditions type II diabetics may develop diabetic ketoacidosis (DKA).[2] This is due to the inability of these individuals to respond to the increased insulin demands imposed by infection, inflammation, trauma, or other endocrine disorders. In these situations, the insulin that is available is antagonized by "stress hormones" such as catecholamines, cortisol, glucagon, and growth hormone.

DKA, characterized by hyperglycemia and ketonemia, still carries a mortality rate of 5–15% despite advances in treatment. These deaths often are due to concurrent infection, myocardial infarction, vascular thrombosis, or acute pancreatitis, all of which may have precipitated the DKA.[2,3]

In order to recognize and treat DKA, it is important to understand its pathophysiology. Insulin is the major anabolic hormone in humans. Without insulin, the liver produces glucose via gluconeogenesis and glycogenolysis. The substrates for these metabolic pathways are amino acids and lactic acid from muscle cells, and glycerol from adipocytes. Insulin deficiency is the major stimulus for the mobilization of free fatty acids. The increased circulating free fatty acids are taken up by the liver and converted to keto acids rather than triglycerides. Keto acids are produced preferentially by the liver in response to an elevated glucagon to insulin ratio in the portal vasculature.[4]

The stress-induced release of counterregulatory hormones (catecholamines, cortisol, and growth hormone) promotes further secretion of glucagon, directly stimulates gluconeogenesis, and antagonizes the effects of circulating insulin on peripheral glucose utilization.[5,6]

The combination of hyperglycemia and ketonemia causes a significant osmotic diuresis. The anionic ketones promote the obligatory excretion of cations, such as sodium and potassium, which results in volume depletion and hypokalemia, respectively. Other inorganic solutes, including calcium, phosphate, and magnesium, also are depleted in association with the diuresis.

CLINICAL PRESENTATION

It is not uncommon for a previously undiagnosed diabetic to first present with DKA, although most patients have a history of diabetes.[2] Symptoms of DKA include thirst, polyuria, weakness, weight loss, vomiting with or without abdominal pain, and altered sensorium. Although cessation of insulin is often the cause of DKA, there should always be a careful search for a precipitating event, especially infection.[2,3] Medications, such as glucocorticoids, beta adrenergic blockers, and thiazides, can all exacerbate DKA.

On examination, patients are usually tachypneic with Kussmaul's respirations occurring when the arterial pH falls below 7.20. A fruit-like odor is generally present on the patient's breath, reflecting ketone production. Blood pressure is usually in the normal range despite volume depletion. Hypotension, when present, portends a poor prognosis.[3] Because hypothermia is common, a normal or even subnormal temperature can occur in the presence of infection. Moreover, an elevated temperature is highly suggestive of an underlying infection. Abdominal pain, with mild abdominal tenderness and hypoactive bowel sounds, is common, and may be due to the ketoacidosis or to pancreatitis. The majority of patients will be drowsy or will have difficulty thinking clearly, with 10% of patients in DKA developing frank coma.[7]

Initial laboratory assessment should include urinalysis, serum electrolytes, glucose, BUN, creatinine, amylase, calcium, phosphate, CBC, blood cultures, electrocardiogram, chest radiograph, and arterial blood gases. Much of the initial diagnostic laboratory measurements can be performed at the bedside. Blood glucose can be measured quickly by using one of the many available glucose oxidase reagent strips. In general, blood glucose levels average 500 mg/dl in patients with DKA. However, in younger individuals the blood glucose can be nearly normal, and with severe dehydration, it can be over 1000 mg/dl. The determining factor for the degree of hyperglycemia appears to be the severity of volume depletion, rather than the degree of acidosis.[4] When a diabetic cannot keep up with urine loss, glomerular filtration rate decreases with a subsequent decrease in glucose excretion. Patients with DKA can have a dramatic decrease in their serum glucose concentration when treated solely with fluids in the absence of insulin.[4] As a consequence of volume depletion, the hematocrit, BUN, and creatinine are often elevated. The serum creatinine can be falsely elevated, because acetoacetate interferes with the creatinine assay in autoanalyzers.

The metabolic acidosis that occurs in DKA is due to excess accumulation of acetoacetate and beta hydroxybutyrate in plasma. Urine ketones will invariably be present. However, if sodium nitroprusside tablets are used, the reaction may be nondiagnostic, because sodium nitroprusside does not react with beta hydroxybutyrate, the principal ketone formed in DKA.

Serum sodium is usually low despite volume depletion and plasma hypertonicity.[3] This is due, in part, to obligatory sodium loss with the ketonuria. The intravascular glucose also acts as a nonpenetrating solute, with sodium entering the intracellular space to equalize the osmotic forces. Severe hypertriglyceridemia also can contribute to a low plasma sodium concentration.

On admission, the patient's plasma potassium level tends to be elevated if there is profound acidosis.[3] However, the potassium level also depends on previous nutritional intake, renal function, and the degree of dehydration. It should be kept in mind that plasma potassium levels do not accurately reflect total body stores of potassium, which are invariably depleted. The initial ECG can be very helpful in assessing tissue potassium levels.[8]

Another laboratory finding that is often present is an elevated amylase level.[3] This may occur in association with acute pancreatitis, but it can be a nonspecific finding as a result of decreased renal clearance of pancreatic and salivary gland amylase.

Leukocytosis is a common finding in DKA. This can be a result of elevated catecholamine and cortisol secretion, although underlying infection still must be investigated.

TREATMENT

The major goals in treatment of DKA are to correct the volume depletion, the insulin deficiency, and the metabolic abnormalities. The osmotic diuresis produced by the hyperglycemia and ketonemia causes significant extracellular volume depletion that should be replaced initially with isotonic saline. Approximately 50% of the estimated fluid loss should be restored over the first 6–8 hours. The remaining fluid deficit can be replaced over the next 12–24 hours. If the patient becomes hypernatremic during the course of therapy, 0.45% saline can be used.

Although fluids will lower plasma glucose concentrations even in the absence of insulin, insulin is needed to halt the continuing catabolic processes. Insulin blocks the release of glucagon and enhances peripheral utilization of glucose. Initially, extremely high doses of insulin were used to treat DKA. In the 1970s, it was discovered that there is a finite plasma insulin concentration at which maximum effect is achieved. At low concentrations, lipolysis, glycogenolysis, and gluconeogenesis are inhibited. At insulin levels of 100 μU/ml, hepatic ketogenesis is blocked. With a concentration of 200 μU/ml, there is maximum stimulation for glucose uptake into cells.[1] Excessive administration of insulin is unnecessary and may cause an increased incidence of hypoglycemia and hypokalemia. The current standard of practice is the so-called low-dose insulin regimen.[4,5,6] An example of this regimen is as follows: A small initial intravenous bolus of 10–20 U crystalline (regular) insulin is given. This is followed by an infusion of insulin piggybacked into the main fluid line at the rate of 5–10 U/hour or 0.1 U/kg/hour. Thus, both the fluid and insulin can be adjusted separately, depending on the patient's requirements. The exact rate of insulin infusion is determined by measuring the blood glucose level every 1–2 hours using reagent strips. After an initial rapid decrease in serum glucose as a result of fluid replacement, the ideal decrease in blood glucose should be 50–100 mg/dl/hour. Rarely, insulin resistance is encountered, often secondary to underlying infection. If the blood glucose level does not fall accordingly, the infusion rate should be doubled every hour until a satisfactory result is achieved. The insulin infusion should not be discontinued until the patient's ketosis and acidemia have resolved. It is not uncommon for the hyperglycemia to resolve in 4–8 hours, whereas the acidosis may take 10–20 hours to correct and ketonuria can persist for 24–48 hours. When the serum glucose concentration has fallen to approximately 250 mg/dl, a 5% dextrose infusion should be initiated, and the insulin infusion can be decreased to 0.03 U/kg/hour. In most patients with DKA, insulin given as an intramuscular injection every 1–2 hours can work as effectively as a continuous infusion.[9] However, this route of therapy should not be utilized if there is any evidence of severe hypovolemia with decreased tissue perfusion.

Although total body potassium stores are invariably depleted in patients with DKA, the initial serum potassium concentration is usually normal or elevated.[3,4] Thus, potassium should not be administered initially, unless the patient is hypokalemic on presentation. With fluid and insulin therapy, potassium moves into the intracellular compartment. There is also continuing urinary potassium loss. Potassium supplementation at the rate of 20–40 mM/hour of potassium chloride can be instituted when serum potassium is in the normal range.

Treatment of the metabolic acidosis with bicarbonate is generally not necessary. It is often used when profound acidosis (pH less than 7.0 or bicarbonate less than 8 mM) is present, because of the common occurrence of myocardial depression and arrhythmias with this degree of acidosis. When used, sodium bicarbonate should be added to the fluid-electrolyte solution until the arterial pH is 7.2 or the plasma bicarbonate is 12 mM. Bicarbonate therapy should not be given indiscriminately, because rapid alkalinization can exacerbate hypokalemia, potentiate lactic acidosis, and possibly worsen cerebral acidosis.[10]

Most patients with DKA have pronounced phosphate depletion with an average deficit of 0.5–1.5 mM/kg, yet the initial plasma values may range anywhere from supranormal to subnormal.[5] With routine treatment of DKA, plasma phosphate usually falls as a result of the intracellular movement of phosphate. With severe hypophosphatemia, rhabdomyolysis, muscle weakness, depressed myocardial function, respiratory failure, hemolysis, and altered consciousness can occur. However, these events appear to be quite rare in patients with DKA.[4] Studies that compare patients treated with, and without, phosphate supplementation have shown no effect on morbidity or mortality.[11,12] In addition, treatment with phosphate can induce hypocalcemia, and too rapid an infusion of phosphate even can cause tetany.[11] If the pretreatment phosphate level is low (less than 1.0 mg/dl) or if complications as a result of hypophosphatemia are suspected, cautious replacement with potassium phosphate at 20–40 mM over 8–12 hours can be infused. Oral phosphate in the form of milk can be administered safely as soon as the patient is tolerating fluids by mouth.

Patients with DKA are at increased risk for developing arterial thrombosis, particularly in the cerebral vasculature. This occurs because of the combination of underlying atherosclerosis, hyperosmolality, increased blood viscosity, and alterations in circulating coagulation factors.[4] Fatal cerebral edema has been reported in children, but fortunately it is quite rare. The cause is not yet known, but it may be related to rapid changes in plasma oncotic pressure. Infection commonly complicates DKA but only rarely is a cause of death. Pneumonia and pyelonephritis are the most common infections,[3] but mucormycosis is a rare infection that has a unique association with ketoacidosis. It usually presents as a sinusitis with a bloody nasal discharge that, if not promptly treated with amphotericin, can lead rapidly to orbital swelling, proptosis, altered consciousness, and death. However, recovery from DKA is usually not problematic if patients are given appropriate treatment. Special care should be taken if the patient is elderly or has underlying cardiovascular disease (especially congestive failure or acute myocardial infarction) or renal failure.

KEY FEATURES

Diabetic ketoacidosis (DKA) is caused by an absolute insulin deficiency and is characterized by hyperglycemia and ketonemia.

A thorough search for a precipitating event should always be undertaken.

Physical examination should be directed at alterations in temperature, breathing pattern, and blood pressure. Signs of volume depletion, cardiac status, neurologic changes, and possible sources of infection need to be assessed.

Laboratory abnormalities include mild to severe hyperglycemia, metabolic ketoacidosis; and elevated BUN, creatinine, hematocrit, and amylase. Total body depletion of potassium and phosphate are invariably present. Leukocytosis is frequently observed, even in the absence of infection.

Treatment is aimed at correcting volume depletion, uncontrolled catabolism, and metabolic disturbances. This is initially accomplished with isotonic saline infusion, a continuous intravenous insulin infusion, and bicarbonate when indicated. Potassium and phosphate depletion should be corrected judiciously.

REFERENCES

1. Padilla AJ, Loeb JN: "Low dose" versus "high dose" insulin regimens in the management of uncontrolled diabetes. Am J Med 63:843, 1977.
   Editorial review of low-dose and high-dose insulin regimens. Discusses the physiologic basis for various insulin regimens and the arguments in favor of and against various doses of insulin.

2. Johnson DD, Palumbo PJ, Chu C: Diabetic ketoacidosis in a community-based population. Mayo Clinic Proc 55:83, 1980.
   Retrospective study of 92 cases of DKA. Discusses presentation, morbidity, and mortality.

3. Beigelman PM: Severe diabetic ketoacidosis (diabetic "coma"), 482 episodes in 257 patients; experience of three years. Diabetes 20:490, 1971.
   Extensive study of 482 episodes of DKA. Presents admission patient profile and laboratory examination, causes of DKA, and associated medical problems. Special reference is given to characteristics of the 32 fatal cases.

4. Foster DW, McGarry JD: The metabolic derangements and treatment of diabetic ketoacidosis. N Engl J Med 309:159, 1983.
   Excellent review of biochemical pathophysiology. Cogent discussion of presentation and treatment of DKA.

5. Kreisberg RA: Diabetic ketoacidosis: New concepts and trends in pathogenesis and treatment. Ann Intern Med 88:681, 1978.
   Good general review of pathophysiology and treatment of DKA. Brief discussion about alcoholic ketoacidosis (AKA).

6. Baruh S, Sherman L, Markowitz S: Diabetic ketoacidosis and coma. Med Clin North Am 65:117, 1981.
   General review of DKA. Includes table of differential diagnosis: DKA, AKA, nonketotic hyperosmotic coma, lactic acidosis, and hypoglycemia.

7. Guisado R, Arieff AI: Neurologic manifestations of diabetic comas: Correlation with biochemical alterations in the brain. Metabolism 42:665, 1975.
   In-depth discussion concerning neurologic changes associated with DKA and nonketotic hyperosmotic coma. Reviews biochemical alterations in the CNS and proposed mechanisms for cerebral edema.

8. Chaua RR: ECG in diabetic ketoacidosis. Arch Intern Med 144:2379, 1984.
   Brief paper on electrocardiographic changes observed with DKA.

9. Sacks HS, et al: Similar responsiveness of diabetic ketoacidosis to low-dose insulin by intramuscular injection and albumin-free infusion. Ann Intern Med 90:36, 1979.
   Prospective, randomized trial of 30 patients with DKA. There was no difference between the two groups in terms of control of DKA, morbidity, or mortality.

10. Lever E, Jaspan JB: Sodium bicarbonate therapy in severe diabetic ketoacidosis. Am J Med 75:263, 1983.
    Retrospective study of 95 episodes of DKA, comparing those treated with bicarbonate (73) with those without bicarbonate (22). There was no difference in any of the parameters measuring recovery from DKA.

11. Fischer JN, Kitabchi AE: A randomized study of phosphate therapy in the treatment of diabetic ketoacidosis. J Clin Endocrinol Metab 57:177, 1983.
    Prospective study of 30 patients with DKA, half of the study group receiving phosphate therapy. There was no difference in any of the recovery indices, and the ionized calcium levels were lower in those patients given phosphate.

12. Wilson RK, et al: Phosphate therapy in diabetic ketoacidosis. Arch Intern Med 142:517, 1982.
    Prospective study of 44 patients with DKA, randomized into three groups consisting of no phosphate therapy, 15 mM of potassium phosphate, and 45 mM of potassium phosphate. Only the last group maintained normal serum phosphate levels. There was no difference between groups in terms of recovery indices, morbidity, or mortality.

Hypoglycemia

Karen Henley, M.D.

Hypoglycemia is the most frequently encountered metabolic emergency. It should be considered in all patients with altered mental status, bizarre behavior, obtundation, or coma.

The most common cause of acute hypoglycemia is excess exogenous insulin. Factors that may contribute to insulin-induced hypoglycemia include decreased or delayed food intake, increased exercise, early pregnancy, excessive alcohol consumption with reduced carbohydrate intake, and an erroneous or accidental change in insulin regimen. Sulfonylurea-induced hypoglycemia is encountered less frequently, but it is more life-threatening than insulin-induced hypoglycemia because low blood glucose levels can persist for more than 24 hours despite treatment. The incidence of hypoglycemia is greater when large doses of sulfonylureas are used, but even small doses have been reported to cause hypoglycemia. Insulin levels are high during tbe hypoglycemic episodes and can remain elevated for more than 24 hours, irrespective of the reported half-life of that particular oral agent. Further insulin secretion often is stimulated with glucose therapy. In addition, other drugs can interact with sulfonylureas and produce hypoglycemia. These drugs include sulfonamides, chloramphenicol, salicylates, phenylbutazone, probenecid, dicumarol, beta adrenergic blockers, anabolic steroids, MAO inhibitors, and a decrease in glucocorticoid dosage.[1]

In the susceptible, nondiabetic individual, alcohol ingestion, coupled with a low-calorie, low-carbohydrate intake, also can result in hypoglycemia. Alcohol impairs hepatic glucose production by directly inhibiting gluconeogenesis via a decreased NAD:NADH ratio. With starvation, glycogen stores become depleted and hypoglycemia ensues.[2]

Other causes of profound hypoglycemia, such as insulinomas, adrenal insufficiency, panhypopituitarism, ectopic production of insulin-like growth factors, renal failure, severe liver failure, and profound congestive heart failure, are rare but should be considered in the appropriate situation.[2]

Hypoglycemia below 35–45 mg/dl usually produces a feeling of weakness, light-headedness, palpitations, and sweating. The autonomic response to hypoglycemia results in significant cardiovascular changes, including tachycardia, a rise in systolic blood pressure, a decrease in diastolic blood pressure, and an increase in peripheral blood flow.[3] Often there is hypothermia secondary to vasodilation and sweating. In conjunction with the release of catecholamines, hypoglycemia initiates the release of glucagon, cortisol, and growth hormone.[4] These hormones counteract the effects of insulin by promoting hepatic gluconeogenesis and peripheral lipolysis and by inhibiting glucose utilization in muscle. Glucagon and catecholamines are the most important hormones in promoting recovery from hypoglycemia. In individuals who have type I diabetes mellitus for greater than 2 years, there is usually a reduced glucagon secretory response to hypoglycemia.[5] These patients are then dependent on epinephrine for prevention of and recovery from hypoglycemia.[6,7] Thus, administration of beta adrenergic antagonists can blunt the warning symptoms of hypoglycemia, as well as prevent normal glucose recovery.[8] Some patients with long-standing type I diabetes also have deficient epinephrine secretion in response to hypoglycemia. These individuals are at 25 times greater risk for profound hypoglycemia than those with an intact epinephrine secretory response.[6]

The neuroglycopenic symptoms of confusion, lethargy, and frank coma may actually be protective, because there is less glucose and oxygen utilization by muscle and brain cells in the comatose state. However, seizures can occur if hypoglycemia is of rapid onset or is prolonged.

The initial treatment of hypoglycemia is standard, irrespective of etiology. Blood should be drawn for plasma glucose and, if possible, immediately measured with a glucose oxidase reagent strip. However, if the strips are not available and hypoglycemia is suspected, treatment should be initiated prior to obtaining the laboratory results. If the patient is conscious, oral administration of concentrated simple carbohydrates is preferred. If the patient is unconscious, intravenous administration of 50 cc of 50% dextrose in water (D50) should be given. If D50 is not available or an intravenous line is difficult to institute, subcutaneous glucagon (1 ml) may be given. As mentioned previously, sulfonylureas can produce severe and prolonged hypoglycemia for greater than 24 hours. It is imperative that these individuals be admitted to the hospital for observation and either oral or intravenous carbohydrate supplementation. Patients who have severe and prolonged hypoglycemia may remain comatose for an extended period of time. However, ingestion of other toxins, hypothermia, head trauma, and postictal obtundation also can complicate hypoglycemic coma and should be considered if the patient does not awaken promptly.

KEY FEATURES

Consider the diagnosis of hypoglycemia in any person who has altered mental function.

Common causes of hypoglycemia include excess insulin, sylfonylureas, and drug interactions with insulin or oral agents.

Type I diabetics without a normal secretory response of glucagon and epinephrine are at increased risk for hypoglycemia.

Patients can exhibit tachycardia with wide pulse pressures, hypothermia, and variable degrees of obtundation.

Treatment is composed of oral or intravenous glucose. Any person who has taken sulfonylureas should be hospitalized for extended observation.

REFERENCES

1. Seltzer HS: Drug-induced hypoglycemia. A review based on 473 cases. Diabetes 21:955, 1972.
   Review of major predisposing factors for drug-induced hypoglycemia. Compilation of all case reports of drug-induced hypoglycemia and their associated clinical presentations.

2. Fajans SS, Floyd JC: Fasting hypoglycemia in adults. N Engl J Med 294:766, 1976.
   Review of normal maintenance of euglycemia with fasting and extensive differential diagnosis of fasting hypoglycemia based on pathophysiology.

3. Hilsted J, et al: Haemodynamic changes in insulin-induced hypoglycemia in normal man. Diabetologia 26:328, 1984.
   Seven normal subjects were made hypoglycemic with IV insulin. Hemodynamic parameters were measured, including plasma volume, cardiac output, heart rate, blood pressure, and peripheral vascular resistance.

4. Cryer PE, Gerich JF: Glucose counter-regulation, hypoglycemia and intensive insulin therapy in diabetes mellitus. N Engl J Med 313:232, 1985.
    Good review of normal glucose homeostasis, counterregulatory mechanisms in non-diabetic and diabetic persons, and therapeutic implications.

5. Bolli G, et al: Abnormal glucose counter-regulation in insulin-dependent diabetes mellitus. Diabetes 32:134, 1983.
    Comparison of 21 diabetic patients and their counterregulatory hormone response to hypoglycemia, with reference to the duration of their diabetes.

6. White NH, et al: Identification of Type I diabetic patients at increased risk for hypoglycemia during intensive therapy. N Engl J Med 308:485, 1983.
    Intravenous infusion of insulin was administered to 22 patients with insulin-dependent diabetes mellitus (IDDM) to study their ability to recover from hypoglycemia and the relationship between their counterregulatory hormone response and recovery. Those patients with combined deficiencies in epinephrine and glucagon had the poorest recovery.

7. Bolli GB, et al: Abnormal glucose counter-regulation after subcutaneous insulin in insulin-dependent diabetes mellitus. N Engl J Med 310:1706, 1984.
    The response of 20 patients with IDDM to hypoglycemia was studied. Seventeen patients had more prolonged and severe hypoglycemia than controls. Those with rebound hyperglycemia had deficiencies in glucagon, epinephrine, norepinephrine, and cortisol response, as well as higher insulin-antibody binding.

8. Bolli G, et al: Important role of adrenergic mechanisms in acute glucose counter-regulation following insulin-induced hypoglycemia in Type I diabetes. Diabetes 31:641, 1982.
    Response of eight patients with IDDM and eight control subjects to insulin-induced hypoglycemia with and without alpha and/or beta adrenergic blockade.

Nonketotic Hyperosmolar Coma

Karen Henley, M.D.

Nonketotic hyperosmolar coma (NKHC) is discussed separately in this text, yet it has considerable biochemical overlap with diabetic ketoacidosis (DKA) and the two entities probably represent the extremes of a continuous spectrum.[1] As its name implies, NKHC is characterized by marked hyperglycemic hyperosmolarity without ketosis. Although patients with hyperosmolar coma may not appear acutely ill, they actually have a higher mortality rate than do patients with DKA.[2] Individuals who develop NKHC are older and may have no history of having diabetes mellitus or have only mild type II diabetes mellitus (noninsulin-dependent diabetes mellitus [NIDDM]).[3,4] In most patients, a precipitating event can be identified, such as sepsis, infection, myocardial infarction, stroke, or renal insufficiency.[3,4] Rarely, other endocrine diseases (thyrotoxicosis, acromegaly, Cushing's syndrome) are associated with NKHC. Various drugs, notably glucocorticoids, thiazide diuretics, beta adrenergic blockers, and phenytoin, also can precipitate NKHC.

Patients with NKHC have symptoms of hyperglycemia that develop slowly, over days to weeks.[3] These symptoms include polydipsia, polyuria, weakness, weight loss, and progressive mental dysfunction.

The physical examination is not as striking as in patients with DKA. Patients with NKHC generally demonstrate signs of severe dehydration and volume depletion (orthostatic hypotension, dry mucosa, poor skin turgor, tachycardia, shock) and various stages of obtundation ranging from lethargy to coma. They also may have transient focal neurologic findings and may be misdiagnosed as having had a stroke.[4,5]

As mentioned previously, the hallmark of NKHC is extreme hyperglycemia and hyperosmolarity without ketoacidosis. The plasma glucose concentration is often over 1000 mg/dl, reflecting profound fluid losses. Because there is usually more free water loss than sodium loss during the osmotic diuresis, sodium concentrations are often greater than 150 (mM) mEq/L.[4] If these values are corrected for intravascular osmotic glucose load, the calculated serum sodium concentration is even greater (the serum sodium level should be corrected by adding 1.6 mEq Na^+/L for every 100 mg/dl excess glucose). There is an obligatory sodium loss in the urine as a result of the "washout" of the renal tubule concentration gradient from the glycosuria. The sodium loss is reflected, primarily, in contraction of the extracellular space, rather than in hyponatremia. The increased intravascular oncotic pressure from the hyperglycemia usually protects the patient from hypovolemia. However, if the patient becomes severely volume depleted, signs of hypovolemia will be seen, including tachycardia, hypotension, and oliguria. Patients with NKHC also have a total body potassium deficit, although not to the same degree as in DKA. The potassium loss in these patients is due to the effects of aldosterone, secreted in response to sodium and volume depletion. By definition, individuals with NKHC do not have severe ketosis, although they may have a mild metabolic acidosis from accumulation of lactate, acetoacetate, and beta hydroxybutyrate.

The treatment of NKHC is similar to that of DKA. Immediate fluid replacement is essential. Isotonic saline is usually used, because hypovolemic shock with decreased tissue perfusion is more life-threatening than is hyperosmolarity. The rate of repletion depends upon the degree of fluid loss, cardiovascular status, and renal function, but in general the patient should receive at least one liter per hour for the first 3–4 hours. Once the patient's vital signs have stabilized and urine output is adequate, 0.45% saline can be instituted if the serum sodium concentration is greater than 155 mEq/L. Insulin therapy is often initiated simultaneously with fluid replacement, although the hyperglycemia can often be corrected with fluids alone.[6] The use of a low-dose insulin drip at 0.05–0.1 U/kg/hour can hasten recovery.

Again, it should be emphasized that an underlying and often precipitating illness is a frequent cause of the high mortality rate encountered in patients with NKHC and needs to be identified and treated aggressively.

KEY FEATURES

Nonketotic hyperosmolar coma (NKHC) is characterized by profound hyperglycemia without significant ketosis.

A precipitating or contributing event can usually be found. This includes infection, renal insufficiency, stroke, myocardial infarction, other endocrine disorders, and drug interactions.

Physical examination should focus on assessing the degree of volume depletion, neurologic deficits, and associated conditions.

Laboratory examination will usually reveal a markedly elevated blood glucose level, hypernatremia, mild hypokalemia, and occasionally a mild metabolic acidosis. Evidence of volume depletion will be reflected in an elevated hematocrit, BUN, and creatinine.

The mainstay of treatment is fluids, with care being taken in any patient who has impaired cardiac or renal function. Initially, isotonic saline is used until vital signs stabilize, then hypotonic saline can be substituted, depending upon the serum sodium concentrations. A low-dose insulin infusion can be used to hasten recovery.

REFERENCES

1. Malchoff CD, et al: Determinants of glucose and ketoacid concentrations in acutely hyperglycemic diabetic patients. Am J Med 77:275, 1984.

   There are a wide spectrum of serum glucose and ketoacid concentrations in diabetic patients. Ketoacid levels correlated best with high free fatty acid levels, low C-peptide levels, and increased body mass index.

2. Khardori R, Soler N: Hyperosmolar hyperglycemic nonketotic syndrome. Am J Med 77:899, 1984.

   Report of 22 patients in NKHC with discussion of pathophysiology, clinical presentation, and treatment.

3. Gerich JE, Martin MM, Recant L: Clinical and metabolic characteristics of hyperosmolar nonketotic coma. Diabetes 20:228, 1971.

   Comparison of characteristics of 20 patients with NKHC versus 10 patients with DKA. Treatment is somewhat outdated.

4. Arieff AI, Carroll HJ: Nonketotic hyperosmolar coma with hyperglycemia: Clinical features, pathophysiology, renal function, acid-base balance, plasma-cerebrospinal fluid equilibria and the effects of therapy in 37 cases. Medicine 51:73, 1972.

   Very detailed prospective study of 37 episodes of NKHC. Special attention is focused on clinical features, presentation, and precipitating factors. Some patients classified as having NKHC may have had DKA. (Outdated treatment section.)

5. Guisado R, Arieff AI: Neurologic manifestations of diabetic comas: Correlation with biochemical alterations in the brain. Metabolism 24:665, 1975.
    In-depth discussion concerning neurologic changes associated with DKA and NKHC.
    Reviews biochemical alterations in the CNS and proposed mechanisms for cerebral edema.

6. Mather HM: Management of hyperosmolar coma. J Royal Soc Med 73:134, 1980.
    General review of treatment of NKHC with special reference to diagnosis and treat-
    ment of associated or precipitating illnesses.

Alcoholic Ketoacidosis

Karen Henley, M.D.

Prolonged starvation causes mild ketoacidosis. Yet, when poor nutrition is combined with heavy alcohol use, severe ketoacidosis may ensue. The pathophysiology underlying the development of alcoholic ketoacidosis (AKA) is not understood fully. It is known that with alcohol consumption, gluconeogenesis and ketogenesis are inhibited. Both these changes result from an increased NADH:NAD ratio, induced by the metabolism of ethanol.[1,2] The effects of starvation, coupled with alcohol ingestion, produce a number of hormonal changes. Insulin secretion is suppressed, and serum levels of cortisol, glucagon, catecholamines, and growth hormone are elevated.[1,3] The increased levels of circulating stress hormones lead to mobilization of free fatty acids from adipocytes. Severe abdominal pain, accompanied by nausea and vomiting, often occurs under these conditions, and alcohol consumption may cease. When the ingested alcohol has been metabolized fully, ketogenesis is no longer inhibited. The high level of circulating free fatty acids is then rapidly oxidized to ketone bodies in the liver. As in diabetic ketoacidosis (DKA), the principal ketone formed is beta hydroxybutyrate (owing to the high NADH:NAD ratio). Low levels of circulating insulin may decrease peripheral ketone body utilization.[1]

Most patients with AKA have a history of poor nutritional intake and heavy alcohol consumption until 24–72 hours prior to their hospital admission. At that time, both alcohol and food intake is severely curtailed, owing to the development of nausea, vomiting, and abdominal pain. The physical examination is not specific, but it often reveals signs of volume depletion, tachypnea, and a distinct ketone odor on the patient's breath. Abdominal findings of mild to moderate tenderness may reflect the effects of ketoacidosis or underlying alcohol-related diseases. Signs of alcohol withdrawal may or may not be observed.

Although most patients with AKA demonstrate mild hyperglycemia (secondary to low insulin levels), some manifest frank hypoglycemia, if glucagon stores are completely depleted and gluconeogenesis is inhibited.[4] Ketoacidosis will be evident, often to a striking degree, owing to the mechanism described previously.[5] Frequently, severe magnesium and phosphate depletion is demonstrable.[2] These depletions arise from the combined effect of poor nutrition and urinary losses. Hypocalcemia may also result from the severe magnesium deficiency.

Treatment is similar to that of DKA, with fluid replacement the primary therapeutic intervention. This is usually in the form of D5NS* to correct the volume deficit and replenish carbohydrate stores.[6] A very small amount of insulin is often helpful to correct the ketosis, although there are no studies that show a beneficial effect on outcome with insulin therapy. Magnesium and phosphate replacement is usually warranted, and bicarbonate should be used if indicated by extreme acidosis. Importantly, thiamine, 100 mg intramuscularly or intravenously, should be given prior to institution of glucose therapy to preclude precipitation of Wernicke's encephalopathy. Other complications of alcohol abuse—withdrawal syndrome, pancreatitis, upper gastrointestinal tract hemorrhage, hepatitis, and/or hepatic failure, pneumonia, and peritonitis—must be considered, sought, and treated as indicated.

KEY FEATURES

Alcoholic ketoacidosis (AKA) is characterized by significant ketoacidosis and serum glucose levels that can vary from mild hyperglycemia to frank hypoglycemia.

Patients usually have a history of poor nutritional intake and heavy alcohol use until 24–72 hours prior to hospitalization. At that time, abdominal pain, nausea, and vomiting intervene and further curtail the intake of food, fluids, and alcohol, resulting in the biochemical and clinical syndrome of AKA.

Physical examination is notable for signs of volume depletion, abdominal tenderness, and other alcohol-related diseases (cirrhosis, pancreatitis, alcohol-withdrawal syndromes).

Laboratory examination is significant for glucose levels ranging from mild hyperglycemia to frank hypoglycemia, a combination of ketoacidosis and lactic acidosis, and magnesium and phosphate deficiency.

The key to treatment is fluids that contain glucose. Small amounts of insulin may be used but often are not necessary. Bicarbonate therapy usually is not indicated, but magnesium and phosphate should be repleted. Thiamine must be given prior to any form of therapy.

---

*D5NS = 5% dextrose in normal saline.

REFERENCES

1. Williams HE: Alcoholic hypoglycemia and ketoacidosis. Med Clin North Am 68:33, 1984.
   Very brief review of pathophysiology, clinical characteristics, and treatment of alcoholic hypoglycemia and ketoacidosis.

2. Isselbacher KJ: Metabolic and hepatic effects of alcohol. N Engl J Med 296:612, 1977.
   The effects of alcohol on carbohydrate, protein, and lipid metabolism, as well as the interactions of alcohol with other important functions (hematologic changes, drug interactions, magnesium and phosphate depletion and autonomic nervous system alterations).

3. Levy LJ, et al: Ketoacidosis associated with alcoholism in nondiabetic subjects. Ann Intern Med 78:213, 1973.
   Clinical study of six episodes of AKA. Discussion of clinical presentation and measurement of ketoacids, lactate, free fatty acids, stress hormones, and insulin.

4. Fulop M, Hoberman HD: Alcoholic ketoacidosis. Diabetes 24:785, 1975.
   Clinical study of 24 patients admitted with suspected AKA. Three patients who continued to drink alcohol shortly prior to admission had lactic acidosis. Clinical presentation and treatment are discussed.

5. Halperin ML, et al: Metabolic acidosis in the alcoholic: A pathophysiologic approach. Metabolism 32:308, 1983.
   Extensive review of acid-base alterations observed in patients with acute and chronic alcohol ingestion. Clinical features, laboratory findings, and treatment also are discussed briefly.

6. Miller PD, Heinig RE, Waterhouse C: Treatment of alcoholic acidosis: The role of dextrose and phosphorous. Arch Intern Med 138:67, 1978.
   Prospective study of 18 episodes of AKA, comparing treatment with 5% dextrose in water versus normal saline. There was more rapid clearing of the acidosis in the glucose-treated group. Authors also studied serum and urinary phosphate recovery in patients on a low versus normal phosphorous diet.

Adrenal Insufficiency

Ravin Davidoff, M.D.

Adrenal insufficiency may be defined as the state in which adrenal steroid production falls below the body's requirements. Normally, 13–20 mg of cortisol per day is produced by the zona fasciculata and zona reticularis of the adrenal gland. However, this is a dynamic process with fluctuations according to the body's needs. Corticotropin-releasing factor (CRF), a 41 amino acid peptide, is released from the hypothalamus and travels via the hypophyseal portal system to the anterior pituitary. There, adrenocorticotropic hormone (ACTH) is secreted as part of a large 31,000-dalton precursor molecule, pro-opiomelanocorticotropin (POMC). ACTH is cleaved from this substrate and acts rapidly on the adrenal gland to produce an increased concentration of steroid hormones in the blood. This appears to be mediated via membrane bound adenyl cyclase with the resultant increase in intracellular cAMP, protein kinase, and protein phosphorylation.

The normal unstressed person has about seven to ten biologic secretory episodes of ACTH per day. These episodes probably result from episodic CRF secretion. The resultant increase in cortisol exerts negative feedback control on the anterior pituitary and probably also on the hypothalamus and higher brain centers (e.g., hypocampus and reticular activating system). Under stress (e.g., fever, surgery, hypoglycemia, exercise, and severe emotional trauma), ACTH secretion increases rapidly. This too appears to be regulated by CRF as well as by other hormones, such as vasopressin, oxytocin, and the catecholamines.[1]

Adrenal insufficiency may thus be divided into two categories (Table 1):
1. Primary adrenocortical insufficiency (Addison's disease)
2. Secondary adrenocortical insufficiency as a result of ACTH deficiency

This article is divided into discussions of chronic adrenal insufficiency and acute adrenal insufficiency.

CHRONIC ADRENAL INSUFFICIENCY

Chronic adrenal insufficiency presents insidiously in most patients, with signs of cortisol and aldosterone deficiency. Anorexia, nausea, vomiting, and abdominal pain are common, and postural hypotension is a very useful physical finding. Signs of severe mineralocorticoid deficiency and hyperpigmentation are not seen in secondary adrenal insufficiency, whereas hypoglycemia and features of other endocrine deficiencies are more common.[2]

Thus, the diagnosis of chronic adrenal insufficiency requires awareness of the subtle presentation because many of the clinical features are so nonspecific. It is important to consider this diagnosis in patients who have been on long-term steroid therapy, as the hypothalamic-pituitary-adrenal axis may be suppressed for up to 12 months after cessation of treatment.[3] These patients may even appear cushingoid, but their pituitary does not release ACTH appropriately at times of stress and they may have adrenal atrophy resulting from a loss of endogenous ACTH

Other than iatrogenic adrenal insufficiency, autoimmune destruction of the adrenal gland is today the most common cause of adrenal insufficiency in the United States. There is a strong association with Hashimoto's thyroiditis (Schmidt's syndrome), hypoparathyroidism, diabetes mellitus, pernicious anemia, and premature ovarian failure.[4] There may be hereditary

TABLE 1.   CAUSES OF ADRENOCORTICAL INSUFFICIENCY

Primary
Acute
Hemorrhage (adrenal trauma, bleeding diathesis)
? Fulminant infection
Chronic
Congenital adrenal hyperplasia
Iatrogenic
　Drugs, especially glucocorticoids
　Mitotane, metyrapone
　Ketoconazole
　Surgery
Immunologic
Infection
　Granulomatous, especially tuberculosis, histoplasmosis, coccidioidomycosis;
　　also, cytomegalovirus
Neoplasm
　Adrenocortical carcinoma
　Metastatic
Miscellaneous
　Sarcoidosis, amyloidosis
　AIDS
　Adrenoleukodystrophy

Secondary
Acute
Hemorrhage/infarction
Infection
Chronic
Congenital
Iatrogenic
　Glucocorticoids rarely
　Radiation
　Surgery
Immune/idiopathic
Infection
　Tuberculosis
Neoplasm
　Pituitary adenoma
Vascular
　Postpartum, post-hemorrhage
Miscellaneous
　Sarcoidosis

factors as well. Most of these patients have adrenal antibodies and many also have antibodies to thyroid, parietal cells, and/or gonadal tissue.

In previous years, tuberculosis was the cause of Addison's disease in up to 90% of cases. Even today, tuberculosis must be considered and the presence of adrenal calcification should alert one to this cause. Extra-adrenal tuberculosis is usually evident (76–97%).[5,6] However, idiopathic atrophy may coexist with extrapulmonary tuberculosis. Another useful pointer toward tuberculous adrenal insufficiency is the presence of enlarged adrenal glands. Adrenal enlargement on CT scan may also be seen with fungal diseases, adrenal hemorrhage, sarcoidosis, amyloidosis, neoplasm, Hodgkin's disease,[5] and non-Hodgkin's lymphoma.[7]

There have been several reports of primary adrenal insufficiency associated with AIDS.[8,9] This is an important consideration, because many of the other diseases these patients have manifest clinical findings identical to those of adrenal insufficiency.

The approach to diagnosis is fairly simple. In suspected cases of chronic adrenal insufficiency, a baseline plasma cortisol concentration is measured and 0.25 mg synthetic ACTH (Cortrosyn) is administered IV or IM. Plasma cortisol is measured 30 minutes and 60 minutes later; the cortisol level should increase by at least 50%, or by greater than 7 μg/100 ml,[10] or to a level of 18 μg/100 ml.[11] If this rise does not occur, the functional adrenal reserve is deficient and a similar test is performed after 0.25 mg CRF is given. On this occasion, baseline and 30-minute ACTH and aldosterone are measured. If ACTH is high with a subnormal aldosterone increment, primary adrenal insufficiency is suggested; however, if ACTH is low-normal with a normal aldosterone increment, secondary adrenal insufficiency is likely. If there is doubt, more definitive testing is performed via a 24-hour ACTH infusion. Normal individuals are able to increase urinary 17-hydroxycorticosteroid excretion to greater than 25 mg/24 hours, and their plasma cortisol levels exceed 40 μg/dl. Patients with primary adrenal insufficiency have the smallest increases. There is a suggestion that the CRF stimulation test may differentiate pituitary from hypothalamic causes of secondary adrenal insufficiency. These patients have low baseline cortisol and plasma ACTH concentrations. One group shows a normal early increase in ACTH, and it is believed they have a hypothalamic disorder. The other patients show no increase in ACTH and have clinical evidence of pituitary disease.[12] Metyrapone[12] and insulin-induced hypoglycemia also test the intact nature of the entire hypothalamic-pituitary-adrenal axis, but the latter should be performed with caution. It is important, however, to exclude other hormone deficiencies in patients with secondary adrenal insufficiency.

ACUTE ADRENAL INSUFFICIENCY

Acute adrenal insufficiency can occur in any patient with chronic adrenal insufficiency who is unable to mount an appropriate response to stress. Thus again, the largest group at risk are the 5 million people in the United States on steroid doses sufficient to suppress the hypothalamic-pituitary-adrenal axis. Of course, all causes of adrenal insufficiency listed in Table 1 may be associated with adrenal crisis. The diagnosis should be suspected if there is a suggestive past medical history; also, it should be suspected in patients who become hypotensive with infection, during induction of anesthesia, or after a prolonged episode of nausea, vomiting, and diarrhea. Coma is rare, but patients may be hypothermic or hyperpyretic. Craving for salt and increased pigmentation point toward primary adrenal insufficiency, and in this group marked hypotension, azotemia, and hyperkalemia may result from aldosterone deficiency.

Acute adrenal insufficiency requires rapid diagnosis, prompt institution of intravenous fluids and intravenous steroids, and correction of the underlying precipitating factors. Baseline blood should be drawn for serum cortisol, electrolytes, glucose, and urea nitrogen. An intravenous bolus of 100–200 mg soluble hydrocortisone (phosphate or succinate) is given initially and followed by a constant infusion of hydrocortisone at 15 mg/hour. Some authors favor simultaneous administration of 100 mg cortisone acetate intramuscularly.[2] This allows for a reservoir if the intravenous infusion is interrupted. These patients may be 20% volume depleted, and the first liter of 5% dextrose in normal saline should be infused over 30–60 minutes (provided there are no contraindications). A clue to adrenal insufficiency may in fact be the presence of hypotension each time the saline infusion is decreased. Electrolyte disorders and hypoglycemia may need to be specifically treated. Occasionally, a vasopressor may be required when the hypotension is refractory to treatment.

Once the emergency is over, the underlying precipitant should be sought and treated. The steroid dose can be tapered and given orally or intramuscularly every 6–8 hours. The usual maintenance dose for these patients and for those with chronic adrenal insufficiency is as follows: hydrocortisone 20 mg or prednisone 5 mg orally in the morning, and hydrocortisone 10 mg or prednisone 2.5 mg orally in the afternoon. Fludrocortisone 0.05–0.1 mg orally in the morning is required in patients with primary adrenal insufficiency. Changes in body weight and blood pressure are useful parameters in adjusting the dose of this mineralocorticoid.

KEY FEATURES

Adrenal insufficiency results from a primary adrenal disorder or secondary to a lack of ACTH.

The clinical features are those of cortisol deficiency. Primary adrenal insufficiency is also associated with mineralocorticoid deficiency.

The most common cause is chronic steroid therapy with hypothalamic-pituitary-adrenal axis suppression.

Other common causes are autoimmune, infectious, and neoplastic disorders.

The *diagnosis* of chronic adrenal insufficiency is confirmed by the lack of cortisol increase to synthetic ACTH injection. High serum ACTH with no aldosterone increase implies primary adrenal insufficiency.

The hallmark of the acute crisis is *hypotension* precipitated by stress.

TREATMENT OF THE ACUTE CRISIS

1. Hydrocortisone phosphate (or succinate) 100 mg IV bolus, followed by a constant infusion of 15 mg/hour
2. Five per cent dextrose in normal saline with first liter given over 30–60 minutes
3. Treat precipitating factors
4. Taper to maintenance dose of:
    a. Hydrocortisone 20 mg po q AM, 10 mg po q afternoon; *or*
    b. Prednisone 5 mg po q AM, 2.5 mg po q afternoon
5. If mineralocorticoid deficiency is present, use fludrocortisone 0.05–0.1 mg po q AM

REFERENCES

1. Chrousos GP: Introduction, pp 344–345. *In* Chrousos GP (moderator): Clinical applications of corticotropin-releasing factor. Ann Intern Med *102*:344–358, 1985.
    An extensive review of the clinical utilization of CRF stimulation testing. This introductory section reviews the physiology feedback control and metabolism of steroid production (ref. 117).

2. Thorn GW, Lauler DP: Clinical therapeutics of adrenal disorders. Am J Med 53:673–684, 1972.
    This review briefly highlights the clinical features of adrenal disorders. The authors then extensively detail the acute and chronic management of these problems.

3. Axelrod L: Glucocorticoid therapy. Medicine 55:39–65, 1976.
    Extensive review of the risks of glucocorticoid therapy and the prolonged suppression of the hypothalamic-pituitary-adrenal axis that may follow chronic steroid use (ref. 188).

4. Turkington RW, Lebovitz HE: Extra-adrenal endocrine deficiencies in Addison's disease. Am J Med 43:499–507, 1967.
    Forty-one per cent of patients with Addison's disease have evidence of a second endocrine deficiency. The association is almost invariably with idiopathic/autoimmune adrenal insufficiency.

5. Vita JA, et al: Clinical clues to the cause of Addison's disease. Am J Med 78:461–466, 1985.
    The clinical findings in 8 patients with Addison's disease and a further 31 autopsied cases are reviewed. Adrenal calcification is very suggestive of tuberculosis and was seen in 53% of patients. Early adrenal tuberculosis, carcinoma, fungal diseases, amyloidosis, sarcoidosis, and adrenal hemorrhage are also associated with adrenal enlargement.

6. Alvarez S, McCabe WR: Extra-pulmonary tuberculosis revisited: A review of experience at Boston City and other hospitals. Medicine 63:25–55, 1984.
    Four patients (3%) were found to have adrenal tuberculosis. All had evidence of old pulmonary tuberculosis and responded to replacement steroid and antituberculous therapy.

7. Shea TC, et al: Non-Hodgkin's lymphoma limited to the adrenal gland with adrenal insufficiency. Am J Med 78:711–714, 1985.
    The first reported case of non-Hodgkin's lymphoma apparently limited to the adrenal gland and associated with adrenal insufficiency.

8. Tapper ML, et al: Adrenal necrosis in the acquired immunodeficiency syndrome. Ann Intern Med 100:239–241, 1984.

   Autopsy findings in ten patients with AIDS revealed cytomegalovirus adrenalitis in seven homosexuals and lipid depletion in the remaining three patients.

9. Greene LW, et al: Adrenal insufficiency as a complication of the acquired immuno deficiency syndrome. Ann Intern Med 101:497–498, 1984.

   Four of 20 patients referred for suspected adrenal insufficiency were found to have primary adrenal insufficiency. Treatment with corticosteroids resulted in clinical improvement.

10. Wood JB, et al: A rapid test of adrenocortical function. Lancet 1:243–245, 1965.

    A description of the ACTH stimulation test. In normal subjects, 250 mg of ACTH caused the mean plasma cortisol level to rise from 14.7 to 31.4 mg/100 ml, and individual increments were 7.5 to 27.5 mg/100 ml.

11. Cunningham SK, et al: Normal cortisol response to corticotropin in patients with secondary adrenal failure. Arch Intern Med 143:2276–2279, 1983.

    The authors stress that a normal response to synthetic ACTH (cortrosyn) does not necessarily imply a normal hypothalamic-pituitary-adrenal axis. Eleven of thirty-two patients with normal response to ACTH had abnormal results with metyrapone. Four of these eleven patients tested by means of insulin-induced hypoglycemia showed concordant abnormal results.

12. Schulte HM: Corticotropin-releasing factor stimulation test in adrenal insufficiency, pp 350–352. In Chrousos GP (moderator): Clinical applications of corticotropin-releasing factor. Ann Intern Med 102:344–358, 1985.

    This section of this previously cited review deals with the use of CRF in adrenal insufficiency. It is proposed that those patients with secondary adrenal insufficiency who show no increase in ACTH after CRF infection have a pituitary abnormality. The remaining patients with secondary adreanal insufficiency show a normal rise in ACTH, and they appear to have a hypothalamic disorder.

Cushing's Syndrome

Ravin Davidoff, M.D.

Cushing's syndrome results from excess glucocorticosteroids. Cushing's syndrome not associated with exogenous steroid administration is a rare clinical entity. However, it is of importance because the syndrome comprises a constellation of signs and symptoms seen frequently in the general medical population, e.g., hypertension, obesity, diabetes mellitus, and osteoporosis. It is important thus to differentiate these "normal" patients from those with Cushing's syndrome, because in many instances the hypercortisolemic state is curable.

Cortisol secretion by the adrenal gland is normally regulated by pituitary adrenocorticotropic hormone (ACTH). The ACTH level, in turn, is determined by corticotropin-releasing factor (CRF), a 41 amino acid peptide produced by the hypothalamus. There appears to be a negative feedback loop to both the pituitary gland and the hypothalamus.[1] Under certain circumstances, this homeostatic control is lost and hypercortisolemia results. There are three major pathogenetic mechanisms that cause Cushing's syndrome:

1. Pituitary Cushing's syndrome or Cushing's disease. This accounts for 2 of 3 cases of spontaneous Cushing's syndrome, results from excessive ACTH, and is associated with bilateral adrenal hyperplasia.
2. Adrenal Cushing's syndrome is secondary to autonomous production of cortisol by an adrenal adenoma or more rarely by adrenal carcinoma. This accounts for approximately 15% of cases of adult Cushing's syndrome.
3. The remaining cases of spontaneous Cushing's syndrome result from ectopic ACTH production or, as more recently documented, ectopic CRF.[2]

There is some variation in clinical presentation, depending on the cause of cortisol overproduction. In particular, adrenal carcinoma is associated with marked virilization, whereas ectopic ACTH production is dominated by mineralocorticoid effect, e.g., hypertension and hypokalemic alkalosis. A composite study has shown that the most common clinical features of Cushing's syndrome are obesity, especially truncal (88%); hypertension (74%); hirsutism (64%); weakness (60%); bruising (42%); and backache from osteoporosis (40%).[3] A clinical diagnosis, based on a florid presentation, is found only 50% of the time.[4]

DIAGNOSIS

It is thus apparent that the diagnosis of Cushing's syndrome is generally made in the laboratory. The principles of diagnosis, again, are 3-fold (Fig. 1):

1. Confirm the diagnosis of Cushing's syndrome.
2. Presumptively identify the cause of hypercortisolism by provocative and suppressive biochemical tests.
3. Confirm the anatomic localization by radiographic studies.

Confirmation of Cushing's Syndrome

The most reliable screening test for hypercortisolism is the 24-hour urine-free cortisol determination. There are few false positives (3.3%) and false negatives (5.6%), but the reliability depends on the adequacy of the 24-hour urine collection.[5] Because of the problem of patient compliance, the overnight dexamethasone suppression test has gained in popularity. One

17-OHCS = 17-hydroxycorticosteroids
CRF = Corticotropin releasing factor

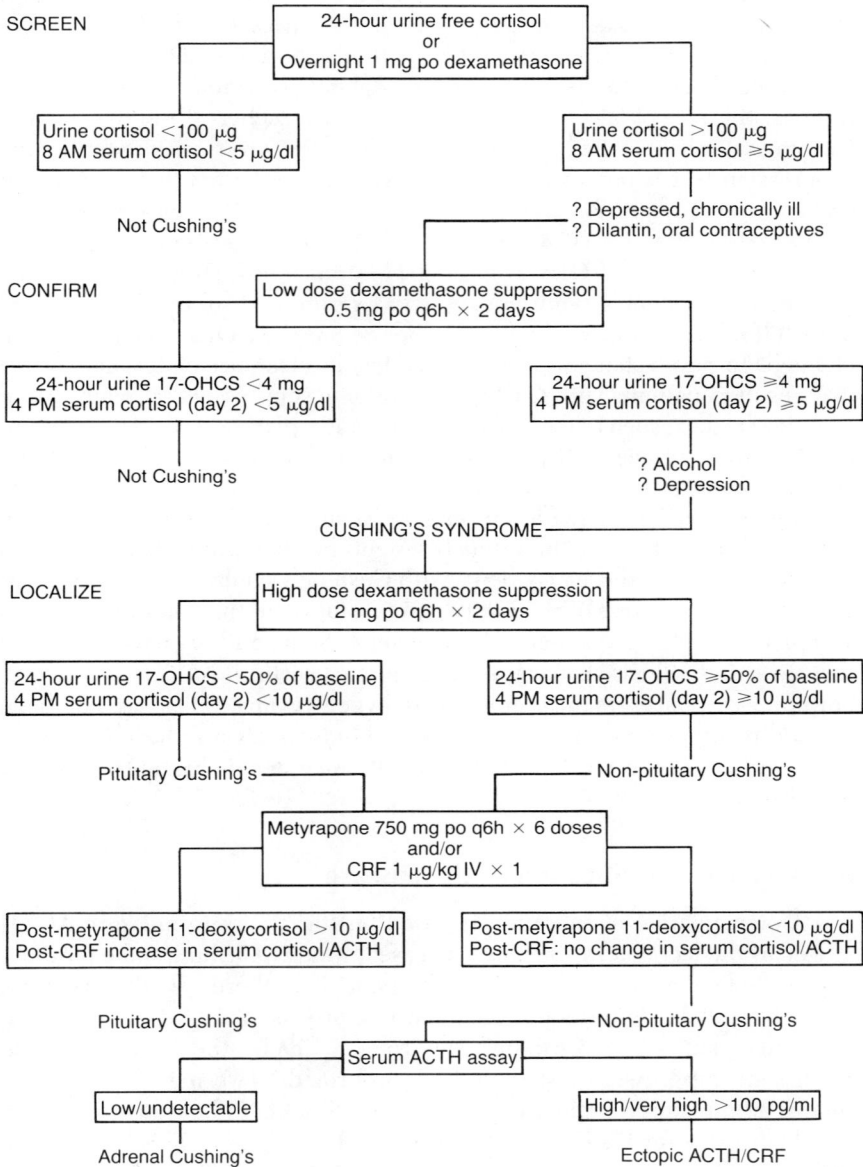

SCREEN

> 24-hour urine free cortisol
> or
> Overnight 1 mg po dexamethasone

Urine cortisol <100 µg
8 AM serum cortisol <5 µg/dl

Urine cortisol >100 µg
8 AM serum cortisol ≥5 µg/dl

Not Cushing's

? Depressed, chronically ill
? Dilantin, oral contraceptives

CONFIRM

> Low dose dexamethasone suppression
> 0.5 mg po q6h × 2 days

24-hour urine 17-OHCS <4 mg
4 PM serum cortisol (day 2) <5 µg/dl

24-hour urine 17-OHCS ≥4 mg
4 PM serum cortisol (day 2) ≥5 µg/dl

Not Cushing's

? Alcohol
? Depression

CUSHING'S SYNDROME

LOCALIZE

> High dose dexamethasone suppression
> 2 mg po q6h × 2 days

24-hour urine 17-OHCS <50% of baseline
4 PM serum cortisol (day 2) <10 µg/dl

24-hour urine 17-OHCS ≥50% of baseline
4 PM serum cortisol (day 2) ≥10 µg/dl

Pituitary Cushing's

Non-pituitary Cushing's

> Metyrapone 750 mg po q6h × 6 doses
> and/or
> CRF 1 µg/kg IV × 1

Post-metyrapone 11-deoxycortisol >10 µg/dl
Post-CRF increase in serum cortisol/ACTH

Post-metyrapone 11-deoxycortisol <10 µg/dl
Post-CRF: no change in serum cortisol/ACTH

Pituitary Cushing's

Non-pituitary Cushing's

> Serum ACTH assay

Low/undetectable

High/very high >100 pg/ml

Adrenal Cushing's

Ectopic ACTH/CRF

Figure 1. Approach to the diagnosis of Cushing's syndrome.

mg dexamethasone is taken by mouth at 11 PM or 12 midnight, and plasma cortisol is measured at 8 AM the next morning. The upper limit varies but is generally accepted as being less than 5 μg/100 ml. This too is an excellent screening test with a false negative rate of less than 2% and a false positive rate, among normal individuals, of 1%.[5] In obese, depressed, hospitalized, or chronically ill patients, or in subjects taking phenytoin (dilantin) or estrogens, the rate of false positivity may be much higher. If the diagnosis of Cushing's syndrome has not been excluded, the low-dose dexamthasone suppression test is performed. In this test, 0.5 mg dexamethasone is given orally every 6 hours for 2 consecutive days, and a 24-hour urine for 17-hydroxycorticosteroids (17-OHCS) is collected on the second day.

Suppression of 17-OHCS to 4 mg/24 hours almost always excludes the diagnosis of Cushing's syndrome. A 4 PM serum cortisol level on day 2 of 5 μg/100 ml correlates well with a 24-hour urinary 17-OHCS concentration of 4 mg.[6] In rare instances, decreased metabolic clearance of dexamethasone may result in patients with Cushing's syndrome suppressing normally. More complex studies, such as cortisol production rate, plasma cortisol fluctuation, and insulin tolerance testing, have not sufficiently increased the sensitivity and specificity to justify their routine use.

Pseudo-Cushing's syndrome may be seen in alcoholic patients and in depressed patients. The clinical features and biochemical tests of alcoholics may be identical to those of patients with Cushing's syndrome. The diagnosis is based on knowledge of the entity and resolution of the abnormal findings within 1–6 weeks of abstinence from alcohol. Some authors have suggested that these individuals show appropriate plasma cortisol, ACTH, and growth hormone responses to insulin-induced hypoglycemia. This has not been verified by other investigators.[7] Depressed individuals may have laboratory tests very similar to Cushing's. The significance of this has not been fully established.

Biochemical Identification of the Disease

Determination of causation is based on the ability to measure ACTH as well as the fact that in Cushing's disease (pituitary Cushing's) the pituitary appears to be functioning at a higher set point. Thus there is feedback control of the hypothalamic-pituitary-adrenal axis, but it is at a different set point. Once the diagnosis of Cushing's syndrome is made, the high-dose dexamethasone suppression test should be performed.[8] Two mg of dexamethasone is administered orally every 6 hours for 2 days, and on the second day a 24-hour urine for 17-OHCS and free cortisol is collected. This is compared with a baseline 24-hour urine 17-OHCS and cortisol. Suppression by at least 50% from the basal state is highly suggestive of pituitary Cushing's. The diagnostic accuracy varies from 94%[5] to 81%.[9] This correlates well with a

4 PM serum cortisol level on day 2 of less than 10 µg/dl.[6] The intact nature of the axis in pituitary Cushing's is further substantiated by the metyrapone test. Such patients uniformly demonstrate a normal post-metyrapone 8 AM serum 11-deoxycortisol concentration (greater than 10 µg/dl).[9]

In centers where it is available, the CRF stimulation test further contributes to the differentiation of pituitary Cushing's from the other forms. The former group shows marked elevation in ACTH and free plasma cortisol after CRF administration. This implies intact pituitary receptors for CRF as well as appropriate subsequent events leading to ACTH production. Only 5% of patients with pituitary Cushing's do not show this response, and 98% of patients with ectopic ACTH do.[10,11]

More recently, two forms of pituitary Cushing's have been documented—a hypopulsatile group in which 24-hour cortisol profiles show decreased pulsatility, and a hyperpulsatile group in which the cortisol profile shows abnormally large spike increments.[12] This may be significant in terms of therapy, as the former group may represent true pituitary Cushing's, whereas the latter may result from excessive pulsatile production of hypothalamic CRF. This hypothesis requires further investigation.

If, however, the axis is not suppressible, measurement of plasma ACTH can help to differentiate adrenal Cushing's (low or undetectable ACTH) from ectopic sources of ACTH or CRF (frequently very high levels of ACTH). Further delineation of adrenal Cushing's syndrome is possible. Adrenal carcinomas generally produce large amounts of androgens as well as cortisol, and thus urinary ketosteroids tend to be very high (>50 mg/24 hours).[13] Adrenal adenoma is suggested by the presence of a low baseline serum dehydroepiandrosterone sulfate concentration in patients with nonsuppressible Cushing's syndrome.[6] Nodular adrenal hyperplasia, an unusual variant of Cushing's syndrome may be a primary adrenal disorder or may be secondary to ACTH hypersecretion, and thus it is difficult to classify definitively.

The most common sources of ectopic ACTH are tumors of the lung, thymus, pancreas, and kidney. Despite the extremely high levels of ACTH, there is frequently a paucity of cushingoid features and many tumors appear to secrete a biologically inactive "big ACTH." Signs of mineralocorticoid excess often dominate this syndrome.

With all biochemical testing, it is important to realize that Cushing's syndrome is an episodic disease and a single normal evaluation does not necessarily exclude the diagnosis.

Anatomic Localization of the Cause

Anatomic localization is guided by the laboratory evaluation. Computerized tomography (CT) of the sella turcica is the most practical technique for detecting pituitary adenomas. However, the vast majority (± 80%) of cases of pituitary Cushing's result from pituitary microadenomas, and these are frequently not visible on CT. The diagnosis of adrenal Cushing's syndrome is confirmed by CT, ultrasound, or isotope scintigrams of the adrenal glands. Here, too, because of diagnostic accuracy, cost efficiency, and radiation exposure, CT is the radiographic technique of choice.[14] Intravenous pyelography, arteriography, adrenal venography, and adrenal venous sampling have little place in the diagnostic and anatomic work-up of patients with Cushing's syndrome.

TREATMENT

Treatment is directed toward the biochemically and anatomically identified cause of Cushing's syndrome. Ideally, treatment should restore the patient to normal, but this is not always the case.

Cushing's syndrome is always curable, but the metabolic and other consequences of certain therapeutic options may be too great to justify their use. It is for this reason that bilateral adrenalectomy is rarely performed today. The operative mortality rate of 4–10%, the rapid postoperative growth of pituitary neoplasms with hyperpigmentation (Nelson's syndrome) in 10–20% of cases, and life-long dependency on replacement adrenocortical hormones have made this an unacceptable form of therapy in most instances.[1]

The preferred treatment for adults with pituitary Cushing's syndrome is transsphenoidal pituitary microsurgery.[15] However, the early optimism of the 1970s has been somewhat tempered by longer follow-up, and cure rates of 70% are the rule.[16] Failure of this procedure may be technical or may implicate the hypothalamus as the underlying cause of hypercortisolemia in these cases of "pituitary Cushing's" patients.[12] Some of these patients respond to cyproheptadine, but irradiation and 6 months of mitotane may be necessary if transsphenoidal microsurgery fails.

Adrenal adenomas and nodular adrenal hyperplasia are cured by adrenal surgery. Adrenal carcinoma responds poorly to surgery, and aminoglutethimide, metyrapone, mitotane, and trilostane have been tried with limited success. Survival is usually brief, with death occurring most often in a year or two.[17]

Treatment of Cushing's syndrome resulting from ectopic ACTH or CRF is directed at the underlying neoplasm. Hypercortisolemia can be controlled with metyrapone or aminoglutethimide, but again, survival is brief because these patients usually have unresectable malignant tumors.

KEY FEATURES

Cushing's syndrome results from excess glucocorticosteroids.
Typical features include obesity, hypertension, virilization, muscle weakness, and backache.

The syndrome may result from pituitary (most common) or ectopic sources of ACTH, or from primary adrenal hypercortisolemia.

Step-wise biochemical evaluation requires initial *screening*; low-dose dexamethasone *confirmation*; and high-dose dexamethasone, metyrapone, and/or CRF *localization*.

Anatomic localization is confirmed most efficiently by computerized tomography.

Treatment is directed at the underlying cause. Transsphenoidal removal of pituitary microadenomas is the most common intervention, but pituitary irradiation, adrenalectomy, and various drugs are used where appropriate.

REFERENCES

1. Gold EM: The Cushing syndromes. Changing views of diagnosis and treatment. Ann Intern Med 90:829–844, 1979.
    An extensive review of the pathogenesis, clinical features, diagnostic objectives, confirmatory biochemical tests, anatomic localization, and treatment of Cushing's syndrome (234 ref.).

2. Carey RM, Varma SK, et al: Ectopic secretion of corticotropin-releasing factor as a cause of Cushing's syndrome. A clinical morphologic and biochemical study. N Engl J Med 311:13–20, 1984.
    Description of a patient with prostatic carcinoma and Cushing's syndrome secondary to ectopic corticotropin-releasing factor production.

3. Ross EJ, Marshall-Jones P, Friedman M: Cushing's syndrome: Diagnostic criteria. Quart J Med 35:149–192, 1966.
    A review of the clinical features of 50 patients with Cushing's syndrome and a comparison with 551 previously reported cases. The following findings were noted: obesity 88%, moon face 75%, muscular weakness 61%, bruising 42%, psychological difficulty 42%, acne 45%, hirsutism 65%, menstrual irregularity 60%, and backache 40%.

4. Nugent CA, Warner HR, Dunn JT, Tyler FH: Probability theory in the diagnosis of Cushing's syndrome. J Clin Endocrinol 24:621–627, 1964.
    This study reviews the incidence of clinical findings in Cushing's syndrome. Using probability values, the authors show how these findings can be applied in patients suspected of having Cushing's syndrome. Fifty per cent of patients had the diagnosis made clinically. Careful physical examination appears more useful for excluding the diagnosis.

5. Crapo L: Cushing's syndrome: A review of diagnostic tests. Metabolism 28:955–977, 1979.
    A very extensive review of the diagnostic tests for Cushing's syndrome. The author reviews and combines the studies through 1978 by detailing an approach to (1) the definitive diagnosis of Cushing's syndrome, and (2) the biochemical localization of the source of the hypercortisolemia.

6. Ashcroft MW, et al: Serum cortisol levels in Cushing's syndrome after low- and high-dose dexamethasone suppression. Ann Intern Med 97:21–26, 1982.
    A well-designed study correlating 24-hour urinary 17-OHCS with 4 PM serum cortisol levels on day 2 of low- and high-dose dexamethasone suppression tests. Nonsuppressible Cushing's syndrome correlated with 4 PM serum cortisol levels of >5 mg/dl and >10 mg/dl after low- and high-dose dexamethasone, respectively. Baseline dehydroepiandrosterone sulfate level of >0.4 mg/ml indicates adrenal adenoma.

7. Lamberts SWJ, et al: Hormone secretion in alcohol-induced pseudo-Cushing's syndrome: Differential diagnosis with Cushing's disease. JAMA 242:1640–1643, 1979.

   A description of two patients with alcohol-induced pseudo-Cushing's syndrome. These individuals showed normal increases in cortisol and ACTH after insulin-induced hypoglycemia and were thus biochemically different from patients with Cushing's syndrome.

8. Liddle GW: Tests of pituitary-adrenal suppressibility in the diagnosis of Cushing's syndrome. J Clin Endocrinol Metab 20:1539–1560, 1960.

   A classic article describing the low-dose dexamethasone suppression test and its utility in screening out normal individuals. The author also describes the ability of high-dose dexamethasone to identify patients with pituitary Cushing's syndrome.

9. Sindler BH, Griffing GT, Melby JC: The superiority of the metyrapone test versus the high-dose dexamethasone test in the differential diagnosis of Cushing's syndrome. Am J Med 74:657–662, 1983.

   This study prospectively compares the metyrapone test with the high-dose dexamethasone test in 25 patients with Cushing's syndrome. The authors conclude that the diagnostic accuracy of the metyrapone test was 100% in differentiating pituitary Cushing's from adrenal Cushing's. This compared with an accuracy of 81% for the high-dose dexamethasone suppression test.

10. Chrousos GP: Differential diagnosis of Cushing's syndrome, pp 346–347. In Chrousos GP (moderator): Clinical applications of corticotropin-releasing factor. Ann Intern Med 102:344–358, 1985.

    An extensive review of the clinical utilization of CRF. Ninety-five per cent of patients with pituitary adenomas show an appropriate increase in ACTH and cortisol after intravenous CRF, whereas patients with adrenal or ectopic ACTH do not show this response. Depressed patients show a blunted ACTH response but a normal cortisol increase to CRF. Bilateral inferior petrosal sinus assays of ACTH after CRF infusion can help to localize nonvisualizable pituitary microadenomas. CRF infusion may also be useful in differentiating pituitary from hypothalamic causes of secondary adrenal insufficiency (ref. 117.)

11. Chrousos GP, et al: The corticotropin-releasing factor stimulation test: An aid in the evaluation of patients with Cushing's syndrome. N Engl J Med 310:622–626, 1984.

    Thirteen patients with pituitary Cushing's syndrome showed an increase in serum cortisol and ACTH after intravenous CRF. This resolved after successful surgery. Nine patients with ectopic or adrenal Cushing's syndrome showed no response to CRF (ref. 117).

12. Van Cauter E, Refetoff S: Evidence for two subtypes of Cushing's disease based on the analysis of episodic cortisol secretion. N Engl J Med 312:1343–1349, 1985.

    The authors analyzed episodic cortisol secretion in 51 normal subjects, 14 patients with adrenal adenoma, and 46 patients with Cushing's disease. In adrenal adenoma, the episodic secretion is greatly dampened. Two thirds of patients with Cushing's disease have "hypopulsatile" patterns, and this may reflect an underlying pituitary abnormality, whereas the remaining hyperpulsatile patients may have a hypothalamic disorder.

13. King DR, Lack EE: Adrenal cortical carcinoma: A clinical and pathologic study of 49 cases. Cancer 44:239–244, 1979.

    Forty-nine patients with adrenal carcinoma are presented. The main age was 34 years, and 37% presented with recognizable endocrine excess. The only cures occurred in patients whose tumors were totally resected, and 36 of 49 (73%) patients died of metastatic disease an average of 7–8 months after diagnosis.

14. Guerin CK, et al: Computed tomographic scanning versus radioisotope imaging in adrenocortical diagnosis. Am J Med 75:653–657, 1983.

    A comparative study of 28 patients with Cushing's syndrome, 58 patients with primary aldosteronism, and 13 patients with nonfunctioning adrenal tumors. Computerized tomographic scanning and iodocholesterol isotope scanning are of comparable diagnostic accuracy, but the former is cheaper, faster, and involves less radiation, and thus is the imaging technique of choice.

15. Bigos ST, et al: Cushing's disease: Management by transsphenoidal pituitary microsurgery. J Clin Endocrinol Metab 50:348–354, 1980.

A follow-up of 24 patients after transsphenoidal pituitary surgery. With a median follow-up of 12 months, 16 patients were cured; 2 apparent "cures" relapsed, and 6 patients were never cured.

16. Burch W: A survey of results with transsphenoidal surgery in Cushing's disease. N Engl J Med 308:103–104, 1983.

A survey of 30 endocrinologists across the United States illustrating extremely variable results depending on the institution and the size of the adenoma. Cure rates ranged from a low of less than 60% to 100%. Recurrence rates of greater than 50% were noted by several institutions.

17. Bertagna C, Orth DN: Clinical laboratory findings and results of therapy in 50 patients with adrenocortical tumors admitted to a single medical center (1951 to 1978). Am J Med 71:855–875, 1981.

A comparison of 26 patients with adrenal adenoma and 32 with adrenal carcinoma. Confirms previous findings that both groups showed no response to metyrapone and no suppression with dexamethasone. Adenomas took longer to diagnose and were uniformly cured by surgery. Adrenal carcinoma was associated with higher levels of urinary 17-ketosteroids and responded poorly to surgical and drug therapy.

Pheochromocytoma

Jon Pehrson, M.D.
Ravin Davidoff, M.D.

Pheochromocytomas are chromaffin tumors that synthesize and secrete excessive quantities of catecholamines; these catecholamines produce hypertension, paroxysms, and hypermetabolism. Hypertension is present in the vast majority of patients with pheochromocytomas; it is sustained in 60% of patients and paroxysmal in 30–40%.[1,2,3] The hypertension is usually severe and responds poorly or paradoxically to commonly used antihypertensive agents. Orthostatic hypotension may also be present and is due to decreased plasma volume, increased basal venous tone, and down-regulation of catecholamine receptors. Paroxysms, which occur in over one half of the patients with pheochromocytomas, usually consist of the sudden onset of headache, palpitations, and sweating. Tachycardia and severe hypertension are usually present during a paroxysm. Marked apprehension, abdominal or chest pain, nausea, and vomiting may also occur. Patients with pheochromocytomas may have adverse reactions to various drugs, resulting in severe paroxysms. Opiates, histamines, glucagon, sympathomimetics, and tricyclic antidepressants have all been associated with precipitation of paroxysms in patients with pheochromocytomas. Cardiac manifestations of pheochromocytomas include arrhythmias, angina, myocardial infarction, congestive heart failure, and cardiac hypertrophy. Signs and symptoms of hypermetabolism are also common and include weight loss, heat intolerance, sweating, and abnormal carbohydrate tolerance. The diagnosis of a pheochromocytoma rests on the demonstration of elevated urinary or plasma levels of catecholamines or their metabolites (metanephrine and vanillylmandelic acid) by a reliable assay. This can usually be accomplished by a 24-hour urine collection, especially if it is initiated immediately after a paroxysm has occurred. Carefully collected plasma catecholamine levels (with an IV line in place 30 minutes prior to sampling and the patient resting in the supine position) also yield comparably reliable results. In equivocal cases, the plasma catecholamine response to clonidine or glucagon may be quite useful in confirming or ruling out the diagnosis of a pheochromocytoma.[2,3,5]

Most pheochromocytomas occur as single intra-adrenal tumors; 10% are bilateral, 10% are extra-adrenal (usually near sympathetic ganglia),[4] and 10% are malignant. A contrast CT scan is usually adequate to demonstrate the tumor. Nuclear imaging with ^{131}I-iodomethylbenzylguanidine has also proved to be quite accurate at localizing pheochromocytomas.[6,7]

TREATMENT

Treatment of pheochromocytomas involves antagonism of catecholamine effects with medications and careful removal.[3,8–10] Alpha adrenergic blockade should be initiated before beta adrenergic blockade to avoid worsening of the hypertension. Phenoxybenzamine, initially at 10 mg every 12 hours orally, is titrated slowly over several days until the blood pressure is controlled, usually at 40–100 mg/day. Paroxysms of hypertension can be controlled during this phase with the more rapid-acting drug phentolamine, 1–5 mg IV. Beta blockade with propranolol starting at 10 mg four times a day is used during alpha blockade to control tachycardia, arrhythmias, and sweating. Doses of alpha and beta blockers must be individualized according to the patient's response. A minimum of 2 weeks treatment is usually necessary to establish a stable blood pressure and restore plasma volume to normal. Treatment with calcium channel blockers has been reported to be quite efficacious in patients with pheochromocytomas; however, experience is still too limited to warrant generalized recommendations.

Surgical resection of pheochromocytomas must include close cooperation and communication among an experienced surgeon, an anesthesiologist, and the attending endocrinologist or internist. Perioperative and postoperative monitoring of blood pressure with an arterial line, volume status with a central venous pressure catheter or Swan-Ganz catheter, and continuous ECG monitoring is mandatory. Marked changes in blood pressure, heart rate, and arrhythmias occur most commonly during anesthesia induction, surgery, and the immediate postoperative period. Manipulation of the tumor during the operation should be kept to a minimum, to limit swings in catecholamine levels. Hypotension may occur intraoperatively, presumably owing to immediate lowering of catecholamine levels, treatment with alpha and beta adrenergic blockers, and volume contraction. Hypotension is best managed by volume expansion; occasionally, direct-acting vasopressors are required. Intraoperative and perioperative arrhythmias usually respond to intravenous propranolol. Large rises in blood pressure can usually be controlled with carefully titrated doses of intravenous phentolamine. Postoperatively, patients should be carefully monitored in an ICU setting because changes in volume status, blood pressure, heart rate, and arrhythmias must be carefully monitored and treated. Urinary or plasma catecholamines should be in the normal range by 10–14 days postoperatively unless postoperative complications have occurred. Persistently elevated excretion of catecholamines or their metabolites suggests an incomplete tumor resection or another pheochromocytoma. Screening of patients with suspected or confirmed pheochromocytoma for the possibility of multiple endocrine adenomatosis is probably indicated only for patients with a very suspicious family history.

KEY FEATURES

Pheochromocytoma is a rare disorder in both the normal and hypertensive population. Pheochromocytoma should be suspected in patients with severe hypertension that responds poorly or parodoxically to antihypertensive medications, hypertensive patients with paroxysms, or hypertensive patients with signs of hypermetabolism.

The diagnosis of pheochromocytoma can almost always be confirmed or excluded by a reliably collected and assayed 24-hour urine collection for catecholamines and catecholamine metabolites. Plasma catecholamine levels and response to clonidine or glucagon may be useful in equivocal cases if the tests are performed under carefully controlled circumstances. CT scanning with contrast medium is usually adequate and reliable for localization of a pheochromocytoma. The large majority of pheochromocytomas occur in the adrenal gland.

Management of pheochromocytomas involves alpha adrenergic blockade followed by beta adrenergic blockade; doses must be individually tailored.

Surgical resection of pheochromocytomas should be preceded by at least 2 weeks of stabilization of the blood pressure, heart rate, and plasma volume.

Successful resection of pheochromocytomas requires close cooperation and communication among an experienced surgeon, anesthesiologist, and an endocrinologist or internist. Meticulous monitoring of the patient's cardiovascular status is of paramount importance during the intraoperative and postoperative period.

REFERENCES

1. Tucker RN, Labarthe DR: Frequency of surgical treatment for hypertension in adults at the Mayo Clinic from 1973–1975. Mayo Clinic Proc 52:549–555, 1975.
   A review of surgical treatment for hypertension performed at the Mayo Clinic between 1973 and 1975. The estimated incidence of diagnosed pheochromocytoma was 0.04% of all hypertensive patients.

2. Grossman E, et al: Diagnosis of pheochromocytoma (letter). N Engl J Med 312:722, 1985.
   This letter questions the conclusions found in the following reference. Grossman and colleagues found that 6 of 12 patients with surgically documented pheochromocytoma did not demonstrate any of the classic triad of symptoms—sweating, tachycardia, and headache.

3. Bravo EL, Gifford RW: Pheochromocytoma: Diagnosis, localization and management. N Engl J Med 311:1298–1303, 1984.
   An excellent overview of the clinical features, biochemical diagnosis, provocative studies, anatomic localization, and treatment of pheochromocytoma. The authors state that the absence of sweating attacks, tachycardia, and headaches in a hypertensive patient rules out the diagnosis of pheochromocytoma 99.9% of the time.

4. Clinicopathologic conference: Micturition induced hypertension in a 58-year-old woman. Am J Med 78:307–316, 1985.
   The discussion of the case focuses on a woman with a bladder mass and paroxysmal hypertensive episodes. The discussant reviews the physiology of adrenergic receptors, the common clinical features of pheochromocytoma, the differential diagnosis, laboratory diagnosis (stressing the value of controlled plasma norepinephrine levels), and localization (CT scan can detect 90% of pheochromocytomas).

5. Bravo EL, et al: Clonidine-suppression test: A useful aid in the diagnosis of pheochromocytoma. N Engl J Med 305:623–626, 1981.
   In ten patients with proven pheochromocytoma, 0.3 mg po clonidine showed no effect on plasma norepinephrine. In every patient with essential hypertension (15), plasma norepinephrine was significantly suppressed 3 hours after clonidine administration.

6. Sisson JC, et al: Scintigraphic localization of pheochromocytoma. N Engl J Med 305:12–16, 1981.
   Describes the successful localization of adrenal and extra-adrenal pheochromocytoma in eight patients. The agent used was ^{131}I-metaiodobenzylguanidine (MIBG). This tracer was able to detect benign and malignant neoplasms and four tumors not detected by computerized tomography.

7. Editorial: Iodobenzylguanidine for location and treatment of pheochromocytoma. Lancet 2:905–907, 1984.
   This editorial reviews the ±500 patients who have been examined by MIBG. Similar results of 85% sensitivity, 98% specificity and 92% clinical accuracy have been found.

Large doses of labeled MIBG have been used to treat malignant metastatic pheochromocytoma. Thirteen of nineteen patients appear to have responded to this treatment.

8. Nigholson JP, et al: Pheochromocytoma and prazosin. Ann Intern Med 99:477–479, 1983.

Prazosin appears to be effective in the long-term management of pheochromocytoma. However, intraoperatively prazosin was not an effective single agent in controlling blood pressure in four patients with pheochromocytoma. Theories proposed include the fact that beta₂ receptors are unopposed, receptor affinity may change with time, and, lastly, the enormous secretion of catecholamines at surgery may overwhelm the competitive antagonism of prazosin.

9. Levine SN, McDonald JC: The evaluation and management of pheochromocytomas. Adv Surg 17:281–313, 1984.

An extensive review of the physiology, clinical features, diagnosis, and localization of pheochromocytoma. Particular attention is paid to surgical technique, the role of the anesthesiologist, and preoperative and postoperative care (ref. 58).

10. Metyrosine for pheochromocytoma. Med Lett Drug Ther 22:28, 1980.

Metyrosine inhibits tyrosine hydroxylase and thus blocks the conversion of tyrosine to DOPA. It decreases catecholamine synthesis by 50–80% and is useful preoperatively and in inoperable patients.

SECTION 3
GASTROINTESTINAL DISEASE

Acid Peptic Disease

Charles Michael Bliss, M.D.

Acid peptic disease can involve all parts of the upper gastrointestinal tract, either acutely or chronically. Although the disease is fairly common (lifetime incidence for duodenal ulcer is 10% for men, 4% for women), the rates of hospitalization, surgery, and mortality have fallen dramatically in the past 20 years, especially for duodenal ulcers. This is not entirely explained by improved therapy.[1]

Patients usually present with the complaint of epigastric pain. Although not diagnostic, the pain pattern in a typical patient with duodenal ulcer will be episodic, both during the day and over the year, often occurring in clusters of symptomatic periods lasting a few weeks. Generally the pain is consistent—presenting in the same fashion every time and rarely increasing in intensity—and relieved by food or anti-ulcer medication. Gastric ulcer pain is similar, but it may be accompanied by nausea, vomiting, and weight loss. Other than in the identification of a succussion splash with gastric outlet obstruction, the physical examination is usually not helpful. Diagnosis of peptic ulcer is made by (1) response to therapy, (2) air contrast upper GI series, or (3) endoscopy. Of the three, endoscopy is by far the most accurate,[2] and it is also the most invasive and expensive. In young patients with recent onset of typical pain who are otherwise healthy, a reasonable argument can be made to treat for 2 weeks and reassess. If symptoms persist, endoscopy should then be performed. If symptoms clear, treatment for an additional 2 weeks is indicated. For older patients with recurrent symptoms not otherwise diagnosed or with persistent vomiting, weight loss, or signs of bleeding, a more precise diagnosis, including biopsy of gastric lesions, should be pursued.

TREATMENT

Although the etiology of the lesion is the same, i.e., "no acid, no disease," the pathophysiology of gastric and duodenal lesions is different. For this reason, therapies may differ.

Gastritis and gastric ulcer occur predominantly in the presence of decreased mucosal resistance to injury. Gastric mucus, a viscous gel that coats the entire stomach surface, acts as a barrier to back diffusion of luminal contents toward the mucosa. In addition to the mucus, bicarbonate is secreted by the surface epithelial cells. This establishes a stable pH gradient from the acidic luminal contents to the neutral surface of the mucosal cell.[3] Prostaglandins appear to play a role in maintaining this gastric mucosal barrier. Thus, therapy is directed not only toward reducing luminal acid-pepsin concentration but also toward maintaining this natural barrier and creating artificial barriers.

Duodenal peptic disease, on the other hand, is clearly related to an increased secretion of acid and pepsin.[4] Patients with duodenal ulcers have more acid-secreting parietal cells than normals, and each cell is more responsive to a given stimulus. Furthermore, following a meal the stimulus to secrete acid is greater, because serum gastrin levels are higher and the inhibitory feedback mechanism that suppresses gastrin release is impaired. Therapy is, therefore, primarily directed toward decreasing gastric acid levels, although protecting the duodenal ulceration from further acid-peptic digestion has also proved to be beneficial.

Buffers. Buffers of gastric acid have been the mainstay of medical therapy for years. Food *per se* is now recognized to be a poor buffer, and there is no benefit to be had in pain relief or ulcer healing from a so-called bland diet. However, food is beneficial in slowing gastric emptying, thus allowing for longer activity of antacids. The degree of acid reduction that is necessary for ulcer healing is not entirely clear. Low-dose antacids, i.e., 1 tablespoon postprandially and at night, were found to heal duodenal ulcers no better than placebo, whereas high-dose (144 mEq of neutralizing capacity) antacids at one and three hours after meals and at bedtime were significantly better.[5] Although antacids have only minor side effects (osmotic diarrhea from the magnesium overload or phosphate depletion with aluminum hydroxide) even with the high concentrate formulations, many patients and physicians do not rely solely on antacids because of the inconvenience and large volume required.

Anticholinergics. Anticholinergics are vagolytic, thus inhibiting basal and some forms of stimulated acid secretion. By themselves, acid reduction is suboptimal, and ulcer healing in carefully controlled trials has been disappointing. Perhaps by reducing gastric and duodenal motility, anticholinergics have found their biggest use in treating duodenal ulcers, by reducing pain and prolonging the intragastric buffering effect of antacids.

H₂-Blockers. H₂-blockers, such as cimetidine and ranitidine, have proved to be very successful. Because of the interaction between the histamine receptor and the cholinergic and gastrin receptors, H₂-blockers have been found to be impressive inhibitors of acid secretion and have become the mainstay of medical management, particularly of duodenal ulcer disease. The healing of gastric ulcers has been less impressive, probably because acid overproduction does not play such a major role in the pathophysiology of gastric ulcer disease. Both cimetidine and ranitidine heal peptic ulcers at similar rates. Because the experience with cimetidine has been greater, side effects, although rare, are recognized to occur. As expected, similar side effects have been noted with ranitidine as experience is gained with this drug.[6] Recently, efficacy has been demonstrated at longer dosing intervals than were originally utilized, even when administered once daily at bedtime.

Sucralfate. Sucralfate is a basic aluminum salt of a sulfated disaccharide that was developed to treat peptic ulcer. When exposed to gastric acid, it turns into a viscous adhesive substance that forms stable complexes with protein. This gel complex contains some acid-buffering capacity, absorbs and resists the proteolytic action of pepsin, absorbs bile salts, and promotes endogenous prostaglandin release. The sum of these activities provides protection against acid, pepsin, and bile salts and has been shown to heal duodenal and gastric ulcers at a rate comparable with H₂-blockers or high-dose antacids.[7] The drug is not absorbed, and mild constipation is the only reported side effect to date. The 1 gm tablet is best taken four times a day, one hour before meals and at bedtime. It can be added to a regimen of antacids or cimetidine, provided the drugs are not taken simultaneously.

Bismuth Salts. *Campylobacter pylori,* a gram-negative bacterium, has been associated with antral gastritis and peptic ulcer disease. Debate regarding this organism and a causal relationship with ulcer disease continues. The organism appears to be sensitive to bismuth salts, such as bismuth subcitrate, and various antibiotics.[8]

Surgery. Most patients with peptic disease are easily treated as outpatients; hospitalization is required only for complications. Active bleeding, gastric outlet obstruction, perforation, and failure of medical therapy to manage the disease effectively are well-recognized complications that frequently require surgery. Bleeding from an acute duodenal ulcer carries a 40% chance of recurrence, and gastric outlet obstruction, even though relieved by continuous nasogastric suction and IV therapy, also carries a high likelihood of eventual surgery. Most physicians believe that two episodes of such complications indicate surgery as evidence of medical therapy failure. Acute perforation is a surgical emergency frequently treated by a simple omental patch closure; further acid-reducing surgery is often not necessary.

Persistent symptoms that interfere with the patient's lifestyle, in spite of full medical therapy, are also best treated surgically.

KEY FEATURES

Duodenal Ulcers
Increased acid secretion
More common in men, but difference decreasing

Risk Factors
Known
    Smoking
    Family history
    Sex

Associated diseases: hyperparathyroidism, chronic obstructive pulmonary disease, chronic renal failure, cirrhosis

Unproven
    Diet
    Aspirin and other nonsteroidal anti-inflammatory drugs
    Stress

Unrelated
    Alcohol
    Caffeine
    Personality

Gastric Ulcers
Decreased mucosal resistance
Equal frequency between sexes

Known
    Smoking
    Family history
    Aspirin and other nonsteroidal anti-inflammatory drugs

Unproven
    Diet
    Stress
    Sex
    Associated disease

Unrelated
    Alcohol
    Caffeine
    Personality

Diagnosis
Best by endoscopy

Treatment
Antacids: full dose—7 times/day
H_2-blockers: cimetidine, ranitidine
Sucralfate

All heal about 70–80% at 4–6 weeks.
Little to choose between cimetidine and ranitidine, as side effects and costs are similar.
Sucralfate perhaps best for elderly patients on multiple medications.

REFERENCES

1. Kurata J: What in the world is happening to ulcers. Gastroenterology 84:1623–1625, 1983.
    Editorial review of worldwide ulcer statistics pointing out changing trends in mortality and hospitalization and an increase of women with acute duodenal ulcers.

2. Dooley CP, et al: Double-contrast barium meal and upper gastrointestinal endoscopy: A comparative review. Ann Intern Med 101:538–545, 1984.
   Endoscopy: Sensitivity 92%, specificity 100%
   UGI: Sensitivity 54%, specificity 91%
   *   Poor patient cooperation and perceptual and technical failures contribute significantly to radiologic failures.*

3. Kauffman GL Jr: Gastric mucus and bicarbonate secretion in relation to mucosal protection. J Clin Gastroenterol 3(suppl 2):51–56, 1981.
   *   Review of endogenous gastric mucosal protection factors.*

4. Feldman M, Barnett C: Gastric bicarbonate secretion in patients with duodenal ulcer. Gastroenterology 88:1205–1208, 1985; Hirschowitz B: Apparent and intrinsic sensitivity to pentagastrin of acid and pepsin secretion in peptic ulcer. Gastroenterology 86:843–851, 1984.
   *   Both articles confirm older observations that gastric acid output is greater in people with duodenal ulcers than in controls.*

5. Fordtran JS, et al: In vivo and in vitro evaluation of liquid antacids. N Engl J Med 288:923–928, 1973; Peterson WL, et al: Healing of duodenal ulcer with an antacid regimen. N Engl J Med 297:341, 1977.
   *   The two classic papers on antacids. The first documents the efficacy of the buffering capacity of various antacids; the second shows that large-dose therapy is effective in healing duodenal ulcer. Thirty cc of Mylanta II, one and three hours after meals and at bedtime, healed duodenal ulcer 76% at four weeks (placebo only 45%).*

6. McCarthy D: Ranitidine or cimetidine? Ann Intern Med 99:551–553, 1983.
   *   Editorial review of two H_2-blockers outlining the reported side effects of each; side effects become more similar as further experience with ranitidine is gained.*

7. Hollander D: Efficacy of sucralfate for duodenal ulcers: A multi-center, double-blind trial. J Clin Gastroenterol 3(suppl 2):153–157, 1981; Hollander D, et al: Protective effect of sucralfate against alcohol-induced gastric mucosal injury in the rat. Gastroenterology 88:366–374, 1985.
   *   Two studies demonstrating the efficacy of sucralfate in gastric and duodenal lesions. Four-week duodenal ulcer healing rates: 82% with sucralfate, 53% with controls.*

8. Blaser M: Gastric Campylobacter-like organisms, gastritis, and peptic ulcer disease. Gastroenterology 93:371–383, 1987.
   *   A review of this hot topic.*

Upper Gastrointestinal Tract Bleeding

Claudia McClintock, M.D.

Upper gastrointestinal hemorrhage accounts for as many as 200,000 hospital admissions a year in the United States; the mortality rate is about 10%. Most patients who are admitted are still bleeding (passing blood or melena, vomiting blood, or showing blood on gastric lavage) or have recently bled enough to cause orthostatic hypotension. In such acutely ill patients, the early goals are aggressive resuscitation, close monitoring, stabilization, and *then* diagnosis. Most patients (80–90%) stop bleeding in the first 24 hours with no specific therapy.

There are several clinical signs of GI bleeding. Melena usually results from bleeding above the ileocecal valve, but with slow transit time colonic blood can turn black. Hematemesis indicates an upper source. Hematochezia is not a good localizing sign; it usually results from a lower GI lesion, but massive upper GI bleeding may also cause hematochezia. Gastric lavage gives the most accurate information. If lavage fluid is free of blood and is bile stained, no upper GI bleeding is occurring. Testing clear lavage fluid with chemical indicators is misleading and unnecessary. If no bile appears in the lavage, bleeding may be continuing from a duodenal lesion associated with pylorospasm.

Laboratory tests are not helpful in evaluating active bleeding. The hematocrit lags behind the clinical state at two points: it remains artificially high during acute bleeding, before extravascular fluid shifts to maintain volume; and it remains low after transfusion, before the same fluid returns to the extravascular space. Chemical tests for occult bleeding are affected by trauma (difficult passage of a nasogastric tube) and by transit time (blood may take 7 days to evacuate the GI tract).

Initial management should include placement of more than one large-bore intravenous catheter; type-and-cross for more units of blood than the estimated amount of loss; correction of coagulopathy, if demonstrated; intubation if bleeding is massive and uncontrollable (to prevent aspiration and adult respiratory distress syndrome); and GI and surgery consults. If a small-bore nasogastric tube returns blood, gastric lavage is begun via a large-bore orogastric tube. The larger the tube, the more efficient the lavage. Neither ice nor saline is better than room temperature tap water for gastric lavage.[1,2]

The most accurate way to identify the source of upper GI bleeding is endoscopy (90–95% successful). Double-contrast radiographs detect 80–85% of lesions, and single-contrast radiographs detect fewer than half; neither radiographic modality pinpoints which lesion is actually bleeding. Several controlled trials have failed to demonstrate any benefit from early diagnosis in patients who stop bleeding spontaneously.[3] However, such patients should undergo some diagnostic procedure, electively, for the following reasons:

1. If a gastric ulcer is detected, it is biopsied and followed to healing.
2. Active peptic ulcers are treated for 6 weeks, but duodenitis/gastritis is treated for only 2 weeks.
3. Patients who show "stigmata of recent hemorrhage" from varices are often treated with sclerotherapy.
4. Identifying peptic disease as the source of bleeding influences decisions about surgery during subsequent bleeds.

Elective endoscopy in stable, nonbleeding patients is a benign procedure (complication rate about 1 in 800).

Patients who continue to bleed, or rebleed within 72 hours, should undergo early endoscopy. Localization of the source of bleeding is important if surgery is required. Endoscopy can provide therapy in addition to diagnosis. Electrocoagulation, heater probe, and laser photocoagulation are all used; a recent study demonstrated that multipolar electrocoagulation of actively bleeding lesions was successful in arresting hemorrhage.[7] Endoscopic sclerosis has been shown in controlled trials to stop or diminish acute variceal bleeding and to reduce the incidence of rebleeding.[8] Patients who are actively bleeding at the time of endoscopy experience greater morbidity (1 in 200) and mortality (1 in 700) than patients who have stopped bleeding.

Causes of upper GI bleeding vary with patient population. In the United States, ulcers (duodenal, gastric, and marginal) account for 40–50% of bleeds. Lesions responsible for upper GI bleeding at Boston City Hospital in 1984 are given in Table 1.

Gastritis is usually due to alcohol, rarely to drugs. Most patients stop

TABLE 1.   LESIONS RESPONSIBLE FOR UPPER GI BLEEDING

Lesion	% of Cases
Gastritis	21
Varices	18
Mallory-Weiss tear	15
Duodenal ulcer	12
Gastric ulcer	12
Miscellaneous and no diagnosis	16

Data from Boston City Hospital, 1984.

bleeding spontaneously; the mortality rate is low. Acid reduction therapy that keeps the gastric pH above 5.0 reduces the risk of rebleeding.[4] Many regimens for acid reduction have been tested on the principle that if a pH of 5.0 is "good," 7.0 is "better." The most effective regimen (maintaining gastric pH at 7.0 more than 95% of the time) is cimetidine 100 mg/hour (continuous infusion) with antacids 30 ml/hour.[9] Surgery should be avoided if possible.

Patients with bleeding esophageal or gastric varices have a high mortality rate (20–30% during hospitalization) and a high rebleeding rate (30% within 6 months). Both are reduced by sclerotherapy. Long-term mortality depends chiefly on the degree of underlying liver failure. Two other therapies are in use. The Sengstaken-Blakemore tube stops bleeding 75–80% of the time, though the complication rate is high unless the patient is intubated, a fourth lumen is used to suction the esophagus, and the balloons are deflated at intervals.[5] Vasopressin (at infusion rates of 0.4–0.8 U/minute) has many dangerous side effects, and one controlled trial failed to demonstrate efficacy in stopping even variceal bleeds.[6] It should be used only as a last resort.

A Mallory-Weiss tear occurs during retching (usually alcohol-related); bleeding often stops spontaneously. If hemorrhage continues or recurs, the tear should be electrocoagulated or oversewn.

Patients with bleeding peptic ulcers are treated with a full (6-week) course of medical therapy. Cimetidine 300 mg qid is an effective ulcer-healing regimen when given for 6 weeks. There is no treatment regimen for duodenitis/gastritis; general practice is to treat for 2 weeks. However, if the patient has hemorrhaged enough to need admission, a full course should be given.

Lower gastrointestinal bleeding is responsible for far fewer admissions than upper tract bleeding. The mortality rate is under 5%, even though the population is generally older than those with upper GI hemorrhage. Initial management is the same as that of upper bleeds, including passage of a nasogastric tube to exclude an upper source. Most patients stop bleeding spontaneously with no specific therapy. In such cases, an elective work-up is undertaken, using either colonoscopy or sigmoidoscopy and barium enema. Single-contrast radiographs detect 40–50% of colonic lesions and are useful for excluding large lesions only. Double-contrast radiographs are as accurate as colonoscopy in detecting lesions (including small polyps and mucosal irregularities). Colonoscopy allows biopsy of lesions, removal of polyps, and visualization of angiodysplasia.

Patients who do not stop bleeding should undergo early colonoscopy. Electrolyte solutions via nasogastric tube provide quick preparation. If a bleeding site is identified, it can be electrocoagulated. This often is not effective permanently, but it may "buy time." If the patient is bleeding too fast to allow colonoscopic visualization, angiography should be utilized to localize the source. Scintigraphic techniques utilizing technetium-99m sulfur colloid or labeled erythrocytes may allow localization at lower rates of hemorrhage than standard angiography.

Common causes of brisk lower GI bleeding include diverticulosis; angiodysplasia; and, in 10% of instances, upper tract sources. Bleeding from diverticulosis or angiodysplasia usually stops spontaneously, but it often recurs. Cautery or surgery may be successful for several months, but bleeding often resumes. Other causes of lower GI bleeding include ischemic bowel, inflammatory bowel disease, neoplasms, and anorectal disease.

KEY FEATURES

I. Goals
  1. Estimate amount of loss
  2. Resuscitate and replace blood loss
  3. Locate and control bleeding
  4. Prevent recurrence
II. Clinical features
  1. Orthostatic signs
  2. Melena
  3. Hematemesis
  4. Nasogastric aspirate
III. Causes of upper GI bleeding
  1. Gastritis: 21%
  2. Varices: 18%
  3. Mallory-Weiss: 15%
  4. Peptic ulcers
    a. Duodenal: 12%
    b. Gastric: 12%
IV. Management
  1. Large-bore IVs and flow sheet
  2. Blood replacement
  3. Gastric lavage
  4. Intubate if bleeding is massive
  5. GI/surgery consults
V. Prognosis of upper GI bleeding
  1. Overall mortality rate 10% (2% in those who stop; 15% in those who continue)
  2. Alcoholic gastritis, Mallory-Weiss: self-limited, surgery rare
  3. "Stress" gastritis: severe, often recurrent, high mortality
  4. Peptic ulcers: 20–30% rebleed, 10%–15% need surgery
  5. Varices: 30% rebleed; 20–30% mortality
VI. Causes of lower GI bleeding
  1. Diverticulosis: 20% rebleed, surgery rare
  2. Angiodysplasia: often rebleed, surgery rare
  3. Ischemic bowel

4. Inflammatory bowel disease
5. Tumor, hemorrhoids, upper source

REFERENCES

1. Ponsky et al: J Surg Res 28:204, 1980; Bryand et al: Am J Surg 124:570, 1972.
   Evidence in favor of room temperature tap water lavage

2. Kiselow and Wagner: Arch Surg 107:387, 1979; Wapnick et al: NY State J Med 76:1963, 1976.
   Articles discuss Levofed in the lavage (uncontrolled).

3. Peterson et al: Routine early endoscopy in upper gastrointestinal tract bleeding. N Engl J Med 304:925, 1981.
4. Hastings et al: Antacid prophylaxis of bleeding in the critically ill. N Engl J Med 298:1041, 1978.
5. Chokjier and Conn: Esophageal tamponade in the treatment of bleeding varices. Dig Dis Sci 25:267, 1980.
6. Fogel et al: Continuous intravenous vasopressin in active upper gastrointestinal bleeding. Ann Intern Med 96:565, 1982.
   Pitressin no better than placebo. For the pro side, see Johnson et al in Ann Surg 186:389, 1977.

7. Laine L: Multipolar electrocoagulation in the treatment of active upper gastrointestinal tract hemorrhage. N Engl J Med 316:1613, 1987.
8. Terblanche et al: Surgery 85:239, 1979; Clark et al: Lancet 2:552, 1980.
   Articles discuss sclerotherapy.

9. Peterson et al: Sustained fasting achlorhydria: A comparison of medical regimens. Gastroenterology 88:666, 1985.

Intestinal Ischemia

William Hale, M.D.

Reduced blood flow to the intestines can result in organ damage at any level of the intestinal tract but typically evolves into two distinct clinical syndromes. Involvement of the superior mesenteric artery leads to small intestinal and right colonic damage and is commonly known as acute mesenteric ischemia. Segmental involvement of the left hemicolon, or ischemic colitis, results from a reduction in the inferior mesenteric circulation. Although overlap may occur, for simplicity these syndromes are discussed separately in the following review.

Despite increased recognition and improved supportive care, acute small intestinal or mesenteric ischemia still carries a very high mortality rate. This results from the nonspecific clinical and laboratory findings in the pre-infarction stage, the occasional progressive nature of the process despite correction of initiating events, and the rising occurrence of nonocclusive ischemia. Twenty-five to fifty per cent of cases result from occlusion of the superior mesenteric artery (SMA) or its branches by thrombus or emboli.[1,2] Nonocclusive ischemia that is due to intense vasoconstriction, with or without underlying atherosclerosis, accounts for 40%–70% of cases.[1,2,5] Occlusion of the superior mesenteric vein causes approximately 10% of cases, and vasculitis of the abdominal vessels is a rare cause of ischemia.[1,2]

Regardless of etiology, the tissue response to reduced blood flow is similar. Initial mucosal damage (edema, hemorrhage, and slough) is followed by muscular atony with dilation and ileus. In severe cases, full-thickness perforation results.[1]

Early diagnosis of acute mesenteric ischemia in the pre-infarction stage is extremely important and requires careful monitoring of high-risk patients, i.e., those with congestive heart failure, acute myocardial infarction, systemic embolization, hypotension, and sepsis. The clinical presentation is nonspecific, but abdominal pain is the outstanding symptom. Colicky and periumbilical at onset, the pain soon becomes diffuse, steady, and, classically, out of proportion to physical findings. Examination typically reveals abdominal distention, often with preserved bowel sounds. Peritoneal signs, if present at all, are a late finding and are indicative of infarction or perforation. Occult GI bleeding is seen in the majority of cases.[1,2,3] Metabolic acidosis, leukocytosis, and hyperkalemia indicate significant tissue necrosis, and evaluation of mesenteric ischemia should not be delayed until they occur.[1,3] Plain films of the abdomen are useful primarily in excluding other diagnoses, such as perforation, volvulus, and obstruction.

Management of acute mesenteric ischemia is based on correction of potential precipitating conditions, aggressive supportive care, and early angiographic evaluation. Documentation of arterial occlusion, either thrombotic or embolic, necessitates surgical intervention with revascularization and possibly resection. A "second look" procedure at 12–24 hours is used to assess viability of remaining bowel. Mortality rates from 30% to 85% are reported, primarily dependent on the amount of bowel involved and the duration of ischemia.[1,2]

Superior mesenteric vein occlusion may complicate polycythemia, portal hypertension, trauma, and oral contraceptive use or may occur spontaneously. Symptoms typically develop over 3–5 days, and early surgical resection has reduced mortality to approximately 20%.[1,2]

Nonocclusive mesenteric ischemia is characterized by its occurrence following low-flow states or the use of intestinal vasoconstrictors and by the absence of major vascular occlusion at angiography. Boley has described several typical angiographic findings in nonocclusive ischemia.[5] These in-

clude narrowing of the take-off of major branches of the SMA, beading of
the vessels as a result of intermittent spasm, and dilation and diffuse pruning
of the arterial circulation.[1,4,5] The infusion of the vasodilating agent papaverine through a SMA catheter has been recommended by some authors,
and uncontrolled studies report a reduction in mortality to approximately
40%.[5] Surgical intervention is required if clinical findings suggest intestinal
necrosis or if there is no clinical or angiographic response to papaverine.

Ischemic colitis typically involves the left colon or splenic flexure and
occurs either spontaneously or following inferior mesenteric artery interruption during aortic surgery. Patients are almost invariably over 50 years
of age, and symptoms consist of lower abdominal pain and bloody diarrhea.[6,7]
The diagnosis can be confirmed by proctosigmoidoscopy showing edematous,
inflamed mucosa, often with submucosal hemorrhage. Low-pressure barium
enema can also be used. Infectious and antibiotic-associated colitis must be
excluded. Biopsy may be helpful in excluding inflammatory bowel disease
if coagulation necrosis is demonstrated. The clinical course is more indolent
than small intestinal ischemia, and resection is usually reserved for those
patients with progressive peritoneal findings. Mortality rates of 38%–55%
have been reported.[6,7] Healing occurs over 2–6 weeks and may result in the
development of stricture or the formation of adhesions.[1]

KEY FEATURES

I. Acute mesenteric ischemia
   A. Etiology
      1. Thrombotic/embolic: 25–50%
      2. Nonocclusive: 40–75%
      3. Venous occlusion: 10%
      4. Vasculitis: rare
   B. High-risk patients:
      1. Low-flow state
      2. Systemic hypotension
      3. Arterial embolization
      4. Diffuse atherosclerotic vascular disease
      5. Vasoconstrictors
   C. Manifestations
      1. Abdominal distention
      2. Diffuse abdominal pain without localizing signs
      3. Occult GI bleeding
      4. Acidosis, leukocytosis, hyperkalemia: late findings
   D. Management
      1. Plain radiographs
      2. Aggressive supportive care
      3. Surgical consultation

    4. Early angiography
        a. Occlusive disease: surgical intervention
        b. Nonocclusive disease: consideration of papaverine in-
           fusion; delayed surgical intervention
II. Segmental ischemic colitis
    A. Etiology
        1. Acute inferior mesenteric artery occlusion
        2. Spontaneous: ?nonocclusive
    B. High-risk patients
        1. Elderly
        2. Systemic hypotension
        3. Low-flow state
        4. Aortic surgery
    C. Manifestations
        1. Abdominal pain
        2. Bloody diarrhea
        3. Fecal leukocytes
    D. Management
        1. Supportive care
        2. Stool cultures and *Clostridium difficile* toxin assay
        3. Proctosigmoidoscopy/barium enema
        4. Surgical consultation

REFERENCES

1. Williams LF: Vascular insufficiency of the intestines. Gastroenterology 61:757–777, 1971.
   Extensive review of the subject with 237 references. Pathophysiology, diagnosis, and management discussed for each type of lesion.

2. Ottinger LW: Mesenteric ischemia. N Engl J Med 307:535–537, 1982.
   Subject review emphasizing more recent survival data, and the importance of early angiographic studies.

3. Cooke M, et al: Diagnosis and outcome of bowel infarction on an acute medical service. Am J Med 75:984–996, 1983.
   Retrospective study of 20 patients with proven small intestinal infarction. Clinical findings: acute abdominal pain, 15 of 20; distention, 15 of 20; occult blood in stool, 13 of 20. Initial findings were nonspecific, and significant delay occurred before surgical evaluation. Angiography was not performed. Twelve of twenty patients had nonocclusive ischemia. Overall survival was only 2 of 20 patients.

4. Siegelman SS, et al: Angiographic diagnosis of mesenteric arterial vasoconstriction. Radiology 112:533–542, 1974.
   Experimental and clinical study into angiographic findings in nonocclusive mesenteric ischemia. Papaverine was effective in two of four cases.

5. Boley SJ, et al: Initial results from an aggressive roentgenological and surgical approach to acute mesenteric ischemia. Surgery 82:848–855, 1977.
   Early angiography was performed in 50 patients considered at risk for acute mesenteric ischemia (AMI). Thirty-five of fifty patients (70%) had diagnosis of AMI made on initial angiogram. Findings: nonocclusive ischemia, 15; SMA embolus, 16; SMA thrombosis, 3; SMV thrombosis, 1. Papaverine was infused in all patients with nonocclusive ischemia and

3 patients with SMA embolus. There was an overall survival rate of 54% (60% in non-occlusive ischemia group).

6. Williams LF, et al: Ischemic colitis: A useful clinical diagnosis, but is it ischemia? Ann Surg 182:439–448, 1975.
    Review of 55 cases of segmental colitis. Pain and bloody diarrhea were present in 75% and 61%, respectively. Average age was 70 years. Forty-two per cent of patients required surgery with a 61% survival rate, whereas the nonoperated group had a 63% survival rate. The left colon and/or the splenic flexure was involved in all but 2 cases. Surgery was reserved for those with significant peritoneal signs or a protracted course.

7. Abel ME, et al: Ischemic colitis: Comparison of surgical and nonoperative management. Dis Colon Rectum 26:113–115, 1983.
    Retrospective review of 18 cases of spontaneous ischemic colitis with 9 managed operatively and 9 nonoperatively. Survival rates were 45% and 55%, respectively.

Inflammatory Bowel Disease

William Hale, M.D.

Crohn's disease (CD) and ulcerative colitis (UC) are chronic inflammatory diseases of the gut that appear principally in adolescents and young adults with clinical courses characterized by remissions and exacerbations. The inflammatory process in UC is confined to the mucosa and submucosa with edema, vascular engorgement, exudation, and shallow ulcerations. The rectum is involved in 90–95% of cases with a variable degree of proximal extension. In contrast, CD is a transmural process characterized by fibrosis and luminal narrowing, formation of fissures, submucosal thickening (creating a "cobblestone" appearance), and segmental involvement of the bowel rather than the continuous involvement typically seen in UC. Noncaseating granulomas are found in 30–50% of cases.

Whereas UC is confined to the colon and rectum, CD may involve any level of the gastrointestinal tract. Data compiled from two studies of CD show that isolated small intestinal involvement occurs in 29% of cases, small intestinal and colonic involvement in 50%, colonic disease alone in 19%, and isolated anorectal disease in 2%.[1,2] Involvement of the terminal ileum, the development of fistulous tracts, and recurrent perianal lesions are hallmarks of CD. Despite the seemingly clear separation into different clinical and pathologic entities, a clear distinction can be made in only 70–80% of cases when the inflammatory process is limited to the colon.[3] Both diseases may be complicated by extraintestinal manifestations such as arthritis, iritis, skin lesions, and liver disease.[4,5,6]

Acute UC typically presents with bloody diarrhea, crampy lower abdominal pain, and variable signs of systemic toxicity. The assessment of clinical severity is based on the frequency of bowel movements; the amount of rectal bleeding; and the presence of anemia, volume depletion, systemic toxicity, and hypoalbuminemia. Mild disease accounts for nearly 60% of cases, whereas 25% of patients have disease of moderate severity and 10–15% manifest severe disease with high fevers, colonic distention, profuse bloody diarrhea, significant volume depletion, and low serum albumin.

Although acute Crohn's colitis can be indistinguishable from UC, CD more typically begins with chronic abdominal pain involving the right lower quadrant and periumbilical area, watery diarrhea, fatigue, and low-grade fevers. Fistulous tracts, chronic perianal disease, and malabsorption are also part of the clinical picture. Growth failure may be the only manifestation of CD in the adolescent.

The initial diagnostic evaluation varies with the clinical presentation. All cases of acute colitis should be carefully screened with repeated stool cultures for bacterial pathogens; assay for *Clostridium difficile* enterotoxin; and early flexible sigmoidoscopy to assess the degree, character, and extent of mucosal inflammation. Barium studies of the colon and small intestine and full colonoscopy with biopsies are essential in the complete evaluation of the patient with inflammatory bowel disease but should generally be deferred until the acute inflammatory process has subsided.

Toxic megacolon complicates 2–5% of cases of acute colitis and is characterized by sudden colonic dilatation, severe systemic toxicity, and often a decrease in stool frequency. Serial abdominal films are important in following patients with moderate and severe colitis. Early barium studies and the use of anticholinergic agents have been linked to the development of toxic megacolon. Aggressive medical support and early surgical intervention have reduced the mortality rate to less than 15%.[7,8]

Treatment of acute inflammatory bowel disease is based on bowel rest, fluid and electrolyte replacement, and drug therapy. Most patients with only mild disease activity can be managed on an outpatient basis, but more severe disease generally requires hospitalization with careful monitoring to detect clinical deterioration.

Acute UC responds to both corticosteroids and sulfasalazine, with more severe cases requiring intravenous steroids initially followed by conversion to oral (or rectal) steroids and the addition of sulfasalazine.[9] Both steroids and sulfasalazine are effective in maintaining disease remission, but side effects limit prolonged steroid use.[10] Newer agents, such as beclomethasone proprionate, tixocortal pivolate, and 5-aminosalicylate, have fewer systemic actions and are currently under study.

Therapy of CD is more complex because of the more diverse clinical manifestations. Active CD responds to therapy with corticosteroids, with sulfasalazine usually reserved for patients with colonic involvement; however, some patients with ileitis alone may respond to sulfasalazine. Unfortunately, neither agent aids in sustaining remission or in preventing postoperative relapse.[11] Immunosuppressive agents (azathioprine and 6-mercaptopurine) are of limited value when used alone but allow for reduction of steroid dose and may have an independent effect in promoting healing of fistulous tracts and perianal disease.[12] However, because of potential hazards, these agents are reserved for patients with persistent severe disease unresponsive to medical and resective therapy. One controlled trial indicated that metronidazole (800 mg daily) is as effective as sulfasalazine in controlling active CD and that larger doses (20 mg/kg daily) may induce healing of resistant perianal disease. Unfortunately, relapse of the perianal disease appears to be common when the dose is tapered.[13]

Maintenance of adequate nutrition in inflammatory bowel disease can be extremely difficult, especially in patients with extensive CD. Although aggressive alimentation often dramatically improves nutritional status and can reverse growth retardation in children, there is little evidence that the overall course of the disease is altered significantly.[14,15] Vitamin and mineral replacement is indicated in patients with extensive small bowel involvement, and a lactose-free diet may be helpful.

The surgical management of inflammatory bowel disease is beyond the scope of this article.

KEY FEATURES

Pathology
Ulcerative colitis (CD): mucosal inflammation
Crohn's disease (CD): full-thickness involvement, fistula formation, granulomas
    30–50%

Extension

UC: Rectal involvement	90–95%
CD: Small intestine (especially terminal ileum)	29%
Small intestine and colon	50%
Colon alone	19%

Manifestations
UC: Bloody diarrhea, fever, toxic megacolon 2–6%
CD: Abdominal pain, fistulous tracts and perianal disease, weight loss, watery diarrhea

Management

UC:	Acute:	Corticosteroids
		Sulfasalazine
	Remission:	Sulfasalazine
CD:	Acute:	Corticosteroids
		Sulfasalazine (colonic involvement)
		Metronidazole (perianal disease)
	Remission:	None

REFERENCES

1. Farmer R, Hawk W, et al: Clinical patterns in Crohn's disease. Gastroenterology 80:66, 1981.
2. Melchjian H, Switz D, et al: Clinical features and natural history of Crohn's disease. Gastroenterology 77:898, 1979.
3. Schacter H, Kirsner J: Definitions of inflammatory bowel disease of unknown etiology. Gastroenterology 68:591, 1975.
4. Greenstein A, Janowitz H, et al: The extraintestinal complications of Crohn's disease and ulcerative colitis: A study of 700 patients. Medicine 55:401, 1976.
5. Eade N: Liver disease in ulcerative colitis. I. Analysis of operative liver biopsy in 138 consecutive patients. Ann Intern Med 72:475, 1970.
6. Thornton J, Teague R, et al: Pyoderma gangrenosum and ulcerative colitis. Gut 21:247, 1980.
7. Binder J, Patterson J, et al: Toxic megacolon in ulcerative colitis. Gastroenterology 66:909, 1974.
8. Present D, Wolfson D, et al: The medical management of toxic megacolon: Technique of decompression with favorable long term following. Gastroenterology 80:1255, 1981.
9. Peppercorn M: Sulfasalazine: Pharmacology, clinical use, toxicity and related new drug development. Ann Intern Med 101:377, 1984.
10. Dissanayake A, Truelove S: A controlled therapeutic trial of long-term maintenance treatment of ulcerative colitis with sulfasalazine. Gut 14:923, 1974.
11. Summer R, Svetz D, et al: National cooperative Crohn's disease study: Results of drug treatment. Gastroenterology 77:1847, 1979.
12. Present D, Korelitz B, et al: Treatment of Crohn's disease with 6-mercaptopurine. A long-term randomized double-blind study. N Engl J Med 302:981, 1980.
13. Ursing B, Alan T, et al: A comparative study of metronidazole and sulfasalazine for active Crohn's disease. Gastroenterology 83:5550, 1982.
14. Dickinson R, Ashton M: Controlled trial of intravenous hyperalimentation and total bowel rest as an adjunct to the routine therapy of acute colitis. Gastroenterology 79:1199, 1980.
15. Morain C, Segal A, et al: Elemental diet as primary treatment of acute Crohn's disease: A controlled trial. Br Med J 288:1859, 1984.

Hepatic Failure

Raymond S. Koff, M.D.

Acute hepatic failure is a devastating syndrome with a variable case fatality rate approaching 95%. The etiology includes disorders associated with extensive or massive hepatic necrosis, such as viral hepatitis, drug-induced and chemical hepatotoxicity, severe hypoperfusion syndromes, exacerbations of chronic active hepatitis, and, infrequently, Wilson's disease. Acute hepatic failure also may occur in syndromes in which hepatocellular necrosis is less prominent but in which fatty change is a salient feature. These include Reye's syndrome, acute fatty liver of pregnancy, and intravenous tetracycline-induced and sodium valproate–induced hepatic failure.

In patients in whom prior liver disease has not been recognized, the syndrome of acute hepatic failure usually develops within 8 weeks of the onset of illness. In an occasional, especially older, patient, hepatic failure may develop as long as 6 months after the onset of symptoms of liver disease.[1]

Hepatic encephalopathy, a cardinal feature of hepatic failure, is accompanied by hypoprothrombinemia and usually progressive jaundice, a diminution of liver size, and in many patients failure of other organ systems. Other causes of encephalopathy must be considered and excluded by appropriate clinical, laboratory, and radiologic assessment. The pathogenesis of hepatic encephalopathy in acute hepatic failure remains poorly understood. Abnormalities in ammonia metabolism, short-chain fatty acid accumulation, and elevated levels of mercaptans have been described, but their role remains uncertain.[2] Alterations in CNS neurotransmission as a result of abnormalities in amino acid neurotransmitters, increased permeability of the blood-brain barrier, and altered functional properties of neural membranes may be critical elements in the pathogenesis of hepatic encephalopathy.[3] Increased numbers of receptors for inhibitory amino acid neurotransmitters and decreased receptors for excitatory amino acid neurotransmitters have been hypothesized. Increased CNS sensitivity to drugs such as the benzodiazepines may be mediated by increased numbers of drug receptors in neural membranes.[3] Hence, use of CNS depressant drugs is best avoided.

Effective treatment to end ongoing hepatocellular necrosis, prevent further necrosis, or stimulate hepatic regeneration is not yet available. Antiviral chemotherapy for fulminant viral hepatitis and experimental procedures designed to eliminate noxious materials from the circulation have no demonstrable benefit and may be dangerous. A series of trials have provided convincing evidence that corticosteroids are of no utility.[4,5] Aggressive maintenance of life functions and the early identification and vigorous treatment of life-threatening complications are believed to increase the likelihood of survival. In large part, survival may be dependent on our ability to support these patients until hepatic necrosis and dysfunction resolve and hepatocyte mass is restored through hepatic regeneration. Prognostic epidemiologic, clinical, and laboratory factors remain poorly defined. However, advanced age and the coexistence of malignancy or debilitating disease appear to impede recovery. Absence or loss of the oculovestibular reflex is associated with a reduced survival rate.[6]

Management is directed by intensivists in a unit familiar with the syndrome. Continuous observation and monitoring of vital signs are essential and should not be hindered by isolation procedures that are necessary, nonetheless, to avoid nosocomial transmission of viral hepatitis. Laboratory assessment includes daily measurement of serum electrolytes, acid-base balance, glucose, prothrombin time, platelet counts, and urine volume. Careful intake and outflow measurements, daily weights, and mental status alterations are recorded. Respiratory function is monitored by frequent measurement of arterial blood gases.

Oral protein intake is restricted, and protein in the lumen of the colon is removed with enemas. Administration of intravenous glucose with supplements of thiamine and vitamin B complex is necessary when oral intake is reduced and if hypoglycemia is recognized. Hypertonic glucose may be given into a central vein to provide additional calories. The efficacy of parenteral hyperalimentation fluids formulated to contain high concentrations of branched-chain amino acids and reduced levels of aromatic amino acids has yet to be demonstrated. Supplemental potassium and phosphorus may be necessary if serum levels decline. The efficacy of lactulose, neomycin, or combined lactulose-neomycin therapy is uncertain in this disorder.

Fluid restriction and judicious administration of small volumes of hypertonic saline may be necessary if severe hyponatremia supervenes, since hyponatremia may contribute to encephalopathy. Hypernatremia, associated with infusion of fresh-frozen plasma, also may lead to deterioration of mental status and should be corrected. Defects in polymorphonuclear granulocyte locomotion and adherence may contribute to the increased risk of bacterial infection associated with contamination of intravenous lines.[7] Early diagnosis of bacterial infection requires a high index of suspicion and obsessive attention to infusion sites.

Respiratory failure is treated by intubation and mechanical ventilation to maintain arterial blood gases and prevent aspiration. The adult respiratory distress syndrome may be recognized in this setting; positive end-expiratory pressure with increased O_2 concentrations may be helpful.

Functional renal failure (the hepatorenal syndrome), acute renal tubular necrosis, and prerenal azotemia may be responsible for azotemia in patients with hepatic failure. Management is difficult; loop diuretics are rarely useful, and fluid challenges must be undertaken with great care.

Cerebral edema and brain stem involvement are major complications and contribute importantly to mortality. Neurosurgically implanted intracranial pressure monitoring devices may permit assessment of therapy, e.g., administration of osmotic diuretics (reported to be beneficial), but their role has not yet been completely defined.[8] Corticosteroids are ineffective in the management of this form of cerebral edema. Intravenous diazepam may interrupt recurrent seizures but must be used cautiously because of enhanced CNS sensitivity.

Bleeding from erosions in the upper gastrointestinal tract may be potentiated by abnormalities in the hemostatic mechanism as a result of decreased levels of coagulation proteins, thrombocytopenia, functionally abnormal platelets, and disseminated intravascular coagulation. Control of bleeding and transient correction of the hemostatic abnormalities may be achieved by infusion of fresh-frozen plasma, packed red cells, and platelet concentrates. Vitamin K is of no known value in this setting. Prophylaxis of stress-induced bleeding may be achieved with sucralfate or intravenous administration of a histamine type 2 (H_2) blocker.

Artificial liver support systems remain theoretical possibilities. Liver transplantation has been attempted in a small but increasing number of patients with acute hepatic failure.[9] This extraordinarily complex and expensive procedure is available in many major medical centers. Unfortunately, most patients with acute hepatic failure succumb before an appropriate donor can be found.

KEY FEATURES

Acute hepatic failure is a consequence of disorders associated with extensive hepatic necrosis or fatty change, such as the following:
- Viral hepatitis
- Drug or chemical hepatotoxicity
- Severe hypoperfusion syndrome
- Exacerbations of chronic active hepatitis
- Wilson's disease
- Reye's syndrome
- Acute fatty liver of pregnancy

Hepatic encephalopathy and hypoprothrombinemia are the cardinal features; multiple organ failure often complicates the course.

Major complications include the following:
- Cerebral edema

- Electrolyte, acid-base, and fluid balance disturbances
- Respiratory and renal failure
- Bacterial infection
- Hypoglycemia
- Gastrointestinal bleeding
  Management requires these steps:
- ICU monitoring
- Correction of electrolyte, acid-base, and fluid balances
- Nutritional support with glucose
- Maintenance of oxygenation
- Prompt recognition and treatment of bacterial infection
- Infusion of blood/blood products for bleeding
- Consideration of intracranial pressure monitoring in treatment of cerebral edema
- Consideration of liver transplantation

Despite vigorous management, the case fatality rate remains unacceptably high.

REFERENCES

1. Gimson AES, O'Grady J, Ede RJ, et al: Late onset hepatic failure: Clinical, serological and histological features. Hepatology 6:288, 1986.
   An important review of hepatic failure occurring relatively late (average 9 weeks) after the onset of symptoms of hepatitis.

2. Hoyumpa AM Jr, Schenker S: Perspectives in hepatic encephalopathy. J Lab Clin Med 100:477, 1982.
   A critical review of selected aspects of the pathogenesis, clinical characteristics, and treatment of hepatic encephalopathy, with 72 references.

3. Schafer DF, Jones EA: Potential neural mechanisms in the pathogenesis of hepatic encephalopathy. Prog Liver Dis 7:615, 1982.
   A provocative discussion of abnormalities of neurotransmission and the putative role of amino acid neurotransmitters in hepatic encephalopathy. Essential reading for an understanding of the likely direction of future research.

4. Acute Hepatic Failure Study Group: A double-blind, randomized trial of hydrocortisone in acute hepatic failure. Gastroenterology 76:1297, 1979.
5. European Association for the Study of the Liver (EASL): Randomised trial of steroid therapy for acute liver failure. Gut 20:620, 1979.
   These multicenter studies from the United States and Europe, taken individually or together, strongly discourage further use of corticosteroids in acute hepatic failure. Of interest, the frequency of complications usually attributed to corticosteroids was no greater in the steroid-treated groups than in the control groups.

6. Hanid MA, Silk DBA, Williams R: Prognostic value of the oculovestibular reflex in fulminant hepatic failure. Br Med J 1:1029, 1978.
   Nine of 10 patients in whom the oculovestibular reflex was present and remained present throughout the duration of coma recovered. In contrast, 4 of 4 patients without the reflex on admission died and all 16 in whom the reflex disappeared died.

7. Altin M, Rajkovic IA, Hughes RD, et al: Neutrophil adherence in chronic liver disease and fulminant hepatic failure. Gut 24:746, 1983.
   Despite elevated white blood cell counts (in 7 of 13 patients with fulminant hepatic

failure) and elevated neutrophil counts (in 8 of 13), reduced neutrophil adherence was detected in 6 of the 13. Parenthetically, leukocytosis is so common in this syndrome that its value as a marker of bacterial infection is very limited.

8. Canalese, J, Gimson AES, Davis C, et al: Controlled trial of dexamethasone and mannitol for the cerebral edema of fulminant hepatic failure. Gut 23:625, 1982.

   In this double-pronged controlled trial, dexamethasone was shown to be ineffective in the prevention of cerebral edema and not to influence survival in treated patients. Treatment of cerebral edema with mannitol, with or without intracranial pressure monitoring, led to more frequent resolution of edema and an enhanced survival rate.

9. Bismuth H, Samuel D, Gugenheim J, et al: Emergency liver transplantation for fulminant hepatitis. Ann Intern Med 107:337, 1987.

   In this French series, 12 of 17 patients with fulminant hepatitis treated with liver transplantation were alive 2 to 15 months after transplantation. Because the experience is uncontrolled, the efficacy of liver replacement in this setting remains uncertain.

Hepatitis

Raymond S. Koff, M.D.

At least six distinct agents are believed to be responsible for viral hepatitis. These compose the hepatitis A virus (HAV), the hepatitis B virus (HBV), the hepatitis D (delta agent) virus (HDV), and two blood-borne and one enterically transmitted non-A, non-B hepatitis viruses. All produce clinically similar acute infections ranging from asymptomatic infections to fulminant, fatal hepatitis with symptomatic hepatitis in the middle. Symptomatic hepatitis can be associated with jaundice, but jaundice is not invariably present. In the United States, symptomatic hepatitis with jaundice appears to be fairly evenly divided between HAV, HBV, and probably non-A, non-B hepatitis virus infections.[1] HDV, a defective virus that requires the helper function of HBV and is therefore seen only when HBV is also present, appears to play an important role in fulminant hepatitis among HBsAg-positive persons.[2]

Asymptomatic infection can be subclinical or inapparent. In subclinical infection, no symptoms are present, but biochemical features of hepatitis, e.g., elevated serum aminotransferase levels, are detected. In inapparent infection, neither symptoms nor biochemical abnormalities are present; serologic studies are required to identify inapparent infection. In suspected viral hepatitis, serologic diagnosis is essential. Serologic diagnosis of hepatitis A requires detection of antibody to HAV of the IgM class (IgM anti-HAV); hepatitis B requires detection of the hepatitis B surface antigen (HBsAg) and/or antibody to the hepatitis B core antigen of the IgM class (IgM anti-

HBc); hepatitis D requires detection of HBsAg and total or IgM antibody to HDV (IgM anti-HDV).[1-3] Unfortunately, serologic markers to identify non-A, non-B hepatitis are not yet available.

Management of subclinical and inapparent infection is limited to measures designed to prevent the spread of infection. Management of symptomatic disease includes supportive therapy as well as preventive measures.

SUPPORTIVE THERAPY

Nearly all patients may be managed at home with weekly visits to the office or clinic. Between visits, telephone contact may be used to assess the evolution of the illness. Hospitalization is reserved for rare patients with pernicious vomiting and dehydration and for those with evidence of fulminant hepatitis. Isolation procedures in the household are of no value, since patients are infectious during the presymptomatic phase. Enteric precautions in the hospital are reserved for patients in the early phase of HAV infection in whom diarrhea or fecal incontinence is noted. Blood and needle precautions are used in patients with HBV or HBV/HDV or suspected non-A, non-B infections.

Maintenance of oral fluid and calorie intake is encouraged; if dehydration is evident, intravenous fluids containing glucose, vitamin B complex, thiamine, and electrolytes may be given to maintain fluid and electrolyte balance and caloric intake. Parenteral feedings with commercially available amino acid solutions have no clear therapeutic value. Antiviral chemotherapy is not available, and corticosteroids have no therapeutic value in this setting. Because drug metabolism may be adversely affected by hepatitis, only essential medications are continued and careful monitoring of clinical response and plasma drug levels may be necessary.[5] Alcohol is avoided during the acute and convalescent phase of the illness.

Vigorous physical activity is restricted during the acute phase. Bed rest is best left to the direction of the patient but is not encouraged. As the illness wanes, limitations in activity are reduced and normal activities are gradually resumed. Aminotransferase elevations or HBsAg-positivity persisting for 6 or more months requires further evaluation.

PREVENTIVE MEASURES

Hepatitis A Virus

Immune globulin, given within 2 weeks of exposure to HAV, is highly effective in the prevention or modification of infection to an inapparent/silent form. The recommended dose is 0.02 ml per kg body weight, administered intramuscularly, to all household contacts of the infected patient. Passive immunoprophylaxis with immune globulin is not necessary for casual contacts in the classroom, workplace, or hospital setting in whom fecal-oral transmission is unlikely. Prophylaxis may be effective for individuals exposed to a common-source vehicle of infection and for workers exposed to HAV in daycare centers and in institutions for the mentally retarded. Susceptible tourists planning to visit HAV endemic regions for less than 2 months should receive immune globulin just prior to departure. For extended travel, a dose of 0.06 ml/kg should be given and repeated at 4–5 month intervals while the individual is in residence in high-risk areas. Transient pain at the injection site is the major adverse reaction to immune globulin administration. A HAV vaccine is under development but will not be available for several years.[6]

Hepatitis B Virus

Both passive and active immunoprophylaxis regimens are available for HBV. Active immunization with the subunit HBV vaccines, composed of either purified and treated plasma-derived HBsAg particles or yeast-derived recombinant HBsAg, is the key preventive measure for individuals with a high risk of HBV infection.[7] In healthy populations, intramuscular (deltoid) injection of 1 ml of the plasma-derived vaccine, containing 20 μg of HBsAg protein, or 1 ml of the yeast-derived vaccine, containing 10 μg of HbsAg protein, given in a three-dose schedule at 0, 1, and 6 months, will induce the formation of anti-HBs (antibody to the HBsAg) in 90–100% of recipients. Response rates are highest in the young and poorest in the elderly and in the immunosuppressed. No important adverse reactions to the HBV vaccine have been identified, and anti-HBs may persist for at least 4–5 years in 80–90% of responders.

Specifically targeted populations for vaccination include health care workers regularly exposed to blood or blood-contaminated secretions, homosexual men, parenteral illicit drug users, multiply transfused patients (hemophiliacs, thalassemics), mentally retarded individuals residing in large institutions, susceptible household contacts of HBsAg carriers, and neonates of HBsAg-positive women. In the last-cited setting, HBV vaccine and hepatitis B immune globulin may be given together at different sites in the anterolateral muscle of the thigh because passive immunization does not interfere with the immunogenicity of the vaccine and combined active and passive immunization is more effective than either agent alone.[8,9]

Hepatitis B immune globulin, a preparation containing a known quantity of anti-HBs, has been used for post-exposure prophylaxis in nonvaccinated health care workers exposed to HBV through needlestick accidents or accidental mucous membrane contamination. Protective efficacy in these settings approaches but does not exceed 75–80%; hence, active immunization is the preferred preventive measure. In the susceptible unvaccinated health care worker exposed to HBV, hepatitis B immune globulin is given in an intramuscular dose of 0.06 ml/kg and is repeated 1 month later. Vaccination should be offered as early as possible in this setting. Despite this recommendation, it should be recognized that the efficacy of combined active and passive immunization in reducing the risk of HBV infection from needlestick or mucous membrane exposure, or in limiting spread of HBV from acutely infected patients to their susceptible sexual contacts, is not yet known.

Neither HBV vaccine nor hepatitis B immune globulin has any therapeutic value in individuals with established HBV infection.[9]

Hepatitis D Virus

Neither passive nor active immunization against HDV is available. HBV vaccination of susceptible high-risk individuals such as parenteral drug abusers, hemophiliacs, and male homosexuals who have not yet experienced HBV infection will prevent both HBV and HDV infection. For HBsAg-positive individuals, avoidance of needle-sharing and reduced use of high-risk blood products contaminated with HDV may prevent transmission of HDV.

Non-A, Non-B Viral Hepatitis

Immune globulin has been given to household and intimate contacts of patients with acute non-A, non-B viral hepatitis. In these very limited experiences, evidence of efficacy has been difficult to assess and recommendations for use of globulin are made without enthusiasm. Active immunization will require isolation, identification, and characterization of the responsible blood-borne agents. Immune globulin prepared in countries experiencing enterically transmitted non-A, non-B hepatitis may be effective in the prophylaxis of this infection, but only very limited supporting data are available.

KEY FEATURES

Viral hepatitis infections may be symptomatic, subclinical, or inapparent. Serologic diagnosis is essential:
- IgM anti-HAV in HAV infection
- HBsAg or IgM anti-HBc in acute HBV infection
- HBsAg and anti-HD or IgM anti-HD in HDV infection

- IgM anti-HAV, HBsAg, and IgM anti-HBc absent in non-A, non-B infections

Supportive therapy of symptomatic hepatitis:
- Management at home without isolation procedures
- Maintenance of fluid and caloric intake
- Avoidance of nonessential drugs and alcohol
- Restriction of vigorous physical activity
- Bed rest at patient's discretion

Preventive measures:
- Immune globulin for household contacts of HAV patients
- Pre-exposure prophylaxis with immune globulin for travelers to high-risk HAV areas
- HBV vaccine as pre-exposure prophylaxis for high-risk populations:
    Homosexual men
    Health care workers exposed to blood
    Parenteral drug users
    Recipients of multiple blood transfusions or blood products
    Neonates of HBsAg-positive women
    Household contacts of HBsAg carriers
    Residents of institutions for the mentally retarded
- Hepatitis B immune globulin as postexposure prophylaxis: limited efficacy
- Use of HBV vaccine to prevent HDV infection
- Uncertain role of immune globulin for prophylaxis of non-A, non-B hepatitis

REFERENCES

1. Francis DP, Hadler SC, Prendergast TJ, et al: Occurrence of hepatitis A, B, and non-A/non-B in the United States. CDC sentinel county hepatitis study. Am J Med 76:69, 1984.
    Among 800 cases of viral hepatitis collected in five counties, 41% were serologically identified as HAV infection, 33% were classified as HBV infection, and 26% were attributed to non-A, non-B hepatitis. HAV predominated in patients less than 15 years of age, whereas non-A, non-B predominated in those older than 44 years. Epidemiologic risk factors associated with each type of hepatitis were identified.

2. Saracco G, Macagno S, Rosina F, et al: Serologic markers with fulminant hepatitis in persons positive for hepatitis B surface antigen. A worldwide epidemiologic and clinical survey. Ann Intern Med 108:380, 1988.
    This collection of fulminant hepatitis in HBsAg-positive persons demonstrates that only half the cases could be attributed to acute hepatitis B. Thirty per cent were caused by HBV and HDV coinfections or HDV superinfection of HBsAg carriers. In the remainder, superinfection of HBsAg carriers with a non-A, non-B hepatitis virus was postulated to be responsible.

3. Decker RH, Kosakowski SM, Vanderbilt, AS, et al: Diagnosis of acute hepatitis A by HAVAB-M, a direct radioimmunoassay for IgM anti-HAV. Am J Clin Pathol 76:140, 1981.
    In this study, direct radioimmunoassay for IgM anti-HAV was shown to be highly specific for the diagnosis of HAV infection with no false positives. Although the test is designed so that the antibody is no longer detectable 3 months after onset of infection, in a few patients a rheumatoid factor–like substance may provide false positive results for as long as 2–3 years (Bucens MR, Pietroboni GR, Harnett GB: False positive results

occurring in a radioimmunoassay for hepatitis A antibody of the IgM class. J Virol Meth 7:287, 1983).

4. Chau KH, Hargie MP, Decker RH, et al: Serodiagnosis of recent hepatitis B infection by IgM class anti-HBc. Hepatology 3:142, 1983.
    Detection of IgM anti-HBc permits detection of HBV infection in patients with HBsAg-negative acute hepatitis; it may be useful in distinguishing between recent and remote HBV infection and in excluding HBV as responsible for episodes of hepatitis in previously asymptomatic HBsAg carriers.

5. Williams RL: Drug administration in hepatic disease. N Engl J Med 309:1616, 1983.
    A superb review of current knowledge of the influence of liver disease, including acute hepatitis, on pharmacokinetics and hepatic disposition of drugs.

6. Provost PJ, Conti PA, Creja PA, et al: Studies in chimpanzees of live, attenuated hepatitis A vaccine candidates. Proc Soc Exp Biol Med 172:357, 1983.
    Employing HAV propagated in cell culture, attenuated HAV variants have been developed that can induce anti-HAV in chimpanzees and provide complete protection against challenge with virulent HAV. Studies in human subjects are not yet available.

7. Seeff LB, Koff RS: Passive and active immunoprophylaxis of hepatitis B. Gastroenterology 86:958, 1984.
    An extensive review of active and passive immunity to hepatitis B, with 142 references.

8. Beasley RP, Hwang L-Y, Lee GC-Y, et al: Prevention of perinatally transmitted hepatitis B virus infections with hepatitis B immune globulin and hepatitis B vaccine. Lancet 2:1099, 1983.

9. Stevens CE, Taylor PE, Tong MJ, et al: Yeast-recombinant hepatitis B vaccine: Efficacy with hepatitis B immune globulin in prevention of perinatal hepatitis B virus transmission. JAMA 257:2612, 1987.
    The efficacy of hepatitis B immune globulin alone in the prevention of HBsAg carrier states in neonates of Taiwanese HBsAg-positive, HBeAg-positive carrier mothers was 71%, that of hepatitis B vaccine alone was 75%, and regimens combining globulin with vaccine had an efficacy of 94%. In a second study performed in the United States, the yeast-recombinant vaccine combined with hepatitis B immune globulin was as effective as the plasma-derived vaccine with hepatitis B immune globulin.

10. Dienstag JL, Stevens CE, Bhan AK, et al: Hepatitis B vaccine administered to chronic carriers of hepatitis B surface antigen. Ann Intern Med 96:575, 1982.
    Repeated administration of HBV vaccine to 16 HBsAg carriers failed to eliminate the carrier state; no important adverse effects were observed.

Diverticular Disease

William Robinson, M.D.

Diverticula of the colon are herniations of the mucosa and submucosa through the muscle wall of the bowel, generally at the site of a nutrient artery. They occur primarily on the lateral surface of the colon between the teniae coli. Their development is felt to be influenced by at least two factors: (1) points of diminished resistance of the bowel wall, i.e., alterations in connective tissue associated with aging; and (2) an increased pressure gradient between lumen and peritoneal cavity, thought to be influenced by fiber deficiency resulting in hypersegmentation and excessive intraluminal pressures from diminished fecal flow.[1-4] Diverticulosis might be a consequence of the segmented hypercontractility seen in some patients with the irritable colon syndrome. It is an acquired deformity of the colon, extremely common in Western societies, rarely noted in normals before the age of 40, and its prevalence is correlated with advancing age. The most common site of diverticula is the sigmoid colon (involved in 95% of cases) and, less frequently, the proximal colon.[1,2] Approximately 80% of those affected will remain symptom-free throughout life.[3] Of the remaining 20%, the clinical manifestations of diverticular disease of the colon will be (1) uncomplicated diverticulosis with associated abdominal pain, (2) diverticular hemorrhage, or (3) diverticulitis (inflammation of diverticula). Because diverticulosis is more common in the elderly, attributing signs or symptoms to the diverticula must be avoided until other conditions have been excluded, e.g., colonic neoplasm.

UNCOMPLICATED DIVERTICULOSIS

Clinically, uncomplicated diverticulosis presents as recurrent left lower quadrant colicky pain without evidence of acute diverticulitis on physical examination or laboratory tests. Associated symptoms include constipation, diarrhea, flatulence, or postprandial exacerbation of pain. This collection of symptoms is probably not due to diverticulosis *per se*, but to the progenitor, irritable colon syndrome. Barium enema shows diverticula and varying degrees of colonic spasm. Sigmoidoscopy is of value chiefly in the differential diagnosis, which includes irritable bowel syndrome, carcinoma of the distal colon/rectum, lactose intolerance, and gynecologic and urologic disorders. Acute treatment generally involves (1) restriction of food; (2) analgesics: meperidene is the agent of choice for severe pain; (3) antispasmodics/anticholinergics, which have not been proved clinically effective, although their effects vary and they are generally employed; and (4) bulk laxatives/high residue diet. Antibiotics and surgical intervention are not indicated.

DIVERTICULAR HEMORRHAGE

Diverticular hemorrhage is usually severe and occurs predominantly in elderly patients with otherwise uncomplicated diverticulosis.[5,6] Diverticular bleeding is painless, sudden in onset, and occurs without signs or symptoms of diverticulitis. Seventy per cent of instances of massive diverticular bleeding occur in the right colon, with the source of bleeding attributed to a minute rupture of one of the intramural arterial branches, asymmetrically placed on the wall adjacent to the lumen of the diverticulum. Evaluation of a patient should include nasogastric tube to rule out an upper gastrointestinal tract bleeding source, proctosigmoidoscopy to rule out other bleeding lesions in the distal colon, and coagulation studies. If rectal bleeding continues to be severe (greater than 0.5 ml/minute), angiography should be performed. If bleeding is mild to moderate (greater than 0.1 ml/minute), bleeding scans are sometimes obtained to define the approximate location of active bleeding and to guide selective arterial studies. If bleeding is minimal, colonoscopy may be useful. Barium studies should be deferred, especially if bleeding is intermittent, because they can interfere with subsequent angiographic studies for 1–7 days thereafter.

Bleeding stops spontaneously in about 80% of patients; the chance of a second hemorrhage is approximately 25%. However, following a second bleed, the risk of recurrent hemorrhage increases to 50%. Guaiac positive stools without evidence of substantial bleeding should not be attributed to diverticular disease.

Treatment generally consists of medical measures: transfusion, correction of coagulation defects, administration of intravenous fluids, restriction of oral intake, bed rest, and surgical consultation. Selective intra-arterial infusion of vasopressin has been used with favorable results; however, if bleeding persists, surgical intervention is indicated, with subtotal colectomy used as a last resort for those patients with persistent severe bleeding without an angiographically identifiable source.

DIVERTICULITIS

Diverticulitis is the most frequent complication of diverticulosis. It is estimated that 10–20% of people known to have colonic diverticula will develop diverticulitis at some time in their lives. The initial pathologic change in diverticulitis is focal inflammation at the diverticular apex felt to develop in response to inspissated fecal material.[7] Peridiverticulitis results when the intramural process in the apex progresses to cause necrosis, micro- or macroperforation, and fecal contamination in the surrounding tissues. Commonly, only one diverticulum is involved; most often, it is in the sigmoid colon.

With microperforation, a small paracolonic abcess forms and with repeated episodes this can lead to a fibrotic response within the colonic wall that can cause segmental narrowing. It follows that the secondary complications associated with diverticulitis, accounting for most of the morbidity, are: (1) intra-abdominal abscess; (2) peritonitis; (3) bowel obstruction; and

(4) formation of fistulae.[8] The last-named complication develops from direct extension of the abscess into the surrounding structures. The most common fistula is a colovesical fistula (commonly between the sigmoid colon and posterior bladder) that results in (1) recurrent urinary tract infections with multiple enteric pathogens; (2) pneumaturia; and (3) fecaluria. It is diagnosed by barium enema, cystography, or intravenous pyelography. In addition, coloenteric fistulae must be considered when evaluating malabsorption or bacterial overgrowth of unknown etiology in middle-aged or elderly patients.

Clinically, patients with diverticulitis generally present with acute onset of persistent, localized abdominal pain accompanied by rigors with or without fever. Anorexia, nausea, vomiting, and changes in bowel habits ranging from diarrhea to constipation may occur. Physical examination may reveal diminished bowel sounds; abdominal tenderness; involuntary guarding; and a palpable, fixed mass. Rectal examination may reveal tenderness with a mass in the cul-de-sac. Laboratory tests reveal an elevated white blood cell count with a left shift; urinalysis may indicate a urinary tract infection.

The diagnosis is frequently suspected on the basis of the findings just described. Other considerations include colon carcinoma, irritable bowel syndrome, ulcerative colitis, Crohn's colitis, and ischemic colitis. Initially, plain supine and upright abdominal radiographs should be obtained to assess the degree of ileus, intestinal obstruction, and free air in the peritoneal cavity or bladder. All patients should have an initial surgical evaluation in the event that resection becomes indicated. Urgent surgical intervention is indicated in patients with (1) generalized peritonitis; (2) persistent intestinal obstruction; (3) enlarging mass; or (4) evidence of abscess. However, surgery should be deferred unless urgently required in view of the difference in surgical mortality rates (5% vs. 1%) when comparing acute vs. elective intervention.[9] Blood, stool, and urine cultures should be obtained. In most instances, proctosigmoidoscopy should be performed with minimal bowel preparation and no air insufflation to rule out distal carcinoma and ulcerative or granulomatous colitis. The diagnostic use of a low-pressure barium enema in the presence of acute diverticulitis remains controversial. The risk of extending an inflamed localized perforation must be weighed against the diagnostic value of the procedure. In any event, all investigators agree that at some point a barium enema should be performed. In addition, any findings on physical examination, radiographic studies, or clinical course suggesting abscess formation should be further evaluated by ultrasound or CT scan.[10]

The initial therapy of diverticulitis is usually medical. It is estimated that 75% of patients will recover on medical treatment alone. The remainder will require surgical intervention. Of those with a first episode who are successfully managed medically, the majority will not have subsequent attacks requiring hospitalization. Medical therapy consists of bed rest; NPO; nasogastric suction if nausea, vomiting, or abdominal distention is present;

intravenous fluids; and broad-spectrum antibiotics. Early surgical evaluation is appropriate, and the patient should then be carefully followed with frequent examination of the abdomen and appropriate radiograph and ultrasound studies to assess the therapeutic response.

KEY FEATURES

A. Definition
   1. Diverticula are acquired herniations of the colonic mucosa and submucosa protruding through the muscular wall of the colon.
B. Etiology
   1. Thought to be twofold:
      a. Increased intraluminal pressure
      b. Points of colonic wall weakness
C. Incidence/location
   1. Common in Western societies
   2. Rarely occurs before age 40, and increases progressively with age
   3. Overall distribution: males/females equal
   4. Most common site of involvement: sigmoid colon
   5. Eighty per cent of those affected remain symptom-free
D. Clinical presentation/complications
   1. Uncomplicated diverticulosis: can be associated with abdominal pain, constipation, diarrhea
   2. Diverticular hemorrhage: majority of episodes of severe bleeding occur in the right colon
   3. Diverticulitis: secondary complications include the following:
      a. Intra-abdominal abscess
      b. Peritonitis
      c. Bowel obstruction
      d. Fistulae
E. Diagnosis/management
   1. Correct diagnosis/treatment depends upon previously mentioned clinical presentation
   2. Evidence of fever, leukocytosis, or abdominal tenderness suggests the need for antibiotics/surgical evaluation
   3. Secondary complications of diverticulitis should be surgically evaluated
   4. Barium studies/endoscopy requiring insufflation of air should not be performed when there are signs of acute inflammation
   5. Attributing signs or symptoms to diverticular disease must be avoided until other conditions have been excluded, e.g., colon neoplasm

REFERENCES

1. Parks TG: Natural history of diverticular disease of the colon. Clin Gastroenterol 4:53, 1975.
2. Almy TP, Howell DA: Diverticular disease of the colon. N Engl J Med 302:324, 1980.
3. Gear JSS, Ware A, et al: Symptomless diverticular disease and intake of dietary fiber. Lancet 1:511, 1979.
4. Fleischner FG: Diverticular disease of the colon—new observations and revised concepts. Gastroenterology 60:316, 1971.
5. Meyers MA, Alonso DR, Gray GF, Baer JW: Pathogenesis of bleeding diverticulosis. Gastroenterology 71:577, 1976.
6. Cosarella WJZ, Kanter IE, Seaman WB: Right-sided colonic diverticula as a cause of acute rectal hemorrhage. N Engl J Med 286:450, 1972.
7. Morson BC: Pathology of diverticular disease of the colon. Clin Gastroenterol 4:37, 1975.
8. Hughes LE: Complications of diverticular disease: Inflammation, obstruction, and hemorrhage. Clin Gastroenterol 4:147, 1975.
9. Lason AM, Masters SS, Spiro HM: Medical and surgical therapy in diverticular disease—a comparative study. Gastroenterology 71:734, 1976.
10. Hulnick DH, Megibow AT, Balthazar EJ, et al: Computerized tomography in evaluation of diverticulitis. Radiology 152:491, 1984.

Diarrhea

Frank E. Murray, M.B., M.R.C.P.I., M.R.C.P.

Diarrhea is an abnormal increase in stool liquidity and weight usually associated with an increase in stool frequency and sometimes accompanied by urgency, incontinence, and discomfort. The etiology of diarrhea varies, and it may be classified as in Table 1.

CLINICAL FEATURES

Important aspects of the history include the duration of the diarrhea (whether it is acute or chronic); the stool volume and frequency; and whether it has characteristics of steatorrhea (pale, bulky, oily, foul-smelling, and difficult to flush), infection (acute onset, frequently following/during foreign travel, high frequency of bowel motion, possibly in association with pain or other systemic features), inflammatory bowel disease (bloody diarrhea, systemic symptoms, or rheumatologic features), cholestasis (jaundice, pruritus, right upper quadrant pain, abnormal liver function tests), or pancreatic dysfunction (pain, oily diarrhea, history of pancreatitis, diabetes mellitus).

Certain categories of diagnosis are apparent. There are four major groups of acute diarrhea. Infectious diarrhea is frequently of abrupt onset,

TABLE 1. ETIOLOGY OF DIARRHEA

I. Osmotic
   A. Disaccharidase deficiency
   B. Lactulose therapy
   C. Magnesium salts
   D. Malabsorption

II. Secretory
   A. Associated with adenyl cyclase activation
      1. Vasoactive intestinal polypeptide
      2. Prostaglandins
      3. Theophylline/caffeine
      4. Bacterial enterotoxins (*Escherichia coli*, cholera)
   B. Not associated with adenyl cyclase activation
      1. Cholecystokinin
      2. Serotonin
      3. Laxatives
      4. Villous adenomas
      5. Bacterial enterotoxins

III. Malabsorption/maldigestion
   A. Mucosal: tropical sprue, celiac sprue, Whipple's disease, amyloidosis
   B. Structural: gastric or intestinal surgery, inflammatory bowel disease, lymphoma, arterial insufficiency
   C. Infection: acute gastroenteritis, traveler's diarrhea, parasites, tuberculosis
   D. Iatrogenic: surgery, drugs, radiotherapy
   E. Maldigestion: pancreatic enzyme deficiency, bile salt deficiency
   F. Systemic: endocrine disorders (Addison's disease, thyrotoxicosis, hypoparathyroidism); vasculitis; malignant disease; severe, widespread skin disease

IV. Abnormal motility
   A. Stasis syndromes: bacterial overgrowth results in malabsorption
   B. Small intestinal hurry: e.g., Zollinger-Ellison syndrome, post-vagotomy diarrhea, post-gastrectomy diarrhea, carcinoid syndrome
   C. Early colonic emptying: irritable bowel syndrome, inflammatory bowel disease, colonic carcinoma, diverticular disease, bile salt diarrhea

V. Inflammatory exudation: inflammatory bowel disease, dysentery, gastroenteritis

VI. Spurious: fecal impaction

following dietary indescretion or foreign travel, and may obtund the patient because it usually is secretory in nature. Common infections include viral (echoviruses, Coxsackie viruses, rotaviruses), bacterial (*Escherichia coli*, Salmonella, Shigella, Yersinia, Campylobacter, *Vibrio cholerae*), and parasitic (amebic dysentery, *Giardia lamblia*, nematode and trematode infections).

Diarrhea in homosexual men represents an increasing medical problem and includes a broadening range of diseases. The most common organisms traditionally have been *Entamoeba histolytica*, Shigella, Campylobacter, Giardia, trepanosomes, Gonococcus, herpes simplex, and Chlamydia; however, with the increasing prevalence of AIDS in this population, the incidence of intestinal cryptosporidiosis, *Isospora belli*, cytomegalovirus (CMV), and *Mycobacterium avium–intracellulare* (mimicking Whipple's disease) has also increased. (See article in Section 5 on AIDS.)

Chronic or recurrent diarrhea suggests inflammatory bowel disease (IBD), irritable bowel syndrome, "lower-grade" infections (especially parasitic), malabsorption syndromes, diverticular disease, or carcinoma. The likelihood of organic disease is strikingly increased if the patient had nocturnal episodes of diarrhea, episodes of incontinence, or blood in the stool.

Secretory diarrhea characteristically is voluminous; has an osmolarity similar to that of plasma; persists even during fasting (e.g., 1–3 days); and is not accompanied by the presence of blood, pus, or fat in the stool.

INVESTIGATION AND MANAGEMENT

Careful clinical history taking and physical examination are the cornerstones of management. Primary emphasis should be placed on assessing the fluid and electrolyte status and the nutritional status of the patient. Clues to the cause of diarrhea, e.g., fever, marked weight loss, flushing, pigmentation, skin rashes, arthritis, uveitis, evidence of liver disease, peptic ulcerations, or lymphadenopathy, should be sought. Initial investigations should include a CBC, BUN, creatinine, electrolyte analysis, urinalysis, and basic stool analysis. Stool examinations for white blood cells (indicating inflammation), occult blood, fat (Sudan stain), and alkalinization (to rule out phenolphthalein use) are the best first-line tests. Further evaluation should depend on the clinical setting; selectivity of tests, based on clinical assessment, is of primary importance. Stool culture is important in acute or traveler's diarrhea. Culture may be performed where indicated for Salmonella, Shigella, Campylobacter, Yersinia; ova and parasite examination is performed to exclude *E. histolytica, Giardia lamblia,* and Strongyloides. Previous antibiotic therapy may suggest antibiotic-associated colitis and a search for *Clostridium difficile* toxin.

Sigmoidoscopy without prior enema is indicated in most cases of chronic diarrhea. Mucosal smears or rectal biopsy may provide additional information, especially regarding inflammation. Appropriate rectal cultures are important in the homosexual patient.

Stool volume determination may be useful, both as an indicator of the need for aggressive fluid replacement and as a diagnostic indicator; stool fat, electrolyte, glucose, pH, and osmolality analysis may be determined as necessary.

Bile salt absorption is best assessed by the C^{14} bile salt breath test (best avoided in children and young women) or by a therapeutic trial of cholestyramine.

Severe, persistent secretory diarrhea in the absence of drug abuse or apparent organic alimentary disease should be evaluated to exclude a secretagogue-secreting tumor, e.g., vasoactive intestinal polypeptide or calcitonin.

The urgency with which investigation should be initiated and followed depends firmly on the clinical manifestations. The investigation and treatment of a patient with a short history of bloody diarrhea who presents in shock are obviously different from those of an anxious young adult with a history of intermittent diarrhea and abdominal pain but otherwise in apparently good health. Where present, any identifiable underlying cause should be treated appropriately.

The most important aspect of management of acute attacks is fluid and salt replacement. Oral ingestion of liquids and salty foods or glucose-saline solution is usually adequate, despite their tendency to temporarily worsen the diarrhea. No agents are yet known to reliably increase absorption or reduce secretion by the intestine. Opiates, e.g., codeine, morphine, diphenoxylate (with atropine), and loperamide, are used to reduce frequency, urgency, and volume of the stool in a wide variety of circumstances; their mode of action appears to be an inhibitory effect on intestinal motility. Opiates should be avoided in patients with severe IBD and in patients with salmonellosis, shigellosis, or pseudomembranous colitis. Bismuth subsalicylate, through uncertain mechanisms, provides symptomatic relief in patients with acute infectious diarrhea. The role of dietary fiber in the treatment of diarrhea is unclear. Traveler's diarrhea is best prophylaxed with trimethoprim/sulfamethoxasole (TMP/SMX) in patients in special risk categories, e.g., achlorhydria, IBD, and those in whom electrolyte disturbances may have dangerous consequences. Recent trials have shown that antibiotics early in the course of an attack may help to abort it. The current treatment of choice is TMP 160 mg/SMX 800 mg bid for 3–5 days in addition to oral rehydration. Doxycycline or trimethoprim alone are appropriate alternatives to TMP/SMX in sulfa-allergic patients. Steroids (either topically, systemically, or both) may be indicated in acute attacks of IBD.

KEY FEATURES

Definition
Abnormal increase in stool liquidity and weight, usually with an increase in stool frequency

Etiology
Osmotic (disaccharidase deficiency, malabsorption syndrome)
Secretory (infectious, hormones, drugs)
Malabsorption/maldigestion (acute and chronic, post-surgical, infectious, systemic)
Motility abnormalities (stasis syndrome, post–gastric surgery, colonic disease)
Inflammatory exudation
Spurious
Idiopathic

Clinical Manifestations

Accurate history taking is the single most important evaluation of patients with diarrhea. The pattern of diarrhea alone frequently narrows the differential diagnosis. There are four major types of *acute* diarrhea:

1. Infectious
2. In the homosexual patient
3. Chronic and recurrent
4. Secretory

Investigation and Management

Investigation and management are primarily directed by the clinical manifestations. Stool examination is important. Correction of fluid and electrolyte abnormalities is pivotal; this can usually be done orally. Absence of good pharmacologic agents to reduce intestinal secretion or to increase absorption is a major drawback. Agents that reduce GI motility should be used with caution and avoided altogether in patients with severe IBD, Salmonella or Shigella infection, and pseudomembranous colitis. Effective antibiotics are available for traveler's diarrhea and certain severe dysenteries. Prophylactic antibiotics should be avoided except in special circumstances.

BIBLIOGRAPHY

1. Binder HJ: The pathophysiology of diarrhea. Hospital Pract *19*:107–118, 1984.
   Excellent summary of the current state of knowledge of normal and abnormal intestinal secretion and absorption.

2. Geddes AM: "I have been back from holiday for a week and still have diarrhea." Br Med J *287*:513, 1983.
   Short summary on the management of this common problem.

3. Cook GG: Traveler's diarrhea—an insoluble problem. Gut *24*:1105–1108, 1983.
   Clear outlines of the current management guidelines for this problem.

4. Fedorak RN, Field M, Chang EB: Treatment of diabetic diarrhea with clonidine. Ann Intern Med *102*:197–199, 1985.
   Describes the use of this alpha-2 adrenergic blocking agent in the treatment of diarrhea in patients with autonomic neuropathy.

Acute Pancreatitis

Frank E. Murray, M.B., M.R.C.P.I., M.R.C.P.

A new classification of pancreatitis (1984) has replaced the previous Marseilles classification, and it separates pancreatitis into either the acute or the chronic form.

Acute pancreatitis is a clinical syndrome diagnosed on the basis of an acute episode of abdominal pain, usually accompanied by nausea and vomiting, in the presence of increased levels of pancreatic enzymes (amylase, lipase, or trypsin) in the blood or the urine.[1] Because the only accurate methods of diagnosing pancreatitis are by biopsy or autopsy, the true incidence is unknown, but it is recognized that about half of the total number of cases is misdiagnosed and that the incidence is probably increasing.

Three etiologic factors are responsible for 90% of episodes of acute pancreatitis. Alcoholic pancreatitis, most commonly seen in men aged 30–50, is characterized by a severe first attack and milder subsequent attacks. It has a better prognosis than gallstone pancreatitis, which is more frequently seen in women aged 50–70, the age associated with the peak incidence of gallstones. It is more likely to develop in patients with small stones and a wide cystic duct. This type of pancreatitis tends to be severe, has a high mortality rate, and usually is not associated with chronic pancreatitis. Idiopathic pancreatitis is the third major cause of acute pancreatitis. Other important etiologic headings include post-trauma (including surgery and ERCP*), drug-related (antibiotics, diuretics/antihypertensives, immunosuppressives, and estrogens), metabolic causes (hypercalcemia, hypertriglyceridemia, hypothermia), infections (various viruses, *Mycoplasma pneumoniae*, and *Ascaris lumbricoides*) connective tissue diseases, and anatomic anomalies.

The spectrum of pathologic changes ranges from mild (peripancreatic fat necrosis, interstitial edema) to severe (intrapancreatic fat necrosis, hemorrhage). These changes may be localized or diffuse. The severity of the clinical attack and the morphologic changes do not necessarily correlate. The retroperitoneal location and the lack of a well-defined capsule allow the inflammatory process to spread freely and affect adjacent organs.

The severity of attacks varies. The most prominent feature is pain, classically of sudden onset, epigastric in location with frequent radiation through to the back, and associated with tenderness. Nausea, vomiting (rarely hematemesis), and a transient ileus are usual. The degree of hypovolemia generally relates to the severity of the attack. "Third-space" losses that are due to the pancreatic "burn" are a major source of fluid loss.

Diagnostic findings include an elevated serum amylase in approximately 80% of patients; characteristically, this occurs in the first 2–12 hours of an attack and returns to normal in 3–5 days in 90% of the cases.[2-4] It is a nonspecific test, though elevation of pancreatic enzymes to over twice the upper limit of normal is generally indicative of acute pancreatitis. Although serum lipase is similarly nonspecific, serum trypsin (an assay not widely available) is derived only from the pancreas and a raised level strongly suggests pancreatitis. Urinary amylase estimations probably offer no advan-

---

*ERCP = endoscopic retrograde cholangiopancreatography.

tage over serum levels. Emergency investigations should include CBC, BUN, creatinine, electrolytes, arterial blood gases, serum transaminases, serum amylase, and abdominal plain films. Evaluation of the biliary tree and the pancreas should probably be performed at an early stage with ultrasonography.[5] A kidney, ureter, and bladder (KUB) radiograph may reveal evidence of ileus or a "sentinel loop" and rule out evidence of a perforated viscus.

The major differential diagnoses are perforated peptic ulcer, acute cholecystitis, mesenteric infarction, and leaking abdominal aortic aneurysm. Occasionally an exploratory laparotomy is required if the diagnosis is seriously in doubt in an ill patient.

Local complications are frequent in severe attacks. Pancreatic pseudocysts, which consist of an accumulation of tissue debris, pancreatic juices, blood, and adipose droplets, may present with persistent pain and hyperamylasemia, ascites, hemorrhage, or a palpable mass. About half resolve spontaneously. Pancreatic phlegmon, consisting of a mass of pancreatic tissue with patchy areas of necrosis, is less frequent. Pancreatic abscess formation, which frequently presents 4–8 weeks after the initial attack, is characterized by fever, pain, and the presence of an abdominal mass; mortality is high, despite antibiotics and surgery. Pancreatic hemorrhage is less common but can be massive and life-threatening. Hepatobiliary obstruction may arise as a result of obstruction of the common bile duct by pancreatic pseudocyst formation or edema or as a result of accompanying biliary stone disease. Hepatocellular disease is more common in pancreatitis of alcoholic origin. Intestinal obstruction, where present, is usually the result of a transient ileus rather than peritonitis. Gastrointestinal hemorrhage may arise as a result of erosion into a large blood vessel, gastritis, or duodenitis and may be made worse by any associated bleeding tendency.

Metabolic complications are frequent. Hyperglycemia (50%) and glycosuria are associated with an elevated glucagon level; hypocalcemia (20–30%) is rarely severe enough to manifest clinically; the hypertriglyceridemia seen frequently in acute attacks is more often a result of the pancreatitis rather than its cause. Lactic acidosis and hypoglycemia are less common. Renal manifestations include acute renal failure; renal vein thrombosis; and mild, reversible renal tubular defects. Pulmonary complications are common and frequently serious or fatal. Pleural effusions (frequently blood-stained exudates with a high amylase content), atelectasis, pneumonitis, and acute respiratory failure as a result of adult respiratory distress syndrome (ARDS) may be seen and are the most common causes of death in the first week of attack. The cardiologic manifestations include hypovolemia, hypotension, pericarditis, and ECG changes that may mimic myocardial ischemia or infarction. Grey Turner's sign, Cullen's sign, and subcutaneous fat necrosis are uncommon. Other infrequent complications include disseminated intravascular coagulation (DIC), eosinophilia (with fat necrosis), anemia, organic delirium (commonly 3–5 days after the beginning of an attack), arthritis, and lytic bone disease.

The prognosis of individual attacks varies; 20–50% are severe. Usually an individual's first attack is the most severe. Overall, the mortality rate is less than 10%. Half of those who die do so in the first week, mainly from pulmonary complications. Following resolution of an acute attack, the pancreas returns to normal. Except for alcoholic pancreatitis, acute pancreatitis rarely evolves into chronic pancreatitis. About half of patients develop further attacks. Poor prognostic features in an attack include increasing age (>55 years), elevated WBC (>16,000/mm³), hyperglycemia (>200 mg/dl), elevated LDH (>350 U/L) and SGOT (>250 U/L) levels, hypoxemia (PaO$_2$ <60 mmHg), a falling hematocrit (<10%), hypocalcemia (<8 mg/dl), the development of a metabolic acidosis (base deficit >4 mEq/L), and hypovolemia. There is preliminary evidence to suggest that a diagnostic peritoneal tap may help prognosticate, especially if hypoxemia is present.

The management of acute attacks involves initial assessment (as described before), intensive care for high-risk patients, "pancreatic rest," and supportive care. Restoring intravascular volume with intravenous fluids is most important: hemodynamic monitoring is required in severe cases. Shock is managed with intravenous fluids, blood, and fresh-frozen plasma. Oral intake is eliminated, and nasogastric aspiration is performed until vomiting and paralytic ileus resolve. Pain relief is best obtained with parenteral opiates (meperidine). The role of peritoneal lavage is controversial. Despite some encouraging initial results, few if any patients seem to benefit from peritoneal lavage. No benefit was seen in the largest controlled study performed so far.[6] It is clear that biliary pancreatitis responds better to early resolution of the ampullary obstruction than to peritoneal lavage. Total parenteral nutrition should be commenced if the patient cannot take nourishment by mouth for a prolonged period. Pulmonary complications are managed by close monitoring of PaO$_2$, oxygen therapy for hypoxia, and drainage of possible pleural effusions. Ventilation support is required occasionally. Hyperglycemia is sometimes severe enough to require insulin administration. Prophylactic antibiotics, aprotinin, cimetidine, and peritoneal dialysis are not routinely indicated. The management of a pseudocyst includes observation (with serial ultrasound), ultrasound-guided puncture and soft pigtail catheter drainage, and occasionally surgery (usually cystgastrostomy). Surgery, combined with antibiotics, is the management of choice for pancreatic abscess. Surgery may be indicated if the initial diagnosis is unclear and there is concern regarding visceral perforation. It may also be necessary in cases in which pancreatitis is secondary to trauma, or in patients with choledocholithiasis. The role of early operative intervention versus endoscopic sphincterotomy for gallstone pancreatitis is an area of intense controversy. Preliminary data suggest that endoscopic sphincterotomy may improve the prognosis in severe gallstone pancreatitis. Ductoplasty of the minor duct has been recommended in patients with pancreas divisum.[7] Similarly, the role of pancreatic enzyme supplementation in acute pancreatitis awaits clarification.

Many causes of acute pancreatitis may persist and should be addressed with a view to preventing further attacks. These include diseases of the biliary and pancreatic ducts, drug-induced (including alcohol) pancreatitis, hypertriglyceridemia, and pancreas divisum.[7]

KEY FEATURES

Definition of Acute Pancreatitis
An acute clinical syndrome of abdominal pain, nausea, and vomiting in the presence of significantly elevated pancreatic enzyme levels

Etiology
The most common causes are the following:
1. Alcohol
2. Biliary tract disease
3. Post-surgery/trauma
4. Others: including metabolic causes, drugs, infections, anatomic abnormalities

Pathology
Localized or diffuse inflammation, generally reversible

Clinical Features
1. Constant, severe epigastric pain, often with radiation to the back, often disproportionate to the relatively benign abdominal examination
2. Nausea and vomiting
3. Transient ileus

Complications
Most important are the following:
1. Pancreatic: pseudocyst, abscess, hemorrhage
2. Intestinal: ileus, hemorrhage
3. Metabolic: hyperglycemia, hypocalcemia
4. Pulmonary: atelectasis, pleural effusions, ARDS

Diagnosis
1. Elevated serum amylase (greater than twofold is virtually diagnostic)
2. KUB
3. Ultrasound important

Management
1. Supportive: Nasogastric aspiration for ileus and relief of nausea and vomiting; intravenous fluids; pain relief
2. Correction of shock and complications (usually pulmonary)
3. Surgery infrequently required
4. Prevention of further attacks

REFERENCES

1. Geokas MC, Baltaxe HA, Banks PA, et al: Acute pancreatitis. Ann Intern Med 103:86–100, 1985.
    Excellent review of the major aspects of the discussion at a conference.

2. Steinberg WA, Goldstein SS, Davis ND, et al: Diagnostic assays in pancreatitis. Ann Intern Med *102*:576–580, 1985.

3. Moossa AR: Diagnostic tests and procedures for acute pancreatitis. N Engl J Med *311*:639–643, 1984.

4. Bouchier IAD (ed): Biochemical tests for acute pancreatitis. Br Med J *291*:1669–1670, 1985.

   Articles 2, 3, and 4 discuss the merits and demerits of many of the biochemical tests used in the diagnosis of acute pancreatitis.

5. Van Dyke JA, Stanley RJ, Berland LL: Pancreatic imaging. Ann Intern Med *102*:212–217, 1985.

   Discusses the best sequence of imaging procedures in pancreatitis.

6. Mayer AD, McMahon MJ, Corfield AP, et al: Controlled trial of peritoneal lavage for the treatment of severe acute pancreatitis. N Engl J Med *313*:399–404, 1985.

   Concludes that the outcome of severe pancreatitis was not greatly, if at all, influenced by the regimen of peritoneal lavage (two liters per hour for three days) used in this large, well-designed, controlled study.

7. Cotton PB: Pancreas divisum: Curiosity or culprit? Gastroenterology 89:1431–1435, 1985.

   Excellent classification of this controversial topic. This summarizes that pancreas divisum (PD) is a common variant and that most people with PD have no pancreatic problem; PD alone is not important. It is the coexistence of PD and stenosis of the accessory orifice that is important and results in obstructive pathology. The author suggests that most patients with "idiopathic" pancreatitis and PD should be managed conservatively. Surgical duct drainage should be considered only when attacks are frequent and disabling and following careful assessment for evidence of obstruction.

Chronic Pancreatitis

Frank E. Murray, M.B., M.R.C.P.I., M.R.C.P.

Chronic pancreatitis is diagnosed when clinical features (abdominal pain, diabetes, steatorrhea) suggest destruction of acinar and ductal tissues by inflammation and progressive fibrotic destruction resulting in irreversible morphologic abnormalities of the pancreas.

The etiology varies. As in acute pancreatitis, alcohol abuse is the most common underlying cause found; this type most often occurs in males in their fourth decade; the incubation time is somewhat shorter than that for alcoholic cirrhosis. Pancreatic calcification is common. Tropical/malnutritional pancreatitis has an earlier age of onset (second decade), is equally common in males and females, and is also frequently associated with gland calcification. Common metabolic causes include hypercalcemia, hyperlipidemia, parenteral alimentation, and $alpha_1$-antitrypsin deficiency. Less common causes include hereditary pancreatitis (which may also be associated with pancreatic calcification), trauma, Zollinger-Ellison syndrome, and anatomic anomalies (including pancreas divisum). Since the 1984 reclassification of pancreatitis, idiopathic hemochromatosis and fibrocystic disease are no longer classified as causes of chronic pancreatitis.

The gross pathologic changes seen in this condition may include irregular sclerosis, destruction and loss of acini with dilation of the extraductal segments, and associated strictures and intraductal calculi. Microscopically, an inflammatory cell infiltrate, edema, focal necrosis, and cyst and pseudocyst formation may be seen. The islets of Langerhans may be relatively spared. The major changes seen may be obstructive in nature.

The clinical manifestations of the condition are characterized by a wide spectrum of symptoms. Symptomatic episodes, similar to acute pancreatitis, may occur, especially in association with alcohol abuse. Pain is a feature in 95% of cases; it tends to be constant and severe, and it is associated with the development of pyschiatric problems and drug addiction. About 10% of patients present with evidence of exocrine insufficiency; the severity of diarrhea, steatorrhea, and weight loss varies. Ten to twenty per cent of patients develop diabetes mellitus; it is suggested that complications of diabetes may be less common in these patients than in those with idiopathic diabetes. Jaundice may occur and is generally due to fibrosis and edema of the pancreas and is transient in duration. Associated liver disease is most commonly alcoholic in origin (steatosis, hepatitis, cirrhosis); cirrhosis secondary to large bile duct obstruction is uncommon. Rare complications include ascites and splenic vein thrombosis (which may lead to portal hypertension).

The diagnostic tests available are imperfect, and their number attests to their individual inadequacies. The secretin/pancreozymin test detects impaired pancreatic secretion (especially bicarbonate concentration or volume) during duodenal intubation. It is most useful as a test of exclusion: a negative test makes a diagnosis of chronic pancreatitis unlikely. The most useful test of exclusion appears to be the bentiromide test, which is a simple, inexpensive, well-tolerated test of chymotrypsin function.[1] The serum trypsin-like immunoreactivity (TLI) is a reliable test of chronic pancreatitis in assocation with steatorrhea.[2] Tests for stool fat, stool protease and triolein, glucose tolerance test, and the Schilling test, though frequently abnormal, are too nonspecific to be reliable. Radiologic studies may be useful in the diagnosis of chronic pancreatitis. An abnormal radiograph may reveal diffuse parenchymal calcification (which indicates destruction of 80% of the parenchyma). Endoscopic retrograde cannulation of the pancreas (ERP) may demonstrate dilated, tortuous, or stenotic ducts. Computed tomographic (CT) or ultrasound scanning may reveal dilated ducts as well as an enlargement of the gland. On the basis of the radiologic changes, chronic pancreatitis may be graded as normal (1), equivocal (2), mild (3), moderate (4), or marked

(5). Serum pancreatic enzyme levels are of little value; they are rarely elevated.

The disease tends to run a course characterized by a gradual deterioration in exocrine function associated with variable (in number and severity) attacks of abdominal pain that tend to decrease as the disease progresses. The outlook is better in patients who refrain from alcohol. At five years following onset, 50% of patients have symptoms for less than one month per year. Overall 20-year survival is 40–50%.[3]

The cornerstone of management is the avoidance or correction of any precipitating factor, e.g., alcohol, hypercalcemia, hyperlipidemia. Pain relief is a major problem. Opiate analgesia is required in 20% of patients; up to 8% become addicted. Pancreatic enzyme replacement may have a role to play. It has been shown that such replacement improves fat absorption and may reduce pain, especially in patients with evidence of malabsorption.[4] It may best be given with meals as tablets or enteric-coated microsphere formulations (at least three with each meal), perhaps with sodium bicarbonate tablets (300 mg at start and end of meal).[5] Fat-soluble vitamins are not usually required, though vitamin D should be administered if there is clinical evidence of osteomalacia. A trial of medium-chain triglycerides may be worthwhile. Although diet and oral hypoglycemic agents are frequently successful in the management of diabetes mellitus when it occurs in this condition, insulin is required in some cases; administration of insulin is difficult because of variable absorption of food products and reduced glucagon response. Ultrasound-guided drainage of pseudocysts or abscesses is rarely required. Surgery may also be required for the management of such complications, for relief of bile duct obstruction, or for control of pancreatic ascites. The final role of surgery for the control of intractable pain has not yet been defined.[6] Ductal drainage (especially if the pancreatic duct is dilated), usually a modified Puestow procedure (side-to-side or lateral pancreatic pancreaticojejunostomy), or pancreatectomy (partial or subtotal) is associated with mortality and morbidity and a variable relief of pain. Surgery is generally reserved for the most intractable cases, and even here, its role is not firmly established.

KEY FEATURES

Definition of Chronic Pancreatitis
Pain and endocrine and exocrine pancreatic dysfunction in the presence of irreversible morphologic abnormalities of the pancreas

Etiology
1. Alcohol
2. Tropical/malnutrition
3. Metabolic
4. Others, including heredity, trauma, pancreas divisum

Pathology
Sclerosis, destruction and loss of acini and islets of Langerhans, ductal dilation, strictures, and calculi

Clinical Features
1. Abdominal pain
2. Steatorrhea, weight loss
3. Diabetes mellitus
4. Obstructive jaundice
5. Others (liver disease, ascites, splenic vein thrombosis)

Diagnosis
1. Secretin/pancreozymin test
2. Bentiromide test
3. Fecal fat analysis
4. Radiology (KUB; ERCP; CT; ultrasound)

Prognosis
Fifty per cent mortality rate at 20 years

Treatment
1. Alcohol avoidance
2. Pain relief
3. Pancreatic enzyme preparations
4. Oral hypoglycemics/insulin, if required, for diabetes mellitus
5. Ultrasound-guided drainage of abscess/pseudocyst
6. Surgery: for pain relief/management of complications

REFERENCES

1. Toskes PP: Bentiromide as a test of exocrine function in patients with pancreatic exocrine insufficiency: Determination of appropriate dose and urinary collection interval. Gastroenterology 85:565–569, 1983.
   Suggests that the optimal conditions for separation of normal from abnormal is to administer a 500-mg dose of bentiromide and to make a 6-hour post-dosing urinary collection for arylamine excretion.

2. Jacobsen DG, Curington C, Connery K, Toskes PP: Trypsin-like immunoreactivity as a test for pancreatic insufficiency. N Engl J Med 310:1307–1309, 1984.
   Suggests that this serum assay may be a reliable test of pancreatic exocrine function once a marked degree of pancreatic insufficiency occurs (enough insufficiency to product steatorrhea).

3. Amman RW, Arcobiantz A, Largiader F, et al: Course and outcome of chronic pancreatitis. Longitudinal study of a mixed medical-surgical series of 245 patients. Gastroenterology 86:821–828, 1984.
   Longitudinal study of over 20 years of 245 patients with chronic pancreatitis.

4. Slaff J, Jacobson D, Tillman CR, et al: Protease-specific suppression of pancreatic exocrine secretion. Gastroenterology 87:44–52, 1984.
   This study demonstrated that pancreatic extract decreases abdominal pain and that

long-term administration to patients with chronic pancreatitis decreased both basal and stimulated pancreatic exocrine secretion.

5. Graham DY: Pancreatic enzyme replacement: The effect of antacids or cimetidine. Dig Dis Sci 27:485–487, 1982.
   Discusses varying regimens available for enzyme administration.

6. Warshaw AS (ed): Pain in chronic pancreatitis. Gastroenterology 86:987–989, 1984.
   Discusses the management of this difficult problem from a surgical viewpoint.

Biliary Tract Disease

Frank E. Murray, M.B., M.R.C.P.I., M.R.C.P.

CHOLECYSTITIS

Acute cholecystitis implies acute inflammation of the gallbladder wall. It is associated with gallstones in over 90% of cases (though not all gallstones produce symptoms[1]). It usually follows impaction of a stone in the cystic duct, leading to outlet obstruction of the gallbladder. Acalculous cholecystitis is usually associated with sudden starvation and immobility and is common in patients on total parenteral nutrition (TPN). Other causes (e.g., polyarteritis nodosa, torsion of the gallbladder, adenocarcinoma, choledocholithiasis) are rare.

Clinically, acute cholecystitis is most common in obese, middle-aged females. Acute attacks are frequently precipitated by a fatty meal. Sudden onset of severe, continuous, right upper quadrant or epigastric pain is characteristic. The pain usually lasts 12–18 hours and precedes any vomiting. Flatulence and nausea often occur. Persistent vomiting is less common and suggests choledocholithiasis. Fever (99–102°F) is common. Jaundice usually indicates choledocholithiasis but may accompany uncomplicated cholecystitis; ductal stone obstruction becomes more likely when the bilirubin level is higher. Physical examination may show an abdomen that moves poorly with respiration. Right upper quadrant tenderness, exaggerated by inspiration (Murphy's sign), is often seen. The gallbladder is usually impalpable, especially in those who have had previous attacks.

Laboratory investigation typically shows an elevated white blood cell count with a left shift and modest rises in bilirubin, transaminases, alkaline phosphatase, and amylase. Abdominal plain films demonstrate gallstones in about 10% of the patients. Blood cultures are positive in about 25% in the first few days of an attack. HIDA scan may demonstrate cystic duct obstruction (though this investigation is less useful in acalculous cholecystitis).

The major differential diagnoses include acute appendicitis, acute pancreatitis, pyelonephritis, urolithiasis, peptic ulceration, acute hepatitis, hepatic abscess, pneumonia, pleurisy, and gonococcal or chlamydial perihepatitis (Fitz-Hugh-Curtis syndrome).

The major complications are gangrene of the gallbladder (with localized perforation, free perforation, or cholecystenteric fistulae, all of which usually require surgical intervention), cholangitis, and gallstone ileus (usually in older patients). Empyema may develop with formation of pus in the gallbladder. Emphysematous cholecystitis is relatively common in men and in diabetics and is due to infection by gas-producing organisms usually in the absence of gallstone disease; it may be the result of ischemia that is due to obstruction of the cystic artery. Chronic cholecystitis may develop later.

The mortality rate in acute cholecystitis is approximately 5% and is highest in elderly patients and those with a complicating medical condition, choledocholithiasis, gangrene of the gallbladder, or perforation. Most attacks of acute cholecystitis subside in a few days with conservative treatment.

Hospital admission is mandatory in all cases of acute cholecystitis. Fluid and electrolyte abnormalities must be corrected. No oral intake is allowed, and nasogastric suction is initiated. The administration of intravenous meperidine may be required to achieve adequate analgesia. Intravenous antibiotics are given in nearly all cases (usually ampicillin, a first-generation cephalosporin, or cefoxitin). Close clinical and laboratory evaluation is required during the attack.

The timing of surgical intervention depends primarily on the severity of the attack and the general condition of the patient. When complications seem imminent, or have already occurred, the patient should be brought to surgery when hemodynamically and metabolically stable. If the diagnosis is uncertain and there is concern about a perforated viscus, surgery may be indicated. For uncomplicated cases, there are two options regarding timing of surgery. Expectant management followed by surgery 6–8 weeks later in uncomplicated cases is favored by some. Other investigators favor surgery early in the attack, especially in older patients without a medical contraindication, who tend to have a higher mortality rate when managed conservatively. It has been suggested that early surgery may result in lower mortality and morbidity and may be more cost effective.

At surgery, cholecystectomy is performed in approximately 90% of cases. Exploration of the common bile duct should be carried out if the patient has had cholangitis, significant jaundice, pancreatitis, dilation of the common bile duct, palpable stones in the common bile duct, or multiple small stones in the gallbladder at the time of surgery. In the critically ill patient, cholecystostomy may be performed as the initial procedure, followed later by an elective cholecystectomy.

Chronic cholecystitis is the most common type of gallbladder disease. Symptoms tend to be less dramatic and more insidious in onset. This condition may be complicated by acute cholecystitis, choledocholithiasis, pancreatitis, cholecystenteric fistulization, gallstone ileus, hydrops of the gallbladder, and, rarely, gallbladder adenocarcinoma. Cholecystectomy is the treatment of choice in most cases. Small cholesterol stones in subjects with "functioning" gallbladders may be dissolved by oral administration of bile acids chenodeoxycholic or ursocholic acid.[2] This form of therapy should be reserved for the poor operative risk patient, because long-term treatment may be required to prevent recurrences.

There is now renewed interest in the treatment of symptomatic gallstones without surgery, using extracorporeal shock wave lithotripsy or contact dissolution with MTBE (methyl-tert-butyl-ether). The final role of these modalities of treatment is not yet clear.

CHOLANGITIS

There are two major types of cholangitis: infective (either bacterial or helminthic) and sclerosing. Sclerosing cholangitis may be secondary to recurrent bacterial cholangitis or primary; the latter, most commonly found in males with ulcerative colitis, usually presents as cholestatic liver disease and may progress to biliary cirrhosis. There appears to be a role for liver transplantation in these patients. Bile duct infestation with *Ascaris lumbricoides* or *Clonorchis sinensis* occurs mainly in the Far East. Bacterial (suppurative) cholangitis is usually associated with choledocholithiasis and benign biliary strictures and occasionally malignant strictures, Caroli's syndrome, sclerosing cholangitis, and biliary-enteric fistulae. The most common organisms isolated include aerobic (*Escherichia coli*, Klebsiella, Pseudomonas, *Streptococcus faecalis*, Proteus, and Staphylococci) and anaerobic (Bacteroides, Clostridia) species. The characteristic clinical features are rigors, fever, pain, jaundice, nausea, vomiting, and pruritus; dark urine and pale stools may also be seen. Recurrent attacks are common. The severity of individual attacks varies greatly. Blood cultures are usually positive during the acute attack. Specific treatment consists of intravenous antibiotic therapy (usually ampicillin, cefoxitin, or the combination of ampicillin and gentamicin with clindamycin or metronidazole) and decompression of the biliary tree. The timing of decompression depends on the clinical condition and the response to antibiotic therapy.[3-5] In the severely toxic or nonresponsive patient, it should be performed urgently. Decompression may be performed by either endoscopic sphincterotomy or surgery.

KEY FEATURES

Cholecystitis
Acute Cholecystitis
1. Acute inflammation of the gallbladder wall
2. ~10% acalculous (especially with sudden starvation, TPN, and immobility)
3. ~90% have associated gallstones
4. Most common in obese, middle-aged females
5. Attacks characterized by right upper quadrant pain and tenderness, vomiting, and fever
6. Laboratory data include elevated white blood cell count and abnormal liver biochemistries, positive HIDA scan, and frequently stones in gallbladder at ultrasonography
7. Amylase frequently elevated
8. Five per cent mortality, mainly in the elderly and debilitated
9. Most attacks subside on conservative regimen of NPO, IV fluids, antibiotics, and analgesia
10. Surgery may be performed early (in first 48 hours) or after 6–8 weeks

Chronic Cholecystitis
1. More insidious than acute cholecystitis
2. Cholecystectomy remains the treatment of choice in the majority of cases

Cholangitis
Sclerosing
May be secondary to repeated infections or primary (most common in patients with ulcerative colitis)

Infective
A result of parasitic or bacterial infections, both aerobic and anaerobic. Bacterial infection is characterized by fever, pain, obstructive jaundice, and vomiting. Blood cultures are usually positive. Management includes antibiotics and decompression of the biliary tree (endoscopically or surgically).

REFERENCES

1. Gracie WA, Ransohoff DF: The natural history of silent gallstones: The innocent gallstone is not a myth. N Engl J Med 307:798–800, 1982.
2. Editorial (NCGSG and Way LW): National cooperative gallstone study and current management of cholesterol cholelithiasis—two views. Gastroenterology 84:644–655, 1983.
   Discusses the role of bile acid dissolution of cholesterol gallstones.

3. Hatfield ARW, Terblanche J, Fataar S, et al: Preoperative external drainage in obstructive jaundice: A prospective controlled clinical trial. Lancet 2:896–899, 1982.
   Study failed to show any advantage associated with prior routine percutaneous biliary drainage.

4. Lam SK: A study of endoscopic sphincterotomy in recurrent pyogenic cholangitis. Br J Surg 71:262–268, 1984.
5. Cotton PB, Bourney PA, Mason RR: Transnasal bile duct catheterization after endoscopic sphincterotomy: Method of biliary drainage, perfusion, and sequential colangiography. Gut 20:285–287, 1979.

SECTION 4
HEMATOLOGY AND ONCOLOGY

Acute Complications of Chemotherapy

Roberta M. Falke, M.D.

The role of cytotoxic drugs in antineoplastic therapy is well established; toxicity often results, especially when combinations of several agents or treatment modalities are used. However, reducing the doses of chemotherapy in an effort to reduce morbidity may compromise response and survival rates. Hence, life-threatening adverse effects will be occasionally encountered in any institution in which significant numbers of cancer patients are treated with the hope of cure or lasting remission. Nonetheless, mortality can be minimized if complications are promptly recognized and treated. Chemotherapy administration and follow-up care should always be performed under the supervision of an experienced oncologist. The drug package insert and, wherever possible, formal treatment protocols should also be consulted.

THE FIRST FORTY-EIGHT HOURS

Hypersensitivity. Severe anaphylactoid (type I) reactions, including hypotension and bronchospasm, may be caused by L-asparaginase (10% of courses), bleomycin (2%), and teniposide (VM-26) (5%). Test doses are usually given and careful monitoring is needed.[3] Episodes should be managed as detailed elsewhere in this text, and the drug discontinued. Hypotension during etoposide (VP-16) infusion is rarely of clinical significance, and it may be avoided by slowing the rate of drug delivery.

Lesser reactions include fever (bleomycin) and urticaria (cisplatin). These can be managed with antihistamines and anti-inflammatory drugs while the drug is continued.

Gastrointestinal

Nausea and Vomiting. Many agents irritate the chemoreceptor trigger zone in the area postrema of the fourth ventricle and/or the vomiting center in the medulla. Cisplatin, dacarbazine (DTIC), the nitrosoureas, and nitrogen mustard are the worst offenders. This side-effect tends to worsen as patients are treated repeatedly with the same agents. Thus, it is important to try to prevent it. When strongly nauseating drugs are used, antiemetics should be started at least one half-hour before treatment and continued on a fixed schedule for 24–48 hours.[4] Effective antiemetics include metoclopropamide, 1–2 mg/kg IV q2h for four doses;[5] dexamethasone, 10–20 mg IV q4h;[6] droperidol, 0.5–2.0 mg/hour infusion; and perphenazine, 5 mg IV bolus and 1–2 mg/hour. Two or more of these drugs may be combined in some protocols. Patients should be watched for excessive central nervous system depression, although some sedation is inevitable and desirable. Extrapyramidal side effects of phenothiazines may be treated with diphenhydramine, 25–50 mg IV. Tetrahydrocannabinol is helpful, especially for anticipatory symptoms: 2.5–5.0 mg PO qid. Milder symptoms may be controlled with oral or rectal perphenazine or prochlorperazine.

Diarrhea. Diarrhea may occur shortly after antimetabolite administration; it is usually self-limited, but may be severe after combinations of fluorouracil and methotrexate or leucovorin.

When gastrointestinal toxicity is severe, fluid and electrolyte losses must be replaced. Parenteral nutrition may be indicated if nausea persists. Hypovolemia may delay the excretion of drugs such as cisplatin and methotrexate, resulting in enhanced toxicity. Hence, patients should be followed closely, and intravenous hydration provided if necessary.

Acute Cardiovascular Toxicity. Arrhythmias may occur immediately following the administration of anthracycline drugs.[7] They are usually not of clinical significance, and neither contraindicate use of the drugs nor predict future cardiotoxicity. Acute myocarditis/pericarditis is rare, may be severe, and is usually reversible. Less than 1% of patients receiving the experimental agent *m*-AMSA have developed fatal arrhythmias. Acute myocardial ischemia and cerebrovascular accidents have been reported following fluorouracil infusion. These complications are unpredictable and fortunately rare. If symptoms suggestive of cardiovascular disease occur following administration of cytotoxic drugs, serious consideration should always be given to the possibility of drug toxicity and to discontinuation of the regimen.

Acute Tissue Necrosis. Extravasation of the many vesicant drugs may lead to the sloughing of large areas of skin.[7,8] This complication should be suspected if pain or erythema occurs during drug administration. Infusion should be stopped, and one should aspirate through the needle before removing it, to remove as much drug as possible. Hydrocortisone, 50 mg, may be locally instilled. Ice may help reduce extension of the injury and serve as a local anesthetic. The consulting oncologist should be contacted immediately, and may recommend a specific antidote. If pain and inflammation persist for more than a few days, surgical excision of necrotic tissue may be necessary.

Renal and Metabolic Disorders. Tumor lysis syndrome is the predictable onset of renal insufficiency when effective drugs cause the sudden destruction of rapidly growing tumor cells (e.g., Burkitt's lymphoma) with release of intracellular solutes such as potassium, phosphates, and uric acid into the bloodstream. Although hydration, allopurinol, and urinary alkalinization may help prevent this complication, it may still occur, and if so, dialysis is indicated.[9]

Renal failure as a result of cisplatin is usually mild and often prevented when intensive hydration and diuresis are used.[10] However, serum creatinine must be followed carefully so that changes in renal function are detected before other renally excreted drugs are given.

Hypercalcemia may occur in 10% of patients treated for breast cancer with hormone therapy for the first time. Treatment should proceed as outlined elsewhere, but the drug is not discontinued, because this complication is usually transient and followed by a tumor response. Hypomagnesemia is a frequent consequence of prolonged cisplatin administration. Supplementation should be given in an effort to prevent it, and levels monitored after therapy.

Neurologic. Neurotoxicity is usually gradual, but acute onset of cerebellar ataxia (high-dose cytosine arabinoside, fluorouracil), seizures (cisplatin), or confusion (L-asparaginase) may occur.[11,12] Differential diagnosis includes brain or meningeal metastases and metabolic disturbance, e.g., hypercalcemia.

More commonly, the administration of vinca alkaloids (vincristine, vinblastine, vindesine) may be followed by severe neuropathic pain, often in the jaw. This symptom abates spontaneously. These drugs may cause paralytic ileus, occasionally requiring hydration and nasogastric suction. Once bowel sounds are present, cathartics such as lactulose and sorbitol may help relieve bowel hypomotility.

ACUTE ILLNESS IN THE WEEKS FOLLOWING CHEMOTHERAPY

Bone Marrow Suppression. Nadir white blood cell (WBC) counts occur between 7 and 14 days after most commonly used drugs and combinations. Oral alkylating agents (busulphan, melphalan), nitrosoureas, and mitomycin C may cause delayed myelotoxicity (6–8 weeks) as a result of stem cell destruction. Patients who become febrile while neutropenic should be admitted to hospital, cultured rapidly, and treated promptly with broad-spectrum antibiotics, usually including a beta-lactam drug and an aminoglycoside. Treatment is continued until any documented infection is appropriately treated, or until absolute neutrophil count is above 1000. Hand washing is the most effective reverse isolation technique.

Thrombocytopenia may appear after leukopenia, and it is usually less profound. Spontaneous bleeding may occur when the count is under 20,000/mm³, and platelet transfusion is advised at that level. In the event of a markedly low platelet count without WBC depression, immune thrombocytopenia or sepsis should be considered. A bone marrow examination may then be needed to distinguish among these possibilities.

Anemia is less common. Many agents cause megaloblastosis. Patients receiving cisplatin usually develop a hypoproliferative anemia requiring transfusion after several cycles. Coombs-positive immune hemolytic anemia has also been described with this drug. However, in general, if persistent anemia is noted, conditions other than chemotherapy-induced myelosuppression must be considered, including gastrointestinal bleeding as a result of disease or other drugs, malignant marrow infiltration, and microangiopathic hemolytic anemia that is due to extensive tumor.

Gastrointestinal. Injury of rapidly growing mucosal cells by cytotoxic agents may affect any site between mouth and anus.[13] Common offenders include methotrexate, fluorouracil, doxorubicin, and bleomycin. Ulcerations usually occur within 7–10 days. Herpes simplex or Candida may superinfect the lesions. Treatment includes systemic analgesics and soothing local solutions such as diphenhydramine, Kaopectate, and lidocaine, or a suspension of sucralfate. Specific antimicrobial therapy may include antifungal agents or acyclovir. If lesions are extensive, hydration and nutrition must be parenteral and the possibility of infection should be anticipated, owing to loss of the protective mucosal barrier. Finally, these patients must be watched very closely, since mucositis is often followed shortly by comparable myelosuppression.

Pulmonary. The insidious onset of interstitial fibrosis may occur after large cumulative doses of most alkylating agents and bleomycin.[14] However, acute respiratory insufficiency and hypoxemia have been described when individuals previously treated with bleomycin are given high-flow oxygen.[15] Acute respiratory difficulty with infiltrates may occur after long-term methotrexate administration, but it is usually reversible. Differential diagnosis includes infection, pulmonary embolism or congestive heart failure. Effective management of interstitial pneumonitis requires early recognition by serial DLCO* measurement. If respiratory insufficiency occurs, oxygen therapy must be used with extreme caution.

---

*DLCO = diffusing capacity of the lungs for carbon monoxide.

Hepatic. Liver necrosis, cholestasis, or veno-occlusive disease may occur following L-asparaginase, mithramycin, and high-dose cytosine arabinoside administration. These events are usually reversible, but may be severe. It is important to be aware of the complications, as they may impair the excretion of other drugs such as vincristine and doxorubicin.

Cardiac. Cardiomyopathy seems to be due to lipid peroxidation of cardiac cell membrane by free radicals. It occurs primarily in patients treated with cumulative doses of doxorubicin exceeding 500 mg/m^2. It is more frequent in individuals with prior heart disease or those who have received mediastinal irradiation. Serial determinations of ejection fraction may help detect this complication before it is clinically apparent. Once cardiomyopathy is manifested, the drug should be stopped immediately. The syndrome may respond to digoxin and diuretics, but it is sometimes relentless and has a high mortality rate.[16]

Acute Renal Failure. Hemolytic-uremic syndrome is an unusual but frequently fatal event after therapy with mitomycin-C.[17] Treatment with plasmapheresis is sometimes successful.

OVERVIEW

Patients who experience severe chemotherapy toxicity often have life-threatening disease in multiple organ systems. Treatment requires hospitalization and extensive support: hydration, correction of electrolytes, alimentation, antibiotics, and blood products may be needed; as well as compassionate control of symptoms such as pain, nausea, fever, and fear.

KEY FEATURES

A. *First 48 hours*
   1. Avoid *extravasation*. If it occurs, remove drug, apply ice, consider local steroids, and inquire about specific antidotes to drugs given.
   2. Prevent *nausea* and *vomiting* with IV antiemetics. If they occur, maintain hydration and urinary output.
   3. If *ileus* is present, hydrate.
   4. Watch for unusual *hypersensitivity* or *cardiovascular* events.
   5. *Creatinine* must be followed after cisplatin and after treatment of bulky, rapidly growing tumors such as Burkitt's lymphoma.
B. *Several days or weeks later*
   1. When *stomatitis* or *esophagitis* occurs, treat pain with analgesics and topical remedies. Maintain hydration and nutrition, and treat fungal or viral superinfection. Severe mucositis may herald severe myelosuppression.
   2. *Myelosuppression*

    a. *WBCs:* Fever and infection common with a granulocyte count of 1000. Culture quickly and treat aggressively.

    b. *Platelets:* Transfuse as needed, usually at counts below 20,000/mm³.

    c. *RBCs:* Transfuse as needed, but rule out other causes of anemia.

  3. *Pulmonary.* DO NOT GIVE HIGH-FLOW O_2 TO PATIENTS WHO HAVE RECEIVED BLEOMYCIN. Rule out infection, pulmonary embolus, congestive heart failure.

REFERENCES

General References

1. Calabresi P, Parks RE: Antiproliferative agents and drugs used for immunosuppression. *In* Gilman AS, et al (eds). The Pharmacologic Basis of Therapeutics. New York, Macmillan, 1985, pp 1247–1306.
2. DeVita VT, et al (eds): Cancer: Principles and Practice of Oncology, 2nd ed. Philadelphia, JB Lippincott, 1985, pp 2008–2032.

Specific References

3. Weiss RB, Bruno S: Hypersensitivity reactions to cancer chemotherapeutic agents. Ann Inter Med 94:66–72, 1981.
   Comprehensive but concise review of occurrence and pathophysiology of hypersensitivity reactions to commonly used chemotherapeutics.

4. Siegel LJ, Longo DL: The control of chemotherapy-induced emesis. Ann Intern Med 95:352—359, 1981.
   Reviews pathophysiology as well as the mechanism of action of some frequently used antiemetics.

5. Gralla RJ, Itri LM, et al: Antiemetic efficacy of high dose metoclopropamide: Randomized trials against placebo and prochlorperazine in patients with chemotherapy-induced nausea and vomiting. N Engl J Med 305:905–909, 1981.
   Only metoclopropamide produced significant decrease in emesis in patients treated with drugs like cisplatin.

6. Aapro MS, Alberts DS: Dexamethasone as an antiemetic in patients treated with cisplatin. N Engl J Med 305:520, 1981.
7. Young RC, Ozols RF, Myers CE: The anthracycline antineoplastic drugs. N Engl J Med 305:139–153, 1981.
   This extensive review discusses the mechanism of action and clinical utility of these drugs. Clinical toxicity syndromes are well delineated, and the etiologies are considered.

8. Larson D: Treatment of tissue extravasation by anti-tumor agents. Cancer 49:1796–1799, 1982.
   Article reviews available remedies.

9. Cohen LF, Balow JE, Magrath IT, et al: Acute tumor lysis syndrome. Am J Med 68:586–591, 1980.
   Hyperkalemia, hyperphosphatemia, and renal failure characterize this dramatic complication. Acute dialysis may be needed.

10. Blachley JD, Hill JB: Renal and electrolyte disturbances associated with cisplatin. Ann Intern Med 95:628–632, 1981.
   Pharmacokinetics, nephrotoxicity, and magnesium wasting are described, as well as efforts to prevent them.

11. Kaplan RS, Wiernik PH: Neurotoxicity of antineoplastic drugs. Semin Oncol 9:103–130, 1982.
   Inclusive review of neurotoxic agents, syndromes, and mechanisms.

12. Herzig RH, Herzig GP, et al: Central nervous system effects of high-dose cytosine arabinoside. Semin Oncol 14(suppl 1):21–24, 1987.

13. Adrian RM, Hood AF, Skarin AT: Mucocutaneous reactions to antineoplastic agents. CA 30:143–156, 1980.
   Article describes cutaneous and mucosal injuries. Illustrated.

14. Bennett JM, Reich SD: Bleomycin. Ann Intern Med 90:945–948, 1979.
   Indications for this agent and toxicity: allergic, mucocutaneous, and pulmonary.

15. Ginsberg SJ, Comis RL: The pulmonary toxicity of antineoplastic agents. Semin Oncol 9:34–51, 1982.
   Most agents lead to interstitial pneumonitis. Roles of drug dose, radiation, and oxygen in potentiating pulmonary toxicity are emphasized.

16. Von Hoff DD, Rozencweig M, Piccort M: The cardiotoxicity of anticancer agents. Semin Incol 9:23–33, 1982.
   Article lists drugs, mechanisms, detection, and management.

17. Jackson AM, Rose BD, et al: Thrombotic microangiopathy and renal failure associated with antineoplastic chemotherapy. Ann Intern Med 101:41–44, 1984.
   One of several case reports describing renal failure, thrombocytopenia, and microangiopathic hemolytic anemia in patients treated with regimens that included mitomycin-C.

Acute Complications of Hemoglobinopathies and Thalassemias

Juan Carlos Vera, M.D.

An awareness of the natural history and morbidity associated with the hemoglobinopathies provides the physician with valuable clues in the prompt recognition and treatment of the acute complications seen in these diseases. Institution of continuous, supportive, and, in certain circumstances, specific therapy has undoubtedly contributed to decreasing the associated morbidity and mortality. These therapeutic advances are even more striking in the thalassemias, in which the use of transfusion and chelator agents in patients with thalassemia major has improved the longevity of these individuals. Without treatment, patients often die by the age of 2 or 3 with hematocrits as low as 5% or 6%.[1] In sickle cell anemia, the use of pneumococcal vaccine and the appropriate treatment of acute complications have similarly improved survival.

GENERAL CONSIDERATIONS

Hemoglobinopathies are usually caused by the production of an abnormal protein molecule, i.e., the substitution of an amino acid in a polypeptide chain; in thalassemia, there is a reduction of the amount of normal protein synthesized, resulting in unbalanced globin synthesis. The list of abnormal hemoglobins or variants is extensive, but the more common abnormalities associated with significant clinical manifestations in the United States are hemoglobin S, C, and the beta thalassemias. In black Americans,[2] the incidence of sickle cell anemia is at least 1 in 600 births for the hemozygous condition (SS), and 1 in 1000 for SC hemoglobinopathy, a condition potentially as severe as SS disease. The sickle cell gene may also be inherited with beta thalassemia, resulting in one other variant of the sickle cell syndromes, sickle thalassemia disease. Hemoglobin S trait is seen in 10% of American blacks, hemoglobin C trait in 2–3%, and beta thalassemia trait in about 0.8%. Sickle cell disease thus constitutes a major public health problem and is frequently encountered as an acute emergency. Individuals carrying the trait (AS) are asymptomatic, except for occasional hematuria.

SICKLE CELL ANEMIA

Sickle cell anemia is the most important of the abnormal variants of hemoglobin, and the clinical manifestations, although variable for each individual, are ultimately determined by (1) intracellular concentration of hemoglobin S, (2) the amount of hemoglobin F (high F levels are protective), and (3) the interaction between hemoglobin S and other hemoglobins.[3-6] The history of patients with homozygous SS disease usually reveals a continuously aggressive illness with chronic hemolytic anemia, punctuated by repeated acute episodes, mainly of the vaso-occlusive type; by infections; and occasionally by a temporary failure of the marrow to maintain erythropoiesis. The sickle cell syndromes, commonly seen in black Americans, are, in order of decreasing severity, homozygous SS, $S\beta^0$ thalassemia, $S\beta^+$ thalassemia, and hemoglobin SC disease. Individuals with $S\beta^0$ thalassemia[7] are often indistinguishable from those with the homozygous state except for their hematologic parameters, as there is no detectable level of hemoglobin A in the red cells.

Painful crisis is the most common emergency in sickle cell anemia, with infarction caused by cells occluding the microcirculation. Certain organs are especially vulnerable to vaso-occlusion (Table 1); others, such as spleen and kidney, are more predisposed to functional impairment. Painful crisis may occur without an obvious precipitating factor, but bacterial or viral infection, hypoxia, acidosis, dehydration, pregnancy, strenuous exercise, anesthesia, surgery, or transfusion reactions may precipitate an episode. In a painful crisis, the discomfort may be generalized or may affect more than one area of the body; on other occasions, the pain is localized to one area, giving rise to a more specific clinical syndrome (abdominal crisis, acute chest syndrome). Adult patients with acute painful crisis often present with fever, unassociated with infection. This phenomenon is best illustrated in the acute chest syndrome,[8,9] in which the distinction between a pneumonitis and an infarct may be difficult because they both frequently present with fever and pulmonary

Table 1. ACUTE SYNDROMES IN SICKLE CELL ANEMIA

Symptoms or Syndrome	Involvement	Pathogenesis
Painful crisis (generalized or localized)	Bone Organs	Microinfarction
Acute chest syndrome	Lung parenchyma Pleura Pulmonary vessels	Local thrombosis Fat embolism
Abdominal crisis	Mesenteric Intestinal vessels	Bowel ischemia
Hand-foot syndrome (children)	Epiphysis	Dactylitis with bone infarction
Hip or shoulder pain	Femoral or humeral head	Avascular necrosis
Seizure, stroke, or subarachnoid hemorrhage	Brain vessels	Hemorrhage or infarct
Aplastic crisis	Bone marrow	Bone marrow failure (transient)
Hematuria	Kidney	Occlusion of vasa recta
Priapism	Penis	Engorgement or stasis of corpora cavernosa
Right upper quadrant syndrome (jaundice)	Liver Biliary tree	Cholecystitis, lithiasis Cholestasis
Splenic sequestration crisis (acute anemia)	Spleen	Acute sequestration of blood in the spleen
Acute arthropathy (pain, effusion)	Joints	Microvascular thrombosis
Monocular blindness	Retinal vessels	Retinal infarct, neovascularization Vitreous hemorrhage
Pneumococcal sepsis	Lungs, blood meninges	Blood-borne infection

infiltrates. Noncardiogenic pulmonary edema may develop in the acute chest syndrome.[10]

Management of a painful crisis is directed at hydration, pain control, and treatment of a precipitating factor or infection. In order to achieve pain control, liberal use of narcotics may be required. Meperidine 50–100 mg and hydroxyzine 50 mg SC q3h is a common and effective combination. This schedule should be continued until control is obtained, but it can be modified as the intensity of the pain decreases over the 48–72 hours: painful crises are self-limited episodes, and the use of narcotics should be restricted to these situations in order to avoid the risk of addiction. Vigorous fluid replacement is a rational form of therapy in sickle cell anemia, because the state of hydration (patients with sickle cell anemia cannot produce a concentrated urine) and cell water content appears to be important in the pathogenesis of sickling.[11] Parenteral hydration with hypotonic solutions, D5W,* or ¼ normal saline can be given at a fast rate (275–300 ml/hour) during the first several hours and continued during the next 24–48 hours as necessary.[12] The most recent attempts at inducing hyponatremia with DDVAP have not shown reproducible results,[13] and a safe and effective antisickling agent is not yet available. Patients with sickle cell anemia are susceptible to infections, particularly with pneumococci and salmonella species,[14] and whenever appropriate, suspected infection should be treated with antibiotics. Use of pneumococcal vaccine is recommended.

Aplastic Crisis

A patient with sickle cell anemia usually maintains a stable hemoglobin and reticulocyte count, reflecting a delicate balance between the accelerated rate of blood destruction and an increased erythropoietic activity in the bone marrow. Expected hemoglobin levels are in the range of 7–8 gm/dl, with a reticulocyte count in the range of 10–20%. Episodes of severe anemia can be seen, particularly in children, and are usually associated with an infection[15] in which the bone marrow is temporarily aplastic, requiring the use of transfusion as an emergency measure. Marrow recovery occurs in 2–6 days.

Splenic Sequestration

Occasionally, massive splenic trapping of red cells develops in children, presenting with acute splenomegaly and anemia; immediate restoration of intravascular volume with transfusion of red cells is indicated.[16]

---

*D5W = 5% dextrose in water.

Other Complications

Hematuria is relatively common in patients with sickle cell anemia, but it seldom requires transfusion or more aggressive treatment. Priapism is seen less commonly and may require exchange transfusion or drainage, if refractory to conservative treatment.[17] Acute ocular complications,[18] owing to retinal or vitreous hemorrhage, can lead to acute monocular blindness with permanent visual loss if not treated promptly with photocoagulation; these complications are largely prevented by the treatment of early lesions. Finally, acute neurologic complications may develop.[19] Cerebral thrombosis, hemorrhage, and subarachnoid bleeding are events that may occur suddenly and are manifested by headaches, seizures, hemiparesis, or loss of consciousness. Strokes tend to recur, and long-term transfusion has been advocated for prevention. Not infrequently, painful swelling of one or more joints,[20] particularly the knees, occurs as an isolated event or accompanying a sickle cell crisis; other joints or bones can also be involved, causing the hand-foot syndrome or aseptic necrosis of the hip or humerus.

Pneumococcal Sepsis

Pneumococcal septicemia[21] is the primary cause of death in patients under the age of 5, and blood-borne infection should be suspected in patients with fever, changes in mental status, pneumonia, or meningitis. Early diagnosis and prophylaxis with pneumococcal vaccine or penicillin are vital.

THE UNSTABLE HEMOGLOBINS

The unstable hemoglobins constitute a rare cause of congenital hemolytic anemia of varying severity.[22] Unstable hemoglobin precipitates inside the red blood cell, causing red blood cell membrane damage and hemolysis; as a result of the precipitation of hemoglobin, intracellular inclusions of denatured hemoglobin (Heinz's bodies) can be demonstrated.

Patients with unstable hemoglobins may present either with an acute hemolytic episode following drugs or infection, or with a chronic hemolytic anemia. Because the patients may be susceptible to oxidant hemolysis, the clinical and hematologic investigations may be indistinguishable from those associated with G-6-PD deficiency. Splenectomy may be helpful in controlling hemolysis, and transfusion should be reserved for hemolytic crisis.

BETA THALASSEMIAS

The beta thalassemias are a heterogeneous group of conditions, but in this article only the management of acute complications associated with the homozygous state is discussed. In blacks, the clinical state is generally that of thalassemia intermedia, which requires minimal or no transfusion and nonhematologic complications generally develop over decades. In the white population, beta thalassemia is mainly found in Italian and Greek immigrant populations; thalassemia major is characterized by profound anemia, hepatosplenomegaly, and bone deformities, requiring regular transfusion to maintain hemoglobin concentration at a level consistent with reasonable activity and growth.[23]

In the second decade of life, cardiac complications occur frequently and are the major cause of death. This is almost entirely due to iron overload resulting in hemochromatosis; sudden death from cardiac arrhythmia or recurrent bouts of congestive heart failure characterize the development of this complication. It appears that regular chelation therapy may reduce the incidence of cardiac death in thalassemia.[1]

KEY FEATURES

Sickle Cell Anemia
A. Sickle cell crisis: diagnosis and management
    1. Bone pain; usually involves more than one site
    2. Intensity of the pain characteristically increases after onset of crisis
    3. Duration of painful crisis: usually 3–6 days
    4. Fever and leucocytosis usually present with or without infection
    5. Hemolytic or aplastic crisis may be associated with this event
    6. Treatment of a crisis
        a. Vigorous hydration
        b. Pain control (narcotics)
        c. Prompt recognition and treatment of an associated infection or precipitant
B. Acute infections: patients susceptible to pneumococcal and Salmonella infections
    1. Pneumococcal sepsis: primary cause of death in children less than 5 years of age (pneumonia, meningitis, septicemia)
        a. Early diagnosis a key to the treatment of this complication
        b. Pneumococcal vaccine effective
        c. Penicillin prophylaxis may be effective in infants
    2. Other causes of infection
        a. Salmonella osteomyelitis, septicemia
        b. Urinary tract infections
C. Cerebrovascular events
    1. Symptoms: sudden onset of headaches, seizures, hemiparesis, changes in mental status
    2. Occurs more commonly in children and young adults
    3. Strokes tend to recur within 3 years
    4. Prophylactic transfusions may be effective in preventing recurrences

Unstable Hemoglobins (Congenital Heinz's Body Hemolytic Anemia)

A. Unstable hemoglobins cause hemolysis by intracellular precipitation of hemoglobin (Heinz's bodies)
B. Substitution of an amino acid or deletion of one or more amino acids results in an unstable molecule
C. Large number of variants with marked variation in the expression of the disease
D. Drugs may produce oxidant hemolysis and increased levels of met-sulfahemoglobin (dusky cyanosis)
E. Heat denaturation is the most helpful test for the detection of unstable hemoglobins
F. Heinz's body preparation frequently positive (if positive, must rule out drug-induced hemolysis, enzyme deficiencies)

THALASSEMIAS

A. Thalassemia major (homozygous beta thalassemia) is characterized by severe anemia, hepatosplenomegaly, and bone deformity.
B. There is heterogeneity in the clinical expression of the disease as well as in the molecular defect.
C. Typically, only a mild form of the disease, thalassemia intermedia, characterized by mild anemia (Hgb of 7–12 gm/dl, Hgb F levels of 25–60%), is seen in the black population.
D. In thalassemia intermedia, children survive into adulthood with minimal complications.
E. Acute complications may be related to the underlying disease or to the treatment (transfusion).
   1. Acute anemia (aplastic crisis) can be seen in untransfused patients.
   2. Cardiac complications are seen in the second decade in patients on chronic transfusion (iron overload).
   3. Bleeding is rare but may occur in patients with thrombocytopenia and hypersplenism.
   4. Acute infections (usually post-splenectomy).
   5. Compression from extramedullary masses in untransfused or poorly transfused patients.
   6. Transfusion reactions.
   7. Acute secondary gout, cholecystitis, and cholelithiasis.

REFERENCES

1. Benz EJ, Propper R, Corash L, French AW, Henry W, Borer J: Thalassemia major: Molecular and clinical aspects. Ann Intern Med 91:883, 1979.
   A detailed discussion of advances in the understanding of the molecular pathology of beta thalassemia, of the role of hypertransfusion, and of iron chelation in the management of these patients. Clinical aspects of the cardiac complications and their management are also discussed, as well as newer approaches to transfusion therapy.

2. Motulsky AG: Frequency of sickling disorders in US blacks. N Engl J Med 288:31, 1973.
   Estimates of the frequency of these hemoglobinopathies in American blacks are presented here based on calculations from heterozygote frequencies.

3. Eaton WA, Hofrichter J, Ross PD: Delay time of gelation: A possible determinant of clinical severity in sickle cell disease. Blood 47:621, 1976.

   Using an in vitro model (time course of gelatin reaction), the authors demonstrate an inverse correlation between the thirtieth power of total deoxyhemoglobin concentration and the delay time; as the solubility of intracellular hemoglobin decreases, the delay time also decreases. It is postulated that this phenomenon could be a determinant of the clinical severity of sickle cell disease.

4. Stevens MCG, Hayes RJ, Vaidya S, Serjeant GR: Fetal hemoglobin and clinical severity of homozygous sickle cell disease in early childhood. J Pediatr 9837, 1981.

   The clinical features of homozygous patients less than 2 years of age and their relationship to hemoglobin F levels are described. Children with hemoglobin F levels less than 21% had more frequent episodes of dactylitis and splenic sequestration; in addition, their death rate was higher.

5. Perrine RP, Pembrey ME, Peter J, Perrine S, Shoup F: Natural history of sickle cell anemia in Saudi Arabia. Ann Intern Med 88:1, 1978.

   Although collected retrospectively by chart review, the data from 270 patients with sickle cell anemia from Saudi Arabia suggest that the high fetal hemoglobin levels observed (22–26%) may account for the milder disease observed in these patients.

6. Ranney H: Interaction of other hemoglobin variants with sickle hemoglobin. N Engl J Med 283:1462, 1970.

   Editorial comment and brief review of the interaction of hemoglobin ^{O}Arab ($\beta^{121\ lys}$), hemoglobin C ($\beta^{6\ lys}$), hemoglobin D ($\beta^{121\ gln}$), ^{C}Harlem ($\beta^{6val,\ 73\ asp}$), and hemoglobin Korle Bu ($\beta^{73\ asn}$) with hemoglobin S. Possible interaction sites are discussed (β^6, β^{73}, β^{122}).

7. Serjeant GR, Sommereux AM, Stevenson M, Mason K, Serjeant BE: Comparison of sickle-β thalassemia with homozygous sickle cell disease. Br J Haematol 41:83, 1979.

   Splenomegaly and higher hemoglobin levels are more commonly seen in Sβ^0 patients, but clinical features are quite similar to those of SS patients. Red blood cells in Sβ patients are invariably microcytic.

8. Charache S, Scott JC, Charache P: Acute chest syndrome in adults with sickle cell anemia. Microbiology, Treatment and Prevention. Arch Intern Med 139:67, 1968.

   No pneumococcal organisms were identified in sputum cultures of 28 adult patients with fever and pulmonary infiltrates. Bacterial organisms were isolated in less than half of these episodes: normal respiratory flora represented a large percentage of them. The data suggest that the majority of these episodes are not infectious.

9. Poncz M, Kane E, Gill FM: Acute chest syndrome in sickle cell disease: Etiology and clinical correlates. J Pediatr 107:861, 1985.

   Prospective study of 102 episodes of the acute chest syndrome (ACS). An infectious cause was identified in only 36% of cases, but those with bacterial infection tended to be sicker.

10. Hayne J, Allison RC: Pulmonary edema. Complication in the management of sickle cell pain crisis. Am J Med 80:833, 1986.

    Description of four episodes of pulmonary edema complicating sickle cell pain crisis. Clinical features and hemodynamic studies suggested a noncardiogenic basis for pulmonary edema.

11. Clark MR, Gratelli JC, Mohandas N, Shohet S: Influence of red cell water content on the morphology of sickling. Blood 55:823, 1980.

    In vitro studies with sickled cells demonstrated that after reoxygenation, the deoxygenated dehydrated cell retained the sickled morphology more readily than well-hydrated cells. It is also shown in these experiments that these cells can be unsickled with hypotonic media. The role of calcium is also tested in this model. The observations support the contention that the morphologic changes associated with sickling are strongly influenced by cell water content.

12. Guy RB, Gavrillis PK, Rothenberg SP: In vitro and in vivo effect of hypotonic saline on the sickling phenomenon. Am J Med Sci 266:267, 1973.

    Aggressive administration of 0.45% saline intravenously can produce amelioration of painful crisis, particularly in patients with mild crisis, although the changes observed in serum sodium osmolarity were variable. In this study, some decreases in the number of circulating sickled cells were also observed.

13. Charache S, Walker WG: Failure of desmopressin to lower serum sodium or prevent crisis in patients with sickle cell anemia. Blood 58:892, 1981.

    DDAVP, an analogue of vasopressin, was evaluated for prevention of sickle cell crisis and induction of hyponatremia in three patients with sickle cell anemia. No beneficial effects were reported, although the study was inconclusive because a state of chronic hyponatremia was not achieved.

14. Barrett-Connor E: Bacterial infection and sickle cell anemia. Medicine (Baltimore) 50:97, 1971.

    An analysis of the pattern of infection in 166 patients with sickle cell anemia (250 episodes). Eighty-five episodes were confirmed bacteriologically; common presentations were pneumonia, meningitis, septicemia, osteomyelitis, and urinary tract infections. Pneumococcus was the most common cause of bacteremia in this series.

15. Mann JR, Cotter KP, Walker RA, Bird GW, Stuart J: Anemic crisis in sickle cell disease. J Clin Pathol 28:341, 1975.

    Description of hemolytic and aplastic crisis occurring in 13 children with sickle cell anemia. Sudden, profound anemia with low hemoglobin levels (2.7–4.6 gm) and low reticulocyte count was seen in 10 of the 16 episodes. Infection was frequently associated with these complications.

16. Seeler RA, Shwiaki ZM: Acute splenic sequestration crisis in young childen with sickle cell anemia. Clin Pediatr 11:701, 1972.

    Article discusses this life-threatening complication in young children (age less than 6) with profound anemia and splenomegaly. The outcome and clinical features of 20 episodes were observed in 14 children. There were 4 deaths (3 before transfusion), and 4 children had recurrent episodes (2 required splenectomy).

17. Baron M, Leiter E: The management of priapism in sickle cell anemia. J Urol 119:610, 1978.

    Case report and review of the management of priapism. Early nonsurgical measures with hydration, analgesia, sedation, and exchange transfusion are advocated as the initial approach: shunting procedures can be reserved for patients who are unresponsive to these modalities.

18. Armaly, MF: Ocular manifestation in sickle cell disease. Arch Intern Med 133:670, 1974.

    The stages of vascular lesions in the eye and their prognosis are described in detail here. Neovascularization of the retinal vessels or of the vitreous can lead to retinal detachment or vitreous hemorrhage, lesions that require photocoagulation. Earlier lesions are asymptomatic but may evolve to a more advanced stage.

19. Powars DR, Wilson B, Imbus C, Pegelow C, Allen J: The natural history of stroke in sickle cell anemia. Am J Med 65:461, 1978.

    The occurrence and progression of stroke in 35 untreated patients—33 were SS, and 2 were SC patients. Children were more at risk for cerebral infarction, whereas adults had intracranial hemorrhage. Cerebral infarct was associated with a high risk of recurrence

244 HEMATOLOGY AND ONCOLOGY

(more than 50%) within the first 3 years. No predictive (or prognostic) factors were identified.

20. Espinoza LR, Spilberg I, Osterland CK: Joint manifestations of sickle cell disease. Medicine 53:295, 1974.

    Joint manifestations are seen almost exclusively in SS patients. In the majority of patients, the joint manifestations are accompanied by symptoms of sickle cell crisis. More than one joint, particularly large joints, is involved in at least 80% of the cases. Fluid examination is usually nonspecific (except for the presence of sickle cells). Small joint involvement is seen more commonly in children (hand-foot syndrome).

21. Powars DR: Natural history of sickle cell disease in the first ten years. Semin Hematol 12:267, 1975.

    Data collected from 422 patients with sickle cell anemia; the morbidity and mortality during the first decade are described. Forty-nine patients died, most of them SS patients and most during early childhood. Pneumococcal sepsis was the leading cause of death, occurring usually within 48 hours of the illness.

22. White JM: The unstable hemoglobin disorders. Clin Hematol 3:333, 1974.

    This article describes the molecular pathology of the unstable hemoglobins as well as the mode of inheritance. The degree of hemolysis is variable; jaundice or methemoglobinemia may be present. Heinz's bodies and increased reticulocyte counts are usually present. Complications are similar to those of other hemolytic anemias. Heat denaturation is a very helpful test in the detection of these abnormalities.

23. Weatherall DJ, Clegg JB: The Thalassaemia Syndromes. 3rd ed. St. Louis, CV Mosby, 1981.

    A thorough review of all variants of the thalassemia syndromes, with detailed description of the genetic, prevalence, clinical, and laboratory features of these inherited disorders. In other chapters, the structure, function, and synthesis of hemoglobin are discussed, as well as developments in the management of thalassemias.

Hemolytic Syndromes

Mark J. Brauer, M.D.

Although hemolysis is not usually thought of as a medical emergency, instances of hemolysis secondary to drug ingestion, hereditary hemolytic disorders, immune-related phenomena, and sepsis constitute a unique and serious group of disorders. The characteristic feature of hemolytic syndromes is a shortening of the normal red blood cell life span. Mature erythrocytes normally survive 4 months (120 days) and must withstand severe mechanical and metabolic stresses as they traverse the circulation. Intrinsic cellular alterations of hemoglobin (sickle cell anemia) and enzyme systems (G-6-PD*

---

*G-6-PD = glucose-6-phosphate dehydrogenase.

deficiency) and membrane cytoskeletal defects (hereditary spherocytosis) may act as signals to reticuloendothelial macrophages, causing them to remove damaged red blood cells from the circulation prematurely. Extrinsic events such as antibody or complement fixation, vasculitis, tumor invasion, and faulty heart valves can produce similar results. An imbalance between early destruction and bone marrow compensation determines the severity of hemolytic anemia. The occurrence of anemia, jaundice, or both is dependent upon the capacity of the bone marrow to increase red blood cell production and upon the ability of the reticuloendothelial system and the liver to process breakdown products of hemoglobin and excrete bilirubin. Acute bone marrow compensation can reach two to three times normal and may then increase to eight to ten times normal if hemolysis is prolonged and chronic.[1]

The diagnosis of anemia that is due to hemolysis involves a series of inductive observations. An anemia, not explained by blood loss or bone marrow suppression associated with evidence of increased bone marrow production and reticulocytosis, is the rule. Although no rigid protocol exists for the study of patients with hemolytic disorders, it is very important to ascertain the chronicity of the process, whether a familial pattern exists, drug or chemical exposure, recurrent episodes of jaundice, presence of pigment gallstones, and finally evidence of underlying disease.[2]

Examination of the peripheral blood film is critical in the evaluation of hemolytic syndromes. Although it may be nonspecific, showing only polychromatophilic, nucleated red blood cells, macrocytes, and occasionally leukocytosis and thrombocytosis, specific erythrocyte morphologic aberrations may be evident. Spherocytosis is observed in many hemolytic states, including hereditary spherocytosis and autoimmune hemolytic anemia. Elliptocytosis may or may not be associated with hemolysis. Cells with spiculated margins (acanthocytes) have been described in severe liver disease, kidney disease (burr cells), and congenital lipid disorders. Fractured red blood cells (schiotocytes), fragmented in a variety of sizes and shapes from small triangular forms to helmet cells, may be seen in heart valve hemolysis, vasculitis, severe hypertension, disseminated intravascular coagulation, and widespread neoplasia. Inclusions within red blood cells suggest hemolysis; malarial and babesial parasites may be seen, and basophilic stippling is observed in a variety of anemias, including lead poisoning.

Additional laboratory data allow for a broader assessment of hemolysis. Acute intravascular hemolysis, most often associated with complement-mediated incompatible transfusion reactions[3] and drug or fava bean ingestion in Mediterranean type G-6-PD deficient individuals (Table 1),[4] is defined by the demonstration of free hemoglobin in the plasma, which at levels of higher than 25 mg/dl colors the plasma pink to the naked eye. Lesser concentrations of free hemoglobin cause a reduction in the serum haptoglobin

Table 1.   DRUGS ASSOCIATED WITH HEMOLYTIC ANEMIA

Agent	Pathogenesis
Those that Work by Immune Mechanism (Coombs Positive)	
Quinine, phenacetin	Immune complex formation
Penicillin, cephalosporins	Drug absorbed to RBC membrane
Cephalosporin	Nonimmune absorption
Methyldopa	Unknown
Those that Work by Nonimmune Mechanism *(Glucose-6-Phosphate Dehydrogenase Deficiency)*	
Acetanilid	
Chloramphenicol	
Naphthalene	Heinz body formation because of
Nitrofurantoin	"redox-stress"
Primaquine	
Sulfonamides	

level and within 48 hours, the appearance of hemosiderin in renal tubular cells then exfoliated into the urine and confirmed by the Prussian blue stain. Extravascular hemolysis, observed in hereditary spherocytosis and autoimmune hemolytic anemia, is more frequent in occurrence and often harder to diagnose. The serum haptoglobin may be depleted regardless of where erythrocytes are destroyed.

Certain laboratory tests may reveal the specific cause of hemolysis and usually are obtained as part of the initial evaluation: Coombs test[2] (immune hemolysis); osmotic fragility[1] (hereditary spherocytosis); enzyme screens[4] (G-6-PD deficiency); sugar water test[5] (paroxysmal nocturnal hemoglobinuria); and hemoglobin electrophoresis (sickle cell, the thalassemias).

Hemolytic syndromes may be subclassified into those of congenital origin and those acquired later in life.[1] The congenital disorders are always due to intrinsic defects in the red blood cell leading to premature splenic destruction. In contrast, most acquired hemolytic disorders are caused by factors extrinsic to the erythrocyte itself causing intravascular but more commonly extravascular hemolysis: antibody fixation secondary to blood transfusion, certain medications (methyldopa, penicillin,[6] cold agglutinins,[7] infections,[8] malaria, gram negative sepsis), mechanical trauma (march hemoglobinuria), or abnormal plasma factors seen in advanced liver[9] and renal disease. The Coombs test is useful in evaluating all immune-related hemolytic states for detection of antibody and/or complement affixed to the red blood cell surface.

The management of hemolytic disease takes the form of general supportive measures applicable to all acute anemias combined with specific treatment modalities applicable to individual processes. Patients with hemolytic anemia present frequently with anemia of sufficient severity to require blood transfusion. Prompt and adequate blood replacement is necessary to prevent cardiovascular collapse. Rarely is it necessary or desirable to raise the hemoglobin level above 8 gm/dl with transfusion. Indications for transfusion therapy in congenital hemolytic anemias are as follows: neonatal hyperbilirubinemia; prolonged anemia superimposed upon active hemolysis; aplastic crisis induced by infection; and pregnancy and preoperative preparation for major surgery. Chronic transfusion therapy is rarely indicated. In acquired hemolytic states, transfusion is rarely necessary or desirable at levels of hemoglobin over 8 gm/dl; however, rapidly progressive anemia observed in patients with acute hemolysis and inadequate bone marrow response necessitates immediate transfusion. Patients with autoimmune hemolytic anemia present a difficult dilemma to a blood transfusion service, and they should be given the most compatible units of O negative packed cells available until antibody production is suppressed by steroid therapy or emergency splenectomy is performed.[10] A key concept is treatment of any underlying disorder and removal of exposure to offending drugs or toxic substances. Hereditary spherocytosis is best managed with splenectomy, although afterward spherocytes may persist in the circulation.[11]

KEY FEATURES

Premature destruction (hemolysis) of circulating red blood cells is caused by one or more of four general mechanisms: (1) a decrease in the surface-area/volume ratio (spherocyte), (2) a structural modification of the red blood cell membrane (antibody fixation), (3) an increased internal viscosity (sickle cell hemoglobin), or (4) splenic hyperfunction.

Increased rates of hemoglobin degradation take place with hemolysis, ultimately leading to increased production and excretion of bilirubin. Levels of indirect-reacting (nonglucuronide) bilirubin show a slight to moderate rise in the serum, and there is elevated fecal urobilinogen.

The laboratory findings common to all hemolytic processes include anemia and reticulocytosis. Serum haptoglobin levels are commonly depressed.

Aplastic crisis is defined as a failure of the bone marrow to compensate during hemolysis. Most commonly, this is precipitated by infection and associated with erythroid hypoplasia and reticulocytopenia.

Two commonly encountered forms of acute hemolysis constituting a medical emergency are related to drug ingestion: (1) glucose-6-phosphate dehydrogenase deficiency and (2) Coombs test positivity secondary to drugs.

REFERENCES

1. Forget BG: Hemolytic anemias: Congenital and acquired. Hosp Pract 15:4–67, 1980.

A comprehensive review of the topic, with emphasis on pathophysiology, diagnosis, and treatment of hemolytic anemias. Exceptional photomicrographs of red blood cell aberrations.

2. Todd D: Diagnosis of haemolytic states. Clin Haematol 4:63–81, 1975.
   A discussion concerning the details of history taking and special laboratory features observed in the evaluation of individuals with hemolysis. The entire edition is devoted to the topic.

3. Greenwalt, TJ: Pathogenesis and management of hemolytic transfusion reactions. Semin Hematol 18:84–94, 1981.
   Excellent state of the art review of mechanisms, harmless antibodies, diagnosis, and delayed transfusion reactions.

4. Luzzatto, L: Inherited haemolytic states: Glucose-6-phosphate dehydrogenase deficiency. Clin Haematol 4:83–108, 1975 (see ref. 2).
   Over 100 variants of G-6-PD deficiency have been described. Enzymatic and clinical differences between the Gd^A- form seen in Afro-American blacks and the Gd^med of Southern Europeans are clearly delineated in this review.

5. Rosse W: Treatment of paroxysmal nocturnal hemoglobinuria. Blood 60:1–20, 1982.
   Review of PNH, including treatment of hemolytic crisis, venous thrombosis, and the inherent risks of unwashed blood transfusion. PNH is the only acquired hemolytic state with intrinsic erythrocyte abnormalities.

6. Garratty G, Petz L: Drug-induced hemolytic anemia. Am J Med 58:398, 1975.
   Classic article on drugs causing positive Coombs (antiglobulin) test. Some are associated with hemolytic anemia, e.g., methyldopa; others were not, e.g., cephalosporins.

7. Turtzo D, Ghatak P: Acute hemolytic anemia with *Mycoplasma pneumoniae* pneumonia. JAMA 236(10):1140, 1976.
   Severe hemolysis as a result of cold polyclonal antibodies, treated successfully with antibiotics and corticosteroids. The cold-agglutinin titer peaked at 1:4096.

8. Crisp D, Pruzanski W: B-cell neoplasms with homogenous cold-reacting antibodies (cold-agglutinins). Am J Med 72:915, 1982.
   Among 78 patients with persistent cold-agglutinins, 31 had lymphoma, 13 macroglobulinemia, 6 chronic lymphatic leukemia, and 28 chronic cold-agglutinin disease. Anemia and Coombs positivity was common with monoclonal globulins.

9. Cooper RA: Hemolytic syndromes and red cell membrane abnormalities in liver disease. Semin Hematol 17:103–112, 1980.
   Target and spur cell formation resulting from a selective transfer of cholesterol from plasma proteins to red blood cell membranes resulting in decreased membrane fluidity, spleen injury, and severe hemolysis. Usually associated with far-advanced liver disease.

10. Petz L: Red cell transfusion problems in immunohematologic disease. Ann Rev Med 33:355–361, 1982.
    Describes detection of alloantibodies, what to transfuse, and when.

11. Valentine W (Moderator): Hemolytic anemia and erythrocyte enzymopathies. Ann Intern Med 103:245–257, 1985.
    Comprehensive up-to-date review with special emphasis on enzyme abnormalities of erythrocytes.

Disseminated Intravascular Coagulation

Rita Blanchard, M.D.

Disseminated intravascular coagulation (DIC) is a clinical syndrome in which the usual factors that localize and control coagulation are over-whelmed. It can be initiated by an alteration of any component in the hemostatic mechanism (vessel wall, plasma proteins, or platelets), but the usual mechanisms involve endothelial or tissue injury with release of tissue thromboplastin leading to activation of the extrinsic coagulation system or activation of the kinin, fibrinolytic, and intrinsic coagulation system by active Hageman's Factor (Factor XII).[1] In special cases, such as snake bite or the administration of prothrombin complexes, DIC may be produced by direct activation of Factor X or prothrombin. Factors that can predispose to or augment DIC include leukocyte products, antigen-antibody complexes, impairment of the reticuloendothelial system, inhibition of fibrinolysis, stimulation of the adrenergic system, and reduced levels of clotting factor inhibitors. Thus, DIC may be induced or aggravated by many mechanisms and there are multiple clinical conditions associated with this syndrome (Table 1).

The clinical presentation of DIC is influenced by the speed, severity, and degree of localization of the consumptive coagulopathy. Acute DIC is indeed a disseminated syndrome. The patient presents with petechiae, ecchymoses, and mucosal oozing. In addition to these peripheral manifesta-

Table 1. DISEASES AND DISORDERS ASSOCIATED WITH DIC

1. *Severe infection:* Bacterial (especially meningococcemia), rickettsial (Rocky Mountain spotted fever), protozoan (falciparum malaria), or viral (disseminated varicella, influenza A)

2. *Malignancy:* Acute leukemia (especially acute promyelocytic) and disseminated lymphomas and adenocarcinoma (especially mucin-producing)

3. *Tissue injury:* Blunt trauma to the brain, massive trauma or burns, heat stroke, acute pancreatitis, acute renal hemograft rejection

4. *Obstetric:* Retained products of conception, amniotic fluid embolism, septic abortion, abruptio placentae, hypertonic saline abortion, and toxemia of pregnancy

5. *Hemolytic transfusion reactions*

6. *Miscellaneous:* Anaphylaxis, snake bite, arterial aneurysms, hypothermia, respiratory distress syndrome, cardiac arrest, connective tissue disorder, and giant hemangiomas

tions, there is almost invariably evidence of renal dysfunction as well as decreased mentation and, especially in trauma cases, a component of adult respiratory distress syndrome (ARDS).[2] The laboratory evaluation reveals what might be expected with activation and consumption of coagulation factors. There is a prolongation of the partial thromboplastin time (PTT), the prothrombin time (PT), and the thrombin time. At least 50% of patients have thrombocytopenia, and the fibrinogen level is often reduced.[3] Fibrin degradation products in a level $\geq$10 μg/ml or a titer $\geq$40 are present in most cases, and fragmented red blood cells (schistocytes) are found on the peripheral smear of two thirds of the patients.[4]

This clinical picture can be confused with a more rare syndrome, thrombotic thrombocytopenic purpura (TTP); however, in TTP many of the other laboratory features of DIC, such as an elevated PT, PTT, and thrombin time, are usually absent. This distinction is important because the treatment of TTP involves plasma therapy or plasma exchange. A more complex diagnostic problem is to distinguish consumptive coagulopathy from hepatic disease with decreased production of coagulation factors and platelets. Many of the laboratory parameters are the same, although the absence or very low levels of fibrin split products are points against a diagnosis of DIC. Evidence suggests that the level of Factor VIII coagulant protein, which was at one time thought to be low in consumptive states and normal or high in liver disease does not distinguish between hepatic disease and DIC.[4]

Treatment of acute DIC includes first and foremost basic life support measures and efforts toward correcting the underlying disorders. If the initiating disorder can be reversed or controlled, the coagulopathy is generally self-limited. While the underlying disorder is being attended to, the patient should be given blood component therapy so as to maintain tissue oxygenation and replete blood coagulation proteins and platelets. Packed red blood cells to maintain a hematocrit of 25–30%, platelet concentrates to a level of 20,000–50,000, and fresh-frozen plasma should be infused. Cryoprecipitate can be used to maintain a fibrinogen level of at least 100 mg/dl. Vitamin K 10 mg subcutaneously should be given to prevent or treat subclinical vitamin K deficiency, which often coexists with DIC in these patients. Some authors feel that if replacement therapy is employed with platelets and fresh-frozen plasma and there is little or no rise in posttransfusion platelet count or no improvement in prothrombin time, further replacement therapy should be discontinued or only given in conjunction with heparin.[5]

The use of heparin for interrupting the cycle of intravascular coagulation has a sound theoretical base, but no prospective, randomized trials studying the efficacy of heparin therapy in the treatment of DIC have yet been published. For this reason, the use of heparin to treat severe DIC remains controversial.[3,5,6] However, in certain clinical situations such as DIC with acute promyelocytic leukemia or when DIC is accompanied by predominantly thrombotic complications such as purpura fulminans, gangrene of the digits, or acute renal failure, heparin therapy is indicated. In addition, if the clinical situation deteriorates despite all other efforts, a trial of heparin therapy should be considered. Heparin should be used only in conjunction with vigorous blood component support. After a bolus of 10,000 U, heparin therapy by continuous infusion should be begun. Because heparin affects many of the key tests of coagulation, it is necessary to monitor those tests unaffected by heparin, such as the fibrinogen level, fibrin split products (FSP), and platelet count. In addition, the conversion of fibrinogen to fibrin may be assessed by ordering a reptilase time. This test will not be affected by heparin but will be sensitive to a low fibrinogen level and fibrin split products. Despite adequate replacement therapy and supportive measures with or without heparin, the mortality rate in acute DIC remains as high as 60–85%.

Heparin has no intrinsic anticoagulant activity, but it exerts its anticoagulant effect by combining in vivo with antithrombin III, a plasma protein with a broad spectrum of anticoagulant activity. A recent study suggests that administration of antithrombin III concentrates alone may be effective in reversing DIC in the obstetric patient.[7]

Unlike the acute picture, chronic DIC may be manifested by bleeding from a traumatic wound alone or only by abnormalities in laboratory studies. In some cases, thrombotic manifestations predominate. Often the only abnormality may be an elevation in the level of FSP, mild thrombocytopenia, or prolonged thrombin time, since compensating mechanisms may increase the synthesis of the coagulation proteins. Underlying disorders found with this form of DIC include disseminated malignancy,[8] expanding aortic aneurysm, giant cavernous hemangioma, and retained products of conception. Many of these disorders cannot be reversed or require surgical correction, and heparin therapy has been useful in controlling the process. In one example of a retained dead fetus and viable twin, the mother was maintained on heparin to allow time for the living twin to reach sufficient maturity for delivery.[9]

Acute localized DIC may occur with sudden overwhelming injury to a specific organ, such as hyperacute allograft rejection[10] or head injury with brain tissue destruction.[11] In the latter case, fibrination commonly occurs acutely and during this critical period it is of prime importance to maintain hemostasis. All such patients should be screened for DIC, and while awaiting the results prophylactic replacement therapy with cryoprecipitate, fresh-frozen plasma, and platelet concentrates is given.

KEY FEATURES

The patient with acute DIC presents with petechiae, ecchymoses, and mucosal oozing and may have renal dysfunction, ARDS, and neurologic abnormalities.

In acute DIC, laboratory manifestations include an elevated PT, PTT, and thrombin time, fibrin split products in a level ≥10 μg/ml or titer of ≥40, thrombocytopenia, hypofibrinogenemia, and a microangiopathic picture on blood smear.

In treating acute DIC (1) the underlying disorder should be recognized and corrected; (2) tissue oxygenation should be maintained with hematocrit of 25–30%; (3) vitamin K 10 mg replacement therapy with platelets and fresh-frozen plasma or cryoprecipitate should be given to control bleeding; (4) if heparin is given, it should be in conjunction with replacement therapy.

Chronic DIC may have as its clinical manifestation only isolated bleeding from a traumatic wound or thrombosis. The laboratory tests may be variable, but usually there is an elevated level of fibrin split products, mild thrombocytopenia, and a prolonged thrombin time.

Heparin has been useful in treating DIC associated with acute promyelocytic leukemia, retained products of conception, expanding aortic aneurysm, and disseminated malignancy.

REFERENCES

1. Mason JW, Colman RW: The role of Hageman Factor in disseminated intravascular coagulation induced by septicemia, neoplasia, or liver disease. Thromb Diath Haemorrh 26:325, 1971.

    Human plasma kallikrein system was assayed in patients with DIC as a measure of activated Factor XII because activation of kallikreinogen is a direct effect of activated Factor XII not effected by thromboplasmin or other blood coagulation intermediates. In comparing patients with DIC and liver disease, DIC with neoplasia, and DIC secondary to septicemia, only those with DIC associated with gram negative septicemia showed evidence of Hageman Factor activation.

2. Siegal T, Seigsoh U, Aghai E, Modan M: Clinical and laboratory aspects of disseminated intravascular coagulation (DIC): A study of 118 cases. Thrombos Haemostas (Stuttg) 39:122, 1978.

    A retrospective study of 118 cases of DIC in which the most frequent causes were infection (40%), trauma (17%), malignancy (7%) and post-surgical (7%). In patients with infection, liver and renal dysfunction were frequent, occurring in 27% and 36%, respectively, whereas in trauma patients, respiratory dysfunction was frequently seen (45%) and liver and renal manifestations were less common. Trauma patients had lower overall mortality (30%) than did nontrauma patients (60%).

3. Colman RW, Robboy SJ, Minna JD: Disseminated intravascular coagulation: A reappraisal. Ann Rev Med 30:369, 1979.

    Over 150 articles on DIC were reviewed and the syndrome reappraised. The prothrombin time (abnormal in over 90% of cases), hypofibrinogenemia (≤150 mg/dl in 70%), and thrombocytopenia (90% of cases) are recommended as screening tests, and the measurement of fibrin degradation products is cited as the most useful confirmatory test. Several clinical trials using heparin in DIC are reviewed, and continuous infusion heparin is recommended in acute DIC with thrombotic, thromboembolic, or necrotizing complications and in chronic DIC. However, some cases of DIC may be resistant to heparin. Prolonged heparin retention may be seen in patients with liver disease and renal dysfunction.

4. Spero JA, Lewis JH, Hasiba U: Disseminated intravascular coagulation: Findings in 346 patients. Thromb Haemostas 38:28, 1980.

In this study, 68% of the patients had evidence of microangiopathic process with ≥10% burr cells and/or fragmented cells on peripheral smear. Of the clotting proteins, Factors II, V, VII, and X were frequently decreased but Factor VIII:C levels were decreased in only 9% of patients. The overall mortality rate was 68%.

5. Feinstein DI: Diagnosis and management of disseminated intravascular coagulation: The role of heparin therapy. Blood 60:284, 1982.

This author argues that replacement therapy with platelets and fresh-frozen plasma should be limited to those patients who are actively bleeding or who require a surgical procedure. If there is a failure to effect a rise in the hemostatic factors after transfusion in the patient with DIC, it may be necessary to replace the hemostatic factors under the cover of continuous heparin infusion. Initial coverage with heparin is probably indicated if the patient has evidence of fibrin deposition (dermal necrosis, acral ischemia, or venous thromboembolism); retained products of conception with hypofibrinogenemia; excessive bleeding associated with giant hemangioma; or neoplastic disease, particularly promyelocytic leukemia.

6. Mant MJ, King EG: Severe, Acute Disseminated Intravascular Coagulation. Am J Med 67:557, 1979.

Forty-seven patients with acute DIC (representing less than .05% of total hospital admissions) were evaluated in this study. Common predisposing factors included infection, shock, trauma, hepatic disease, and malignancy. In a nonrandomized manner, 12 patients were treated with heparin; bleeding worsened in 7 and diminished in 5, and 10 patients died (83%). In the 35 patients who did not receive heparin, DIC diminished in 13 and 30 patients (86%) died. The authors concluded that heparin therapy is rarely beneficial and it may exacerbate bleeding.

7. Maki M, Tarao T, Ikenoue T, Tekemura T, Sekiba K, Shirakawa H: Clinical evaluation of antithrombin III concentrates for disseminated intravascular coagulation in obstetrics. Gynecol Obstet Invest 23:230–240, 1987.

A well-controlled prospective clinical trial evaluating 39 women with DIC secondary to abruptio placentae or postpartum hemorrhage. Twenty-four women were treated with AT III concentrates and fifteen were treated with gabexate mesilate (FOY), a synthetic protease inhibitor used in the treatment of DIC in Japan. The subjects were well matched in terms of severity of DIC and clinical features. Patients treated with antithrombin III concentrates showed significantly faster recovery of their platelet count and prothrombin time into the normal range as compared with the patients treated with FOY. Treatment with antithrombin III consisted of a single infusion of 3000 U on day one. No patient required further treatment with AT III after the initial infusion.

8. Sack GH, Levin J, Bell WR: Trousseau's syndrome and other manifestations of chronic disseminated coagulopathy in patients with neoplasms. Medicine 56:1, 1977.

Analysis of 182 patients with chronic DIC and malignancy showed the following common clinical features: migratory thrombophlebitis in 96, hemorrhage in 75, and arterial emboli in 45, with 12 patients having all three. The most prominent hematologic derangements were hypofibrinogenemia and thrombocytopenia. Forty-one patients had lesions of nonbacterial thrombotic endocarditis.

9. Romero R, Duffy TP, Berkowitz RL, Chang E, Hobbins JC: Prolongation of a preterm pregnancy complicated by death of a single twin in utero and disseminated intravascular coagulation. N Engl J Med 310:772, 1984.

A case report of a patient with a twin gestation and death in utero of one of the twins at 26 weeks. Evidence of DIC was detected at 29.5 weeks with a fibrinogen of 95 and fresh-frozen plasma >40 μg/ml. With heparin infusion at 1000 U/hour, fibrinogen rose to 230 after three days, but treatment was discontinued after eleven days. DIC recurred, and heparin was restarted and the fibrinogen level rose to 400 mg/dl. Treatment was discontinued after 2 weeks, and DIC did not recur. The patient delivered at 36 weeks.

The authors stress that in this case the use of heparin reversed coagulopathy associated with fetal death and allowed sufficient time for the maturation of the remaining twin; however, they warn that in the case of monozygotic twins, heparin may not be as efficacious in protecting the circulation of the surviving twin.

10. Starzl TE, Boehmig HJ, Amemiya H, Wilson CB, Dixon FJ, Giles GR, Simpson KM, Halgrimson CG: Clotting changes, including disseminated intravascular coagulation, during rapid renal-homograft rejection. N Engl J Med 283:383, 1970.
    Two cases of hyperacute graft rejection accompanied by DIC in renal transplant recipients are described. By the measurement of gradients across intracorporeal and extracorporeal homografts, the authors demonstrated that the new kidneys sequestered immunoglobulins, platelets, white blood cells, and clotting factors. Moreover, renal venous blood contained fibrinolytic activity. This type of rejection has been characterized as immunologically induced coagulopathy.

11. Goodnight SH, Kenoyer G, Rapaport SI, Patch MJ, Lee JA, Kurze T: Defibrination after brain-tissue destruction. N Engl J Med 290:1043, 1974.
    A prospective study of 26 patients to evaluate defibrination after acute head trauma. In 13 patients in whom trauma apparently did not destroy brain tissue, there was no evidence of DIC, but in 9 of 13 patients with visible brain tissue destruction, evidence of transient DIC (hypofibrinogenemia, low levels of Factor V, VIII, or platelets) was found. The hemostatic abnormalities, although they did not cause systemic sequelae, were severe enough to have effected intracranial bleeding. The authors recommend that cryoprecipitate (12 U) as well as 2–4 U of fresh-frozen plasma be given immediately to patients with visible brain tissue destruction while awaiting the results of the hemostatic tests.

Thrombocytopenia

Rita Blanchard, M.D.

Automated blood cell counting equipment has made thrombocytopenia, defined as platelet count less than 150,000, easy to detect. However, increased hemorrhagic risk with injury or surgery is generally not seen until the platelet count falls below 100,000 and spontaneous hemorrhage is rare above a platelet count of 20,000.[1] These general guidelines apply if platelet function is normal and if there are no associated abnormalities in coagulation. Many conditions and medications can cause platelet dysfunction (Table 1), and the patient can exhibit bleeding despite a normal or only mildly depressed platelet count. Thrombocytopenic bleeding is characterized by bleeding from mucosal surfaces and the presence of petechiae on the mucosa and skin, especially in areas with high hydrostatic pressure. Therapy includes simple precautions so as to avoid disruption of the hemostatic process— avoidance of medications that interfere with platelet function and anticoagulants; and abstinence from all unnecessary invasive procedures, including intramuscular injections and insertion of intravenous lines into large vessels that are not easily compressible.

In the thrombocytopenic patient who is actively bleeding, it is important first to assess the etiology of the thrombocytopenia because the mechanism of thrombocytopenia may alter the survival of transfused platelets. Three basic mechanisms of thrombocytopenia exist: (1) decreased platelet production, (2) hypersplenism, and (3) increased destruction. Clues as to mechanism of thrombocytopenia are found on the peripheral blood smear. In thrombocytopenia associated with decreased platelet production, the platelets on smear appear small and dusty or pale, whereas with increased platelet destruction the blood smear often shows large, dense platelets that may be accompanied by red blood cell fragments. Next, the evaluation should include a bone marrow aspiration and biopsy to assess platelet production. Increased platelet destruction is characterized by a normal marrow with normal or increased numbers of megakaryocytes. With decreased production or marrow replacement, the marrow aspiration will show decreased numbers of megakaryocytes or may produce a "dry" tap. In the latter case, evaluation by marrow biopsy is essential.

If the thrombocytopenia is due to increased destruction, it is important to distinguish whether the low platelet count is the harbinger of a more global coagulation abnormality such as disseminated intravascular coagula-

Table 1.   DRUGS AND CONDITIONS ASSOCIATED WITH PLATELET DYSFUNCTION

Acute viral infections, including HIV
Aspirin and other nonsteroidal anti-inflammatory agents
Antihistamines
Beta blockers
Clofibrate
Collagen vascular disorders, especially SLE
Dextran
Dipyridamole
Extracorporeal bypass
Heparin
Heroin
High-dose penicillin and carbenicillin
Hydroxychloroquine and chloroquine
Nitrofurantoin
Myeloproliferative disorders (polycythemia vera, chronic myelogenous leukemia, sideroblastic anemias, preleukemia)
Paraproteins in certain patients with multiple myeloma
Phenothiazines
Prostacyclin
Prostaglandin E
Sulfinpyrazone
Ticlopidine
Tricyclic antidepressants
Uremia

tion (DIC), thrombotic thrombocytopenic purpura (TTP), hemolytic-uremic syndrome (HUS), or a disorder with isolated platelet destruction.

DIC is always secondary to an underlying disorder, and thrombocytopenia in DIC is generally accompanied by other abnormalities in coagulation tests—a positive test for fibrin split products; a decreased fibrinogen level; and a prolonged thrombin time, partial thromboplastin time, and prothrombin time. Sepsis alone may cause thrombocytopenia by absorption of immune comlexes on the platelet surface, leading to phagocytosis.[2]

In TTP, a rare disorder of unknown etiology, the patient presents with thrombocytopenia, fever, microangiopathic hemolytic anemia, renal dysfunction, and neurologic abnormalities.[3] This classic pentad of symptoms is not always manifested on presentation, and a high degree of clinical suspicion is required. The diagnosis may be confirmed by biopsy of dermal or mucosal purpura. Once the diagnosis is confirmed or considered highly probable, therapy with transfusion of fresh-frozen plasma and/or plasmapheresis with exchange transfusion should be begun immediately.

HUS appears to be a localized form of TTP with a triad of clinical findings, including microangiopathic hemolytic anemia, thrombocytopenia, and renal failure. It is predominantly a disease of infants and children, occurring in both epidemic and sporadic form. In adults, HUS tends to occur in the sporadic form and is associated with pregnancy, oral contraceptive use, and connective tissue disorder. Infants tend to have primarily glomerular involvement, whereas adults tend to have arteriolar pathology or acute cortical necrosis. There is a high spontaneous recovery rate with just supportive care in the epidemic (childhood) form of HUS, but in the sporadic form plasmapheresis has been required to induce remission in most cases.[4]

The most common causes of isolated thrombocytopenia as a result of accelerated platelet destruction are autoimmune thrombocytopenia and drug-related thrombocytopenia. In these conditions, the factors affecting the patient's own platelets will also cause destruction of transfused platelets. Thus, unless the primary process is ameliorated, platelet transfusion may not be effective in controlling bleeding. In patients with idiopathic thrombocytopenic purpura (ITP), antibody coats autologous platelets, leading to destruction by the reticuloendothelial system.[5,6,7] Platelet survival may be reduced to a few hours, and in most patients is less than 1 day. Diagnosis is made primarily on clinical grounds and bone marrow examination. Detection of high levels of platelet-associated IgG is a helpful diagnostic adjunct but is usually not available on an immediate basis. Fortunately, less than 5% of patients with ITP present with life-threatening hemorrhage. These patients seem to tolerate very low platelet counts, theoretically, because a reduction in megakaryocyte maturation produces circulating platelets that are young and "hyperfunctional."

In the treatment of life-threatening bleeding in ITP, therapy must be directed toward reduction of platelet destruction, as well as platelet replacement. Corticosteroids (1 mg/kg/day prednisone) are begun immediately. Alternatively, in pediatric cases or in patients in whom high-dose corticosteroids are contraindicated, high-dose intravenous gamma globulin has proved to be efficacious.[8] Platelet transfusions should be given as often as necessary to control hemorrhage. Even though the transfused platelets are rapidly destroyed and may not cause an increment in the platelet count, they generally protect against catastrophic bleeding. However, if life-threatening hemorrhage is not controlled by transfusion, gamma globulin, or corticosteroids, emergency splenectomy or plasmapheresis should be considered.

Drug-related thrombocytopenias are characteristically self-limited, and resolve with discontinuation of the offending agent. The drugs most commonly implicated include quinine, quinidine, heparin, penicillin, digitoxin, phenytoin (Dilantin), and sulfonamides.[9] The initial step in management is to discontinue the suspected drug(s). Platelet transfusions should be used to control serious bleeding, but the transfused platelets usually are rapidly destroyed and may have to be given frequently. Confirmation of the diagnosis can be made in some cases by demonstrating that the patient's plasma will agglutinate normal donor platelets in the presence of the drug but not in its absence.[10] For most cases, however, absolute confirmation of the role of the drug is never made but only suspected from the clinical course.

An unusual cause of thrombocytopenia occurs 7–10 days after transfusion and is termed post-transfusion purpura. Affected patients generally lack a platelet antigen (PLA-1) and paradoxically destroy their own platelets when exposed to blood containing even trace amounts of PLA-1 antigen. Treatment modalities have included transfusion with PLA-1 negative blood and attempting to remove the offending antibody by plasmapheresis.[11,12]

Conditions associated with decreased platelet production include idiopathic marrow aplasia; bone invasion by tumor; treatment with cytotoxic drugs or radiation; aplasia that is due to drugs, chemicals, insecticides, or viruses; alcoholism; megaloblastic anemias (folate and vitamin B_{12} deficiency); and leukemia. If these patients have not been previously transfused, they have the best response to platelet transfusion because the survival of the transfused platelets is close to normal, i.e., several days.[11] A single unit of random donor platelets will generally raise the platelet count by 5000–10,000/mm³. If the patient is actively bleeding, the platelet count should be maintained in excess of 50,000 until the bleeding stops or the patient's marrow recovers. Factors that decrease platelet survival, such as infection, fever and alloimmunization to platelet transfusion, may necessitate an increased frequency of platelet transfusions.

Within the sphere of thrombocytopenia secondary to decreased production of platelets, alcoholic thrombocytopenia can present a diagnostic problem. Alcohol has a toxic effect on the bone marrow, and binge drinkers may often present with gastrointestinal bleeding and thrombocytopenia. The bone marrow aspiration may reveal a normal number of megakaryocytes, giving the appearance of increased platelet destruction. In uncomplicated cases, the platelet count rises with abstinence in 2–3 days and is usually normal at 10 days. A rebound thrombocytosis is often seen. The transfused platelets in the alcoholic should have a normal half-life provided there is not coexisting hypersplenism.[13]

The spleen normally contains about one third of the platelets produced by the bone marrow. In patients with enlarged spleens, the platelet mass may be normal but the circulating platelet count decreased to the order of 30,000–80,000, depending on the degree of splenomegaly. Platelet survival is normal or only modestly decreased. If platelet transfusions are required, the patient will need more platelets than a normosplenic individual, although the frequency with which the transfusions are given should not be increased.

Platelet transfusions are also used prophylactically. In this case, the physician must balance the need to give platelets to prevent bleeding with the risk of alloimmunization to platelet transfusions. The true threshold to prevent bleeding in thrombocytopenia has not been established, but based on studies of acute leukemic patients many physicians have chosen to maintain the platelet count above $20,000/\mu l$.[1,14] Serious bleeding rarely occurs at platelet counts above $5000/\mu l$ unless there is a complicating feature such as fever, infection, or coexistent platelet dysfunction. In a patient in whom prolonged thrombocytopenia is anticipated, platelet transfusion should be reserved for bleeding that involves more than skin, mucous membrane, or epistaxis.[10]

Rarely, a patient will present with what appears to be severe thrombocytopenia with widely fluctuating platelet counts but with no bleeding manifestations and no detectable underlying disorder. In this case, the clinician must consider the possibility of pseudothrombocytopenia, a phenomena of *in vitro* platelet clumping in the presence of chelating agents. The platelet count of these patients will be shown to be normal if capillary blood samples are taken and diluted directly.

KEY FEATURES

Spontaneous thrombocytopenia bleeding is rare at platelet counts above 20,000 unless there is an aggravating condition.

Three mechanisms of thrombocytopenia—decreased marrow platelet production, hypersplenism, and increased peripheral platelet destruction—can be distinguished by (1) examination for splenomegaly, (2) examination of the peripheral blood smear for platelet size and presence of schistocytes, and (3) bone marrow aspirate and/or biopsy to assess megakaryocyte number.

With platelet destruction, it is important to distinguish global co-agulation disorders (DIC, TTP, and HUS) from disorders causing isolated thrombocytopenia (ITP, drug-induced thrombocytopenia, and post-transfusion purpura), and appreciate that transfused platelets will be susceptible to the same increased destruction unless the cause for plate-let destruction is treated.

Nonalloimmunized patients with thrombocytopenia of decreased production respond to platelet transfusion raising their platelet counts 5000–10,000 per unit of donor platelets given.

Hypersplenic individuals generally have fairly normal platelet sur-vival but require more platelets than normal individuals to sustain the same increment in platelet count.

REFERENCES

1. Gaydos LA, Freireich EJ, Mantel N: The quantitative relation between platelet count and hemorrhage in patients wth acute leukemia. N Engl J Med 266:905, 1962.

   A classic study of 92 patients (both children and adults) with acute leukemia, examining the association between thrombocytopenia and hemorrhage. The frequency of severe hem-orrhage, discounting petechiae, ecchymoses, and epistaxis, was found to be less than 1% above a platelet count of 20,000. In addition low (<10,000) or falling platelet counts generally preceded the onset of gross hemorrhage by several days. Of those patients dying of fatal intracerebral hemorrhage, 50% had intracerebral leukostasis. However, without accompanying intracerebral leukostasis, no patient dying of intracranial hemorrhage had a platelet count in excess of 10,000.

2. Kelton JG, Neame PB, Gauldie J, Hirsh J: Elevated platelet-associated IgG in the throm-bocytopenia of septicemia. N Engl J Med 300:760, 1979.

   Thirty-one of forty-six episodes of septicemia were complicated by thrombocytopenia, with the majority of these patients (16/31) showing elevated levels of platelet IgG. It is postulated that the mechanism of thrombocytopenia is related to coating of platelets with IgG, perhaps in the form of circulating immune complexes.

3. Machin SJ: Thrombotic thrombocytopenic purpura: Clinical annotation. Br J Haematol 56:191, 1984.

   A brief review of the pathogenesis, diagnosis, and therapeutic approach to treatment of TTP with emphasis on the utility of transfusion with fresh-frozen plasma and plasma-pheresis. Prostacyclin infusions and the role of antiplatelet agents are discussed as adjuncts to transfusion therapy in refractory cases.

4. Levin M, Barrat TM: Haemolytic uraemic syndrome. Arch Dis Child 59:397, 1984.

   A review of the epidemiology, histopathology, and pathogenesis of hemolytic uremic syndrome. The syndrome is divided into epidemic and sporadic forms, which the authors feel have different pathophysiologic mechanisms and require different treatment modali-ties.

5. Karpatin S: Autoimmune thrombocytopenia purpura. Blood 56:329, 1980.
6. McMillan R: Chronic idiopathic thrombocytopenic purpura. N Engl J Med 304:1135, 1981.
7. Jacobs PJ, Wood L, Dent DD: Results of treatment in immune thrombocytopenia. Quart J Med 58:153, 1986.

   Three excellent review articles on the clinical presentation, pathogenesis, treatment, and complications of autoimmune thrombocytopenic purpura.

8. Bussel JB, Kimberly RP, Inman RD, Cunningham-Rundles C, Cheung E, Smithwick EM, O'Malley J, Barandun S, Hilgartner MW: Intravenous gamma globulin in the treatment of chronic idiopathic thrombocytopenic purpura. Blood 62:480, 1983.

   Twelve patients, eight children and four adults with chronic ITP, were given intra-venous gamma globulin 400/mg/kg/day for five days. All had been previously treated with prednisone, and half had received additional therapy with vincristine, 6-mercaptopurine, or cyclophosphamide. Half the patients had undergone splenectomy. In all but two cases, platelet counts rose from pretreatment levels (2000–65,000) to over 100,000. Two of the twelve patients had a sustained remission.

9. Hackett T, Kelton JG, Powers P: Drug induced platelet destruction. Semin Thromb Hemost 8:116–137, 1982.

   Allergic drug-induced thrombocytopenia usually presents with an acute hemorrhagic syndrome, often with a chill, and the bone marrow reveals increased megakaryocytes. Stopping the offending agent usually leads to prompt recovery in 4–14 days. The most common offending agents are quinine, quinidine, heparin, penicillin, digitoxin, phenytoin, (Dilantin), and sulfonamide derivatives. Gold salts and methyldopa are exceptions, in that thrombocytopenia may occur several months after the drug is administered and persist for long periods after discontinuation of the drug.

10. Chong BH, Berndt MC, Koutts J, Castaldi PA: Quinidine-induced thrombocytopenia and leukopenia: Demonstration and characterization of distinct antiplatelet and antileukocyte antibodies. Blood 62:1218, 1983.

   Discusses a patient with the rare syndrome of simultaneous quinidine-induced throm-bocytopenia and leukopenia in which a quinidine-dependent antiplatelet antibody was detected in the plasma by platelet aggregometry. This antibody appeared to be directed against one of the intrinsic platelet membrane proteins, GP1b.

11. Abramson N, Eisenberg PD, Aster RH: Post-transfusion purpura—immunologic aspects and therapy. N Engl J Med 291:1163, 1974.

   Article discusses a case of post-transfusion purpura in which treatment with pred-nisone and plasmapheresis was given, with recovery to a normal platelet count in 1 week. It is stressed that plasmapheresis rather than exchange transfusion should be employed to decrease the level of antibody. Although PLA negativity occurs in about 2% of the population, the vast majority of patients with the syndrome are women who have presum-ably been sensitized during pregnancy.

12. Slichter SJ: Controversies in platelet transfusion therapy. Ann Rev Med 31:509, 1980.

   In 23 patients with thrombocytopenia from decreased marrow production, platelet recovery was 56% of the number transfused and survival was 5.2 days. These results are only modestly reduced, since normal subjects had 65% recovery and 9.6 day survival. The efficacy of the transfusion should be documented by obtaining platelet counts at 1 and 4 hours and then daily after transfusion. The increments may be reduced to 20–40% with fever or infection. In a group of leukemic patients, those who achieved a post-transfusion platelet increment of 40,000 had major vessel bleeding controlled 83% of the time, whereas those whose increment was <20,000 had bleeding controlled in only one third of the cases.

13. Cowan DH: Effect of alcoholism on hemostasis. Semin Hematol 17:137, 1980.

   The effects of alcohol in noncirrhotic patients are primarily on the platelet and include decreased platelet survival, ineffective thrombopoiesis resulting in decreased production, and qualitative abnormalities. In 112 relatively stable chronic alcoholics, thrombocytopenia existed in 3% and was unrelated to socioeconomic or nutritional status. In 108 acutely ill alcoholic patients, thrombocytopenia was present in 26% and was not correlated with severity of abnormalities in liver function, anemia, or folate deficiency. Two or three days elapsed after the last drink before platelet counts began to rise and the counts peaked at 10–14 days.

14. Roy AJ, Jaffe N, Dierassi I: Prophylactic platelet transfusions in children with acute leukemia: A dose response study. Transfusion 13:283, 1973.
     *In this study, minor bleeding episodes of skin, mucous membranes, microscopic he-
     maturia epistaxis, and guaiac-positive stools were found in more than 50% of individuals
     with platelet counts less than 40,000 but there was no correlation between frequency of
     bleeding and absolute count. Serious bleeding occurred in 26% of the 62 patients with
     platelet counts between 0 and 10,000, in 10% between 10,000 and 20,000, and in 5% in
     those between 20,000 and 40,000.*

The Prolonged Partial Thromboplastin Time: Anticoagulant Overdose and Common Congenital Factor Deficiencies

Rita Blanchard, M.D.

In the evaluation of a patient with an isolated prolongation of the partial thromboplastin time (PTT), several diagnostic possibilities must be considered: a mild congenital coagulation deficiency, a circulating anticoagulant, or a laboratory error. To eliminate the last possibility, a second sample should be obtained, drawn from lines free of anticoagulant, filling the tube with the proper amount of blood, and taking it immediately to the clinical laboratory. If the results are still abnormal, the next step is to test for a circulating anticoagulant and to request simple mixing studies. Patients who demonstrate the presence of a circulating anticoagulant may be refractory to replacement therapy unless the anticoagulant is removed or treated. In other cases, such as the "lupus" anticoagulant, the inhibitor appears to be directed toward the phospholipid used in the coagulation reagent and the clinical consequence may be a paradoxical "prethrombotic" state and an increased incidence of spontaneous abortion rather than a bleeding diathesis.[1]

Circulating anticoagulants can also be exogenous, and sampling of an arterial line without flushing out the heparin can cause a prolonged PTT. In this case, the thrombin time will also be prolonged but the reptilase time, which utilizes a snake venom protease to convert fibrinogen to fibrin, should be normal. If the patient has serious or life-threatening bleeding while on heparin therapy, the anticoagulant effect should be reversed with protamine sulfate. If the heparin has been given within minutes, generally one gives

1 mg of protamine per 100 U of heparin. This should be given over 10–30 minutes, since rapid injection of protamine may induce hypotension. Heparin has a half-life of about 1 hour and the general therapeutic range is between 0.3 and 0.4 U heparin/ml, so that the dose of protamine to neutralize a continuous intravenous infusion of heparin can be calculated by multiplying plasma volume by 0.3–0.4/100. Because protamine is cleared more rapidly than heparin, the treatment may have to be repeated. To reverse the anticoagulant effect of a subcutaneous injection of heparin, protamine sulfate should be given in a dose equivalent to approximately 50% of the last heparin dose. Again, the protamine may have to be repeated because of prolonged absorption of heparin from the subcutaneous depot.[2]

Sodium warfarin (Coumadin) is an anticoagulant that acts by reducing the circulating levels of the vitamin K–dependent coagulation proteins (Factors X, IX, VII, and II). In patients with warfarin overdose, the PTT as well as the prothrombin time is prolonged but the test for a circulating anticoagulant is negative and the thrombin time is normal. If the patient has potentially life-threatening bleeding and a prolonged prothrombin time, the coagulation defect can be reversed immediately by infusion of Factor IX concentrate, which contains all the vitamin K–dependent factors. If the prothrombin time in a patient with mild bleeding or at risk for bleeding is markedly prolonged (≥4 times control), a judicious combination of vitamin K and fresh-frozen plasma should be employed. The fresh-frozen plasma will partially reverse the defect immediately, whereas vitamin K usually works in 6–12 hours. A small dose of vitamin K (1–2 mg) may be sufficient in combination with cessation of the warfarin in patients with a protime 2–4 times normal. High doses of vitamin K (i.e., 25 mg) may cause the patient to become refractory to anticoagulant therapy. If the bleeding is not severe and the patient is only slightly beyond the therapeutic range, it may be adequate simply to omit the anticoagulant therapy for 2–3 days.

If the test for a circulating anticoagulant is negative, simple mixing studies are performed. In this test, the patient's plasma is mixed in parallel with plasma from patients deficient in Factors VIII, IX, XI, and XII. Complete normalization of the PTT implies at least a 50% level of the factor and effectively rules out a congenital isolated deficiency. Many patients whose PTT is only modestly (5–10 seconds) prolonged will not demonstrate either a circulating anticoagulant or a congenital factor deficiency. If the patient is bleeding and has a normal bleeding time, platelet count, thrombin time, and prothrombin time and a negative test for fibrin split products, a trial of fresh-frozen plasma (15 ml/kg) should be given.

If the bleeding time and PTT are abnormal but all other tests are normal, the possibility of von Willebrand's disease should be considered. This diagnosis can be confirmed by demonstration of abnormal platelet aggregation with ristocetin and low or abnormal Factor VIII antigen in the face of normal results in other platelet function studies. This disorder is caused by a missing or defective plasma protein, the von Willebrand's protein, which is necessary for both platelet activity and Factor VIII stabilization.[3] Therefore, these patients have an abnormal bleeding time and may have prolonged PTT secondary to a low level of Factor VIII. The platelet dysfunction is the most clinically important deficiency, since most patients manifest mucosal bleeding rather than hemarthrosis and intramuscular bleeding. von Willebrand's disease is thought to be the most common coagulation disorder. It is an autosomal trait but with a variable degree of expression within a family. The patients should be treated with cryoprecipitate, a source rich in the missing protein, rather than with Factor VIII concentrates, which contain little of the effective protein. Cryoprecipitate in relatively low doses will cause an increase in Factor VIII levels, but in order to correct the bleeding time much larger doses of cryoprecipitate must be administered (10 U/12 hours). Prophylactic therapy of von Willebrand's disease may involve several new modalities, including DDAVP and estrogens.[4]

Patients with hemophilia A or Factor VIII deficiency will have a prolonged PTT, an abnormal mixing study with Factor VIII deficient plasma, a Factor VIII assay level of <30%, and a normal bleeding time. Because this is an X-linked disorder, the patients are almost always male and may have had multiple episodes of hemarthrosis and intramuscular bleeding. Factor VIII deficient patients who present with minor or moderate bleeding should be given replacement therapy to maintain their Factor VIII levels at 30%; with more serious hemorrhage, levels of 50–60% should be sought. These levels cannot be achieved in most hemophilia A patients using fresh-frozen plasma without fluid overload; therefore, therapy is generally with either cryoprecipitate or Factor VIII concentrates. Each unit of cryoprecipitate contains 80–90% the amount of Factor VIII in 250 ml of plasma. Factor VIII concentrates are even higher in Factor VIII activity. The choice of product depends on the desired factor level and the previous transfusion history of the recipient. For patients with mild deficiency of Factor VIII levels (10–30%) who have not been treated with VIII concentrates in the past, cryoprecipitate is the therapy of choice, because there is less risk of hepatitis and other blood-borne diseases.[5] For bleeding episodes in severe hemophiliacs, Factor VIII concentrates are used. In initiating therapy in hemophilia A, the patient's plasma volume (40 ml/kg) is calculated and one assumes a half-life of 8 hours. Therefore, in a severe hemophiliac (<1% Factor VIII) who weighs 60 kg, an initial dose of 2000 U of Factor VIII should raise the plasma level to about 80% immediately and at eight hours 40% should remain. Alternatively, one can assume that infusion of 1 U of Factor VIII per kg of the patients' weight will raise the plasma concentration by 2 U/dl. In practical terms, a half-life should be determined in each patient, taking timed samples for assay immediately after infusion and at hourly to two-hourly intervals. Most patients will, in fact, have a shorter half-life for infused Factor VIII than the predicted 8 hours. In 10% of severe hemophiliacs, antibodies to the normal infused Factor VIII develop and can neutralize the effect of infusion. Conventionally, these inhibitors are measured in Bethesda units: 1 U of inhibitor/ml will neutralize the amount of Factor VIII in 1 ml of normal plasma. Patients with low-titer inhibitors (1–3 U) can be treated with high-dose pulsed Factor VIII concentrates or continuous infusion of Factor VIII concentrates. Patients with high-titer inhibitors (≥5 U) and those with inhibitors that can be "induced" to high titer by an anamnestic response are special cases. These patients are treated conservatively without factor infusion for minor bleeding episodes; for major bleeds, special products that bypass Factor VIII activity are available.[6,7] Because of the differing regimens of treatment for hemophiliacs with inhibitors, it therefore seems prudent to recommend that each hemophiliac have a test for inhibitor activity prior to beginning replacement therapy and that this should be repeated if an increasing requirement for Factor VIII develops during treatment.

Patients with Factor IX deficiency (Christmas disease), also inherited as a sex-linked disorder, are very similar in clinical presentation to Factor VIII deficient patients. Treatment principles are also quite similar. Differences, however, do exist, since Factor IX is a smaller molecule than Factor VIII and is not present in cryoprecipitate. Therefore, cryoprecipitate is not used to treat these patients, but rather fresh-frozen plasma is used for patients with mild deficiency and prothrombin concentrates for patients with severe deficiency. The distribution of the infused Factor IX is both intravascular and extravascular, and therefore a loading dose consisting of twice the calculated amount must be given when initiating therapy. The decay curve of infused Factor IX is biphasic, with a first phase half-life of 5 hours and a second phase of about 24 hours.[8]

Other less common congenital coagulation factor deficiencies leading to an isolated prolongation of the PTT are Factor XI and Factor XII deficiency. Both are autosomal traits, and Factor XII deficiency carries no increased hemorrhagic risk. The risk of bleeding with severe Factor XI deficiency is generally much less than that of severe Factor VIII or IX deficiency. Although spontaneous hemorrhage is rare, there is an increased risk of bleeding with trauma, dental extractions, or surgical procedures. In these cases, because of the long half-life of Factor XI (>72 hours), the patient can be treated with fresh-frozen plasma.

KEY FEATURES

A. Repeat the test
B. If a second sample also has an abnormal PTT, order the following:

    1. Test for circulating anticoagulant
    2. Simple mixing studies with Factor VIII, IX, XI, and XII deficient plasma
    3. Bleeding time if patient is not thrombocytopenic
C. If a test for a circulating anticoagulant is positive:
    1. Test thrombin time and prothrombin time for presence of circulating anticoagulant
    2. If thrombin time is prolonged, order reptilase, fibrin degradation products, and fibrinogen. Major diagnostic possibilities are DIC, heparin, paraproteinemia, or dysfibrinogenemia
    3. If PTT and/or PT prolongation:
       a. Order mixing studies with deficient plasma to locate factor against which anticoagulant is directed
       b. Thromboplastin dilution test for "lupus" anticoagulant
D. If the mixing studies show a deficiency, perform a specific factor level and in case of severe Factor VIII deficiency a test for Factor VIII procoagulant
    1. Factor VIII deficiency: replace with cryoprecipitate or Factor VIII concentrate
    2. Factor IX deficiency: replace with fresh-frozen plasma or Factor IX concentrate
    3. Factor XI: treat, if bleeding, with fresh-frozen plasma
    4. Factor XII deficiency: no treatment necessary
E. If bleeding time and PTT are elevated, especially if plasma does not correct Factor VIII deficient plasma, consider von Willebrand's disease
    1. Confirm diagnosis by platelet aggregation studies in presence of ristocetin and von Willebrand's factor quantitation in plasma
    2. Treat with cryoprecipitate: for severe bleeding, 10–30 U/kg q9h
F. If bleeding time, test for circulating anticoagulant, or mixing studies are not abnormal, and the patient is bleeding, a trial of fresh-frozen plasma is indicated.

REFERENCES

1. Elias M, Eldor A: Thromboembolism in patients with "lupus"-type circulating anticoagulant. Arch Intern Med *144*:510–515, 1984.
    In 25 patients with the lupus anticoagulant, bleeding occurred in only 5 patients, 4 of whom had severe thrombocytopenia, while no excessive bleeding was noted in 18 operative procedures. No therapeutic regimen tried had any effect in decreasing the lupus anticoagulant, but anticoagulants were successful in treatment and prevention of thrombosis.

2. Kelton JG, Hirsh J: Bleeding associated with antithrombotic therapy. Semin. Hematol *17*:259–291, 1980.
    An excellent review of the uses and indications for antithrombotic therapy, including heparin, warfarin, and fibrinolytic and antiplatelet agents. The treatment of the bleeding patient on anticoagulants is outlined, as are the recommended methods of administering and monitoring both heparin and warfarin so as to prevent bleeding complications.

3. Zimmerman T, Ruggeri ZM: von Willebrand's disease. Prog Hematol *5*:203–236, 1983.
    An in-depth discussion of the molecular basis of von Willebrand's disease in both its

classic and variant forms. Clinical features and diagnostic criteria are outlined, and it is stressed that in certain physiologic states (pregnancy, liver disease) the disorder may be impossible to diagnose. For severe bleeding episodes in von Willebrand's disease a dose of 30–50 U/kg of cryoprecipitate q12h is recommended. Treatment with DDAVP is also reviewed.

4. Gill FM: Congenital bleeding disorders: Hemophilia and von Willebrand's disease. Med Clin North Am 68:601–616, 1984.

    This article offers a concise summary of the general care, treatment of bleeding episodes, and a summary of the various factor replacement products used in the treatment of hemophilia and von Willebrand's disease. Complications of therapy and the acquired immune deficiency syndrome (AIDS) are discussed. Newer approaches to therapy are briefly reviewed.

5. Eyster EM, Gail MH, Ballard JO, Al-Mondhiry H, Goedert JJ: Natural history of human immunodeficiency virus infections in hemophiliacs. Ann Intern Med 107:1, 1987.

    A cohort of 84 hemophiliacs in whom time of seroconversion for HIV antibody could be ascertained was followed with serial T cell subsets, platelet counts, and review of clinical symptomatology. Ten patients developed AIDS at 24–95 months after seroconversion. T cell counts <200, older age at seroconversion, and thrombocytopenia were all associated with an increased risk for developing AIDS.

6. Bloom AL: Clotting factor concentrates for resistant haemophilia. Br J Haematol 40:21–27, 1978.
7. Kasper, CK, Dietrich SL: Comprehensive management of Haemophilia. Clin Haematol 14:489, 1985.

    Treatment of hemophilia A patients with inhibitors by various modalities such as high-dose Factor VIII plasmapheresis, Factor IX concentrates, and activated Factor IX concentrates as well as local and supportive therapy is discussed. It is stressed that no reliable in vitro method exists for monitoring therapy with activated Factor IX concentrates.

8. Mammen E: Congenital coagulation abnormalities. Semin Throm Hemost 9:1–70, 1983.

    This issue outlines both the common and the uncommon congenital coagulation abnormalities, including Factor XI deficiency, Factor X deficiency, and dysfibrinogenemias. Brief synopses are given for the biochemistry, mode of inheritance, and clinical and laboratory features, as well as therapy of each deficiency. In addition, congenital disorders causing thromboses (antithrombin III deficiency, plasminogen deficiency, and protein C deficiency) are reviewed.

Hyperleukocytic and Hyperviscosity Syndromes

Barbara Bjornson, M.D.

HYPERLEUKOCYTOSIS

Patients with leukemia may have extraordinarily elevated concentrations of leukocytes in the blood. Occasionally the leukocyte counts are high enough to produce symptoms and signs resulting from impaired circulation in organs such as the lung and brain.

The hyperleukocytic syndrome occurs more frequently in the myelogenous leukemias than in the lymphatic leukemias. This difference is in part explainable by the smaller cell volume of leukemia lymphocytes and the intrinsic "stickiness" of myeloblasts. Thus, the majority of patients who present with this syndrome have acute myelogenous leukemia (AML) or chronic myelogenous leukemia (CML) and a minority have acute lymphocytic leukemia (ALL). Occasionally, symptoms of the hyperleukocytic syndrome are the presenting complaints that lead the patient to seek medical attention and thus to the diagnosis of leukemia.

The presenting signs and symptoms of the hyperleukocytic syndrome include pulmonary manifestations such as tachypnea, dyspnea, and hypoxia. It should be noted that *in vitro* arterial pO_2 measurements are notoriously inaccurate when the leukocyte count is very elevated because of utilization of oxygen by the large number of leukocytes. Nevertheless, true hypoxia has been observed. The nervous system signs include stupor, delirium, dizziness, tinnitus, deafness ataxia, blurred vision, papilledema, retinal vein distention, and intracranial hemorrhage. Priapism and vascular insufficiency may also be associated with extreme elevations in the leukocyte count. Sudden death may occur, and this is usually as a result of intracranial hemorrhage. Thus, the hyperleukocytic syndrome should be promptly diagnosed and treated, since the manifestations may be quite severe and life threatening.

The symptoms observed with extreme elevations in the numbers of circulating immature cells are related to impaired blood flow in the microcirculation where aggregates of white blood cells may be observed. The leukocytes probably also compete for oxygen in the small vessels of the lung and brain, and invasion of vessel walls by these immature cells has also been observed pathologically.

A specific white blood cell count cannot be used to define hyperleukocytosis. In general, however, these patients have white blood cell counts that exceed 100,000/mm³ as well as a high percentage of blasts in the differential. A quick estimate of the degree of leukocytosis may be obtained by determining the leukocrit, which is performed by measuring the buffy coat fractional volume in the standard microcentrifuge spin hematocrit tube. In addition to the factitious hypoxia mentioned previously, extreme elevation of the white blood cell count may result in other spurious laboratory results. Elevation of the serum potassium concentration may result from release of potassium by the leukocyte. Glucose can be falsely decreased, especially because autoanalyzer techniques do not allow for the use of glycolytic inhibitors such as sodium fluoride in the collection tube. For an accurate glucose determination, the serum should be separated promptly and the specimen should not be allowed to stand.

Because the manifestations of this syndrome are directly related to the large numbers of circulating leukocytes, the therapy is aimed at promptly lowering the leukocyte count. The two methods for lowering the leukocyte count include leukapheresis and cytotoxic therapy. The advantages of leukapheresis include the fact that it works rapidly to reverse the hyperleukocytic syndrome and can be used immediately without having to wait for the effect of allopurinol to reduce the risk of hyperuricemia. It also avoids the other risks of chemotherapy-induced cytolysis, including hyperkalemia and hyperphosphatemia. Hydration, allopurinol, and the appropriate chemotherapy should also be instituted concomitantly. In children too small to have leukapheresis and for adults with severe CNS manifestations, early cranial irradiation has been recommended.

HYPERVISCOSITY SYNDROME

Patients with the plasma cell dyscrasias, including macroglobulinemia and multiple myeloma, may develop circulatory and hemorrhagic disturbances as a result of increased blood viscosity produced by the monoclonal immunoglobulins. These are referred to as the hyperviscosity syndrome. The clinical manifestations of the hyperviscosity syndrome are related to the circulatory disturbances caused by the altered flow characteristics of the blood.

The disturbance in circulation may be readily appreciated by careful examination of the ocular fundi, in which characteristic "link-sausage" effects, consisting of alternating bulges and constrictions, are seen within the retinal veins. Retinal hemorrhages and exudates and papilledema may also be found, and patients may present with blurred vision or even complete loss of vision. The neurologic manifestations tend to fluctuate and include headache, dizziness, vertigo, nystagmus, postural hypotension, somnolence, stupor, and even coma. These symptoms are the result of intracerebral vascular occlusion. Other neurologic manifestations include paresis, and focal or generalized seizures. Cerebrovascular hemorrhage may occur secondarily. Deafness is occasionally seen as a result of hyperviscosity leading to thrombosis of the venous system in the ear. A fairly frequent presenting complaint in the hyperviscosity syndrome is epistaxis. Often these patients have generalized oozing from the mucous membranes of nasopharynx, gastrointestinal tract, and bladder. Following minor trauma or a surgical procedure, prolonged bleeding is often noted. These bleeding manifestations are exacerbated by other effects of the dysproteinemia on the clotting system. Congestive heart failure can be precipitated by an increased serum viscosity, other concomitant problems, including anemia and expanded plasma volume, also contribute to this complication. Finally, the presenting signs and symptoms of the hyperviscosity syndrome may be more subjective, including weakness, fatigue, and anorexia.

The level at which the elevated serum viscosity leads to symptoms as well as the major organ system affected varies greatly from patient to patient. Viscosity is defined as the property of a fluid that resists flow. In blood, the viscosity is related to the presence of the formed elements, such as red blood cells, and to proteins. It is important to note that at any given protein concentration there is a correlation between blood viscosity and hematocrit. The concentration of protein as well as properties intrinsic to the proteins determines the plasma viscosity. Molecular size and shape are important determinants of viscosity. For example, IgM molecules have the highest molecular weight of the immunoglobulins and also a bulky shape. Thus, Waldenström's macroglobulemia, in which there is an increased concentration of IgM monoclonal protein, is most commonly associated with the hyperviscosity syndrome. Multiple myeloma associated with IgA paraproteins is also particularly prone to the hyperviscosity syndrome, presumably because of the tendency of IgA molecules to form polymers. Finally, IgG myeloma is least likely to be associated with the hyperviscosity syndrome; nevertheless, it does occur, particularly with M components of the IgG_3 subclass. This may be explained by the propensity of IgG_3 to form concentration and temperature dependent aggregates.

Serum viscosity determinations are simply performed by measuring the rate of flow of serum through a capillary tube at a given temperature and pressure. This is customarily performed with an Ostwald viscosimeter; however, in the emergency setting one may quickly estimate the serum viscosity by measuring the amount of time it takes for the test serum to pass through a red blood cell pipette versus the time it takes for water to pass through. The results are expressed as the ratio of flow time of serum to flow time of water. The normal range for serum viscosity is between 1.4 and 1.8. Patients with a relative viscosity of 2–4 are rarely symptomatic. Symptoms of the hyperviscosity syndrome may be seen at viscosities between 4 and 8, and patients with levels between 8 and 10 almost always have the clinical manifestations of the hyperviscosity syndrome.

Once a diagnosis of hyperviscosity syndrome is established, plasmapheresis is indicated. Virtually all of the manifestations of this syndrome respond, at least temporarily, to plasmapheresis. Serum viscosity should be monitored before and after plasmapheresis. Prompt initiation of the appropriate chemotherapy is important to control the clonal proliferation responsible for the elevated protein.

KEY FEATURES

Hyperleukocytosis
1. More frequent in myelogenous leukemias than in lymphatic leukemias.
2. No specific WBC count can be used to define syndrome, but most patients have WBC >100,000/m³.
3. May present with respiratory distress, neurologic symptoms, visual disturbance, or peripheral vascular compromise.
4. Leukapheresis is preferable treatment, but cytotoxic therapy and radiation have important roles as well.

Hyperviscosity
1. Usually occurs in patients with plasma cell dyscrasias.
2. Clinical features are due to altered flow characteristics of blood.
3. Common symptoms include neurologic abnormalities, visual disturbances, hemorrhage, and congestive heart failure.
4. Therapy involves plasmapheresis and treatment of the underlying disorder.

BIBLIOGRAPHY

1. Lichtman MA, Rowe JM: Hyperleukocytic leukemias: Rheological, clinical and therapeutic considerations. Blood 60:279–283, 1982.
   An excellent brief review, the emphasis on pathophysiology. The clinical manifestations and therapy are concisely covered.

2. Rowe JM, Lichtman MA: Hyperleukocytosis and leukostasis: Common features of childhood chronic myelogenous leukemia. Blood 63:1230–1234, 1984.
   An analysis of 90 cases of CML, 10 childhood and 80 adult. The childhood cases differed in that hyperleukocytosis was extremely common.

3. Eisenstaedt RS, Berkman EM: Rapid cytoreduction in acute leukemia. Management of cerebral leukostasis by cell pheresis. Transfusion 18:113–115, 1978.
   The method of leukapheresis for rapidly lowering circulating blast count is described.

4. Bloch KJ, Maki DG: Hyperviscosity syndromes associated with immunoglobulin abnormalities. Semin Hematol 10:113, 1973.
   An excellent review of the clinical aspects of the hyperviscosity syndrome.

5. Wright DJ, Jenkins DE: Simplified method of estimation of serum and plasma viscosity in multiple myeloma and related disorders. Blood 36:516, 1970.
   A rapid screening test using the red blood cell pipette as the viscosimeter.

6. Isbister JP, et al: Experience with large volume plasmapheresis in malignant paraprotein-emia and immune disorders. Aust NZ J Med 8:154, 1978.
   Therapy is covered very well in this report.

Superior Vena Cava Syndrome

Teresa A. Nolan, M.D.

Obstruction of the superior vena cava (SVC) produces a constellation of clinical symptoms and signs that may present either insidiously, or abruptly as an acute illness requiring emergency treatment. Prior to the 1950s, the leading causes of this syndrome were aortic aneurysms (particularly syphilitic aneurysms), chronic mediastinitis (frequently as a result of granulomatous infections), and intrathoracic tumors.[1,2] At present, however, the overwhelming majority (80–90%) of cases are caused by malignant intrathoracic tumors. Primary lung carcinomas compose about three fourths of the malignancies. Small cell carcinoma has emerged as the most frequent histologic type, followed by epidermoid (squamous cell) carcinoma. Lymphomas represent 10–15% of malignancies associated with SVC obstruction. Less commonly, cases result from metastatic cancers, germ cell neoplasms, and thymomas. Benign causes of the SVC syndrome include mediastinal fibrosis, goiter, and thrombosis (primary or secondary to instrumentation).[3] A number of reports have implicated central venous catheters and pacemaker wires as causes of venous thrombosis and, occasionally, fibrotic constriction that is due to long-term catheter placement.[4]

A review of the regional anatomy is helpful in understanding the pathophysiology and clinical manifestations of SVC obstruction. The superior vena cava enters the right atrium along the right side of the trachea. It is encircled by several groups of mediastinal lymph nodes that drain the entire right lung and the lower part of the left lung. A major portion of the vessel is enveloped by pericardium, and its posteromedial border is adjacent to the vertebral column. Thus the SVC is relatively fixed and can be displaced only slightly by a growing tumor mass. These factors, together with the thin wall and low intravascular pressure of the SVC, make it especially vulnerable to compression and obstruction.

The clinical features of SVC obstruction are attributable to (1) the development of venous hypertension and engorgement in tissues normally drained by the SVC; and (2) the development of collateral venous channels, both in the superficial veins of the thorax and abdomen and in certain deep venous systems, including the internal mammary, mediastinal, vertebral, abdominal, and intercostal veins. The most common presenting symptoms include a feeling of fullness in the head, dyspnea, cough, swelling of the face or upper extremities, dysphagia, chest pain, and syncope. Physical findings associated with SVC obstruction are plethora and edema of the face, neck, and arms; distention of the neck veins; dilated superficial veins of the chest wall; tachypnea; cyanosis; and CNS abnormalities such as papilledema and lethargy.

The chest radiograph is abnormal in more than 80% of patients with SVC syndrome.[3,12] The most frequent radiographic findings are right superior mediastinal mass and/or right hilar or upper lobe mass; other abnormalities include bilateral hilar adenopathy and pleural effusion. Computer tomographic examination of the chest is an excellent means of identifying mass lesions and defining anatomic relationships in the patient with SVC syndrome.[12]

When a patient exhibits characteristic signs and symptoms, the diagnosis of SVC obstruction is self-evident, and further efforts should be directed toward establishing an etiologic diagnosis. In atypical cases, it may be necessary to confirm the presence of SVC obstruction using conventional or radionuclide venography. In general, such studies are not warranted because they do not provide etiologic information or aid in treatment planning and may delay more definitive investigations.[5]

A tissue diagnosis should be actively sought in all cases of SVC syndrome.[6,7] Investigations should follow a logical sequence, beginning with the least invasive procedures. Sputum or pleural fluid specimens should be obtained for cytologic examination, and biopsy of superficial enlarged lymph nodes should be performed if possible. Bone marrow aspiration and biopsy should be considered prior to more invasive procedures, as these studies will be positive for carcinoma in one fifth to one third of patients with small cell lung cancer and are often positive in patients with lymphoma as well. Biopsy obtained by bronchoscopy, mediastinoscopy, or limited thoracotomy will generally yield a definitive tissue diagnosis; the choice among these procedures should be decided by the availability of experienced endoscopists and surgeons at a particular institution and by the condition of the patient. It should be recognized that invasive diagnostic procedures are potentially hazardous in patients with SVC obstruction and occasionally result in severe bleeding from thin-walled collateral veins or abrupt respiratory decompensation during anesthesia as a result of airway edema. Some authors have recommended that acutely ill patients with advanced signs of SVC obstruction, in whom a tissue diagnosis is not obtainable by noninvasive means, should undergo emergency radiation therapy without further attempts at biopsy by bronchoscopy, mediastinoscopy, or thoracotomy. However, in several studies, invasive diagnostic procedures have been associated with low rates of complications, demonstrating that in most cases of SVC obstruction, a tissue diagnosis can be made prior to initiation of therapy.[8]

The mainstay of therapy for SVC obstruction that is due to malignant tumors is radiation therapy.[9] Some reports have indicated that patients with chemotherapy-sensitive tumors (small cell lung cancer, lymphoma) may respond equally well to chemotherapy alone or to chemotherapy plus radiation.[10] The amount of radiotherapy necessary to relieve symptoms of SVC obstruction depends upon multiple factors, including the type of malignancy, concomitant chemotherapy, and previous radiation. Generally speaking, small cell lung cancers and lymphomas may be effectively palliated at doses of 3000–4000 rad, whereas squamous cell cancers and adenocarcinomas often require 5000–6000 rad for adequate control. Symptomatic relief after treatment occurs in 65–100% of patients reported in various series. The majority of patients die of their malignancies, although some enjoy long-term survival.

Several nonspecific measures may be of value in the management of SVC obstruction, although their efficacy is largely unproved; these include elevation of the head of the bed, corticosteroid therapy, and diuretics. Corticosteroids are frequently used to decrease tumor- or radiation-related edema. These agents also have antineoplastic activity against certain lymphomas. Diuretics may provide rapid, though often transient, relief of edema.

Fibrinolytic agents or heparin may be useful in lysing intravascular thrombi or preventing clot propagation, especially in patients with catheter-related SVC obstruction.[11] However, one must weigh the potential benefits of these drugs against the added risk of bleeding in patients who may already have multiple risk factors for hemorrhage.

Surgical approaches, such as thrombectomy or bypass of the obstruction, are generally reserved for those cases in which the cause is known to be benign, the symptoms progressive, and fibrinolytic therapy is either ineffective or contraindicated.

KEY FEATURES

The vast majority of cases of SVC obstruction are caused by malignant intrathoracic tumors, particularly small cell lung cancer.
Typical features of SVC syndrome include the following:
- Plethora and edema of the face, neck, and arms
- Distention of neck veins and superficial veins of the chest wall
- Tachypnea
- Cyanosis
- Occasionally CNS abnormalities such as lethargy and papilledema
The chest radiograph shows a superior mediastinal and/or right hilar or upper lobe mass in more than two thirds of cases.
Tissue diagnosis should be sought in all cases prior to initiation of radiotherapy, although on rare occasions acutely ill patients may require treatment before definitive diagnosis.

Treatment consists primarily of radiation therapy, occasionally replaced by chemotherapy for small cell lung cancer or lymphoma. Elevation of the head of the bed, corticosteroid therapy, and diuretics may be helpful. Heparin and fibrinolytic agents are occasionally useful, particularly in cases of catheter-associated SVC obstruction.

REFERENCES

1. McIntyre FT, Sykes EM Jr: Obstruction of the superior vena cava: A review of the literature and report of two personal cases. Ann Intern Med 30:925–960, 1949.
   Historical perspective.

2. Schechter MM: The superior vena cava syndrome. Am J Med Sci 227:46–56, 1954.
   Historical perspective.

3. Parish JM, Marschke RF, Dines DE, Lee RE: Etiologic considerations in superior vena cava syndrome. Mayo Clinic Proc 56:407–413, 1981.
   This series of 86 patients with SVC syndrome points out that 16% of patients have a normal chest radiograph. Several cases were caused by central venous catheters and pacemakers. The authors state that acute onset of obstructive symptoms is likely to be caused by malignancy, whereas benign causes (excepting central venous catheters) are associated with chronic, slowly progressive symptoms.

4. Fritz T, Richeson JF, Fitzpatrick P, Wilson G: Venous obstruction: A potential complication of transvenous pacemaker electrodes. Chest 83:534–539, 1983.
   The authors report four cases of SVC obstruction that were due to pacing catheters and review the literature regarding this relatively new cause of SVC syndrome.

5. Lokich JL, Goodman R: Superior vena cava syndrome: Clinical management. JAMA 231:58–61, 1975.
   The authors stress that a major pitfall in management is overzealous attempts to establish the site of obstruction by venography, and suggest that acutely ill patients present an oncologic emergency that often requires radiation therapy without a definitive diagnosis.

6. Perez CA, Presant CA, Van Amburg AL: Management of superior vena cava syndrome. Semin Oncol 5:123–134, 1978.
   Literature review and recommendations based on a series of 84 patients.

7. Schraufnagel DE, Hill R, Leech JA, Pare JAP: Superior vena caval obstruction: Is it a medical emergency? Am J Med 70:1169–1174, 1981.
   The authors found that 15% of their 107 cases were caused by benign disorders and that it frequently took longer to make a diagnosis in benign cases. Because none of their patients experienced serious complications of the SVC obstruction itself or from the diagnostic procedures performed, they question the designation of SVC obstruction as a radiotherapeutic emergency requiring treatment without tissue diagnosis.

8. Lewis RJ, Sisler GE, Mackenzie JW: Mediastinoscopy in advanced superior vena cava obstruction. Ann Thorac Surg 32:458–462, 1981.
   The 15 patients in this series from Rutgers University tolerated mediastinoscopy without complication, and there was a definitive diagnosis in each case, confirming that in experienced hands the procedure is a reasonable alternative when less invasive measures have been unrevealing.

9. Davenport D, Ferree C, Blake D, Raben M: Response of superior vena cava syndrome to radiation therapy. Cancer 38:1577–1580, 1976.

This series of 19 patients documents rapid and effective symptomatic relief with radiation therapy.

10. Maddox AM, Valdivieso M, Lukeman J, Smith TL, Barkley HE, Samuels ML, Bodey GP: Superior vena cava obstruction in small cell bronchogenic carcinoma: Clinical parameters and survival. Cancer 52:2165–2172, 1983.

    This series from the M.D. Anderson Hospital shows combination chemotherapy to be as effective as radiation for emergency treatment of SVC syndrome in patients with small cell lung cancer. The authors point out that the high incidence of systemic metastases at presentation may favor chemotherapy over radiation for this disease.

11. Herrera JL, Willis SM, Williams TH: Successful streptokinase therapy of acute idiopathic superior vena cava thrombosis. Am Heart J 102:1063–1064, 1981.

    Brief report.

12. Levine BW, Mark EJ: A 56-year-old man with diffuse pulmonary disease and the superior vena cava syndrome (CPC). N Engl J Med 318:168–177, 1988.

    Illustrative case of a patient with usual interstitial pneumonitis, rheumatoid arthritis, and SVC syndrome from intercurrent oat cell carcinoma. Excellent description of clinical features, results of diagnostic studies, and postmortem findings.

Transfusion Reactions

Mark J. Brauer, M.D.

Although transfusion of blood and its components is usually a safe and effective form of therapy, untoward effects do occur. These side effects are referred to as transfusion reactions. Some of the adverse complications are avoidable, whereas others cannot be prevented. Physicians must be aware of the possible and preventable risks of blood transfusion therapy and measure these against potential benefits.

When any unusual or unexpected symptom or sign appears while blood is being transfused or shortly after, consider that it may have been induced by the blood product until proved otherwise. As a rule, stopping the transfusion will minimize the adverse effect. The American Association of Blood Banks (AABB) recommends the following steps to be taken for all discernible transfusion reactions:

1. Stop transfusion.
2. Keep intravenous line open with 0.9% saline.
3. Notify attending physician and blood bank.
4. Send freshly collected blood and urine samples to blood bank for analysis.

5. If necessary, send blood unit and administration set to the blood blank for examination.

As a general rule, if urticaria is the *only* adverse effect, infusion of the blood product can be restarted after administration of an antihistamine.

Acute intravascular hemolysis is the most feared and damaging adverse effect of a transfusion.[1,2] It may be heralded by fever, chills, back pain, flushing, hypotension, dyspnea, chest pain, and intense burning at the infusion site. More severe manifestations include hemoglobinemia, hemoglobinuria, oliguria, shock, and disseminated intravascular coagulation (DIC). The physician's first effort should be directed toward this possibility. Prompt diagnosis and therapy can be life saving. To exclude a hemolytic transfusion reaction quickly, a sample of centrifugally anticoagulated blood should be examined for evidence of hemoglobin in the plasma; as little as 50 mg/dl of free hemoglobin will color the plasma pink. A test for antibody coating of the red blood cells (Coombs antiglobulin test) should also be performed immediately. If both these tests are negative, it is most unlikely that the patient is having a hemolytic transfusion reaction. If hemolysis is found, the physician should first check to see that the correct blood was given. Errors somewhere from the initial blood sample drawing for crossmatch to the actual administration of the unit are the leading causes of such reactions.

Adverse reactions to blood transfusion that occur during the transfusion or within an hour or so of its completion are referred to as immediate transfusion reactions. These can be subdivided into those immunologically mediated and those that do not involve immunologic mechanisms (Table 1).

Fever is one of the most common early manifestations of immune hemolysis, being present in 35 of 47 cases reported by Peneda and coworkers.[3]

Table 1.   IMMEDIATE TRANSFUSION REACTIONS

Type	Etiology
Immunologic	
Hemolytic	Erythrocyte incompatibility
Anaphylactic	Antibody to IgA
Febrile	Antibody to donor leukocyte antigens
Urticarial	Antibody to plasma proteins
Noncardiogenic pulmonary edema	Antibody to donor leukocytes
Nonimmunologic	
Congestive heart failure	Volume overload
Hypothermia	Rapid administration of cold blood (may cause cardiac arrest)
Emboli	Microthrombi in stored blood
Massive transfusion effect (10 U acutely or replacement of one blood volume in 24 hours)	Hyperkalemia: banked blood
	Hypocalcemia: citrate
	Thrombocytopenia or clotting factor deficiency: dilution effect
Fever	Bacterial contamination

Chills accompany fever in one half of cases. Rarely, generalized oozing or frank bleeding may be the first signs of DIC triggered by an incompatible (ABO) transfusion. Baseline clotting studies, including platelet count, fibrinogen assay, and fibrin split products are helpful to assess the severity of DIC.[2] To prevent renal failure secondary to hemoglobinuria and shock, 1000 ml of 0.9% saline should be given over 1–2 hours. Then diuretic therapy with furosemide 20–80 mg intravenously is administered. Continued use of fluids and diuretics to maintain urine flow around 100 ml/hour is employed for the first 24 hours.[4]

The prevention of hemolytic transfusion reactions is difficult. For every 6000 U of blood given, one such reaction will occur.[3] Therefore, clinicians should be prepared to diagnose these reactions quickly and know how to avert or minimize severe complications.

Congestive heart failure induced by transfusion is common and preventable. The very young, the elderly, patients with cardiac disease, and those individuals with expanded plasma volumes (long-standing anemias) are most likely to develop heart failure with transfusion. In these patients, the usual transfusion rate of 200 ml/hour may be too rapid because they cannot accommodate for the rapid expansion of blood volume. If congestive heart failure develops, the transfusion should be stopped or the rate slowed dramatically. Rapid-acting diuretics are given intravenously and phlebotomy of 200–400 ml of blood may be necessary. If available, plasmapheresis before transfusion may be employed to reduce the patient's plasma volume. Very rarely, noncardiogenic pulmonary edema may occur on an immunologic basis.[5]

For every 10 U of whole blood or packed cells given for severe trauma or major surgery, a one blood-volume exchange of the recipient's own blood occurs. Infusion of large amounts of refrigerated blood often reduces the core body temperature and may cause cardiac arrest. The use of a blood warmer can prevent this complication.

During massive transfusion, platelet washout may occur and Factor VIII may also be depleted. To avoid this problem, 10 U of platelets should be given for every 10 U of transfused blood products as well as 2 U of fresh-frozen plasma. A coagulation screening battery is helpful.[6]

DELAYED TRANSFUSION EFFECTS

Damaging effects of blood transfusion can occur days to years after completion of the initial event. Again, both immunologic and nonimmunologic factors may be operative. A blood transfusion introduces a large number of "nonself" antigens, all potentially immunogenic. This is true even of perfectly crossmatched blood thought to be totally compatible with the recipient. A delayed transfusion reaction results from the formation of antibodies to such donor cells.[7] Recall formation of antibodies not detectable by current blood bank testing is referred to as an anamnestic reaction. It is not unheard of for a delayed hemolytic reaction to cause symptoms of fever, hemoglobinuria, renal failure, or even death. Usually the onset of a delayed hemolytic reaction is insidious, with the gradual development of anemia; however, serum sickness and posttransfusion thrombocytopenia have been described.[8] Alloimmunization to IgA in IgA-deficient individuals is responsible for many urticarial reactions and even life-threatening anaphylaxis.[9]

Post-transfusion disease transmission, e.g., viral hepatitis and acquired immune deficiency syndrome (AIDS),[10] is beyond the scope of this discussion except to comment that each time a blood product is ordered, the clinician's prime responsibility is making certain the therapy is warranted. In fact, the incidence of non-A, non-B hepatitis may be increasing in spite of improved testing techniques.

In order to guard the blood supply and potential recipients from infection with the human immunodeficiency virus (HIV), described as the causative agent of AIDS, currently a system is in place providing three different forms of protection: voluntary self-exclusion by donors defined by behavior as being at increased risk for HIV infection, confidential unit exclusion by donors who feel under pressure to donate, and HIV-antibody testing that detects most infected units. However, even these stringent measures cannot remove all risk for those in need of blood transfusion.[11] Despite appropriate screening and precautions, as of early 1987, 2% of adults and 12% of children with AIDS had acquired the disease from transfusion of blood or blood products.[12]

KEY FEATURES

Allergic Reactions
In about 1% of transfusions, the recipient may experience pruritus, hives, and urticaria. The transfusion should be stopped and an antihistamine given (diphenhydramine, 50 mg intravenously). Rare IgA-deficient individuals may experience life-threatening anaphylaxis requiring epinephrine and intravenous steroids.

Febrile Reactions
Are common in multiply transfused patients (1–5%). Leukocyte-poor red blood cells virtually eliminate this problem using washed erythrocytes.

Hemolytic Reactions
Are almost always due to mislabeling or faulty identification of the patient or unit because of clerical error. Cardiovascular collapse, renal

shut down, and disseminated intravascular coagulation (DIC) must be anticipated and treated accordingly.

Response to Suspected Hemolytic Transfusion Reaction
1. Stop blood.
2. Keep intravenous line open with 0.9% saline.
3. Notify physician and blood bank.
4. Spin sample to view supernatant for plasma hemoglobin and perform direct Coombs test on patient's cells.
5. If test is positive, send unit to blood bank and institute treatment for shock, renal failure, and DIC.

REFERENCES

1. Goldfinger D: Acute hemolytic transfusion reactions—a fresh look at pathogenesis and considerations regarding therapy. Transfusion 17:85, 1977.
   A comprehensive review of our then-current knowledge of acute hemolytic transfusion reactions. It emphasizes the primary pathogenic mechanisms, namely, disseminated intravascular coagulation and hypoperfusion leading to ischemic tissue necrosis. Therapy of these underlying factors is emphasized.

2. Greenwalt TJ: Pathogenesis and treatment of hemolytic transfusion reaction. Semin Hematol 18:84, 1981.
   Diagnosis and management of renal failure and the use of intravenous heparin are well discussed. Laboratory and clinical findings are given in easy to read tables; also, a discussion of "almost" harmless antibodies.

3. Pineda AA, Byzica SM Jr, Taswell HF: Hemolytic transfusion reaction: Recent experiences in a large blood bank. Mayo Clinc Proc 53:378, 1978.
   Data on 47 cases of hemolytic transfusion reactions are presented, along with a review of the literature. Emphasis is on human error and limitations of then-current technology of compatibility testing.

4. Schmidt PJ, Holland PV: Pathogenesis of acute renal failure associated with incompatible transfusion. Lancet 2:1169, 1967.
   A classic paper describing two patients with acute reversible renal damage following blood transfusion. One had Duffy's incompatibility, the other high-titre anti-Kell. The reaction was attributed to red blood cell stroma complexed to antibody.

5. Carilli AD, Ramanamurty MV, et al: Non-cardiogenic pulmonary edema following blood transfusion. Chest 74:310, 1978.
   When pulmonary angiographic studies and hemodynamic measurements were made, normal wedge pressures were observed and contrast material appeared to extravasate across the alveolar-capillary (a-c) membranes into the alveoli. The mechanism of a-c membrane injury is discussed.

6. Counts RB, Haisch C, Simon TL, et al: Hemostasis in massively transfused trauma patients. Ann Surg 190:91, 1979.
   Massive transfusion was given to 27 patients who were studied prospectively to determine whether blood transfusion was responsible for disturbances in hemostasis. Study was worthwhile and carefully performed.

7. Pineda AA, et al: Delayed hemolytic transfusion reactions. Transfusion 18:1, 1978.
   Twenty-three cases of delayed hemolytic transfusion reactions are reviewed. Nineteen patients had clinical evidence of hemolysis, and fever was the most common symptom.

Death subsequent to delayed transfusion occurred in three cases. The Coombs test was always positive.

8. Morrison FS, Mollison PL: Post transfusion purpura. N Engl J Med 275:243, 1966.
   An example of the rare syndrome of post-transfusion purpura secondary to severe thrombocytopenia is described. As in all previously published cases, the specificity of the antibody was directed against the PI^AI platelet antigen.

9. Vyas GN, Holmdahl L, et al: Serologic specificity of human anti-IgA and its significance in transfusion. Blood 34:573, 1969.
   Persons lacking IgA produce class specific anti-IgA as a result of parenteral exposure to incompatible gamma globulin or blood components. Anti-IgA antibodies were found in 86% of anaphylactic and urticarial transfusion reactions.

10. Curran J, et al: Acquired immuno-deficiency syndrome (AIDS) associated with transfusions. N Engl J Med 310:69, 1984.
    As of August 1, 1983, over 2000 cases of AIDS have been reported to the Centers for Disease Control. About 1.5% of all cases reported appear to follow the administration of blood components within 5 years. The report strengthened the possibility that AIDS may be transmitted in blood.

11. Bove J: Transfusion-associated hepatitis and AIDS: What is the risk? N Engl J Med 317:242, 1987.
    A short state of the art review of (1) post-transfusion hepatitis, including new tests (alanine amino transferase and antibody to hepatitis B core antigen) that should reduce the risk of non-A, non-B hepatitis even further, and (2) transfusion-associated AIDS, especially why new cases continue to be reported, perhaps because of recently infected sero-negative low-risk donors.

12. Friedland GH, Klein, RS: Transmission of the human immunodeficiency virus. N Engl J Med 317:1125–1134, 1987.
    Late-1987 state-of-knowledge review of all known transmission routes. Of note, although whole blood, blood cellular components, plasma, and clotting factors have transmitted HIV, other products prepared from blood, such as immunoglobulin, albumin, plasma protein fraction, and hepatitis B vaccine, have not been implicated.

Cancer Pain: Acute Management

Roberta M. Falke, M.D.

Pain is a dreaded complication of cancer, but even severe episodes can be controlled if managed aggressively. Effective therapy follows from understanding the physiology of pain transmission, perception, and modulation.[1]

PAIN PHYSIOLOGY: FROM INJURY TO INSULT

Pain signals are generated by nociceptors at sites of tissue injury. These receptors are stimulated by extreme temperature and pressure, as well as by chemical mediators of inflammation, including prostaglandins. Therapeutic modalities aimed at interrupting these initial events include nonsteroidal anti-inflammatory drugs[2] and antineoplastic therapy. Pain signals are inhibited at several levels of their transmission. Therapy often seeks to augment this natural modulation. Nociceptors have high thresholds, so that non-noxious stimuli are felt preferentially (gate theory of Melzack and Wall).[3] Transcutaneous electrical nerve stimulation (TENS) is in part an attempt to override painful impulses with frequent innocuous stimuli.[4] Pain afferents synapse with inhibitory neurons. Several neurotransmitters participate in pain modulation, including the endogenous opioid peptides or endorphins.[5] These bind to receptors in the spinal cord, medulla, and periaqueductal gray matter. The arrival of a pain signal at the higher centers activates descending pain modulation pathways. As a result, an inhibitory interneuron dampens the pain message shortly after it reaches the dorsal horn region of the spinal cord. Exogenous opioids produce analgesia by binding to opiate receptors both in the spinal cord and in the brain. The message is subsequently relayed to the limbic system and associative areas, where it acquires an affect that greatly influences its perception. Acute pain is usually associated with anxiety.[6] Reduction of anxiety is, therefore, an important therapeutic step.

MANAGEMENT OF ACUTE CANCER PAIN

Establishing site, radiation, and time course of the pain during the initial evaluation may help distinguish among organ damage, soft tissue invasion, skeletal involvement, and nerve injury. The acute onset of extreme pain suggests acute tissue necrosis, i.e., hemorrhage, ischemia, or fracture, although chronic pain from a previously known site of disease may suddenly become more severe. A reliable estimate of subjective discomfort may be obtained by asking the patient to rate the pain on a numerical scale from 1 to 10. Careful physical and neurologic examinations are mandatory, and the clinician should observe and record accurately the level of function tolerated; voluntary positioning, weight bearing, and range of motion should be documented initially and followed during treatment.

Reassurance that pain will be controlled helps allay anxiety and must be supported by immediate, effective therapy. By addressing the pain first, one may encourage an uncomfortable patient to tolerate diagnostic tests. Narcotic analgesics are the agents of choice: they act at spinal cord and central levels and thus inhibit both the transmission and the perception of painful impulses.

Morphine sulfate (MS) and hydromorphone (Dilaudid) are effective agents (Table 1). MS, 8–10 mg IM or SC, works within 15 minutes and lasts 1–2 hours. An intravenous dose works in 10 minutes and lasts about an hour. By ordering narcotics on fixed schedules that reflect these intervals, rather than PRN, one can prevent episodes of pain and avoid reinforcing "painful" and drug-seeking behaviors. One should ask the patient frequently whether the last dose given was effective, and whether it remained so for the entire prescribed interval. Meperidine (Demerol) works, but toxic metabolites may accumulate in patients with renal insufficiency.[7] Partial antagonists, such as butorphanol (Stadol) and pentazocine (Talwin), should not be used.

Continuous intravenous or subcutaneous infusion provides a steady effect that can be evaluated and adjusted instantaneously.[7,8] The initial hourly dose should approximate one twenty-fourth of the total amount of narcotics used over the previous 24 hours. Infusion rate may be increased every 2 hours if pain persists (in increments of 2–5 mg of MS), until relief or toxicity. Morphine may also be given by epidural route: small doses can provide lasting relief with minimal sedation. Careful monitoring is necessary: side effects include pruritus and, rarely, respiratory depression. Hydromorphone and oxymorphone are also available as suppositories. If excessive sedation is noted, the drug should be held until there is significant improvement or until the patient is awake enough to complain of pain. At this time, therapy is resumed with smaller doses; the use of the antagonist naloxone should be reserved for potentially life-threatening overdose only. Constipation is inevitable; cathartics should be prescribed prophylactically. Nausea may dictate a change of narcotic, although tolerance to this effect may develop rapidly.

An efficient work-up is geared toward treatable problems. In hospitalized cancer patients, pain is due to the cancer in 75% and to treatment in

Table 1.   EQUIANALGESIC DOSES

	Duration of Effect (Hours)	Plasma Half-life (Hours)
Hydromorphone (Dilaudid) 8 mg PO (2 mg SC)	3	
Morphine sulfate 50 mg PO (10 mg SC)	1½	
Levorphanol tartrate (Levo-Dromoran) 4 mg PO (2 mg SC)	4	12
Methadone 20 mg PO (10 mg SC)	4–6	18
Oxymorphone (Numorphan) 1 mg IM (3 mg supp)	3–6	

25%.[9] Common emergencies such as brain and epidural metastatic disease are dealt with elsewhere in this text. Other frequent syndromes include the following:

1. *Bone metastases*. The most sensitive test is the bone scan. Conventional radiographs of "hot" areas may show completed or impending fracture. Patients with back pain and abnormal radiographs should have myelography. Treatment is radiation therapy. Most lesions become less painful with 2000 rad or less. Orthopedic consultations should be obtained concerning the need for prophylactic repair of long bone lesions, as well as for optimal splinting and rehabilitation.

2. *Abdominal pain*. Potential causes include bowel obstruction as a result of cancer; infiltration of liver, pancreas, or retroperitoneum; and chemotherapy- or narcotic-induced ileus. Appropriate tests include plain radiograph and CT scan. Conservative management is best, if possible, with NPO and nasogastric suction if necessary; surgical consultation should be obtained. Antineoplastic therapy should be instituted if possible, and if surgery is not imminent. Liver pain may respond to palliative radiotherapy.

3. *Neuropathic pain*. This syndrome is usually the result of nerve infiltration by tumor; iatrogenic causes include surgery, chemotherapy, and radiation. Neurologic damage may not be reversible despite removal of the offending agent or mass. Lack of "gating" by normal afferent impulses seems to result in hyperesthesia and disorganized activity in higher brain centers that is experienced as pain. Most sensitive tests are history and nerve conduction tests. Tricyclic antidepressants, phenothiazines, and anticonvulsants have all been used with varying success.[1,10] Transcutaneous electrical nerve stimulation (TENS) may be extremely helpful, and has no adverse effects.[11]

Once the acute episode is controlled, the diagnostic evaluation underway, and the patient comfortable, a transition to oral analgesic therapy should be attempted. As shown in Table 1, the oral to parenteral ratio of some commonly used drugs is high. Oral meperidine is, however, erratically absorbed and should be avoided. Owing to their long-half-lives, methadone and levorphanol may accumulate in the debilitated patient, leading to marked toxicity.[12] These difficult agents have largely been supplanted by sustained-release morphine. The effective equianalgesic dose of oral morphine for the previous 24 hours is simply divided into every-12-hour doses. Some patients may need every-8-hour dosing. Immediate-release oral morphine or hydromorphone may be used for "breakthrough" pain until the ideal dose of the sustained-release preparation is reached.[1]

Adjunctive therapies are those aimed at improving mood and have an additive analgesic effect. Antidepressants, phenothiazines, antihistamines, and such behavioral maneuvers as guided imagery and hypnosis may all be considered. Cancer patients need not remain in pain. Safe, effective relief can usually be obtained with aggressive, carefully monitored therapy.

KEY FEATURES

1. Acute pain is accompanied by anxiety. Treat both.
2. Use parenteral narcotic drugs first. Employ fixed dosing, not PRN, and adjust per response. May add major tranquilizers, antidepressants.
3. Rapid, accurate diagnosis may allow control of pain by tumor reduction.
4. Alternate routes: continuous IV or SC; epidural; suppository.
5. Methadone analgesia lasts 4–6 hours, but drug accumulates in plasma if given q6h. Sustained release morphine is effective twice a day.
6. TENS is a safe, effective treatment for all pain; particularly useful for peripheral nerve injuries.

REFERENCES

1. Twycross RG: The management of pain in cancer. A guide to drugs and dosage. Prim Care Cancer 8:15–23, 1988.
   Excellent review of pain management, based on pharmacology, physiology, and psychosocial factors.

2. Robinson DR: Prostaglandins and anti-inflammatory drugs. Disease-a-Month 30(3), 1983.
   Comprehensive review of these agents: biochemistry, pharmacology, and toxicology.

3. Melzack R, Wall PD: Pain mechanisms: A new theory. Science 150:971–977, 1965.
   Classic description of the gate theory.

4. Tyler E, Caldwell C, Ghia JN: Transcutaneous electrical nerve stimulation: An alternative approach to the management of postoperative pain. Anesth Analg 61:449–456, 1982.
   Review of use of TENS in acute postoperative pain: rationale and clinical trials. Eight studies, including 7400 patients, showed 75% of TENS patients significantly reduced their intake of narcotics.

5. Krieger DT: Opioids and pain. In Endorphins and enkephalins. Disease-a-Month 28(10):23–28, 1982.
   Review of opioid peptides: biochemistry, distribution, possible mechanisms of action, and physiologic role.

6. Bonica JJ: Neurophysiologic and pathologic aspects of acute and chronic pain: Arch Surg 112:750–761, 1977.
   Extensive review of neurologic physiology of pain.

7. Foley KM: The practical use of narcotic analgesics. Med Clin North Am 66:1091–1104, 1982.
   Describes the narcotic analgesics: pharmacology and equianalgesic doses. Discusses

individualized therapy: duration of effect and disposition, and side effects of most available drugs.

8. Campbell CF, Mason FB, Weiler JM: Continuous subcutaneous infusion of morphine for the pain of terminal malignancy. Ann Intern Med 98:51, 1983.
    One patient obtained excellent relief from prolonged subcutaneous infusion. Patient and family easily handled line at home: no intravascular access was needed.

9. Kanner RM, Foley KM: Patterns of narcotic use in a cancer pain clinic. Ann NY Acad Sci 362:162, 1981.

10. Taub A, Collins WF Jr: Observations on the treatment of denervation dysesthesia with psychotropic drugs: Postherpetic neuralgia, anesthesia dolorosa, peripheral neuropathy. Adv Neurol 4:309–315, 1974.
    Reviews previous essentially anecdotal experience with tricyclics and phenothiazines. This experience includes 17 patients with postherpetic neuralgia. All but three had "significant relief" and reduction of narcotic intake within 2 weeks.

11. Tasker RR, Organ LW, Hawrylyshyn P: Deafferentation and causalgia, In Bonica JJ (ed): Pain. New York, Raven Press, 1980, p 305.
    Pathophysiologic basis for electrical stimulation in deafferentation syndromes.

12. Ettinger DS, Vitale PJ, Trump DL: Important clinical pharmacologic consideration in the use of methadone in cancer patients. Cancer Treat Rep 63:457–459, 1979.
    Drug accumulates because of long half-life. Case report of iatrogenic overdoses.

SECTION 5
INFECTIOUS DISEASES

Spontaneous Bacterial Peritonitis

James J. Heffernan, M.D.

Spontaneous bacterial peritonitis (SBP) has been recognized as a distinct clinical entity only in the last several decades. It was first described in detail in the French literature in 1958 and in the American literature in 1964; since that time, a number of larger clinical reviews have been published.[1-4,9] The term "spontaneous bacterial peritonitis" has, by general usage, become restricted to adult populations with underlying cirrhosis. Primary peritonitis of childhood and secondary peritonitis, as from bowel perforation, pelvic infection, or trauma, is not discussed here.

Ascites is the *sine qua non* of SBP. Most patients studied to date have been middle-aged male alcoholics with Laennec's cirrhosis.[1-4,9] However, this phenomenon is well described among patients with post-necrotic cirrhosis, Wilson's disease, chronic active hepatitis, alpha-1-antitrypsin disease, and hemochromatosis.[2,5,9] SBP has also been described among those with biliary cirrhosis, cardiac cirrhosis, systemic lupus erythematosus, alcoholic hepatitis, acute viral hepatitis, malignant ascites, and pancreatitis without cirrhosis. The prevalence of this syndrome among all hospitalized alcoholics carrying the diagnosis of cirrhosis has been estimated at 3–5%.[2,9] Among hospitalized patients with cirrhosis and documented ascites, the prevalence of SBP is 8–10%.[2,6] SBP carries an extremely grim prognosis. Only 5% of patients from the extended series of Conn and Fessel in 1971 lived to leave the hospital.[2] More recent data suggest an associated mortality rate still in excess of 60–70%.[4,6,9]

Several mechanisms have been postulated in the pathogenesis of this disease, although none have been proved solely responsible: (1) invasion of edematous bowel mucosa by enteric organisms; (2) more frequent and persistent bacteremic episodes in patients with cirrhosis; (3) inadequate clearance of bacteria in the portal circulation in the setting of cirrhosis, portal hypertension, and portosystemic shunts; (4) poor clearance of organisms from gastrointestinal lymphatics; and (5) diminished bactericidal activity of ascitic fluid in cirrhotics.[12]

The clinical features of SBP include fever and chills, abdominal pain, deteriorating mental status, hypoactive bowel sounds, and nonlocalizing abdominal tenderness, with or without rebound, in a cirrhotic patient with pre-existing ascites.[2,4,9] Obvious considerations in the differential diagnosis include pancreatitis, cholangitis, cholecystitis, peptic ulcer disease with perforation, diverticulitis, ischemic bowel, pelvic inflammatory disease, intraabdominal abscess, and tuberculous or secondary peritonitis. Although the typical features occur in 60–90% of cases, atypical presentations with minimal symptoms are reported in all clinical series. The vast majority of cases have been shown to have laboratory evidence of pre-existing hepatic dysfunction, with a worse prognosis for those patients with evidence of acute liver injury.[9] Hypotension and severe encephalopathy are also clinical markers for a poor early outcome,[2,4] as is renal insufficiency.[9]

Once the diagnosis is suspected, the work-up should proceed with alacrity. While evaluation to exclude a surgical cause proceeds, diagnostic paracentesis should be performed without delay in all febrile patients with ascites. A coagulopathy is often present, usually resistant to correction with vitamin K and often to fresh-frozen plasma; an attempt to improve the patient's coagulation status should be made but should not materially slow efforts to obtain ascitic fluid for analysis. Gram's stain of peritoneal fluid is positive in a minority of cases of SBP and should always be included in the evaluation process.[1-4] On the basis of data compiled from numerous clinical series, the ascitic fluid polymorphonuclear leukocyte (PMN) count is the best single predictor of SBP.[2,6,7,12] When one excludes patients with malignant ascites, secondary peritonitis, and culture-negative SBP from consideration, an ascitic fluid PMN count greater than 250 mm^3 is highly sensitive (94%), specific (95%), and accurate (95%) for the diagnosis of SBP.[12] A depressed peritoneal fluid PH and/or elevated peritoneal fluid lactate level are adjunctive findings of high specificity and diagnostic accuracy.[10,12] Standard chemistry studies are not discriminatory, but an elevated peritoneal fluid amylase strongly suggests pancreatitis or a perforation. The early results of ascitic fluid analysis must always be interpreted in the light of the clinical situation; antibiotic coverage before the return of culture results is usually indicated.[7]

The ultimate and unequivocal diagnosis of SBP rests on the results of appropriately obtained cultures. Concurrently obtained blood cultures have been positive in 50–60% of cases in which a bacteriologic diagnosis is obtained from the ascitic fluid.[2-4,9] Infection at other sites is noted in up to a third of cases, most commonly the urinary tract, with *Escherichia coli*, or the lower respiratory tract, with *Streptococcus pneumoniae* or *E. coli*.[2,9] The overwhelming majority of cases of SBP have been caused by single isolates of aerobic gram negative enteric bacilli (55–75%), predominantly *E. coli*; and aerobic gram positive streptococci (20–35%), especially pneumococci and enterococci but also group A and viridans streptococci.[1-4,9] Staphylococci, anaerobic organisms, and Candida species have been isolated infrequently and when recovered are more often part of a mixed flora.[9,11]

Antimicrobial therapy is most often initiated before the return of culture results and must include coverage for the organisms commonly isolated in SBP, specifically gram negative aerobic enteric bacilli and gram positive aerobic streptococci (including the enterococcus). The backbone of empiric therapy is thus ampicillin 1.5–2.0 gm IV q6h and gentamicin or tobramycin 2.0 mg/kg IV load then 1.5 mg/kg IV q8h (if renal function is normal). If resistant gram negative organisms are suspected, amikacin 5 mg/kg IV q8h should be substituted for gentamicin or tobramycin. Aztreonam has also been used successfully, in place of an aminoglycoside, for SBP caused by gram negative organisms. If the peritonitis is felt to be secondary (as in the setting of gut perforation) or if the ascitic fluid Gram's stain reveals a polymicrobial flora or organisms morphologically suggestive of Bacteroides species, clindamycin 600 mg IV q6–8h or metronidazole should be added to the regimen. Single-agent empiric therapy with a later-generation extended spectrum penicillin has diminished activity against gram positive cocci, and sole use of a cephalosporin of any generation will not effectively cover the possibility of enterococcal infection. Once culture and sensitivity results are in hand, a more specific antibiotic regimen may be substituted: (1) high-dose penicillin G (>10 million U/day IV in divided doses) for group A streptococci or *S. pneumoniae*; (2) continuation of ampicillin and an aminoglycoside for enterococcal infection; and (3) an aminoglycoside, aztreonam, extended spectrum penicillin, or later-generation cephalosporin as indicated by sensitivity patterns for gram negative enteric bacilli with an antipseudomonal penicillin in the setting of infection with *Pseudomonas aeruginosa*. Oxacillin, vancomycin, or a first-generation cephalosporin should be included in the unusual setting of staphylococcal infection, whereas clindamycin, metronidazole, or cefoxitin are indicated for anaerobic organisms. Intravenous therapy with standard dosages of commonly used antibiotics produces adequate drug levels in ascitic fluid.[8] Aggressive supportive measures for hepatic failure (reviewed elsewhere in this text) are often necessary.

In the larger series to date, 60% of patients have demonstrated an objective response to therapy.[2,4,9] Those with peritonitis caused by enteric organisms, those with evidence of more acute hepatic injury or of renal dysfunction, and those with hypotension or marked encephalopathy have the bleakest prognosis.[2,4,9] In even the most recent series, only a minority of patients with SBP survive the hospitalization. Most deaths not attributable to sepsis result from accelerated hepatic failure or its complications.

KEY FEATURES

Pre-existing ascites is the *sine qua non* of SBP, generally in the setting of alcoholic cirrhosis.

SBP may also complicate postnecrotic cirrhosis, chronic active hepatitis, Wilson's disease, hemochromatosis, alpha-1-antitrypsin disease, cardiac or biliary cirrhosis, lupus erythematosus, and acute hepatitis.

Major clinical features at presentation:

Fever	54–90%
Abdominal pain	51–87%
New or worsening encephalopathy	51–85%
Rebound tenderness	42–64%
Decreased or absent bowel sounds	21–54%
Hypotension	5–14%
Neither fever nor abdominal pain	5–7%

Differential diagnosis includes pancreatitis, biliary tract disease, ischemic bowel, diverticulitis, pelvic inflammatory disease, gut perforation, and intra-abdominal abscess, all with or without secondary peritonitis; must also consider tuberculous peritonitis.

Suggestive ascitic fluid findings include the following:

PMN > 250/mm^3

pH < 7.31

lactate > 25 mg/dl

Elevated amylase suggests pancreatitis or perforation
Routine chemistries are not discriminatory
Diagnosis rests on positive fluid Gram's stain and/or culture

The overwhelming majority of cases are caused by gram negative aerobic bacilli, especially *E. coli,* and gram positive aerobic cocci, especially group D (enterococcus) and *S. pneumoniae;* staphylococci and anaerobic species are isolated infrequently.

Treatment

Empiric (pending cultures): Ampicillin and gentamicin or tobramycin; substitute amikacin as the aminoglycoside if resistant organisms are suspected, and add clindamycin if anaerobic species are suggested by Gram's stain. Consider aztreonam in place of aminoglycoside.

Culture-Proven Infection

Gram negative aerobic enteric bacilli: Aminoglycoside, aztreonam, extended spectrum penicillin, or cephalosporin as indicated by antibiotic sensitivities, with or without antipseudomonal penicillin for infection with *P. aeruginosa*

S. pneumoniae or group A steptococcci: Penicillin G

Group D streptococci (enterococcus): Ampicillin and an aminoglycoside

Staphylococci: Oxacillin or nafcillin, vancomycin, or a first-generation cephalosporin as indicated by sensitivity pattern
Anaerobic organisms: Clindamycin, metronidazole, or cefoxitin

Intravenous antibiotics achieve acceptable peritoneal fluid levels. Despite aggressive supportive measures and appropriate antibiotic therapy, only 30–40% of patients survive hospitalization.

REFERENCES

1. Conn HO: Spontaneous peritonitis and bacteremia in Laennec's cirrhosis caused by enteric organisms. Ann Intern Med 60:568, 1964.
    Initial American report of six cases in five alcoholic patients with decompensated cirrhosis. All were bacteriologically confirmed with concurrent ascitic fluid and blood cultures positive for E. coli (four episodes), Aeromonas liquefaciens (one episode), and Streptococcus faecalis (one episode). Clinical features and pathogenesis are discussed.

2. Conn HO, Fessel J: Spontaneous bacterial peritonitis in cirrhosis: Variations on a theme. Medicine (Baltimore) 50:161, 1971.
    The definitive review of this topic, including a series of 32 episodes in 28 patients and discussion of another 46 cases from the literature. Detailed description of clinical features, laboratory findings, and bacteriology—gram negative enteric bacilli (54%), pneumococci (20%), and other gram positive aerobic streptococci (17%) were most often implicated. The authors estimate a 3% incidence rate among patients with cirrhosis.

3. Curry N, McCallum RW, Guth PH: Spontaneous peritonitis in cirrhotic ascites. Am J Dig Dis 19:685, 1974.
    Fifteen cases were identified retrospectively, all with ascites and cirrhosis (13 from alcoholic liver disease and 2 from chronic active hepatitis). The diagnosis was confirmed on the basis of ascitic fluid Gram's stain, culture, or both. Blood cultures were positive in 60% of cases. Organisms implicated included E. coli (7 cases), Klebsiella species (3 cases), S. pneumoniae (2 cases), S. faecalis (2 cases), and an alpha streptococcus (1 case).

4. Weinstein MP, Iannini PB, Stratton CW, Eickoff TC: Spontaneous bacterial peritonitis. Am J Med 64:592, 1978.
    Retrospective review of 28 episodes in 25 patients, all with confirmed or presumed cirrhosis. Clinical and laboratory features were similar to those previously reported; mortality was lower, although still substantial (57%). Markers of a poor outcome included increasing encephalopathy, more than 85% granulocytes in blood or ascitic fluid, total bilirubin >8.0 mg/dl, and serum albumin <2.5 gm/dl.

5. Epstein M, Calia F, Gabuzda GJ: Pneumococcal peritonitis in patients with postnecrotic cirrhosis. N Engl J Med 278:68, 1968.
    Six episodes in five patients are described. Three of the patients were children, but all had documented cirrhosis.

6. Kline MM, McCallum HW, Paul HG: The clinical value of ascitic fluid culture and leukocyte count studies in alcoholic cirrhosis. Gastroenterology 70:408, 1976.
    A prospective study of ascitic fluid cell counts and culture results in 63 consecutive male patients with alcoholic cirrhosis. Ascitic fluid cultures were positive in 5 cases, all associated with a peritoneal fluid pleocytosis of >300 WBC/mm³; however, this value was exceeded in 50% of 58 culture negative cases, with differential counts of 2–98% PMN leukocytes.

7. Conn HO: Spontaneous bacterial peritonitis: Multiple revisitations. Gastroenterology 70:455, 1976.
   Editorial response to the last reference cited, stressing the potential problems in interpreting such data.

8. Gerding DN, Hall WH, Schierl EA: Antibiotic concentrations in ascitic fluid of patients with ascites and bacterial peritonitis. Ann Intern Med 86:708, 1977.
   Good penetration into ascitic fluid by eight different antibiotics was demonstrated. Ascitic fluid antibiotic concentration exceeded 50% of the concurrent serum level in 31 of 36 cases.

9. Hoefs JC, Canawati HN, Sapico FL, Weiner J, Montgomerie JZ: Spontaneous bacterial peritonitis. Hepatology 2:399, 1982.
   Retrospective review of 43 cases, all with positive peritoneal fluid cultures and pleocytosis >250 PMN leukocytes/mm³. Clinical features were similar to those of previous studies. Single organisms were identified in 38 cases and multiple organisms in 5. Gram negative aerobic bacilli accounted for 32 and gram positive aerobic streptococci for 14 of 50 isolates; Staphylococcus aureus (1 isolate) and anaerobic species (3 isolates) accounted for the remainder. Twenty-six of forty-three patients survived the episode of SBP, but only thirteen survived the hospitalization. A rapid demise was correlated with acute liver disease, hepatomegaly, serum creatinine >2.1 mg/dl, serum bilirubin >8.0 mg/dl, and WBC >25000/mm³.

10. Gitlin N, Stauffer JL, Silvestri RC: The pH of ascitic fluid in the diagnosis of spontaneous bacterial peritonitis in alcoholic cirrhosis. Hepatology 2:408, 1982.
    Study of ascitic fluid characteristics in a population of 56 male alcoholics with cirrhosis and ascites. Six patients with culture-proven SBP were found to have a mean peritoneal fluid pH of 7.25 (7.12–7.31), with concurrent blood pH of 7.47. Those without SBP had both peritoneal fluid and blood pH of 7.47 (7.39–7.58).

11. Targan SR, Chow AW, Guze LB: Role of anaerobic bacteria in spontaneous bacterial peritonitis of cirrhosis. Am J Med 62:397, 1977.
    Two case reports and review of the literature. Stresses the infrequent occurrence of anaerobic bacteria ascites in SBP (6% of 128 cases reviewed). Anaerobic infection is more commonly polymicrobial and less commonly associated with bacteremia than is SBP caused by aerobic organisms.

12. Wilcox CM, Dismukes WE: Spontaneous bacterial peritonitis. A review of pathogenesis, diagnosis, and treatment. Medicine (Baltimore) 66:447, 1987.
    Excellent review of previously published studies with especially cogent critique of diagnostic criteria and straightforward treatment recommendations.

Tetanus

James J. Heffernan, M.D.

Tetanus is a life-threatening neurologic disorder caused by an exotoxin produced by vegetative forms of *Clostridium tetani*, a ubiquitous, anaerobic, motile, spore-forming gram positive bacillus. Major clinical features of the disease include local or generalized muscular rigidity; severe generalized spasms; frequent autonomic disturbances, especially of the sympathetic system; and, less commonly, neuromuscular blockade most apparent in cranial nerve territories. The case fatality rate was as high as 76% before the availability of antitoxin; even with aggressive supportive care, antibiotics, and the use of antitoxin, mortality may reach 40%, although more recent intensive treatment regimens have yielded survival rates as high as 90%.[3,6,7] Asphyxiation was a common cause of death in the past. Most tetanus deaths in the United States at present result from primary cardiac arrest or other autonomic disturbances, or from secondary complications, especially infections.[3,7,9,10] There have been several reports of striking improvements in survival without intensive care measures in medically indigent areas with the administration of intrathecal antitoxin early in the disease course.[12,13]

Tetanus is largely a disease of undeveloped and developing nations, with as many as 500,000 cases worldwide annually, many of these in the neonatal setting with an attendant mortality rate of 60%.[1] Males predominate in nearly all series. In recent years, the incidence of reported tetanus in the United States has stabilized at a rate of 75–100 cases/year, primarily as a result of active immunization programs, better neonatal care, and shifts in population away from high-risk occupations and settings.[1,8,14] Parenteral drug abusers and the elderly are heavily represented in the current domestic case load, the former on the basis of contaminated drugs or equipment with the development of mixed subcutaneous infections, and the latter as a result of inadequate or absent immunization or of waning immunity.[3,4,14] The overall case-fatality ratio for cases of tetanus in the United States remains in excess of 25%, with most fatalities occurring in those over age 50.[14]

Tetanus occurs as a result of contamination of devitalized tissue by *C. tetani* or its spores, most commonly in the setting of trauma, burns, or as a complication of gut-associated surgical problems or their treatment. Fecal contamination of wounds may arise from endogenous or exogenous sources; the injury itself may be trivial and in more than 20% of recent cases none is identified. Postoperative tetanus has been described following gastrectomy, appendectomy, bowel resection, hemorrhoidectomy, snare removal of polyps, and rubber band ligation of internal hemorrhoids, and as a complication of anorectal abscess.[5] Tetanus has also been reported as a complication of chronic otitis media and cutaneous ulcers. *C. tetani* and its spores are found widely in nature, especially in the soil of warm agricultural areas, but also in the stool of many species, including humans, and prominently in that of larger domesticated animals. Spores have been found in heroin and in house and operating room dust.[2] The vegetative form of the organism is susceptible to heat, antiseptics, and antibiotics; the spores are much more resistant to physical measures and may survive for years when not exposed to light or high heat.

Introduction of the organism, usually in its spore form, into an environment of low oxidation-reduction potential, as in devitalized tissue or an abscess, results in growth and elaboration of both a clinically unimportant hemolysin, tetanolysin, and tetanospasmin, a protein neurotoxin that is, with the exception of botulinum toxin, the most potent poison ever identified, fatal for a variety of mammalian species, including humans, at a total dose as low as .00001–.0001 mg. This toxin is totally responsible for the clinical manifestations of tetanus. In light of the ubiquity of the organism and the potency of its toxin, there is no herd immunity; protection is achieved only with active individual immunization. Table 1 provides tetanus prophylaxis and prevention recommendations.[1,8]

The incubation period from introduction of the organism to onset of symptoms is generally 3–21 days but may be as short as 24 hours with heavy fecal contamination or head wounds or many weeks with a small inoculum in a marginally oxygenated site. Toxin produced locally binds to motor nerve terminals near the site of toxin production and disseminates hematogenously to bind to similar sites throughout the body. The toxin is incorporated into motor nerve terminals, where it inhibits acetylcholine release with the production of some degree of neuromuscular blockade. It is transported in retrograde fashion up the motor axon and into the CNS, where it produces its major clinical effect after crossing to postsynaptic inhibitory neurons in

Table 1. TETANUS IMMUNIZATION

Children less than 7 years of age: DTP at 6 weeks of age or older, with two subsequent doses each at 4–8 week intervals; fourth dose 1 year after the third; booster dose at 4–6 years of age or prior to entering school unless fourth primary dose administered after fourth birthday; Td booster every 10 years thereafter.

Persons 7 years of age and older: Td at first visit, repeated in 4–8 weeks, and then again in 6–12 months; Td booster every 10 years thereafter.

Wound Prophylaxis

Immunization History	Clean Minor Wounds		Other Wounds	
(number of doses)	Td	TIG	Td	TIG
0, 1, or unknown	Yes	No	Yes	Yes
2	Yes	No	Yes	No*
3 or more	No†	No	No‡	No

*Yes, if wound more than 24 hours old.
†Yes, if more than 10 years since last dose.
‡Yes, if more than 5 years since last dose.
DTP = tetanus and diphtheria toxoids and pertussis vaccine absorbed (for pediatric use); Td = tetanus and diphtheria toxoids adsorbed (for adult use); TIG = human tetanus immune globulin.

the spinal cord and brain stem with the subsequent inhibition of glycine release. Motor activity is thus grossly disinhibited, with the subsequent development clinically of rigidity, loss of fine control, and intense generalized spasms of sufficient magnitude to fracture bones and cause asphyxia. The term "tetanic seizure" refers to the most severe generalized spasms with universal recruitment of skeletal muscles. Toxin enters the spinal cord and brain stem most quickly via the shortest and most metabolically active motor neurons, which in fact explains the nearly uniform early appearance of trismus and dysphagia. A similar pattern of interference with inhibitory neurons at the spinal cord level is postulated as the basis for the frequently observed autonomic (especially sympathetic) lability, manifested clinically in wide fluctuations in both pulse and blood pressure, tachydysrhythmias, asystolic cardiac arrests, abnormal sweating patterns, altered bowel and bladder function, and fever even in paralyzed individuals.[1,9,10,15] Increased urinary catecholamines have been frequently described. The toxin also binds to gangliosides throughout the CNS with possible contribution to the various clinical features. The pathologic findings variably reported in brain stem structures of those succumbing to the disease have not clearly been linked to direct effects of toxin; those recovering generally do so completely, although persistent autonomic lability has been described many months after the fact.

Although 80% of tetanus patients develop generalized disease, two clinical variants are recognized: (1) localized tetanus with rigidity and spasm confined to a limited motor distribution, usually one extremity; and (2) cephalic tetanus manifested in cranial nerve dysfunction, which often evolves into severe generalized disease.[1,2,6,7] The former syndrome is felt to represent the disease process in a patient with some level of antibody protection (sufficient to preclude hematogenous spread of toxin), and the latter is believed to reflect the early neuromuscular blockade in a patient with a cephalic source of toxin, as in otitis media.

Tetanus remains a diagnosis made largely on clinical grounds; culture confirms the presence of C. tetani in only 30% of instances. The differential diagnosis includes a number of serious conditions, most rapidly distinguishable from tetanus: hypocalcemic or hypomagnesemic tetany; meningitis; seizures; intracranial catastrophes, especially hemorrhage, with posturing; retroperitoneal hemorrhage; and drug or withdrawal phenomena, especially dystonic reactions associated with major tranquilizers. An extremely important mimic of tetanus among parenteral drug abusers is strychnine poisoning, which indeed produces motor disinhibition at the same spinal interneurons but by the different mechanism of receptor blockade. A variety of local processes, mostly infectious, can produce simple trismus.

TREATMENT

The treatment of tetanus hinges on aggressive supportive care. The lowest case fatality rates are reported from centers that deal regularly with the disease and recognize early on the need for airway control and paralysis in moderate and severe cases.[6,7] By general accord, mild disease is defined by muscular rigidity; moderate disease by the onset of dysphagia and tolerable spasms; and severe disease by the presence of overwhelming, uncontrollable, generalized reflex spasms. A short incubation period and a short period of onset, defined as the time between earliest symptoms and the first major spasm, are both relatively sensitive but not specific markers of severe disease.[1,7]

The most effective regimens base treatment on a rapid and ongoing assessment of severity of disease. Milder cases are closely observed and administered sedative and muscle relaxant medications. Although barbiturates, both short and long acting, were the mainstay of therapy in older series, they have been supplanted largely by diazepam and chlorpromazine administered either orally or, more commonly, parenterally in representative doses of 2–20 mg IV q2–6h and 25–100 mg IV q6h, respectively. The onset of dysphagia presages the considerable risks of asphyxiation and aspiration; intubation or tracheostomy is mandated as quickly as possible, with mechanical ventilation given if spasms or sedative medications interfere with respiratory function. In the setting of severe disease with uncontrollable spasms, pharmacologic paralysis supersedes the use of sedative-muscle relaxants. Both D-tubocurarine and pancuronium have been used effectively, the former with some theoretic advantage because of the risk of exacerbating hypertension and tachycardia with pancuronium.

All patients with tetanus and identified wounds should undergo débridement of devitalized tissue, preferably after receipt of antitoxin. Antibiotics effective against the vegetative forms of C. tetani are routinely administered for 10–14 days, although this is clearly adjunctive to the major thrust of treating the intoxication. Recommended antibiotic regimens include (1) procaine penicillin G 1.2 million U IM qd, (2) aqueous penicillin G 1.0 million units IV q3–6h, (3) erythromycin 500 mg IV q6h, and (4) tetracycline 500 mg IV q6h. At least one study has shown metronidazole to be superior to procaine penicillin.[16] Antitoxin should be administered as early in the disease course as possible. Various studies have suggested no further benefit from doses greater than 500 U of human tetanus immunoglobulin (TIG), although 1000–3000 U IM is the dosage range most commonly recommended. Passive immunization should be repeated every 3 weeks until resolution of disease. Several reports have described striking benefits from the early intrathecal and intracisternal administration of TIG, presumably by preventing fixation of toxin at the most critical sites within the spinal cord and brain stem.[12,13] All patients should receive active immunization with 0.5 ml adsorbed toxoid IM at a location remote from that used for antitoxin.

The management of the often severe associated autonomic disturbances remains somewhat controversial. Intensive care unit observation and monitoring are essential. Sympathetic blocking agents (both alpha and beta), especially propranolol, have proved effective in the management of persistent hypertension and tachycardia; however, patients have frequently demonstrated marked spontaneous lability in sympathetic tone, which reinforces the need for extremely close monitoring after any intervention.[9,10] One case report has described impressive sustained improvement in sympathetic hyperactivity with the administration of high-dose parenteral morphine sulfate, presumably by attenuating central sympathetic efferent outflow.[11] Epidural blockade with bupivacaine has also been shown to be effective in reducing autonomic hyperactivity in isolated cases.[15]

In the management of severe cases of tetanus, paralysis may need to be sustained for up to 4 weeks and full recovery generally takes several months. Complications include cardiopulmonary arrest, long bone and vertebral fractures, rhabdomyolysis, aberrations in fluid and electrolyte homeostasis, decubitus ulcers, contractures, tracheal hemorrhage, thromboembolic disease, malnutrition, and pulmonary and urinary tract infection; much of this morbidity can be prevented, minimized, or effectively treated with intensive supportive care.

One must remember that tetanus is an entirely preventable disease; attention should be directed toward establishing or reinforcing immunization among adults as well as among children.[14]

KEY FEATURES

All clinical features result from effects of neurotoxin.

Short incubation period and short period of onset presage worse disease.

Most cases are of generalized tetanus (80–92%).

All patients should receive human tetanus immunoglobulin, wound débridement, active immunization, and antibiotics.

Treatment is otherwise predicated on severity of clinical features:

1. Mild (muscular rigidity): muscle relaxants, sedatives.

2. Moderate (dysphagia, mild spasms): as for mild disease; also, tracheostomy and, as needed, mechanical ventilation.

3. Severe (uncontrollable, general spasms): as for moderate disease; also, pharmacologic paralysis.

Features of sympathetic hyperactivity may occur with any level of disease but usually with severe cases; require strict monitoring and may respond with adrenergic blockers or morphine sulfate.

Mortality can be limited to 10% with aggressive management.

Tetanus is totally preventable with adequate active immunization.

REFERENCES

1. Martin RR: Clostridium tetani (tetanus). *In* Mandell GL, Douglas RG, Bennett JE (eds): Principles and Practice of Infectious Diseases, 2nd ed. New York, John Wiley and Sons, 1985, pp 1355–1359.
   Comprehensive and well-referenced chapter with limited discussion of treatment.

2. Weinstein L: Tetanus. N Engl J Med 289:1293, 1973.
   Good review of clinical features. Details of pathophysiology and management have been better elucidated subsequently.

3. Faust RA, Vickers OR, Cohn I: Tetanus: 2,449 cases in 68 years at Charity Hospital. J Trauma 16:704, 1976.
   Retrospective review. Mean age of incidence increased from 25 to 40 years over period of study, with persistent although less pronounced male preponderance. Neonatal tetanus was not seen in later years. Case fatality rate among more recent cases (1967–1974) was 58%; cause of death was respiratory failure in 7 of 14 fatal cases, cardiac arrest in 5, and massive tracheal hemorrhage in 2.

4. Heurich AE, Brust JC, Richter RW: Management of urban tetanus. Med Clin North Am 57:1373, 1973.
   Detailed treatment recommendations based on experience with 48 parenteral drug abusers with tetanus at Kings County and Harlem Hospitals. The authors stress the nearly uniform occurrence of severe disease among this population.

5. Myers KJ, Heppell J, Bode WE, et al: Tetanus after anorectal abscess. Mayo Clinic Proc 59:429, 1984.
   Case report of tetanus as a sequela of an aerobic-anaerobic synergistic perineal infection following incision and drainage of an anorectal abscess. Referenced discussion of tetanus complicating other surgical settings.

6. Trujillo MJ, Castillo A, Espana JV, et al: Tetanus in the adult: Intensive care and management experience with 233 cases. Crit Care Med 8:419, 1980.
   Venezuelan series of 233 cases that accounted for 10.4% of admissions to a university hospital ICU during the study period (1969–1979). Age range was 5–75 years, with 2:1 male predominance; 2.5% mild, 5.5% moderate, 92% severe disease; 60% developed autonomic hyperactivity. Excellent results of aggressive management regimen were reported, with case fatality rate of only 11%; cardiac arrest and sepsis each accounted for over 35% of fatalities. Average length of stay in the ICU was 21.7 days.

7. Edmondson RS, Flowers MW: Intensive care in tetanus: Management, complications, and mortality in 100 cases. Br Med J 1:1401, 1979.
   Article describes ICU experience (1964–1977) at a British regional referral unit for tetanus. This is an excellent review of clinical features and aggressive management. Adequate primary immunization was documented in only two patients, neither of whom received a toxoid booster with injury. Ninety patients required paralysis for up to 44 days (avg. 21 days), and 93 underwent tracheostomy. Noteworthy sympathetic hyperactivity was noted in 21 cases. Case fatality rate in the ICU was only 8%, with deaths resulting

from pulmonary infection, cardiac arrest, GI hemorrhage, tension pneumothorax, and anaphylaxis.

8. Immunization Practices Advisory Committee, Centers for Disease Control: Diphtheria, tetanus, and pertussis: Guidelines for vaccine prophylaxis and other preventive measures. Ann Intern Med 95:723, 1981.
   Detailed CDC guidelines including recommendations for primary tetanus immunization and wound prophylaxis.

9. Kerr JH, Corbett JL, Prys-Roberts C, et al: Involvement of the sympathetic nervous system in tetanus. Lancet 2:236, 1968.
   Retrospective review of selected clinical features in a series of 82 patients with tetanus. A syndrome of sympathtic hyperactivity and instability is described, manifested in labile hypertension and tachycardia, dysrhythmias, vascular constriction, sweating, pyrexia, and increased urinary catecholamines; four fatal cases attributed to same.

10. Tsueda K, Olvier PB, Richter RW: Cardiovascular manifestations of tetanus. Anesthesiology 40:588, 1974.
    General discussion of the sympathetic hyperactivity seen in tetanus with brief report of features of nine cases, all in drug addicts. Article emphasizes the extreme lability of this syndrome.

11. Rie MA, Wilson RS: Morphine therapy controls autonomic hyperactivity in tetanus. Ann Intern Med 88:653, 1978.
    Case report describing impressive response of hypertension, tachycardia, and hypoperfusion to high-dose morphine sulfate infusion after failure of alpha blockade (phentolamine). Beta blockers were not used because of low cardiac output.

12. Gupta PS, Kapoor R, Goyal S, et al: Intrathecal human tetanus immunoglobulin in early tetanus. Lancet 2:439, 1980.
    Indian study of 97 patients presenting with mild tetanus who received standard supportive care and human tetanus immune globulin (TIG) either 250 IU intrathecally or 1000 IU intramuscularly. Of 49 patients treated with intrathecal TIG, disease progressed in 3 (6%) and 1 (2%) died; of the 48 patients who received TIG intramuscularly, disease progressed in 15 (31%) and 10 (21%) died.

13. Sanders RK, Joseph R, Martyn B, et al: Intrathecal antitetanus serum (horse) in the treatment of tetanus. Lancet 1:974, 1977.
    Comparison of conservative standard care versus the same care plus intrathecal antitetanus immunoglobulin (horse) at either of two doses in a single blind prospective trial of 322 cases at a rural Indian hospital. Pharmacologic paralysis and tracheostomy were not performed. Overall case fatality rate for controls was 14.5%, whereas that for all patients receiving intrathecal TIG was 7% and that for the lower dose of TIG was 4.5%, the differences from control significant at the $p < .05$ and $p < .01$ levels, respectively.

14. Centers for Disease Control (CDC): Tetanus—United States, 1985–1986. MMWR 36:477, 1987.
    Limited description of 147 cases, 71% in persons $\geq$ age 50. An identified acute injury was noted in 71% of cases, with a median incubation period for those with a known date of injury of 7 days. The case-fatality ratio was 31% overall, 42% for those $\geq$ age 50, and 5% for those $<$ 50 years of age.

15. Southorn PA, Blaise GA: Treatment of tetanus-induced autonomic nervous system dysfunction with continuous epidural blockade. Crit Care Med 14:251, 1986.
    Case report.

16. Ahmadsyah I, Salim A: Treatment of tetanus: An open study to compare the efficacy of procaine penicillin and metronidazole. Br Med J 2:648, 1985.

Prospective, nonrandomized clinical trial comparing procaine penicillin and metronidazole in the treatment of moderate tetanus among 173 patients. The groups were comparable by a number of parameters befroe treatment. The case-fatality ratio for those treated with metronidazole was 7%; for those treated with penicillin 24% (p<.01).

Toxic Shock Syndrome

M. Anita Barry, M.D.

Toxic shock syndrome (TSS) is an acute, potentially fatal multisystem disorder associated with *Staphylococcus aureus*. A syndrome similar to TSS has been described since 1927 under a variety of names, including staphylococcal scarlet fever syndrome. Following a 1978 report on a series of cases in children, increased surveillance activity revealed a prominent association between the occurrence of TSS and menstruation.[1] Further studies have shown that TSS is most commonly reported in young white menstruating females. Of 2815 cases reported to the Centers for Disease Control as of June 1, 1985, 2669 occurred in females.[2] Although a majority of all cases were menstrually associated, the proportion of nonmenstrual cases increased from 7% in 1980 to 27% in 1984. Use of tampons, particularly high absorbency brands, appears to increase risk in menstrually associated cases.[3] However, whether risk can be decreased by using tampons only intermittently is unresolved.[3,4] Nonmenstrual TSS cases have been almost invariably associated with *S. aureus* infections at various sites, including surgical wound infections, focal cutaneous and subcutaneous lesions, deep abscesses, adenitis, bursitis, primary bacteremias, and postpartum infections.[5]

Data from various studies suggest that toxigenic strains of *S. aureus* play a prominent role in the pathogenesis of TSS. Staphylococci have been isolated from menstruating TSS patients at significantly increased rates compared with those found in a healthy population.[6,7] In addition, most nonmenstrual cases have had *S. aureus* isolates recovered.[5] Initial studies identified two toxins, exotoxin C and enterotoxin F, felt to play a significant role in pathogenesis. Exotoxin C was characterized by its ability to induce fever and increase host susceptibility to endotoxin. Enterotoxin F produced hypotension; ascites; rash; conjunctival erythema; and muscle, kidney, and liver abnormalities in laboratory animals.[7,8] These two toxins now have been shown to be identical and are known as toxic shock syndrome toxin-1.[8a] Although the exact pathogenesis of TSS remains unresolved, a leading hypothesis is that a blood-soaked tampon acts as a culture medium in an individual colonized with *S. aureus,* allowing for the proliferation of toxin-producing organisms. Systemic access for the toxin may be provided by cervical or mucosal ulcerations described as a consequence of tampon use.

Information on the clinical manifestations of TSS is based on cases severe enough to be included in epidemiologic surveys, but the occurrence of a milder form of the disease seems likely. Common presenting signs and symptoms include fever, hypotension, and a diffuse sunburn-like rash. In addition, myalgias, arthralgias, nonexudative mucous membrane inflammation (pharyngitis, conjunctivitis, vaginal hyperemia), and periarticular or periorbital edema may be noted. The skin rash typically results in full-thickness desquamation of the hands and feet 5–12 days after the rash has resolved. In addition, transient alopecia and nail loss have occurred. Vomiting and diarrhea, as well as nonfocal neurologic abnormalities, have also been described.[4,6,9] Laboratory findings include leukocytosis with an increase in immature forms, sterile pyuria, elevated prothrombin and partial thromboplastin times, hypocalcemia, low serum protein and albumin concentrations, elevated BUN and creatinine levels, liver enzyme abnormalities, and elevated bilirubin and creatine kinase levels. Mild anemia, thrombocytopenia, and hypophosphatemia have also been described.[4,6,9]

Long-term sequelae of TSS, in addition to skin desquamation and hair or nail loss, include chronic renal failure, late onset rash, and neuromuscular and neuropsychological abnormalities.[10,11] Recurrences in individual patients have clearly been documented but are probably decreasing in frequency as a consequence of increased antistaphylococcal antibiotic therapy and diminished tampon use.[1,4,6,9,12]

Treatment is mainly supportive. Large amounts of intravenous fluids (2.4–20 L over the first 24 hours) and vasopressors may be required to maintain blood pressure. Although antibiotics have not been shown to decrease the duration of illness, available evidence suggests that they may prevent disease recurrence.[1,9] A beta lactamase resistant semisynthetic penicillin is the drug of choice; a first-generation cephalosporin may also be considered. Vancomycin or clindamycin are alternatives for penicillin allergic patients. Prior to the beginning of antibiotic therapy, cultures from nares, vagina, cervix, blood, urine, and pharynx should be obtained on appropriate media with a specific request for *S. aureus* isolation. Possible foci of infection should be identified and removed (e.g., tampon) or drained (e.g., abscess). The benefit of irrigation with antiseptic solutions is unproved. Use of corticosteroids has been suggested, but supporting data are limited.[13]

KEY FEATURES

Toxic shock syndrome (TSS) is an acute, potentially fatal multisystem disorder associated with toxigenic strains of *Staphylococcus aureus.*

Toxic shock syndrome toxin-1 appears to play a major role in pathogenesis.

A majority of cases have been menstrually associated and have occurred in white patients.

Use of tampons, especially those of high absorbency, predisposes to the risk of developing TSS.

Nonmenstrual TSS cases have been associated with staphylococcal infection at a variety of sites.

Major clinical features include fever, hypotension, diffuse erythematous desquamating rash, nonexudative mucositis, myalgias, arthralgias, periarticular and periorbital edema, vomiting, diarrhea, and nonfocal neurologic abnormalities.

Laboratory abnormalities include leukocytosis with left shift; sterile pyuria; azotemia; coagulopathy; hypocalcemia; hypoproteinemia; hypophosphatemia; anemia; thrombocytopenia; and elevations in liver enzymes, bilirubin, and creatine kinase.

Treatment is supportive. Antibiotic use has not convincingly ameliorated the disease course but may reduce the rate of recurrence.

The case fatality rate in 1984 was 2.7%.

Sequelae have included renal failure, neuromuscular and neuropsychologic abnormalities, delayed rash, and hair and nail loss.

REFERENCES

1. Davis JP, Chesney PJ, Wand PJ, et al: Toxic shock syndrome: Epidemiologic features, recurrence, risk factors and prevention. New Engl J Med 303:1429–1435, 1980.
    In this early series of 38 TSS cases, 35 were menstrually associated and all occurred in whites. Use of beta lactamase resistant antibiotics resulted in lower recurrence rates. Results of a case control study on tampon and contraception use are also included.

2. Centers for Disease Control (CDC): Morbidity and Mortality Weekly Report, Annual summary 1984: 3, 9, 63, 64, 124, 125.
    Of 2815 cases reported to the CDC, a majority occurred in non-Hispanic whites and were menstrually associated. Case fatality rates ranged from 2.7% in 1984 to 4.7% in 1980.

3. Osterholm MT, Davis JP, Gibson RW, et al: Tri-state toxic shock syndrome study. I. Epidemiologic findings. J Infect Dis 145:431–440, 1982.
    This case control study matched 80 TSS cases with neighborhood controls to assess risk factors. Women using tampons had an 18 times increased risk of disease compared with nonusers. Risk was most closely associated with degree of tampon absorbency.

4. Shands KN, Schmid GP, Dan BB, et al: Toxic shock syndrome in menstruating women: Association with tampon use and Staphylococcus aureus and clinical features in 52 cases. N Engl J Med 303:1436–1442, 1980.
    In this retrospective case control study of women with TSS and controls who used tampons, the TSS patients were significantly more likely to use tampons continuously during menstruation. Fourteen of forty-four cases had one or more subsequent recurrences.

5. Reingold AL, Hargrett NT, Dan BB, et al: Nonmenstrual toxic shock syndrome: A review of 130 cases. Ann Intern Med 96 (suppl. part 2):871–874, 1982.
    Of 130 nonmenstrual TSS cases, the vast majority were associated with S. aureus infections at different sites. Nonmenstrual cases had clinical features similar to those of

the menstrual type, but demographic characteristics differed. Nonmenstrual cases occurred in a population that mirrored that of the United States as a whole.

6. Tofte RW, Williams DN: Clinical and laboratory manifestations of toxic shock syndrome. Ann Intern Med 96 (suppl. part 2):843–847, 1982.

   S. aureus was isolated in 13 of 19 vaginal cultures and in 8 of 12 cervical cultures obtained from 28 women with TSS. All isolates produced both exotoxin C and enterotoxin F.

7. Schlievert PM, Kelly JA: Staphylococcal pyrogenic exotoxin type C: Further characterization. Ann Intern Med 96 (suppl. part 2):982–986, 1982.

   Using blinded testing, exotoxin C could be detected in all of 44 S. aureus isolates from patients with TSS but only in 5 of 37 controls. Biologic characteristics of the toxin are described.

8. Vergeront JM, Stolz SJ, Cross BA: Prevalence of serum antibody to staphylococcal enterotoxin F among Wisconsin residents: Implications for toxic shock syndrome. J Infect Dis 148:692–698, 1983.

   The prevalence of antibody to enterotoxin F, considered to be a marker for the staphylococci causing TSS, was found to increase with advancing age. Characteristics of enterotoxin F are described.

8a. Bonventre PF, Weckbach L, Saneck J, et al: Production of staphylococcal enterotoxin F and pyrogenic exotoxin C by *Staphylococcus aureus* isolates from toxic shock syndrome–associated sources. Infect Immun 40:1023–1029, 1983.

   Using a variety of techniques, the authors demonstrated that enterotoxin F and exotoxin C appear to be the same protein.

9. Davis JP, Osterholm MT, Helms CM, et al: Tri-state toxic shock syndrome study. II. Clinical and laboratory findings. J Infect Dis 145:441–448, 1982.

   Clinical and laboratory results in a group of nonfatal TSS cases are described. In this series, only 44 of 54 vaginal/cervical isolates were positive for S. aureus, emphasizing that failure to isolate the organism does not rule out the diagnosis. The role of antibiotics and discontinuation of tampon use in decreasing risk of recurrence is discussed.

10. Chesney PJ, Crass BA, Polyak MB, et al: Toxic shock syndrome: Management and long-term sequelae. Ann Intern Med 96 (suppl. part 2):847–851, 1982.

    Dermatologic, neuromuscular, and renal sequelae observed in 36 patients are discussed.

11. Rosene KA, Copass MK, Kastner LS, et al: Persistent neuropsychological sequelae of toxic shock syndrome. Ann Intern Med 96 (suppl. part 2):865–870, 1982.

    Six of twelve women evaluated 2–12 months after recovery from TSS were found to have a variety of neurologic symptoms, including headache, memory lapses, and difficulty in concentrating. EEG abnormalities were found in five of these six. A possible direct effect of S. aureus toxin in the CNS is considered.

12. Helgerson SD, Mallery BL, Foster LR: Toxic shock syndrome in Oregon. JAMA 252:3402–3404, 1984.

    Fifty-three TSS cases followed for a total of 777 person-months revealed only one recurrence. The authors attribute this low rate to increased antibiotic use and infrequent resumption of tampon use among patients.

13. Todd JK, Ressman M, Caston SA, et al: Corticosteroid therapy for patients with toxic shock syndrome. JAMA 252:3399–3402, 1984.

    In this retrospective study of 45 TSS patients, those given steroids early in their course had a shorter duration of fever and more rapid return to clinical stability. However, no significant difference in death rate was observed between treated and untreated groups.

Endocarditis

Howard Libman, M.D.

Endocarditis, a potentially life-threatening illness with a variable and often nonspecific clinical presentation, is a relatively common disease, accounting for one of every thousand medical service admissions.[1-3] Men are more often affected than women, and the majority of patients are over 50 years old. Although a distinction is usually made between "acute" or "subacute" endocarditis, many pathogens can present in either fashion, and treatment and prognosis depend more upon the causative organism than upon the clinical presentation.

PATHOGENESIS AND ETIOLOGY

Experimental endocarditis[4] requires a platelet-fibrin deposit on the endothelial surface of the heart (nonbacterial thrombotic endocarditis [NBTE]) at the time of bacteremia. In the animal model, trauma, turbulence, or metabolic derangements may result in NBTE; in humans, cardiac abnormalities are often, but not always, clinically apparent. Bacteremia, usually the result of a defect in local skin or mucosal defenses, may be associated with dental procedures, surgery, or instrumentation; prophylactic antibiotic therapy[5] is usually recommended in these settings for patients with valvular disease, although there are few scientific data to demonstrate its efficacy. Many cases of endocarditis are not preceded by an invasive event and are probably the result of transient, low-grade, clinically occult bacteremias that occur in the normal host.

Of patients with a structural cardiac abnormality who develop endocarditis, rheumatic heart disease, although decreasing in prevalence as rheumatic fever has become less common, accounts for approximately 40% of cases. Congenital heart diseases, especially ventricular septal defect, patent ductus arteriosus, bicuspid aortic valve, coarctation of the aorta, and tetralogy of Fallot, compose about 20%. Degenerative cardiac lesions, such as calcified mitral annulus, atherosclerotic vascular disease, and mural thrombosis, are responsible for nearly 40%. Other risk factors include the presence of a prosthetic heart valve,[6] a dialysis access site, mitral valve prolapse[7] or idiopathic hypertrophic subaortic stenosis, and a history of intravenous drug abuse[8] or recent invasive procedure. The mitral valve is most commonly affected (especially in rheumatic heart disease), followed by the aortic valve and by a combination of the two. Right-sided endocarditis is unusual except in patients with a history of intravenous drug abuse, in whom it is present with or without left-sided disease over half the time.

Streptococci are responsible for approximately 60% of cases of endocarditis, the majority of which are caused by the viridans group, a diverse collection of organisms that are alpha hemolytic and originate from the mouth. Next most common are the enterococci,[9] which are usually from a genitourinary or gut source. Other streptococci that may result in endocarditis include nonenterococcal group D organisms (e.g., S. bovis), which have been associated with colonic malignancy, and, more rarely, S. pneumoniae and S. pyogenes. Staphylococci are responsible for about 20% of cases, with S. aureus,[10] usually arising from the skin, accounting for the vast majority; coagulase-negative staphylococci have become important pathogens in patients with prosthetic valves. Other causes of endocarditis include aerobic gram negative bacilli[11] (particularly in intravenous drug abusers, patients with prosthetic valves, and cirrhotics), fungi[12] (in intravenous drug abusers, patients with prosthetic valves, and those receiving hyperalimentation and/ or prolonged antibiotic therapy), miscellaneous other bacteria, and rickettsiae and chlamydiae. Approximately 10% of cases represent "culture-negative" endocarditis.[13]

HISTORY AND PHYSICAL EXAMINATION

The symptoms and signs are the result of several different pathophysiologic mechanisms.[14] Patients may present with clinical manifestations relating to infection on the valve itself (e.g., new onset aortic regurgitation), embolization (e.g., a new cerebrovascular accident[15] in left-sided endocarditis), metastatic infection (e.g., pleuritic chest pain and cough representing septic pulmonary emboli in right-sided disease), and/or an immunologic response to the infection[16] (e.g., immune complex glomerulonephritis).[17]

The most common symptoms are nonspecific and, in decreasing order of frequency, are fever, chills, generalized weakness, and musculoskeletal[18] and constitutional complaints; however, if specific organ systems are affected by one or more of the cited mechanisms, the presentation may be localized. Signs include fever (seen in about 90% of patients but sometimes absent in the elderly, in those with chronic illness, and in those receiving previous antibiotic therapy); a heart murmur (85%, but often a nonspecific flow murmur); a changing murmur (5–10%); a new murmur (3–5%, usually regurgitant); and a variety of skin manifestations (up to 50% of patients), including splinter hemorrhages (linear lesions in nailbeds), petechiae (present on conjunctivae, mucosal surfaces, and distal extremities), Osler's nodes (painful nodules on pads of fingers and toes representing septic embolization and/or immune complex deposition), and Janeway's lesions (painless hemorrhagic plaques on palms and soles resulting form septic embolization). Other embolic phenomena, mycotic aneurysms, Roth's spots (round retinal hemorrhages with central pallor), splenomegaly, clubbing, renal failure, and acute polyarticular arthritis may also be seen.

LABORATORY STUDIES

Anemia of chronic disease is common with subacute endocarditis, whereas a leukocytosis and/or a leftward shift is seen more often with acute disease. Other nonspecific findings may include an elevated erythrocyte sedimentation rate, hypergammaglobulinemia, hypocomplementemia, the presence of circulating immune complexes, cryoglobulinemia, and a positive rheumatoid factor and other collagen-vascular and syphilis serologic results. Urinalysis is frequently abnormal, with microscopic analysis revealing erythrocytes, leukocytes, casts, and/or bacteria. The electrocardiogram is unremarkable except when septic involvement (progressive conduction system abnormalities) or pericarditis (ST segment elevation) occurs. The chest radiograph is normal unless congestive heart failure or septic pulmonary emboli (diffuse nodular lesions that eventually cavitate) are present.

Because the bacteremia of endocarditis is generally continuous, two sets of blood cultures from separate venipuncture sites over a short period of time will permit isolation of the etiologic agent in at least 90% of cases.[19] The yield is not significantly enhanced by obtaining more than three to four sets unless the patient has received prior antibiotic therapy. Echocardiography[20] is not a highly sensitive test for detecting vegetations and is not often useful in diagnosing or ruling out endocarditis. Its main utility is in the diagnosis of culture-negative endocarditis or in determining whether surgical intervention might be necessary (e.g., looking for large vegetations, aortic regurgitation, perivalvular abscess), but these issues are usually decided primarily on other clinical grounds.

DIAGNOSIS

If the presentation of endocarditis is acute, the patient will generally appear ill enough to require admission, and a presumptive diagnosis can be made on the basis of positive blood cultures in the appropriate clinical setting. However, if the presentation is subacute, the patient will often delay days to weeks before seeing a physician. The symptoms may be exclusively constitutional and the physical examination unremarkable. Because of the lack of sensitive and specific manifestations, the early diagnosis of endocarditis requires a high degree of clinical suspicion. The diagnosis should be considered in patients with a febrile illness of greater than 1 week's duration without localizing symptoms or signs, particularly in the context of underlying cardiac valvular disease. Patients with positive blood cultures, underlying valvular disease, and no evidence of primary localized infection elsewhere are likely to have the disease; patients with positive blood cultures and a new regurgitant heart murmur and/or embolic phenomena are very likely to have it.

The differential diagnosis of endocarditis is large and includes a variety of systemic infections (e.g., infectious mononucleosis, hepatitis B, tuberculosis, secondary syphilis, disseminated gonococcal infection), collagen-vascular diseases (e.g., systemic lupus erythematosus, rheumatoid arthritis), serum-sickness–like illnesses (secondary to medications or intravenous drugs), atrial myxoma, acute rheumatic fever, and dissecting aortic aneurysm with regurgitation. True culture-negative endocarditis, although unusual, should be considered in the following settings: (1) prior administration of antibiotic therapy;[21] (2) infection with fastidious, slow-growing, or unusual organisms (such as nutritionally deficient streptococci, anaerobes, brucella, mycobacteria, fungi, rickettsiae, and chlamydiae); and (3) subacute or chronic disease involving only the right side of the heart.

INITIAL MANAGEMENT

Patients with possible endocarditis should be admitted to the hospital, cultured as described previously, and observed clinically. If the patient has taken oral antibiotics, additional blood cultures should be obtained during the first several days after admission and antibiotic therapy should be held if possible; the addition of penicillinase to blood culture bottles and/or the use of blood cultures with a resin that binds antibiotics may be useful in this setting. Empirical antibiotic therapy is indicated in patients who appear toxic, in those with a new regurgitant murmur; and in patients with evidence of cardiac decompensation, major systemic embolization, or metastatic infection.

Initial therapy should include a semisynthetic penicillin, such as oxacillin, given intravenously in maximal doses. If there is a history of genitourinary or bowel manipulation, coverage should be directed at the enterococcus (e.g., penicillin and an aminoglycoside). In patients who are allergic to penicillin and in patients with prosthetic valves, vancomycin is substituted. Empirical antibiotic therapy of patients with a history of intravenous drug abuse should be based upon the epidemiology of the local area. Once blood culture results are available, therapy should be made specific based upon disk sensitivity results and minimum inhibitory/bactericidal concentrations; serum cidal levels[22] and antibiotic levels may be useful adjunctively.[23] Clinical response to appropriate therapy is usually gradual, occurring over 3–7 days. In patients with complications,[24] such as congestive heart failure, major embolic disease, or mycotic aneurysm, and in patients with prosthetic valves, early surgical intervention is often necessary.[25] Although diuretics and/or digitalis are useful in the management of congestive heart failure, the use of anticoagulation in the treatment of embolic disease is controversial.

KEY FEATURES

Endocarditis often presents nonspecifically and should be considered in the differential diagnosis of any patient, particularly one with underlying valvular disease or other risk factor, who has fever without a clear source.

Common symptoms include:
- Fever, chills
- Generalized weakness
- Musculoskeletal and constitutional complaints
  Common signs include:
- Fever
- Cardiac murmur (infrequently changing or regurgitant)
- Skin manifestations (including splinter hemorrhages, petechiae, Osler's nodes, and Janeway's lesions)
- Splenomegaly, clubbing in longstanding disease

CLINICAL FEATURES OF ENDOCARDITIS ACCORDING TO PATHOGEN

Pathogen	Important Settings*	valv	Clinical Manifestations† emb	met	imm	Treatment‡	Prognosis
Viridans strep	1,2	+	+/−	−	+	pcn +/− strep	Excellent
Enterococci	1,3	+	+/−	−	+	pcn/amino	Fair
S. aureus	4,5	+	+	+	+/−	semi pcn	Variable
Coagulase-negative staph	6	+	+/−	−	+/−	Vancomycin	Fair
Enteric gram negative rods	1,5,6	+	+	−	+/−	lact/amino	Fair
Fungi	1,5,6,7	+	+	+/−	+/−	ampho/valve	Poor

*1 = underlying valvular disease; 2 = dental manipulation; 3 = genitourinary or pelvic surgery; 4 = dermatitis, cellulitis, or intravascular line; 5 = intravenous drug abuse; 6 = prosthetic valve; 7 = hyperalimentation, antibiotic therapy.

†valv = valvular dysfunction, emb = major embolic disease, met = metastatic infection, imm = immunopathologic phenomena.

‡pcn = penicillin, strep = streptomycin, amino = aminoglycoside, semi pcn = semisynthetic penicillin, lact = beta-lactam antibiotic, ampho = amphotericin B.

Initial laboratory studies in a patient with possible endocarditis should consist of:
- Complete blood and differential counts
- Urinalysis, electrocardiogram, and chest radiograph
- Three to four sets of blood cultures taken over a short period of time from separate venipuncture sites
  Differential diagnosis of endocarditis includes:
- Other systemic infections (mononucleosis, hepatitis, tuberculosis, syphilis, disseminated gonococcal infection)
- Collagen-vascular diseases (systemic lupus erythematosus, rheumatoid arthritis)
- Serum-sickness–like illnesses (secondary to medications or drug abuse)
- Other cardiovascular diseases (atrial myxoma, acute rheumatic fever, dissecting aortic aneurysm)
  Initial management of a patient with suspected endocarditis should consist of:
- Empirical antibiotic therapy directed against the most likely pathogen(s) if there is systemic toxicity or evidence of valvular dysfunction, embolic disease, or metastatic infection
- Early surgical consultation in the presence of congestive heart failure, major embolic disease, progressive conduction system abnormalities, mycotic aneurysm, or prosthetic valve

REFERENCES

1. Pelletier LL, Petersdorf RG: Infective endocarditis: A review of 125 cases from the University of Washington Hospitals, 1963–72. Medicine 56:287, 1977.
   Comprehensive review of experience at urban medical center. Many patients had a history of intravenous drug abuse, had a prosthetic valve, or were referred for acute congestive heart failure. S. aureus was the most common pathogen, complications were frequent, and mortality was high (37%).

2. Van Reyn CF, et al: Infective endocarditis: An analysis based on strict case definitions. Ann Intern Med 94:505, 1981.
   Formal case definitions for "definite," "probable," and "possible" endocarditis are described. Compared with earlier studies, patients were older, underlying valvular disease more common, and mortality lower.

3. Kaye D: Changing pattern of infective endocarditis. Am J Med 78(suppl 6B):157, 1985.
   Discussion of trends in endocarditis. Degenerative cardiac disease and prosthetic valves are becoming increasingly common risk factors.

4. Freedman LR, Valone J: Experimental infective endocarditis. Prog Card Dis 22:169, 1979.
   Description of experimental model in rabbits.

5. Durack DT: Current issues in prevention of infective endocarditis. Am J Med 78 (suppl 6B):149, 1985.
   Newly revised, simplified recommendations for antibiotic prophylaxis are presented.

6. Wilson WR, Danielson GK, Giuliani ER, Geraci JE: Prosthetic valve endocarditis. Mayo Clinic Proc 57:155, 1982.

Endocarditis occurred in 2% of patients with prosthetic valves. Staphylococci were the most common pathogens in early-onset disease, and streptococci in late-onset. Overall mortality rate was 59%.

7. Clemens JD, et al: A controlled evaluation of the risk of bacterial endocarditis in persons with mitral-valve prolapse. N Engl J Med 307:776, 1982.
    Patients with mitral valve prolapse are at increased risk for endocarditis compared with the rest of the population, but the absolute risk appears small.

8. Reisberg BE: Infective endocarditis in the narcotic addict. Prog Card Dis 22:193, 1979.
    Review. Affected population is young, right-sided involvement is frequent, and prognosis is better than in nonaddicts. Important pathogens include S. aureus, aerobic gram negative bacilli, and fungi; there is considerable local variation in bacteriology.

9. Wilkowske CJ: Enterococcal endocarditis. Mayo Clinic Proc 57:101, 1982.
    Enterococcal endocarditis is seen following genitourinary or pelvic manipulation. Clinical presentation is variable; treatment is with penicillin and an aminoglycoside.

10. Thompson RL: Staphylococcal infective endocarditis. Mayo Clinic Proc 57:106, 1982.
    Review of diagnosis and management.

11. Cohen PS, Maguire JH, Weinstein L: Infective endocarditis caused by gram-negative bacteria: A review of the literature, 1945–1977. Prog Card Dis 22:205, 1980.
    Comprehensive review. A relatively uncommon cause of endocarditis but less so than in the past. Treatment is often problematic, and valve replacement is sometimes necessary.

12. Rubinstein E, et al: Fungal endocarditis: Analysis of 24 cases and review of the literature. Medicine 54:331, 1975.
    Comprehensive review. Candida species are the most common pathogen. Treatment consists of amphotericin B and valve replacement, but prognosis is poor.

13. Van Scoy RE: Culture-negative endocarditis. Mayo Clinic Proc 57:149, 1982.
    Review of differential diagnosis and evaluation of patients. Survival is excellent if patient becomes afebrile within a week, but poor (50%) if fever persists longer.

14. Hermans PE: The clinical manifestations of infective endocarditis. Mayo Clinic Proc 57:15, 1982.
    Review of various clinical presentations.

15. Jones HR, Siekert RG, Geraci JE: Neurologic manifestations of bacterial endocarditis. Ann Intern Med 71:21, 1969.
    Neurologic symptoms were common and resulted from embolic cerebrovascular accidents, transient ischemic attacks, toxic encephalopathy, and meningitis.

16. Phair JP, Clarke J: Immunology of infective endocarditis. Prog Card Dis 22:137, 1979.
    Review of immunologic response in endocarditis.

17. Neugarten J, Baldwin DS: Glomerulonephritis in endocarditis. Am J Med 77:297, 1984.
    Review of clinical and morphologic features.

18. Churchill MA, Geraci JE, Hunder GG: Musculoskeletal manifestations of bacterial endocarditis. Ann Intern Med 87:754, 1977.
    Musculoskeletal complaints were common, and included arthralgias, arthritis, low back pain, and myalgias.

19. Aronson MD, Bor DH: Blood cultures. Ann Intern Med 106:246, 1987.

Two or three blood culture sets almost always suffice to establish or rule out bacteremia.

20. Popp RL: Echocardiography and infectious endocarditis. Curr Clin Topics Infect Dis 4:98, 1983.
    Comprehensive clinical review.

21. Pazin GJ, Saul S, Thompson ME: Blood culture positivity: Suppression by outpatient antibiotic therapy in patients with bacterial endocarditis. Arch Intern Med 142:263, 1982.
    Oral antibiotic therapy may suppress positive blood cultures for hours to days.

22. Coleman DL, Horwitz RI, Andriole VT: Association between serum inhibitory and bactericidal concentrations and therapeutic outcome in bacterial endocarditis. Am J Med 73:260, 1982.
    Review of literature of controversial subject. No clear association between serum concentrations and therapeutic outcome has been demonstrated in any study to date.

23. Washington JA: The role of the microbiology laboratory in the diagnosis and antimicrobial treatment of infective endocarditis. Mayo Clinic Proc 57:22, 1982.
    Review of practical aspects of the clinical microbiology of endocarditis.

24. Wilson WR, Giuliani ER, Danielson GK, Geraci JE: Management of complications of infective endocarditis. Mayo Clinic Proc 57:162, 1982.
    Major complications include congestive heart failure, myocardial abscess/rupture, myocardial infarction, pericarditis, systemic embolus, mycotic aneurysm, and metastatic infection.

25. Dinubile MJ: Surgery in active endocarditis. Ann Intern Med 96:650, 1982.
    Review of indications for surgical intervention. Major criteria include congestive heart failure, multiple embolic episodes, persistent bacteremia, fungal endocarditis, development of progressive heart block, and prosthetic valve dysfunction.

Meningitis and Encephalitis

Howard Libman, M.D.

Acute meningitis[1-3] and encephalitis[4] are medical emergencies that require rapid clinical evaluation and treatment. Delay adversely affects the clinical outcome of bacterial meningitis and herpes simplex meningoencephalitis.

PATHOGENESIS AND ETIOLOGY

Streptococcus pneumoniae[5] and *Neisseria meningitidis*[6] are the most frequent causes of bacterial meningitis in adults, whereas *Haemophilus influenzae*[7] is the most common pathogen in young children. Less frequent causes in adults include enteric gram negative bacilli (in chronically ill patients with recent central nervous system trauma or surgery, or in association with bacteremia),[8] *Staphylococcus aureus* (in similar circumstances), *Staphylococcus epidermidis* (in the context of a ventricular shunt), and *Listeria monocytogenes*.[9] Encephalitis is usually viral in origin, with arboviruses, enteroviruses, and herpes simplex virus the most common pathogens. Although meningitis may result from local spread of contiguous infection, hematogenous spread of remote infection, or direct implantation from head trauma[10] or neurosurgery, many patients have no identifiable risk factors.

The aseptic meningitis syndrome refers to meningitis with negative cerebrospinal fluid (CSF) Gram's stain and bacterial cultures. Causes that require antimicrobial therapy include partially treated bacterial meningitis, parameningeal suppurative foci (e.g., brain abscess, subdural empyema, epidural abscess), *Mycobacterium tuberculosis*,[11] syphilis,[12] fungi (e.g., *Cryptococcus neoformans*),[13] herpes simplex virus,[14] and bacterial endocarditis.[15] Other causes include many additional viruses (including human immunodeficiency virus),[16,17] leptospirosis, neoplastic disease, sarcoidosis, and systemic lupus erythematosus.

CLINICAL FEATURES

The patient or his family should be questioned about recent head trauma, local or systemic infection, underlying medical problems, and contact with others who are ill. Meningococcal meningitis affects mainly young adults and may occur sporadically or in outbreaks within a closed population; pneumococcal meningitis is seen primarily in older adults. Viral meningitis is most common in patients 5–20 years of age and occurs most often in summer and fall.

Symptoms of meningitis include fever, headache, vomiting, photophobia, and mental dysfunction ranging from lethargy to coma. Seizures and cranial nerve deficits may also be observed. Papilledema is infrequent, and its presence should prompt the search for brain abscess or tumor. The clinical presentation of encephalitis is similar to that of meningitis, but altered consciousness is always a significant feature.

If meningitis with or without encephalitis is suspected from the history, the initial physical examination is brief and directed. It should include the head and neck (for recent trauma, local infection, and papilledema), heart (for endocarditis), lungs (for pneumonia), and abdomen (for splenectomy), and skin (for petechial or purpuric rashes). A careful neurologic examination is important as well, looking for focal deficits and the presence of meningeal signs.

DIAGNOSIS

Lumbar puncture (LP) should be performed at the conclusion of the physical examination unless a mass lesion is clinically suspected. If evidence of increased intracranial pressure or focal neurologic findings are present, computed tomography (CT) of the head is performed first. At the time of LP, the CSF opening pressure is recorded, and fluid is obtained for cell and differential counts, glucose and protein concentrations, and bacterial culture. A Gram's stain of the sediment is performed; an India ink stain and a stain for acid-fast bacilli should also be prepared. An extra tube of CSF is held for any additional tests that may be suggested by the initial evaluation. A white blood cell count over 1200/μl with a predominance of neutrophils, a protein concentration over 150 mg/dl, and a glucose concentration less than 30 mg/dl suggest a bacterial process. However, because these values are not specific for bacterial meningitis, its definitive diagnosis requires a positive Gram's stain or culture.

If aseptic meningitis is present, attention is directed to ruling out those causes that require antimicrobial or other therapy. In partially treated bacterial meningitis, the Gram's stain and culture are often negative and the remainder of the CSF profile is unaffected.[18] In this setting, counterimmunoelectrophoresis or latex agglutination of the CSF for bacterial antigens is sometimes useful. If a parameningeal focus of infection is suspected, CT scan of the head, sinus or mastoid films, vertebral radiographs, and/or a bone scan are indicated. When tuberculosis is a possibility, a skin test (purified protein derivative [PPD]) is planted and a chest radiograph and sputum examination for acid-fast bacilli are performed. If infection with *Cryptococcus neoformans* is suspected, CSF and urine specimens for cryptococcal antigen are obtained. Blood and CSF serologic tests (e.g., VDRL, FTA-abs) are necessary to evaluate for neurosyphilis. Brain biopsy is required for the early diagnosis of herpes simplex virus meningoencephalitis. CSF cytologic study is indicated if carcinomatous meningitis is suspected.

THERAPY

Once the LP is completed, blood cultures are obtained and the patient is started on empirical therapy[19] with high-dose parenteral penicillin G (2 million U IV q2h). Chloramphenicol (100 mg/kg/day IV in four divided doses) is used if the patient is allergic to penicillin. If the clinical situation suggests infection with an enteric gram negative bacillus, *S. aureus*, or *S. epidermidis*, the appropriate antibiotic is begun (respectively, a third-generation cephalosporin, a semisynthetic penicillin, and vancomycin). Frequent neurologic checks should be performed. Supportive measures in the care of the patient include maintenance of the airway and seizure control.

If the CSF analysis is normal, antibiotic therapy can usually be stopped, although normal results do not absolutely exclude impending bacterial meningitis.[20] If the CSF is abnormal but does not suggest a bacterial etiology, it may be wise to continue empirical therapy pending culture results. A repeat LP 12–24 hours after admission is often helpful in clarifying a nonspecific or confusing profile.[21] Empirical therapy should be changed to definitive therapy if the CSF or blood cultures yield an etiologic agent.

The patient with meningococcal meningitis is kept in respiratory isolation during the first day of therapy, and family and other close contacts should receive antimicrobial prophylaxis (rifampin, 600 mg PO bid × 2 days [adult regimen]). Prophylaxis is not necessary in health care workers, with the exception of an individual who performs mouth-to-mouth resuscitation. Prophylaxis is recommended for young children who have contact with a patient with *H. influenzae* meningitis.

If herpes simplex encephalitis is suspected, a decision is made early in the clinical course whether to obtain a brain biopsy. Antiviral therapy (acyclovir or adenine arabinoside) should be initiated as soon as possible. There is no specific therapy for the other causes of encephalitis.

KEY FEATURES

The most frequent bacterial causes of acute meningitis in the adult are:
- *Streptococcus pneumoniae*
- *Neisseria meningitidis*

The aseptic meningitis syndrome refers to meningitis with negative CSF Gram's stain and bacterial culture. Causes that require antimicrobial therapy include:
- Partially treated bacterial meningitis
- Parameningeal infection
- Tuberculous meningitis
- Neurosyphilis
- Cryptococcal meningitis
- Herpes simplex meningoencephalitis
- Bacterial endocarditis

Lumbar puncture with CSF analysis should be performed promptly in suspected cases of meningitis. Initial studies include a cell count, glucose and protein concentrations, Gram's stain, and bacterial culture. Additional studies may be suggested by these results and the clinical setting.

In the presence of a negative CSF Gram's stain, the following results suggest a bacterial etiology:
- White blood cell count >1200/μl
- A predominance of neutrophils

- Glucose <30 mg/dl
- Protein >150 mg/dl
    Initial management of meningitis consists of:
- Empirical therapy with high-dose penicillin G when a bacterial process is possible (chloramphenicol in the patient who is allergic to penicillin)
- In certain clinical situations, other antibiotic therapy may be appropriate
- Supportive measures, such as maintenance of the airway and control of seizure activity
- Respiratory isolation of the patient with meningococcal meningitis during the first day of treatment
- If N. meningitidis is the suspected pathogen, family and other close contacts require antimicrobial prophylaxis with rifampin
    If herpes simplex meningoencephalitis is suspected, a brain biopsy is performed or empirical antiviral chemotherapy is initiated.

REFERENCES

1. Carpenter RR, Petersdorf RG: The clinical spectrum of bacterial meningitis. Am J Med 33:262, 1962.
    Review of experience with bacterial meninigitis. The vast majority of patients had pneumococcal, meningococcal, or H. influenzae disease. The mortality rate of pneumococcal meningitis (50%) was more than three times that of the others.

2. Swartz MN, Dodge PR: Bacterial meningitis—a review of selected aspects. N Engl J Med 272:725, 842, 898, 954, 1003; 1965.
    Comprehensive review.

3. Karandanis D, Shulman JA: Recent survey of infectious meningitis in adults: Review of laboratory findings in bacterial, tuberculous, and aseptic meningitis. South Med J 69:449, 1976.
    Ninety per cent of cases of bacterial meningitis had a positive CSF Gram's stain. Hyponatremia in conjunction with a negative Gram's stain was highly suggestive of tuberculous meningitis. Almost all patients with viral meningitis had a CSF white blood cell count lower than 2700/μl, a protein concentration less than 250 mg/dl, and a normal glucose level.

4. Kennard C, Swash M: Acute viral encephalitis: Its diagnosis and outcome. Brain 104:129, 1981.
    Review of experience at The London Hospital. Mortality was highest in patients with herpes simplex encephalitis.

5. Olsson RA, Kirby JC, Romansky MJ: Pneumococcal meningitis in the adult: Clinical, therapeutic, and prognostic aspects in forty-three patients. Ann Intern Med 55:545, 1961.
    The overall mortality rate was 65%. Delay in seeking treatment was common.

6. Wolf RE, Birbara CA: Meningococcal infections at an army training center. Am J Med 44:243, 1968.
    Meningococcal infection was classified into four syndromes: (1) bacteremia without sepsis, (2) septicemia without meningitis, (3) meningitis with or without bacteremia, and (4) meningoencephalitis.

7. Merselis JG, Sellers TF, Johnson JE, Hook EW: Hemophilus influenzae meningitis in adults. Arch Intern Med *110*:837, 1962.
   The disease, although unusual in adults, affected patients with chronic underlying medical conditions. Its clinical manifestations were similar to those of the other bacterial meningitides.

8. Berk SL, McCabe WR: Meningitis caused by gram-negative bacilli. Ann Intern Med 93:253, 1980.
   Spontaneously occurring meningitis had an abrupt onset and a relatively fulminant course, whereas post-surgical disease was insidious, more protracted, and commonly caused by multiple resistant organisms.

9. Lavetter A, Leedom JM, Mathies AW, Ivler D, Wehrle PF: Meningitis due to listeria monocytogenes: A review of 25 cases. N Engl J Med *285*:598, 1971.
   This disease primarily affected infants, the elderly, and those with underlying medical illness. The CSF Gram's stain was frequently negative. Ampicillin was the preferred antibiotic.

10. Hand WL, Sanford JP: Posttraumatic bacterial meningitis. Ann Intern Med 72:869, 1970.
    Fifty per cent of patients developed meningitis within 2 weeks of injury, but there was delay of more than a year in 25%. All patients had a skull fracture and/or CSF rhinorrhea. S. pneumoniae was the most common pathogen.

11. Kennedy DH, Fallon RJ: Tuberculous meningitis. JAMA *241*:264, 1979.
    Initial stain for acid-fast bacilli was positive in only 37% of cases. Early treatment was associated with a better prognosis.

12. Hooshmand H, Escobar MR, Kopf SW: Neurosyphilis: A study of 241 patients. JAMA *219*:726, 1972.
    Manifestations were often nonspecific. Response to treatment was variable.

13. Lewis JL, Rabinovich S: The wide spectrum of cryptococcal infections. Am J Med 53:315, 1972.
    Predisposing factors, particularly lymphoma or corticosteroid therapy, were identified in many of the patients.

14. Barza M, Pauker SG: The decision to biopsy, treat, or wait in suspected herpes encephalitis. Ann Intern Med 92:641, 1980.
    Clinical features are reviewed. A decision analysis approach to management is presented.

15. Ziment I: Nervous system complications in bacterial endocarditis. Am J Med 47:593, 1969.
    Review. Neuropsychiatric manifestations are present in up to 50% of patients with bacterial endocarditis. The aseptic meningitis syndrome, occasionally secondary to embolization or mycotic aneurysm, is sometimes seen.

16. Lepow ML, Carver DH, Wright HT, Woods WA, Robbins FC: A clinical, epidemiologic and laboratory investigation of aseptic meningitis during the four-year period, 1955–1958. N Engl J Med *266*:1181, 1962.
    Approximately 50% of patients suffered some degree of disability for weeks to months after the acute illness, but nearly all were fully recovered within one year.

17. Ho DD, et al: Primary human T-lymphotropic virus infection type III infection. Ann Intern Med *103*:880, 1985.
    Aseptic meningitis may be part of the clinical presentation.

18. Blazer S, Berant M, Alon U: Bacterial meninigitis: Effect of antibiotic treatment on cerebrospinal fluid. Am J Clin Pathol 80:386, 1983.

    Two to three days of conventional antibiotic therapy, although rendering the Gram's stain and culture negative, did not significantly affect CSF composition. The white blood cell count, and glucose and protein concentrations were unchanged.

19. McCabe WR: Empiric therapy for bacterial meningitis. Rev Infect Dis 5 (suppl):74, 1983.

    An approach to empirical treatment based upon the clinical setting.

20. Onorato IM, Wormser GP, Nicholas P: "Normal" CSF in bacterial meningitis. JAMA 244:1469, 1980.

    Case reports and a review of the literature. Repeat LP within 24 hours is suggested in all febrile patients in whom the clinical features remain compatible with meningitis.

21. Feigin RD, Shackelford PG: Value of repeat lumbar puncture in the differential diagnosis of meningitis. N Engl J Med 289:571, 1973.

    A brief period of close observation followed by repeat lumbar puncture will often help distinguish bacterial from aseptic meningitis when the initial CSF analysis is abnormal but not strongly suggestive of a bacterial process.

Brain Abscess

Howard Libman, M.D.

Brain abscess is a curable disease with significant mortality. Because its symptoms and signs are nonspecific, delay in diagnosis is common.

PATHOGENESIS AND ETIOLOGY

Pyogenic intracranial infection begins as a focal area of cerebritis, with abscess formation occurring days to weeks later. Organisms may originate from a local or distant site of infection, or may be directly implanted by trauma or surgery. Common contiguous sites include the middle ear, mastoid bone, and sinuses; common distant sites include the lungs and endocardium. In the former case, a solitary abscess is likely to develop in the lobe nearest the primary infection; thus, otitis media and mastoiditis are usually associated with temporal lobe abscess, whereas paranasal sinusitis often results in frontal lobe infection. In the latter case, multiple abscesses that are randomly located are likely to occur.

The bacteriology of brain abscess is complex.[1] Because of lack of uniformity in microbiologic technique, different patterns of primary infection, and variability in prior administration of antimicrobial therapy, the literature is not consistent. In general, streptococci, enteric gram negative bacilli,

Staphylococcus aureus, and anaerobes are isolated with greatest frequency. Polymicrobial infection is found nearly a quarter of the time.

CLINICAL FEATURES

The presentation of brain abscess is usually subacute or indolent.[2-7] Symptoms and signs of increased intracranial pressure predominate. A primary site of infection is sometimes evident. Headache is frequent; altered consciousness, nausea, vomiting, and focal or generalized seizures may occur as well. Fever is often absent. Twenty-five per cent of patients have nuchal rigidity, and a similar percentage have papilledema. Focal neurologic deficits, the nature of which are determined by the location of the abscess, are noted in over a third of cases.

The white blood cell count is normal or mildly elevated. A lumbar puncture, if performed, commonly reveals an abnormal cerebrospinal fluid (CSF) consistent with aseptic meningitis (modest pleocytosis, normal glucose concentration, and a moderately elevated protein level). The CSF Gram's stain and culture are negative unless the abscess has ruptured into the subarachnoid space or ventricles. Lumbar puncture is contraindicated when brain abscess is suspected because of the lack of useful information to be gained and the associated increased risk of brain herniation.

DIAGNOSIS

Brain abscess should be considered in any patient with discrete neurologic deficits or evidence of increased intracranial pressure, particularly when there is fever, leukocytosis, or an identifiable primary site of infection. The diagnosis is supported by the presence of a focal abnormality on radionuclide brain scan or computed tomography of the head (CT scan). Brain scan is very sensitive for early detection and can identify lesions as small as 1 cm.[8] CT scan, although providing a more detailed picture than brain scan, is not as sensitive in the cerebritis stage.[9] Once abscess formation has occurred, the two tests are of equal value.[10] Characteristic CT findings of abscess consist of a central area of decreased attenuation surrounded by a contrast-enhancing ring (the "doughnut sign"). A variable amount of edema, which appears as a zone of decreased attenuation, is present around the lesion. Cerebral angiography, although not necessary for diagnosis, may be helpful preoperatively in some cases in order to define the anatomy of the lesion better.

The differential diagnosis of brain abscess includes tumor, herpes simplex and other viral encephalitides, subdural empyema, epidural abscess, cerebral infarction, and mycotic aneurysm. In the immunocompromised host, toxoplasmosis and fungal infection are additional considerations.

THERAPY

The mortality rate of brain abscess has ranged as high as 30–60% in some series.[2-7] Because death is often from brain herniation, increased intracranial pressure should be treated aggressively. Hyperventilation is effective in the acute setting; mannitol and systemic corticosteroids are useful over a longer period of time. Empirical intravenous antibiotics—penicillin G (24 million U/day) and chloramphenicol (100 mg/kg/day)—are administered pending surgical exploration. Antibiotic therapy in the context of trauma or neurosurgery should include a semisynthetic penicillin to cover for *S. aureus*. Metronidazole may be used if anaerobic infection is suspected. The optimal timing of surgery is not entirely clear. The procedure of choice is excision of the abscess cavity, although incision and drainage are often successful as well. Some brain abscesses, especially small, multiple ones, may respond to antibiotic therapy alone.[11,12]

KEY FEATURES

Bacteria reach the brain in one of the following ways:
- Contiguously (from the middle ear, mastoid bone, or sinuses)
- Hematogenously (from the lungs or endocardium)
- Direct implantation (from trauma or surgery)

The bacteriology of brain abscess is variable. Common isolates include streptococci, the enterobacteriaceae, *S. aureus,* and anaerobes.

The diagnosis is suspected on clinical grounds, supported by brain or CT scan, and established by surgical exploration. Lumbar puncture is not useful and is contraindicated because of the increased risk of herniation.

Initial management of brain abscess consists of:
- Hyperventilation, mannitol, and corticosteroids, as necessary, to decrease intracranial pressure
- Empirical antibiotic therapy with high-dose penicillin G and chloramphenicol
- In the context of trauma or surgery, empirical treatment should include a semisynthetic penicillin

REFERENCES

1. de Louvois J, Gortvai P, Hurley R: Bacteriology of abscesses of the central nervous system: A multicentre prospective study. Br Med J 2:981, 1977.
   Streptococci were isolated from the majority of patients. Anaerobes, staphylococci, and enteric gram negative bacilli were also found with some frequency. The importance of proper culturing of abscess specimens is emphasized.

2. Garfield J: Management of supratentorial intracranial abscess: A review of 200 cases. Br Med J 2:7, 1969.
3. Samson DS, Clark K: A current review of brain abscess. Am J Med 54:201, 1973.
4. Brewer NS, MacCarty CS, Wellman WE: Brain abscess: A review of recent experience. Ann Intern Med 82:571, 1975.
5. Yang S: Brain abscess: A review of 400 cases. J Neurosurg 55:794, 1981.
6. Nielsen H, Gyldensted C, Harmsen A: Cerebral abscess: Aetiology and pathogenesis, symptoms, diagnosis, and treatment. Acta Neurol Scandinav 65:609, 1982.
7. Harrison MJG: The clinical presentation of intracranial abscesses. Quart J Med 204:461, 1982.
    Reviews of the clinical features and treatment.

8. Crocker EF, McLaughlin AF, Morris JG, Benn R, McLeod JG, Allsop JL: Technetium brain scanning in the diagnosis and management of cerebral abscess. Am J Med 56:192, 1974.
    Brain scan was sensitive in the early diagnosis and localization of brain abscess.

9. Whelan MA, Hilal SK: Computed tomography as a guide in the diagnosis and follow-up of brain abscesses. Radiology 135:663, 1980.
    The characteristic CT findings of brain abscess are described, as is their differential diagnosis.

10. Pinsky S, Yum HY, Patel D, Bekerman C, Ryo UY: Comparison of radionuclide brain scan and computerized tomography for the detection of intracranial infections. Clin Nucl Med 6:12, 1981.
    Brain scan was more sensitive than the CT scan in detecting diffuse intracranial infection; the two tests were roughly equal in their ability to detect brain abscess.

11. Heineman HS, Braude AI, Osterholm JL: Intracranial suppurative disease: Early presumptive diagnosis and successful treatment without surgery. JAMA 218:1542, 1971.
12. Kamin M, Biddle D: Conservative management of focal intracerebral infection. Neurology 31:103, 1981.
    Case reports. Some patients with brain abscess may be cured by antibiotics alone.

Pneumonia

Howard Libman, M.D.

Despite the availability of a wide variety of antibiotics, pneumonia remains an important cause of morbidity and mortality, accounting for 10% of general hospital admissions and representing a leading cause of death in the United States. A careful clinical approach to the problem is essential.[1]

PATHOGENESIS AND ETIOLOGY

In the patient with normal lung defense mechanisms, the airways below the larynx and the lung parenchyma are kept essentially sterile. The cough reflex, the presence of tracheobronchial mucus and a ciliary transport system, and humoral and cellular immunity are important in maintaining this state. Compromise of one or more of these defenses may lead to microbial colonization and lower respiratory tract infection. Conditions that interfere with pulmonary defenses include upper respiratory infection, cigarette smoking, chronic obstructive pulmonary disease, altered consciousness, intrabronchial obstruction, and immunosuppressive disease or therapy.

Infecting agents commonly enter the lungs via the airways, although hematogenous spread in the context of endocarditis or another distant focus of infection may also occur. The most common causes of community-acquired pneumonia[2,3,4] in the immunocompetent adult include *Streptococcus pneumoniae,*[5] *Staphylococcus aureus,*[6] *Haemophilus influenzae,*[7] *Klebsiella pneumoniae* and other enteric gram negative bacilli,[8] and mixed anaerobes,[9,10] which cause classic bacterial pneumonia;[11] *Legionella* species,[12] *Mycoplasma pneumoniae,*[13,14] and the influenza virus,[15] which produce the atypical pneumonia syndrome;[16] and *Mycobacterium tuberculosis.*[17,18]

HISTORY

Important history to obtain includes the patient's age (viruses, except for influenza, are an infrequent cause of pneumonia in the normal adult; mycoplasmal pneumonia occurs primarily in older children and young adults), occupational and animal exposures, recent travel, and underlying medical conditions. Immunosuppression resulting from illness or chemotherapy may indicate infection with an opportunistic pathogen. A history of tuberculosis or exposure to someone with the disease may suggest infection with *M. tuberculosis.* Aspiration pneumonia is suspected in the context of poor dentition, altered consciousness, or a neuromuscular disorder affecting the patient's ability to swallow. A history of intravenous drug abuse raises the question of endocarditis with septic pulmonary emboli. Recent hospitalization may indicate infection with a nosocomial pathogen (e.g., enteric gram negative bacilli, *S. aureus*).

Specific symptoms are useful in distinguishing bacterial pneumonia from the atypical pneumonia syndrome. Bacterial pneumonia is characteristically abrupt in onset, beginning with a fever and a shaking chill. Soon thereafter, dyspnea, pleuritic chest pain, and a cough productive of purulent sputum occur. The atypical pneumonia syndrome is manifested initially by constitutional symptoms, such as headache, myalgias, and malaise. A few days later, fever and a cough—generally nonproductive or minimally productive—develop; dyspnea and pleuritic chest pain are commonly absent.

PHYSICAL EXAMINATION

The general appearance of the patient and the vital signs are important indicators of the severity of the illness, although the height of the fever is not useful diagnostically. Examination of the thorax may be normal, reveal nonspecific abnormalities, or show evidence of consolidation. Classic changes associated with pulmonary consolidation include increased vocal fremitus, dullness to percussion, bronchial breath sounds, inspiratory rales, and egophony and whispered pectoriloquy. Although the presence of these changes implies bacterial pneumonia, their absence does not rule it out. Extrapulmonary findings may occasionally suggest a specific pulmonary infection (e.g., bullous myringitis, mycoplasmal pneumonia; endocarditis, hematogenous *S. aureus* pneumonia; meningitis, *S. pneumoniae* or *H. influenzae* pneumonia; periodontal disease and an absent gag reflex, aspiration [mixed anaerobic] pneumonia).

LABORATORY STUDIES

A white blood cell and differential count, chest roentgenogram, sputum examination, and room air arterial blood gases compose the initial laboratory work-up on the patient with suspected pneumonia. Sputum and blood cultures, a diagnostic thoracentesis (if pleural fluid is present), a tuberculin skin test (if tuberculosis is suspected clinically), and a serum sample for acute serologic testing are obtained once the diagnosis of pneumonia is established. If sputum is not expectorated spontaneously, hydration, humidification, and postural clapping and drainage are sometimes helpful. When these are not effective, nasotracheal suctioning should be performed. Transtracheal aspiration[19] is indicated in the seriously ill patient in whom a sputum sample is unobtainable. In the immunocompromised host, needle aspiration or transbronchial or open lung biopsy may be necessary to determine the causative pathogen.

Gross examination of the sputum may reveal a clear, thin specimen, suggesting a nonbacterial etiology, or a mucopurulent or blood-tinged specimen, usually indicating a bacterial process. Microscopic examination is performed with Gram's stain and stain for acid-fast bacilli. The "adequacy" of an individual sample is based upon the presence of polymorphonuclear leukocytes and pulmonary macrophages, and the absence of squamous cells. Samples with fewer than 10 squamous cells and greater than 25 neutrophils per low power field correlate well with those obtained by transtracheal aspiration.[20] An adequate sputum sample reflects the microbiology of the pulmonary process, and procuring such a specimen, particularly in the acutely ill patient, should be given high priority.

The chest radiograph may provide clues regarding the etiology of pneumonia[21] but is not diagnostic of a specific pathogen.[22] Posteroanterior and lateral chest radiographs should be obtained on all patients. The presence of cavitation, pleural effusion, or lobar or segmental involvement suggests a bacterial process. Features more typical of nonbacterial pneumonia include diffuse involvement and a reticulonodular pattern. Specialized radiographic techniques, ultrasonography, or computed tomography may be necessary, on occasion, to provide additional information regarding the nature of difficult-to-interpret infiltrates.

DIFFERENTIAL DIAGNOSIS

Pneumonia can usually be distinguished from upper respiratory tract infection on the basis of symptoms and clinical course. If a patient's "cold" worsens following a period of improvement, if it continues for longer than a week, or if dyspnea becomes prominent, lower tract disease should be suspected. Acute bronchitis may present in a manner similar to pneumonia, but physical examination does not reveal consolidation and the chest radiograph is clear. Although fever with a pulmonary infiltrate generally represents an infectious process, consideration should always be given to alternative diagnoses, such as congestive heart failure; chronic obstructive pulmonary disease; bronchiectasis; pulmonary infarction; neoplastic disease; and hypersensitivity, drug, and radiation pneumonitis.

INITIAL MANAGEMENT

The patient's age, underlying medical problems, respiratory status, ability to take oral antibiotics, and reliability are important considerations in deciding whether admission is required. Because of the potential seriousness of pneumonia, it is wise to be conservative when there is doubt as to whether outpatient management is feasible in a particular case. Initial antibiotic therapy should be based upon the clinical presentation, radiologic findings, and sputum Gram's stain results.[23] If a predominant organism is seen on Gram's stain, treatment should be specific. If no pathogen is identified, empirical therapy with erythromycin (500 mg qid) is reasonable for community-acquired pneumonia in the immunocompetent host but, preferably, only after an adequate sputum sample has been reviewed. Empirical therapy should be changed to definitive therapy if sputum or blood cultures yield an etiologic agent. Clinical response to antibiotics is seen in most uncomplicated bacterial pneumonias within 72 hours.

Supportive measures in management include rest, hydration, supplemental oxygen as required, postural clapping and drainage, and the control of symptoms. In general, the patient's pO_2 is maintained at greater than 60 mmHg. Because cough serves as an effective clearance mechanism, it should not be routinely suppressed. However, if it is nonproductive and bothersome to the patient, codeine is often beneficial. Pleuritic chest pain is controlled with an analgesic or anti-inflammatory agent. Continuous nasogastric suctioning is indicated when there is gastric dilatation or small bowel ileus.

KEY FEATURES

CLINICAL FEATURES OF CLASSIC BACTERIAL PNEUMONIA AND THE ATYPICAL PNEUMONIA SYNDROME*

Feature	Bacterial Pneumonia	Atypical Pneumonia
History	Abrupt onset	Gradual onset
	Fever, chills	Constitutional symptoms
	Pleuritic chest pain, dyspnea	Absence of pleuritic chest pain, dyspnea
	Productive cough	Minimally productive cough
Physical examination	Toxic appearance	Appears less ill
	Evidence of pulmonary consolidation	Nonspecific findings
Laboratory findings	Increased WBC with left shift	Normal or mildly increased WBC
	Radiographic findings of cavitation, pleural effusion, or lobar or segmental involvement	Radiographic findings of diffuse involvement, reticulonodular pattern
	Sputum Gram's stain shows a predominant organism	Sputum Gram's stain without predominant organism

*Common causes of the atypical pneumonia syndrome include Legionella species, *Mycoplasma pneumoniae,* and the influenza virus; uncommon causes include other viruses, psittacosis, Q fever, tularemia, and plague.

Initial laboratory studies in a patient with suspected pneumonia should consist of:
- White blood cell and differential count
- Chest radiograph (PA and lateral: decubitus films if indicated)
- Microscopic examination of an adequate sputum sample (Gram's stain, stain for acid-fast bacilli)
- Room air arterial blood gases
  Once the diagnosis is established, the following are obtained:
- Sputum and blood cultures
- Diagnostic thoracentesis (if indicated)
- Skin test (PPD) for tuberculosis (if indicated)
- Serum for acute serologic testing
  Alternative diagnoses in the patient with fever and pulmonary infiltrate include:
- Congestive heart failure
- Chronic obstructive pulmonary disease
- Bronchiectasis

- Pulmonary infarction
- Neoplastic disease
- Hypersensitivity, drug, and radiation pneumonitis
  Initial management of pneumonia should consist of:
- When possible, specific antibiotic therapy directed at the causative pathogen
- Erythromycin for the empirical therapy of community-acquired disease in the immunocompetent host
- Supportive measures, including hydration, supplemental oxygen, postural clapping and drainage, and control of symptoms

ANTIBIOTICS OF CHOICE FOR COMMON CAUSES OF COMMUNITY-ACQUIRED PNEUMONIA

Pathogen	Antibiotic
Streptococcus pneumoniae	Penicillin
Staphylococcus aureus	Oxacillin or nafcillin
Haemophilus influenzae	Ampicillin*
Enteric gram negative bacilli	A cephalosporin or an aminoglycoside
Mixed anaerobes	Penicillin
Legionella species	Erythromycin
Mycoplasma pneumoniae	Erythromycin
Influenza virus	No specific therapy
Mycobacterium tuberculosis	Isoniazid and rifampin

*A third-generation cephalosporin is indicated for beta-lactamase–producing strains.

REFERENCES

1. Shulman JA, Phillips LA, Petersdorf RG: Errors and hazards in the diagnosis and treatment of bacterial pneumonias. Ann Intern Med 62:41, 1965.
   A description of the most common errors made in the management of pneumonia. Many points are still quite relevant.

2. Fekety FR, et al: Bacteria, viruses, and mycoplasmas in acute pneumonia in adults. Am Rev Resp Dis 104:499, 1971.
   Sixty-two per cent of patients with acute pneumonia admitted to the Johns Hopkins Hospital had pneumococcal infection; the vast majority of the remaining patients had pneumonia of uncertain etiology.

3. Sullivan RJ, Dowdle WR, Marine WM, Hierholzer JC: Adult pneumonia in a general hospital: Etiology and host risk factors. Arch Intern Med 129:935, 1972.
   Fifty-seven per cent of the cases of pneumonia could be attributed to specific bacterial pathogens, with pneumococcus the most frequent etiologic agent, gram negative bacilli the second, and S. aureus the third. Viral infections other than influenza appeared unrelated to adult pneumonias.

4. Dorff GJ, Rytel MW, Farmer SG, Scanlon G: Etiologies and characteristic features of pneumonias in a municipal hospital. Am J Med Sci 266:349, 1973.
   Fifty-three per cent of patients had pneumococcal pneumonia, 10% had gram negative bacillary infection, 7% had staphylococcal pneumonia, and 9% had viral or mycoplasmal disease.

5. Mufson MA: Pneumococcal infections. JAMA 246:1942, 1981.
   Clinical review.

6. Musher DM, McKenzie SO: Infections due to staphylococcus aureus. Medicine 56:383, 1977.
   General review of staphylococcal infection. Of 20 cases of pneumonia, 11 were primary and 9 were hematogenous. All patients with primary pneumonia had at least one underlying medical problem, and approximately one third had antecedent viral respiratory infection.

7. Wallace RJ, Musher DM, Martin RR: Hemophilus influenzae pneumonia in adults. Am J Med 64:87, 1978.
   Eighty-five per cent of patients had at least one chronic medical illness. Bacteremia was common in those over 50 years of age with underlying pulmonary disease. Mortality was high in bacteremic patients (57% versus 11% in the nonbacteremic group).

8. Pierce AK, Sanford JP: Aerobic gram-negative bacillary pneumonias. Am Rev Resp Dis 110:647, 1974.
   Clinical review. Enteric gram negative bacilli have become an increasingly frequent cause of community-acquired pneumonia.

9. Bartlett JG, Finegold SM: Anaerobic infections of the lung and pleural space. Am Rev. Resp Dis 110:56, 1974.
   Comprehensive review of anaerobic pneumonitis, necrotizing pneumonia, lung abscess, and empyema.

10. Bartlett JG: Anaerobic bacterial pneumonitis. Am Rev Resp Dis 119:19, 1979.
    Anaerobic bacterial pneumonitis may be difficult to distinguish from pneumococcal pneumonia on clinical grounds.

11. George WL, Finegold SM: Bacterial infections of the lung. Chest 81:502, 1982.
    Clinical review.

12. Shands KN, Fraser DW: Legionnaires' disease. Disease-a-Month 27(3):1, 1980.
    Review of clinical features, diagnosis, and treatment.

13. Murray HW, Masur H, Senterfit LB, Roberts RB: The protean manifestations of mycoplasma pneumoniae infection in adults. Am J Med 58:229, 1975
    Description of the spectrum of clinical disease, including respiratory manifestations.

14. Clinical conferences at The Johns Hopkins Hospital: Mycoplasma pneumonia. Johns Hopkins Med J 139:181, 1976.
    Case presentation and a clinical review.

15. Stuart-Harris CH: Twenty years of influenza epidemics. Am Rev Resp Dis 83:54, 1961.
    Review of clinical features of uncomplicated and complicated influenza infection.

16. File TM, Tan JS, Murphy DP: Atypical pneumonia syndrome. Primary Care 8(4):673, 1981.
    Clinical review.

17. Glassroth J, Robins AG, Snider DE: Tuberculosis in the 1980's. N Engl J Med 302:1441, 1980.

18. Snider DE, et al: Standard therapy for tuberculosis. Chest 87(Suppl):117, 1985.
    Diagnosis, therapy, and prevention are discussed.

19. Ries K, Levison ME, Kaye D: Transtracheal aspiration in pulmonary infection. Arch Intern Med 133:453, 1974.

Transtracheal aspiration was reasonably safe and was an effective method of determining the etiologic agent.

20. Murray PR, Washington JA: Microscopic and bacteriologic analysis of expectorated sputum. Mayo Clinic Proc 50:339, 1975.
   A method for determining the suitability of expectorated sputum samples for bacterial culture is presented.

21. Scanlon GT, Unger JD: The radiology of bacterial and viral pneumonias. Radiol Clin North Am 11(2):317, 1973.
   Review of characteristic radiologic features.

22. Tew J, Calenoff L, Berlin BS: Bacterial or nonbacterial pneumonia: accuracy of radiographic diagnosis. Radiology 124:607, 1977.
   The specific pattern on chest radiograph was not useful in distinguishing bacterial from nonbacterial pneumonia.

23. Donowitz GR, Mandell GL: Empiric therapy for pneumonia. Rev Infect Dis 5 (suppl.):40, 1983.
   An approach to the empirical treatment of pneumonia based upon the clinical setting and Gram's stain.

Legionnaires' Disease

Howard Libman, M.D.

Legionnaires' disease takes its name from the serious outbreak of pneumonia in 1976 that affected American Legion conventioneers at a Philadelphia hotel.[1] The etiology of the illness, at first unclear, was found in 1977 to be a "new" gram negative bacterium.[2] *Legionella pneumophila* has since been demonstrated serologically to have been the cause of many previous outbreaks of pulmonary infection. The organism is now recognized as a common cause of community-acquired and nosocomial pneumonia,[3] which may occur sporadically[4] or in outbreaks.[5] Another species, *L. micdadei* ("Pittsburgh pneumonia agent"), has also been identified as an important pulmonary pathogen.[6] Several additional Legionella species have been isolated in recent years, but their clinical significance is not yet clear.

L. pneumophila is a fastidious, aerobic bacillus that is weakly staining and does not grow well on most conventional media. It has been isolated from soil and a variety of environmental sites associated with water. Infection is most likely acquired through inhalation of aerosolized organisms by a susceptible host; person-to-person spread has not been demonstrated.

CLINICAL FEATURES

Legionnaires' disease occurs throughout the year but is most common in summer and fall.[7-11] Patients are usually middle aged or elderly, and men are more often affected than women. Approximately 50% of patients have at least one chronic underlying medical condition, and some patients are significantly immunosuppressed.[12] Legionellosis has a wide clinical spectrum, ranging from self-limited upper respiratory infection to fulminant pneumonia.

The presentation of pneumonia is generally acute. The first symptoms are constitutional and include anorexia, malaise, weakness, lethargy, myalgias, and headache; upper respiratory symptoms are usually absent. Fever, chills, and a minimally or moderately productive cough ensue, sometimes in association with pleuritic chest pain. A wide range of mental status abnormalities, from confusion to delirium, and gastrointestinal complaints, including diarrhea, abdominal pain, and vomiting, have also been described but are not consistently present.

Physical examination is remarkable for a high-grade fever, with a pulse-temperature disparity and, initially, no evidence of pulmonary consolidation. The white blood cell count is mildly elevated with a left shift. The chest radiograph[13] most often shows a patchy alveolar infiltrate in a single lobe, usually lower, which may spread and become nodular in appearance over time; small pleural effusions are noted about half the time. The sputum is not grossly purulent, and Gram's stain shows few leukocytes and no predominant bacterium. Urinalysis may reveal proteinuria, hematuria, or other cellular elements. Nonspecific metabolic abnormalities that have been described include elevated liver function tests, hyponatremia, hypophosphatemia, and elevated creatine phosphokinase and aldolase.

The complications of legionnaires' disease, most common in the immunosuppressed patient, include respiratory failure, hypotension, acute renal failure, and disseminated intravascular coagulation.

Prognosis is related to the severity of the underlying illness(es) and the rapidity of institution of appropriate antibiotic therapy. Among hospitalized patients, the mortality rate is approximately 15%, whereas in immunocompromised patients it is significantly higher.

DIAGNOSIS

Legionnaires' disease is one entity of the differential diagnosis of the atypical pneumonia syndrome.[7-11] Illnesses that present in a similar fashion include mycoplasmal pneumonia, viral pneumonia, psittacosis, Q fever, tularemia, and plague. The diagnosis should be seriously considered when atypical pneumonia presents in older adults, in those with underlying medical illness, or in the immunosuppressed. Specific features of the history, physical examination, and initial laboratory evaluation, although suggestive,[14,15] are not pathognomonic. Occasionally, *L. pneumophila* has been identified using conventional or modified Gram's stain techniques.[16,17] However, definitive diagnosis requires one or more of the following: (1) culture of the organism on specially enriched media (e.g., charcoal yeast extract agar), (2) special staining (e.g., Dieterele's silver) of a clinical specimen or demonstration of the organism by the direct fluorescent antibody (DFA) technique, or (3) indirect fluorescent antibody (IFA) testing of acute and convalescent sera.[18] (A positive IFA is defined as a fourfold rise in titer to greater than 1:128 at three weeks, or a single titer of 1:256.) An additional test, which detects urinary antigen specific for Legionella, may also prove to be useful.[19]

THERAPY

Erythromycin (500–1000 mg qid) is the antibiotic of choice and, in ill patients, should be given parenterally; the penicillins, cephalosporins, and aminoglycosides are ineffective.[7-11] Rifampin is added if the clinical response, which is often slow, is unacceptable. As with other types of pneumonia, general supportive measures, such as supplemental oxygen and postural clapping and drainage, are important as well.

KEY FEATURES

Legionnaires' disease is caused by *Legionella pneumophila,* a fastidious aerobic gram negative bacillus that requires specially enriched media for growth. It is a common cause of both community-acquired and nosocomial pneumonia and has a wide clinical spectrum.

Its clinical characteristics include the following:

- An acute onset
- Constitutional symptoms early in the course
- Fever, chills, and a minimally to moderately productive cough later; dyspnea and pleuritic chest pain are less common
- A variety of mental status and gastrointestinal abnormalities in some patients
- The absence of pulmonary consolidation on initial physical examination
- A mildly elevated white blood count with a left shift
- A chest radiograph that shows a patchy alveolar infiltrate in a single lobe, usually lower, which may spread contiguously
- Sputum that does not appear grossly purulent; a Gram's stain that shows few to moderate white blood cells without a predominant organism

- Nonspecific urinary and metabolic abnormalities in some patients
    Legionnaires' disease is one entity of the differential diagnosis of the atypical pneumonia syndrome. Although it may be suggested by the clinical presentation, the definitive diagnosis is based upon one or more of the following:
- Culture of the organism on specially enriched media
- Silver stain or direct fluorescent antibody testing of sputum or tissue
- Indirect fluorescent antibody testing of acute and convalescent sera
    Therapy consists of erythromycin, given parenterally in acutely ill patients, and supportive measures.

REFERENCES

1. Fraser DW, et al: Legionnaires' disease: Description of an epidemic of pneumonia. N Engl J Med 297:1189, 1977.
    Original description of the 1976 Philadelphia outbreak.

2. McDade JE, et al: Legionnaires' disease: Isolation of a bacterium and demonstration of its role in other respiratory disease. N Engl J Med 297:1197, 1977.
    Original description of the isolation of L. pneumophila.

3. Yu VL, Kroboth FJ, Shonnard J, Brown A, McDearman S, Magnussen M: Legionnaires' disease: New clinical perspective from a prospective pneumonia study. Am J Med 73:357, 1982.
    L. pneumophila was the most common cause of pneumonia in this study. Approximately one third of cases were community acquired. Clinical features, apart from hyponatremia, were not helpful in distinguishing legionnaires' diseases from other types of pneumonia.

4. England AC, Fraser DW, Plikaytis BD, Tsai TF, Storch G, Broome CV: Sporadic legion-ellosis in the United States: The first thousand cases. Ann Intern Med 94:164, 1981.
    Description of the epidemiology of sporadic legionnaires' disease.

5. Eickhoff TC: Epidemiology of legionnaires' disease. Ann Intern Med 90:499, 1979.
    Description of the epidemiology of epidemic legionnaires' disease.

6. Muder RR, Yu VL, Zuravleff JJ: Pneumonia due to the Pittsburgh pneumonia agent: New clinical perspective with a review of the literature. Medicine 62:120, 1983.
    Review of pneumonia caused by L. micdadei. The illness affects the chronically ill and the immunosuppressed, has no distinguishing clinical characteristics, and is diagnosed and managed in a fashion similar to legionnaires' disease.

7. Center for Disease Control: Legionnaires' disease: Diagnosis and management. Ann Intern Med 88:363, 1978.
8. Swartz MN: Clinical aspects of legionnaires' disease. Ann Intern Med 90:492, 1979.
9. Shands KN, Fraser DW: Legionnaires' disease. Disease-a-Month 27(3):1, 1980.
10. Keys TF: Legionnaires' disease: A review of the epidemiology and clinical manifestations of a newly recognized infection. Mayo Clinic Proc 55:129, 1980.
11. Ching WTW, Meyer RD: Legionella infections. Inf Dis Clinics North Am 1(3):595, 1987.
    Reviews of the clinical features, diagnosis, and treatment.

12. Saravolatz LD, et al: The compromised host and legionnaires's disease. Ann Intern Med 90:533, 1979.
    The clinical presentation was not distinctive, and lung biopsy was sometimes necessary for diagnosis. Most patients responded favorably to intravenous erythromycin.

13. Fairbank JT, Mamourian AC, Dietrich PA, Girod JC: The chest radiograph in legionnaires' disease. Radiology 147:33, 1983.
    There was no consistent radiographic pattern, and infiltrates were commonly slow to clear.

14. Miller AC: Early clinical differentiation between legionnaires' disease and other sporadic pneumonias. Ann Intern Med 90:526, 1979.
    The early clinical criteria included (1) prodromal "viral" illness, (2) dry cough or confusion or diarrhea, (3) lymphopenia without marked neutrophilia, and (4) hyponatremia. Legionnaires' disease was very likely if any three of these were present on admission.

15. Helms CM, Viner JP, Sturm RH, Renner ED, Johnson W: Comparative features of pneumococcal, mycoplasmal and legionnaires' disease pneumonias. Ann Intern Med 90:543, 1979.
    Patients with legionnaires' disease were more likely to present with unexplained encephalopathy, hematuria, and elevation of liver function tests than were those with pneumococcal or mycoplasmal pneumonia.

16. de Freitas SL, Borst J, Meenhorst PL: Easy visualization of Legionella pneumophila by "half-a-gram" stain procedure. Lancet 1:270, 1979.

17. Liu F, Wright DN: Gram stain in legionnaires' disease. Am J Med 77:549, 1984.
    The Gram's stain of clinical specimens is sometimes positive.

18. Edelstein PH, Meyer RD, Finegold SM: Laboratory diagnosis of legionnaires' disease. Am Rev Resp Dis 121:317, 1980.
    Comparison of sensitivity and specificity of the various "definitive" tests. Performance of all three—culture, DFA, and IFA—improved the diagnostic yield.

19. Kohler RB, et al: Rapid radioimmunoassay diagnosis of legionnaires' disease: Detection and partial characterization of urinary antigen. Ann Intern Med 94:601, 1981.
    The test may be positive even after treatment has been initiated.

Infection in the Immunocompromised Host

Howard Libman, M.D.

The immunocompromised host presents numerous diagnostic and therapeutic challenges to the clinician. A wide spectrum of common and opportunistic pathogens may cause infection at a variety of sites.[1-4] Routine diagnostic evaluation is often unrevealing. Empirical therapy with potentially toxic antimicrobial agents is sometimes necessary. Difficult questions may arise concerning the need for and timing of invasive diagnostic procedures.

CLINICAL APPROACH

In the evaluation of such a patient,[1] the following questions should be asked:
1. In which particular way(s) is the patient immunocompromised?
2. What kind of pathogens and sites of infection should be anticipated?
3. Based upon the initial clinical evaluation, what are the most likely diagnostic possibilities?

Patients are most often immunocompromised on the basis of (1) granulocytopenia, (2) defective humoral immunity, (3) defective cellular immunity, (4) disruption of the skin or mucosa, (5) anatomic obstruction, and/or (6) altered consciousness.

Granulocytopenia is commonly seen in association with acute leukemia, bone marrow transplantation or replacement, myelosuppressive drug or radiation therapy, and aplastic anemia. The risk of infection remains normal until the absolute granulocyte counts falls to 1000 cells/μl. When the count drops below this level, the incidence of infection increases, with the most dramatic rise occurring under 100 cells/μl. The most frequent sites of infection are the skin, oropharynx, esophagus, lungs, and perianal area. Endogenous flora, whether community-acquired or nosocomial, are the usual pathogens. These include enteric gram negative bacilli (especially *Pseudomonas aeruginosa*), *Staphylococcus aureus*, and the fungi Candida and Aspergillus species.

Defective humoral immunity, resulting from a lack of or dysfunction of opsonizing antibodies to encapsulated organisms, is present in several clinical settings. It is most often seen in patients with agammaglobulinemia, multiple myeloma, chronic lymphocytic leukemia, and asplenism. Infection with pyogenic bacteria such as *Streptococcus pneumoniae, Haemophilus influenzae, S. aureus*, and certain enteric gram negative bacilli is most common. Recurrent pneumonia is frequent, but other types of infection may be seen as well.

Because of its complexity, the cellular immune system is influenced by many different disease processes. Examples include Hodgkin's disease, T cell lymphomas, and the acquired immune deficiency syndrome (AIDS). Patients with solid tumors or acute lymphocytic leukemia and those undergoing bone marrow or organ transplantation may be compromised by radiation or chemotherapy that they receive. Common pathogens include the bacteria *Listeria monocytogenes, Nocardia asteroides*, non-typhosa Salmonella species, *Mycobacterium tuberculosis*, and the atypical mycobacteria; varicella-zoster virus, cytomegalovirus, and herpes simplex virus; the fungus *Cryptococcus neoformans;* and the protozoa *Pneumocystis carinii* and *Toxoplasma gondii*.

The skin and mucous membranes, major components of the nonspecific immune system, may be affected in a variety of ways. Patients with dermatitis, burns, skin trauma, and cutaneous malignancy are at increased risk for cellulitis and other soft tissue infections. Intravenous drug abusers may develop endocarditis or osteomyelitis from parenteral injection. Patients with chronic obstructive pulmonary disease are predisposed to bronchitis and pneumonia because of dysfunction of the mucociliary transport system. Diagnostic and therapeutic interventions, such as intravascular catheterization, endotracheal intubation, mechanical ventilation, urinary catheterization, and surgery, may lead to infection by permitting normal flora access to sterile body sites.

Anatomic obstruction results in infection by interfering with normal clearance mechanisms. Common clinical examples include bronchogenic carcinoma leading to postobstructive pneumonia, prostatic hypertrophy resulting in urinary tract infection, and biliary retention secondary to lymphoma or pancreatic carcinoma causing ascending cholangitis. The etiologic agents are usually part of the regional flora.

Altered consciousness, present in many acutely ill patients, may lead to aspiration of nasopharyngeal or gastric contents. Neuromuscular diseases that compromise the gag reflex may do the same. If aspiration pneumonia is community acquired, anaerobic mouth flora are the most frequent pathogens. In the chronically ill or hospitalized patient, enteric gram negative bacilli and S. aureus are common.

INITIAL MANAGEMENT

The acute management of the immunocompromised host with presumed infection involves a careful history and physical examination, and determination of the specific compromising factors.[1,5] Special attention should be directed to those body sites most likely involved. The initial laboratory evaluation consists of complete blood and differential counts, serum creatinine, liver function tests, urinalysis, chest radiographs, multiple blood cultures, and any additional tests suggested by the preliminary clinical data. Extra serum samples should be frozen for acute phase serologic testing. If it is not clear from the initial evaluation in which manner the patient is immunocompromised, a serum protein electrophoresis, quantitative immunoglobulins, and skin tests for delayed hypersensitivity are indicated.

Patients with granulocytopenia and those who are otherwise significantly immunocompromised should be treated with empirical antimicrobial therapy while awaiting culture results. The agents used in a given patient should be based upon determination of the most likely pathogens. Because enteric gram negative bacilli and S. aureus account for most serious infections in granulocytopenic individuals, coverage with a semisynthetic penicillin and an aminoglycoside (with or without an antipseudomonal penicillin) is generally recommended. Empirical therapy with other agents may be indicated if a definitive diagnostic test is unavailable or contraindicated. Once the bacteriology of the infection is known, specific therapy is provided. Modified reverse isolation procedures (e.g., use of a private room, careful handwashing before contact with patient, avoiding contact if infected) and antimicrobial prophylaxis against endogenous flora (e.g., nystatin and trimethoprim/sulfamethoxazole) are usually instituted in the context of granulocytopenia. Different precautions may be indicated in other clinical settings.

A more aggressive diagnostic approach is appropriate if an opportunistic pathogen is considered likely, if the patient is critically ill, if there is deterioration on empirical therapy, or if the initial work-up is inconclusive. The indications for the timing of invasive diagnostic procedures are different for each patient. Because the ultimate prognosis in the severely immunocompromised host depends primarily upon the ability to treat the underlying illness, ethical considerations are often an integral part of the decision making process.

KEY FEATURES

A rational approach to the immunocompromised patient requires asking the following questions:
- In which particular way(s) is the patient compromised?
- What kind of pathogens and sites of infections should be anticipated?
- Based upon the initial clinical evaluation, what are the most likely diagnostic possibilities?

Specific compromising factors include:
- Granulocytopenia
- Defective humoral immunity
- Defective cellular immunity
- Disruption of the skin or mucosa
- Anatomic obstruction
- Altered consciousness

PATHOGENS AND SITES OF INFECTION ASSOCIATED WITH SPECIFIC COMPROMISING FACTORS

Compromising Factor	Pathogens	Sites of Infection
Granulocytopenia	*P. aeruginosa* Enterobacteriaceae *S. aureus* Candida species Aspergillus species	Skin Oropharynx Esophagus Lungs Perianal area
Defective humoral immunity	*S. pneumoniae* *H. influenzae*	Lungs
Defective cellular immunity	*M. tuberculosis* Atypical mycobacteria *L. monocytogenes* *N. asteroides* *C. neoformans* Herpes viruses *P. carinii* *T. gondii*	Dependent upon pathogen
Disruption of skin or mucosa	Regional flora	Skin Lungs GI tract Urinary tract
Anatomic obstruction	Regional flora	Lungs Biliary tract Urinary tract
Altered consciousness	Pharyngeal flora	Lungs

MAJOR MECHANISMS OF COMPROMISED HOST DEFENSE
IN CERTAIN CLINICAL SETTINGS

Diagnosis/References	Mechanism	Basis
Solid tumor[6]*	Disruption of skin or mucosa	Disease, chemotherapy
	Anatomic obstruction	Disease
Acute leukemia[5,7-12]	Granulocytopenia	Disease, chemotherapy
	Disruption of skin or mucosa	Iatrogenic procedures, chemotherapy
Chronic lymphocytic leukemia[13]	Defective humoral immunity	Disease
Lymphoma[14,15]	Defective cellular immunity	Disease, chemotherapy
	Anatomic obstruction	Disease
Multiple myeloma[16]	Defective humoral immunity	Disease
Asplenism[17]	Defective humoral immunity	Impaired opsonic activity
Organ transplantation[18,19]	Defective cellular immunity	Immunosuppressive therapy
	Disruption of skin or mucosa	Iatrogenic procedures
Acquired immune deficiency syndrome[20,21,22]	Defective cellular immunity	Disease
	Disruption of skin or mucosa	Iatrogenic procedures
Substance abuse[23]	Disruption of skin or mucosa	Parenteral injection, trauma
	Altered consciousness	Drug effect
Corticosteroid therapy[24]	Defective cellular immunity	Multiple effects

*References apply to patients with granulocytopenia of any cause.

The initial management of the immunocompromised host with presumed infection includes the following:
- A careful history and physical examination
- Laboratory studies consisting of a complete blood and differential count, serum creatinine, liver function tests, urinalysis, chest radiograph, multiple blood cultures, and any additional tests suggested by the preliminary clinical data
- Patients with granulocytopenia and patients who are significantly compromised in other ways should be treated with empirical antibiotics
- Modified reverse isolation and antimicrobial prophylaxis against endogenous flora may be useful in granulocytopenic patients

REFERENCES

1. Dilworth JA, Mandell GL: Infections in patients with cancer. Semin Oncol 2:349, 1975. *Overview of the problem.*

2. Gold JWM: Opportunistic fungal infections in patients with neoplastic disease. Am J Med 76:458, 1984.

Description of clinical experience with candidiasis, aspergillosis, and cryptococcosis.

3. Wong KK, Hirsch MS: Herpes virus infections in patients with neoplastic disease: Diagnosis and therapy. Am J Med 76:464, 1984.
   Clinical review of herpes simplex virus, varicella-zoster virus, cytomegalovirus, and Epstein-Barr virus infections.

4. Wong B: Parasitic diseases in immunocompromised hosts. Am J Med 76:479, 1984.
   Experience with infections that are due to P. carinii, T. gondii, Strongyloides stercoralis, and the genus Cryptosporidium is reviewed.

5. Wiernik PH: The management of infection in the cancer patient. JAMA 244:185, 1980.
   An approach to the granulocytopenic patient is presented.

6. Inagaki J, Rodriguez V, Bodey GP: Causes of death in cancer patients. Cancer 33:568, 1973.
   Infection was responsible for 47% of deaths in patients wtih solid tumors. Pneumonia, septicemia, and peritonitis were the most common types.

7. Pizzo PA, et al: Duration of empiric antibiotic therapy in granulocytopenic patients with cancer. Am J Med 67:194, 1979.
   Empirical antibiotics should be continued until the white blood cell count is greater than 500 µl in the febrile, granulocytopenic patient who becomes afebrile during treatment.

8. Pizzo PA, Robichaud KJ, Gill FA, Witebsky FG: Empiric antibiotic and antifungal therapy for cancer patients with prolonged fever and granulocytopenia. Am J Med 72:101, 1982.
   Continuation of empirical antibiotics may be indicated in the granulocytopenic patient who remains febrile on therapy. Report recommends the addition of amphotericin B in this group of patients if fever persists for more than 7 days.

9. Pizzo PA, et al: Approaching the controversies in antibacterial management of cancer patients. Am J Med 76:436, 1984.
   Discussion of and an approach to common clinical problems.

10. Clift RA, Buckner CD: Granulocyte transfusions. Am J Med 76:631, 1984.
    Granulocyte transfusions are indicated in severely neutropenic patients with bacterial infection that persists despite maximal antibiotic therapy.

11. Henry SA: Chemoprophylaxis of bacterial infections in granulocytopenic patients. Am J Med 76:645, 1984.
    Discussion of the usefulness of trimethoprim/sulfamethoxazole to suppress endogenous flora in patients with granulocytopenia.

12. Armstrong D: Protected environments are discomforting and expensive and do not offer meaningful protection. Am J Med 76:685, 1984.
    Discussion of the controversies surrounding the utility of protected environments in managing granulocytopenic patients.

13. Shaw RK, et al: Infection and immunity in chronic lymphocytic leukemia. Arch Intern Med 106:467, 1960.
    Over half the patients studied developed bacterial infection, with lungs, upper respiratory tract, and skin the most common sites. There was reasonable correlation between infection and hypogammaglobulinemia.

14. Schimpff SC, et al: Infections in 92 splenectomized patients with Hodgkin's disease: A clinical review. Am J Med 59:695, 1975.

Infection was uncommon except for herpes zoster in radiated patients and bacterial infection in patients with recurrent Hodgkin's disease with persistent granulocytopenia.

15. Bishop JF, Schimpff SC, Diggs CH, Wiernik PH: Infections during intensive chemotherapy for non-Hodgkin's lymphoma. Ann Intern Med 95:549, 1981.
    Granulocytopenia, related to chemotherapy, was the major predisposing factor. The most common sites of infection were lungs, skin, and alimentary tract. Gram negative bacilli and S. aureus *were the most frequent pathogens.*

16. Meyers BR, Hirshman SZ, Axelrod JA: Current patterns of infection in multiple myeloma. Am J Med 52:87, 1972.
    Urinary tract infection and pneumonia were the most common infections. Enteric gram negative bacilli were the most frequent pathogens.

17. Heier HE: Splenectomy and serious infections. Scand J Haematol 24:5, 1980.
    Clinical review.

18. Rubin RH, Wolfson JS, Cosimi AB, Tolkoff-Rubin NE: Infection in the renal transplant recipient. Am J Med 70:405, 1981.
    Post-surgical bacterial infection predominated the first month following transplantation; cytomegalovirus infection, and pyelonephritis 1–4 months post-transplant; and a mixture of conventional and opportunistic infections more than 4 months post-transplant.

19. Winston DJ, Gale RP, Meyer DV, Young LS: Infectious complications of human bone marrow transplantation. Medicine 58:1, 1979.
    Comprehensive review.

20. Fauci AS, et al: Acquired immunodeficiency syndrome: Epidemiologic, clinical, immunologic and therapeutic considerations. Ann Intern Med 100:92, 1984.
21. Fauci AS, et al: The acquired immunodeficiency syndrome: An update. Ann Intern Med 102:800, 1985.
22. Grierson HL, Purtilo DT: New developments in AIDS. Inf Dis Clin North Am 1(3):547, 1987.
    Review articles on a rapidly evolving epidemic.

23. Louria DB: Infectious complications of nonalcoholic drug abuse. Ann Rev Med 25:219, 1974.
    Clinical review.

24. Dale DC, Petersdorf RG: Corticosteroids and infectious diseases. Med Clin North Am 57(5):1277, 1973.
    Corticosteroids affect host defenses in many different ways. Patients who receive chronic steroids are probably at increased risk for infection with a variety of pathogens.

Sepsis

Thomas Treadwell, M.D.

Sepsis, from the Greek word meaning decay, describes a toxic condition secondary to a localized or systemic infection. The word is often improperly used interchangeably with septicemia or bacteremia, because patients who appear septic may not be bacteremic, and conversely, many bacteremic patients are not toxic. Sepsis may result from a localized infection with toxemia, e.g., diphtheria, certain clostridial infections, or toxic shock syndrome; or may be the result of non "bacterial" agents, such as viruses, rickettsia, fungi, or even protozoa. Clearly, in the United States, most septic patients have a systemic bacterial infection, and this is the focus of this article.

A host of endogenous and exogenous mediators have been implicated in the pathophysiology of sepsis and bacteremia.[1] The most well studied of bacterial products is endotoxin, or lipopolysaccharide, found in the outer membranes of gram negative bacteria, which by itself may reproduce many of the clinical and laboratory findings of gram negative sepsis. However, gram positive infections are often clinically indistinguishable from those caused by gram negative bacilli, and other bacterial components or toxins may well be important, such as polysaccharide capsules of pneumococci, intracellular toxins of hemolytic streptococci and *Staphylococcus aureus,* and the exotoxins of *Pseudomonas aeruginosa.* Proposed endogenous mediators of sepsis include endogenous pyrogen (interleukin 1), catecholamines, kinins, tumor necrosis factor (cachectin), complement, endorphins, histamine, prostaglandins, and products of macrophages and white blood cells.

Many of these pathophysiologic mediators have been used to explain the clinical manifestations of sepsis, which unfortunately are similar irrespective of the offending agent. The vast majority of patients have fever, which tends to be higher for bacteremias caused by gram negative organisms. Occasionally, patients with severe bacteremia will fail to mount a fever or will present with hypothermia; such patients have higher mortality rates. The triad of fever, chills, and hypotension, the classic findings of gram negative bacteremia, is seen in one third of such cases. Other findings include tachypnea, respiratory alkalosis, metabolic acidosis, granulocytosis, coagulation abnormalities (including thrombocytopenia and disseminated intravascular coagulation), rashes, and oliguria.[2] Often signs or symptoms that are due to the primary infection site overshadow the systemic findings of sepsis.

Shock remains the most important syndrome associated with sepsis, and after heart disease, infection is the most common cause of shock. Gram negative bacteremia is associated with shock in 40% of cases, compared with lesser rates for gram-positive bacteremia (29% and 14% for *S. aureus* and pneumococcal bacteremia, respectively).[3] Typical hemodynamic changes in early sepsis include marked diminutions in arterial blood pressure, peripheral vascular resistance, central venous pressure, and pulmonary capillary wedge pressure with an elevated cardiac index ("warm shock"), patients late in sepsis may have depressed myocardial function and elevated systemic resistance, resulting in cool, clammy skin ("cold shock").[4,5] Shock dramatically increases mortality rates in all infections, and the major effort in the treatment of sepsis should be the prevention and early treatment of hypotension.

Because most fatalities that are due to sepsis occur within the first 48 hours, early recognition is of the utmost importance. Vigorous attempts to identify a primary source should be made, obtaining material for Gram's stain and culture whenever possible. Although never helpful in acute management, blood cultures should be drawn in an effort to document bacteremia. The "rule of three's" is helpful: that is, three blood cultures (usually drawn 30 minutes apart), incubated for 3 days, will detect more than 90% of bloodstream pathogens.[6] Immunologic methods to detect certain bacterial antigens in body fluids for rapid diagnosis have generally not been helpful except to confirm Gram's stain findings or in patients with meningitis.

The acute management of the septic patient consists of specific (antibiotic) and supportive therapy. Prompt institution of antimicrobial therapy will reduce morbidity and mortality; however, it should always be based, if possible, on results of Gram's stains of appropriate material and subsequently tailored, based on culture results, to the least toxic, narrowest spectrum, and least expensive regimen. In the absence of solid microbiologic data, the clinician must often start antibiotics empirically pending cultures, based on the likely site of infection and suspected pathogens for that site, community vs. nosocomial acquisition, underlying medical conditions, and the expected side effects of antibiotics.

Equally important in the management of sepsis are nonspecific measures, including vigorous volume expansion with crystalloid; careful monitoring of hydration, if necessary, with central venous presssure (CVP), wedged pulmonary artery catheterization and arterial pressure measurements; continuous observation of mental status and urine output; adequate ventilation; correction of acid-base abnormalities; and drainage/removal of purulent accumulations or foreign bodies. If shock is not corrected by volume expansion, vasoactive agents (usually dopamine) should be administered. The use of pharmacologic doses of steroids remains one of the most controversial topics in medicine. However, recent clinical trials of high-dose corticosteroids have failed to show a benefit in septic shock.[7] The opiate antagonist naloxone has been shown to reverse shock in uncontrolled studies in humans;[8] however, the first randomized, prospective controlled trial of this agent has shown no significant difference from placebo.[10] Antiserum to certain lipopolysaccharide antigens has been shown to decrease mortality in shock that is due to gram negative septicemia; currently, this is not a practical approach.[9]

KEY FEATURES

Sepsis results from the toxic manifestations of localized or systemic infection, most commonly as a result of bacteremia. Clinical features include alteration in body temperature, chills, tachypnea, changes in mentation, oliguria, coagulation abnormalities, acidosis, and shock. There are many etiologic agents.

Diagnostic Measures
1. Identification of possible primary site of infection
2. Obtain material for Gram's stain/culture
3. Two or three blood cultures, 30 minutes apart

Special Therapeutic Measures
1. Start antibiotic therapy after cultures are obtained
2. If possible, therapy is based on Gram's stain/culture results
3. Empiric therapy is based on clinical and epidemiologic factors
4. For suspected infection that is due to (by no means a complete list):
   a. Gram negative bacilli: aminoglycoside, aztreonam, or "new" cephalosporin
   b. *S. aureus:* oxacillin, a cephalosporin, or vancomycin
   c. Streptococci (nonenterccoccal): penicillin or cephalosporin
   d. Enterococci: ampicillin or vancomycin
   e. *Haemophilus influenzae:* chloramphenicol or ampicillin, second- or third-generation cephalosporin
   f. *Bacteroides fragilis:* clindamycin, metronidazole, cefoxitin, sulbactam-ampicillin

General Therapeutic Measures
1. Volume expansion, usually with crystalloid
2. Monitor fluid balance with indwelling urinary catheter if necessary
3. Frequent monitoring of arterial blood pressure
4. Monitor volume expansion with CVP catheter or pulmonary artery catheter
5. Adequate ventilation, supplemental oxygen
6. Correction of acidosis
7. Institution of vasoactive agents if volume expansion fails or results in decreased cardiac output
   a. Dopamine 2–20 µg/kg/minute, titrate urine output and systolic blood pressure
   b. Dobutamine 2–15 µg/kg/minute
   c. Norepinephrine 40–200 µg/minute
8. Drainage of purulent collections
9. ? Naloxone
10. ? Antiserum

REFERENCES

1. McCabe WR, Treadwell TL, DeMaria A: Pathophysiology of bacteremia. Am J Med 75: (suppl 1B):7, 1983.
   A review discussing mediators and pathophysiologic events in septicemia.

2. Kreger BE, Craven DE, McCabe WRF: Gram negative bacteremia IV. Re-evaluation of clinical features and treatment in 612 patients. Am J Med 68:344, 1980.
Underlying disease remains the most important determinate of outcome, but appropriate antibiotic therapy reduced mortality in all groups. There was no benefit of (1) steroids or (2) antibiotic combinations vs. single agents demonstrated.

3. McCabe WR, Olans RN: Shock in gram-negative bacteremia: Predisposing factors, pathophysiology, and treatment. *In* Remington JS, Swartz MN (eds): Current Clinical Topics in Infectious Diseases. New York, McGraw-Hill, 1981, p. 121.

4. Gunnar RM, et al: Hemodynamic measurements in bacteremia and septic shock in man. J Infect Dis 128:5295, 1973.
Patients with gram negative bacteremia have an early vasodilatory phase, but in established shock they have depressed myocardial function compared with patients with gram positive septicemia.

5. Morris DL, et al: Hemodynamic characteristics of patients with hypothermia due to occult infection and other causes. N Engl J Med 102:153, 1985.
Patients with hypothermia secondary to infection have decreased systemic vascular resistance and increased cardiac index.

6. Young LS, et al: Gram-negative rod bacteremia: Microbiologic, immunologic and therapeutic considerations. Ann Intern Med 86:456, 1977.
An excellent review with emphasis on the immunology and antimicrobial therapy of gram negative bacteremia.

7. Bone RC, et al: A controlled clinical trial of high-dose methylprednisolone in the treatment of severe sepsis and septic shock. N. Engl J Med 317:653, 1987.
Randomized, prospective, placebo-controlled clinical trial that demonstrated no benefit of steroids in the treatment of severe sepsis/septic shock.

8. Peters WP, et al: Pressor effect of naloxone in septic shock. Lancet 1:529, 1981.
An uncontrolled study in which small doses of this opiate antagonist had a transient pressor effect in septic shock.

9. Ziegler EJ, et al: Treatment of gram-negative bacteremia and shock with human antiserum to a mutant *Escherichia coli*. N Engl J Med 307:1125, 1982.
Antiserum to a rough mutant of E. coli *diminished mortality in patients with gram negative bacteremia, an effect that was most pronounced in patients in shock.*

10. DeMaria AD, Craven DE, Heffernan JJ, McIntosh T, Grindlinger GA, McCabe WR: Naloxone vs placebo in treatment of septic shock. Lancet 1:1363, 1985.
Standard dosage naloxone (0.4–1.2 mg) was no better than placebo in ameliorating hypotension in septic shock.

Acute Sinusitis and its Complications

Rochelle L. Epstein, M.D.

Sinusitis, an infection involving one or more of the paranasal sinuses, is a frequent complication of the single most common infectious disease: the common cold. Other predisposing conditions for this type of infection include dental infections; allergic rhinitis; trauma (surgical or accidental); and any one of several anatomic abnormalities, such as septal deviation, tumors, or nasal polyps. Bacterial sinusitis is the usual form of infection, but rarely, fungal[1] and mycobacterial sinusitis can occur.

The exact pathophysiology of sinusitis is not entirely understood. It has been known for many years that the normal sinuses are sterile.[2] It is believed that this sterile condition is maintained by the ciliary motion of respiratory epithelial cells that line the upper respiratory tract and the sinus cavities. Sinusitis occurs because of a combination of two factors: bacteria or other pathogens invade the sinuses because of a disturbance of normal ciliary motion, and obstruction of the normal drainage of the sinuses allows these organisms to proliferate and cause infection.[3,4] In its most common form, bacterial sinusitis results from superinfection of the sinuses in the setting of viral upper respiratory infection.[11] A variety of respiratory viruses are known to injure respiratory ciliated epithelial cells, with impairment of ciliary motion.[5] Although respiratory viruses have been cultured from sinus aspirates, it has never been shown that they can directly cause sinusitis. Because viral infections also cause inflammation of nasal mucosa, there is also obstruction of sinus drainage; thus, this is an ideal setting for development of sinus infection. Allergic rhinitis predisposes to sinus infection by very similar mechanisms.[3,4] Other conditions predispose to sinusitis for anatomic reasons. Dental infections involve the sinuses by direct spread, anatomic abnormalities such as septal deviation result in obstruction of sinus drainage, and surgical and accidental trauma can result in direct spread of infection to the sinus cavities. Suppurative sinusitis is a not infrequent complication of prolonged nasotracheal or nasogastric intubation.

Sinusitis is predominantly a disease of adults, largely because full development of the maxillary, frontal, and sphenoid sinuses does not occur until adolescence.[3] The ethmoid sinuses develop slightly faster, with significant development by age 7 and complete development by age 12.[6,7] Because colds are the most common predisposing factor, the disease follows the seasonal incidence of upper respiratory disease: peak incidence in late fall, winter, and early spring. Disease in the summer has been associated with swimming.[3] Patients most commonly present with facial pain, usually associated with purulent nasal discharge. Fever, headache, and nasal obstruction are other common complaints. Less commonly, patients may complain of abnormal sense of smell or change in voice quality. On physical examination, patients may have an assortment of physical signs, depending upon the involved sinus(es).[4,8] Maxillary sinusitis is the most common form of isolated sinusitis; the other sinuses usually become involved multiply. In maxillary sinusitis, nasal examination may reveal pus at the middle meatus.

Although classic signs of sinus tenderness or overlying erythema might be present, they are frequently absent. Tearing of the eyes or eyelid edema is very suggestive of ethmoid sinusitis. Transillumination of the maxillary sinuses can be a useful clinical tool when performed correctly in a darkened room but when done incorrectly can provide misleading clinical information. The radiologic finding of a cloudy sinus can be a useful finding when correlated to symptoms, if the patient does not have chronic disease.[3,4,8]

The microbiology of bacterial sinusitis has been studied extensively since the late 1800s.[2] Not surprisingly, the organisms that cause this disease are those bacteria that are ordinarily associated with the upper respiratory tract, predominantly the gram positive cocci.[2,8] A representative study showed that *Streptococcus pneumoniae* and *Haemophilis influenzae* account for slightly less than two thirds of cases, with other cases involving an assortment of organisms, including anaerobes (12%), Neisseria species (8.5%), *Streptococcus pyogenes* (3%), *Staphylococcus aureus* (2%), and some gram negative organisms.[8] There is some evidence that pure anaerobic infection is significantly associated with chronic sinusitis rather than the acute form of the disease.[9]

The therapy of acute sinusitis includes a combination of systemic antibiotic therapy with decongestants. Mechanical drainage of the affected sinus(es) is rarely but sometimes necessary. Topical decongestant therapy with phenylephrine hydrochloride nose drops, $\frac{1}{4}-\frac{1}{2}\%$, is probably the best choice, although a variety of oral agents are probably also effective.[3,4,9] The choice of antibiotics is empirical, since infected material is not usually available for diagnostic cultures. Microbiologic and clinical studies support the use of an agent effective against both *H. influenzae* and *S. pneumoniae*. A ten-day course of any one of the following regimens appears to have equal efficacy: ampicillin, 500 mg q6h; amoxicillin, 500 mg tid; and trimethoprim-sulfamethoxazole (80/400 mg), two tablets bid.[3,4,8] Infections that do not respond to these treatments might contain a significant component of *S. aureus*, which would require therapy with a penicillinase-resistant penicillin.[8]

Sinusitis has been associated with a variety of severe infectious complications, including osteomyelitis (particularly of the frontal bone), subperiosteal abscess, orbital cellulitis, cavernous sinus thrombosis, meningitis, brain abscess, and epidural or subdural empyema.[3] Perhaps the most feared of these complications with a significant clinical incidence is direct spread of the infection to the orbit. In children, this complication usually follows ethmoid sinusitis; in adults, it usually results from frontal or maxillary infections.[6,7,10] Benign edema of the orbit can occur simply as a reaction to sinus inflammation; however, frank infections of the orbit, including orbital cellulitis, orbital abscess, optic neuritis, or cavernous sinus thrombosis, can result in blindness or death. The orbit is susceptible to these infections because of its intimate anatomic contact with the sinuses: a paper-thin bony plate separates the orbit from the ethmoid air cells; the floor of the frontal sinus forms the superior wall of the orbit; the roof of the maxillary sinus contributes to the floor of the orbit; and the medial wall of the orbit includes portions of the maxillary, ethmoid, and sphenoid bones. In addition, there is abundant vascular communication with free flow of blood between the ophthalmic and sinus venous systems, with common drainage into the cavernous sinus.[4,6,10]

Orbital complications are most common in children and young adults, probably because prior to full sinus development there is wide open communication between the nasal cavity and the sinus areas.[6] Most patients present with perioribital swelling and fever, along with a variety of other signs and symptoms, including rhinorrhea, headache, eye pain, proptosis, and purulent nasal discharge. Although studies of the microbiology of the infection have been limited by the relative difficulty of obtaining culture material, it appears that in young children *H. influenzae* is the predominant organism. *S. pneumoniae*, group A streptoccci, and *S. aureus* appear to be the leading pathogens in other age groups.[3,7] Because of the severity of this infection and the disastrous consequences of inadequate treatment, in-hospital therapy with intravenous antibiotics is essential. For children, ampicillin or chloramphenicol therapy is recommended; for adults, therapy with oxacillin is suggested. Some authors believe that combination therapy is safer, adding penicillin G to either of the other regimens for better streptococcal coverage. Treatment should also include decongestants. Surgical drainage is necessary only if an intraorbital abscess is documented.

KEY FEATURES

Pathophysiology
Invasion of normally sterile sinuses by bacteria, owing to failure of protective function of ciliated epithelial cells combined with obstruction of drainage
Usual cause: common cold
Other causes: dental infections, allergic rhinitis, nasal polyps, trauma
Etiology
Mostly upper respiratory bacteria, especially pneumococci, *H. influenzae*, mouth anaerobes, and other streptococci. Rarely: fungi, mycobacteria
Clinical
Occurs more often in adults than in children
Symptoms: facial pain, fever, headache, nasal obstruction, purulent nasal discharge

Physical signs: sinus tenderness, facial erythema, eye tearing or lid edema, pus in the nose at the middle meatus, cloudy sinus on radiograph

Treatment: systemic antibiotics—ampicillin amoxicillin, or tri-methoprim-sulfamethoxazole—in addition to decongestants (topical Neo-Synephrine is best)

Complications

Orbital cellulitis, osteomyelitis, subperiosteal abscess, cavernous sinus thrombosis, meningitis, brain abscess, subdural or epidural empyema

REFERENCES

1. Gass JDM: Ocular manifestations of acute mucormycosis. Arch Ophthal 65:226–236, 1961.
   A detailed review of ophthalmologic fungal infections. The article includes clinical photographs and stained histologic sections.

2. Bjorkwall T: Bacteriologic examination in maxillary sinusitis; bacteriologic flora of the maxillary antrum. Acta Otolaryngol 83:33, 1950.
   This is a very old study, but it contains an extensive review of all bacteriologic studies of both healthy and infected sinuses conducted up until 1950. Although the data are old, the conclusions appear to remain true to the present time.

3. Gwaltney JM Jr: Sinusitis. In Mandell GL, Douglas RG, Bennett JE (eds): Principles and Practice of Infectious Diseases. New York, John Wiley and Sons, 1979, pp 458–466.
   This is a very thorough review of the subject, including an excellent bibliography list.

4. Branch WT Jr, Weinstein L: Disease of the upper respiratory tract. In Branch WT Jr (ed): Office Practice of Medicine. Philadelphia, WB Saunders Co, 1982, pp 3–56.
   An extensive review of all aspects of upper respiratory diseases with a complete bibliography. A superb set of anatomic drawings and illustrations demonstrating correct methods of performing various examinations (such as sinus transillumination or use of the nasal speculum) make this chapter an excellent reference source on the subject.

5. Klein JD, Collier AM: Pathogenesis of human parainfluenza type 3 virus infection in hamster tracheal organ culture. Infect Immunol 10:883–888, 1974.
   This study is one example of several papers in which a tissue organ culture model system was used to demonstrate functional as well as histologic effects of viral infection on ciliated epithelial cells.

6. Chandler JR, Langenbrunner DJ, Stevens ER: The pathogenesis of orbital complications in acute sinusitis. Laryngoscope 80:1414–1428, 1970.
   This article details the anatomic relationship of the orbit to the paranasal sinuses, describes the spectrum of orbital complications with the help of diagrams and photographs, and provides clinical information about diagnosis and treatment.

7. Haynes RE, Cranblett HG: Acute ethmoiditis. Its relationship to orbital cellulitis. Am J Dis Child 114:261–267, 1967.
   A study of 26 patients in whom a clinical diagnosis of orbital cellulitis was directly associated with radiographic or other unequivocal evidence of ethmoid sinusitis. The article emphasizes the occurrence of this disease in children, notes the high complication rate, and encourages early suspicion of this diagnosis so that prompt treatment can be initiated.

8. Hamory BH, Sande MA, Syndor A, Seale DL, Gwaltney JM: Etiology and antimicrobial therapy of acute maxillary sinusitis. J Infect Dis 139:197–202, 1979.
   A microbiologic study in which needle puncture was used to obtain specimens for

culture. Efficacies of several antibiotic regimens were compared, both for clinical resolution of symptoms and for microbiologic cure (by repeat puncture).

9. Frederick J, Braude AL: Anaerobic infection of the paranasal sinuses. N Engl J Med 290:135–137, 1974.
    A relatively recent study documenting significant presence of anaerobic bacteria in culture aspirates of chronically infected nasal sinuses. Unlike previous studies, in which specimens were obtained via external puncture (thus allowing nasal contamination), these specimens were obtained directly during surgical procedures.

10. Jarrett WH, Gutman FA: Ocular complications of infection in the paranasal sinuses. Arch Ophthal 81:683–688, 1969.
    A comparison of clinical features of seven cases of ocular complications of sinus infections, with photographs and comments on pathophysiology and treatment.

11. Katz A, Simpson GT: The nose and paranasal sinuses. *In* Noble J (ed): Textbook of General Medicine and Primary Care, 1st ed. Boston/Toronto, Little, Brown, 1987, pp 827–838.
    Excellent discussion of the anatomy, physiology, and clinical problems of the sinuses and upper airway.

Pyelonephritis

Rochelle L. Epstein, M.D.

Acute pyelonephritis is an infection of the upper urinary tract, including the ureters and the renal parenchyma. The basic mechanism of this infection is the upward spread of infectious organisms from an infected lower urinary tract.[1–4] Hence, pyelonephritis cannot be viewed as a separate disease entity, but must be viewed as one end of the spectrum of acute urinary tract infections (UTIs). Although pyelonephritis turns out to be a relatively rare cause of chronic renal failure in adults,[1,4,5] it remains important because of its association with transient renal dysfunction and a high risk of sepsis. Serious renal complications can occur, such as renal papillary necrosis[6] and perinephric abscess.[7] Pyelonephritis remains a serious complication of pregnancy, with deleterious effects on both the mother and the fetus,[4] and can result in life-threatening infection in infants, and in diabetic, elderly, or chronically ill patients.

Despite many years of study, gaps still remain in our understanding of the pathophysiology of these infections. Some infections can be explained by the presence of anatomic abnormalities that result in obstruction of the normal flow of urine or defects in voiding. This is particularly true of infections in males, which most frequently occur in early childhood (congenital anomalies) or in older age groups (obstruction as a result of prostate enlargement).[4,7] Instrumentation of the urinary tract, especially the use of indwelling urinary catheters, are also well-described causes of UTI's.[8] This article focuses on the "uncomplicated" form of infection, in which defined predisposing conditions do not exist. Traditionally, UTIs have been viewed as bacterial diseases caused predominantly by gram negative enteric bacteria. It now appears likely that nonbacterial pathogens, primarily chlamydia and genital mycoplasmas, also play a role, particularly as causes of urethritis.[4] Because most of our understanding of UTIs stems from studies of bacterial infections, these are emphasized in this limited review.

UTIs are extremely common in the female population, in whom it has been estimated that 10–20% of women experience a UTI at some point in their lifetime.[4,7] Only a very small proportion of these patients develop pyelonephritis. The initial stage of infection involves colonization of the vaginal introitus and periurethral area by pathogenic organisms that are normal inhabitants of the gut. This is followed by colonization of the urethra, passage of organisms into the normally sterile bladder, and, if these organisms become established and proliferate, development of infection. In some patients, organisms then invade the urethers (reflux occurs secondary to incompetent vesicourethral valves) and spread upward to the kidney, causing pyelonephritis.[1–4] *Escherichia coli* causes a major proportion of these infections (80–90%), with Klebsiella, Proteus, and Enterobacter being the other leading pathogens, followed by Pseudomonas, staphylococci, and group D streptococci. Numerous studies have attempted to explain why specific bacteria are prevalent and why some patients develop infections whereas others do not. A variety of characteristics have been identified as contributing factors, including bacterial virulence factors (motility, presence or absence of pili, quantity of K antigen, serum sensitivity, etc.) and host defense factors (local antibody production, serum antibodies, possible differences in ability of vaginal epithelial cells to bind bacteria, etc.).[2,4] Many studies have also demonstrated particular susceptibility of pregnant women to UTIs, the very high incidence of complicating pyelonephritis in these women (20–40%), and the possible physiologic explanations for this high rate of complicating pyelonephritis.[2,4,7]

A clinical syndrome involving dysuria, frequency, urgency, and suprapubic tenderness has been used to identify patients suspected of having UTIs, and diagnostic laboratory criteria exist for distinguishing bladder infections from contamination, "benign" bacteriuria, and the "urethral syndrome."[4,7,9] Because patients with upper tract involvement require more prolonged therapy than those with lower tract disease and are more prone both to relapse and to reinfection,[4,7,9–11] it is essential to determine whether or not an individual patient has upper tract involvement. Although the clinical syndrome described previously with the addition of more serious systemic symptoms including flank pain and/or tenderness, fever, and chills has traditionally been used to identify the subgroup of patients with pye-lonephritis, many studies have now demonstrated that clinical signs and symptoms alone are poor indicators of the presence or location of infection. Invasive studies, including bilateral ureteral catheterization, the "bladder washout" technique, and renal biopsy, have proved to be reliable methods of documenting the presence of upper tract infection.[4,7,9] To date, no entirely satisfactory noninvasive method exists for making this diagnosis.[4,12] A wide variety of methods are under study, including the popularized immunoflu-orescence technique of looking for antibody-coated bacteria in urine. The ultimate utility of this technique has yet to be determined.[12] For treatment purposes, we must therefore continue to use the clinical presentation de-scribed previously, along with microbiologic documentation, to decide which patients have pyelonephritis. Patients with occult upper tract disease (i.e., those not presenting with a classic clinical picture) are unlikely to respond to ordinary outpatient regimens for uncomplicated UTI. Thus, it has been suggested that failure to respond to standard treatment with an appropriate antibiotic (assuming that sensitivity of the infecting organism is known) or rapid relapse with the identical organism be included as criteria for this diagnosis.[4,9]

Although prolonged treatment is recommended for infections involving the renal parenchyma, there are still controversies concerning optimal treat-ment of pyelonephritis, particularly in patients who are clinically not very ill.[4,11] It is generally agreed that patients appearing "toxic," with systemic symptoms including fevers, chills, nausea, or vomiting, and local tenderness, should be admitted to the hospital for treatment with parenteral antibiotics and intravenous fluids. Patients at high risk of sepsis (pregnant women, diabetics, elderly or debilitated patients) and patients suspected to have an anatomic abnormality or obstruction of the urinary system should also receive vigorous in-hospital therapy. Blood and urine cultures should always be obtained prior to initiating therapy, and a Gram's stain of the urine should be examined as a guide to initial therapy. Renal ultrasound is an excellent test for detecting obstruction. Because most infections are caused by E. coli or other community-acquired gram negative organisms, treatment with am-picillin or a cephalosporin is appropriate empiric therapy. In severely ill patients, or if enterococcal infection is suspected (gram positive cocci on Gram's stain), an aminoglycoside should be added. The optimal duration of therapy has not been well defined, but studies showing high relapse and reinfection rates despite appropriate antimicrobial therapy have led some authors to recommend 6 weeks of treatment.[4,10,11] It has certainly been shown that many patients can be cured with courses as short as 2 weeks;[4,11] therefore, therapy must be individualized. Fluid therapy is essential adjunctive treat-ment. In addition to treating dehydration, an expected manifestation of fever and poor fluid intake, it has been demonstrated that water diuresis itself helps to eradicate kidney infection.[4]

Outpatient therapy with oral antibiotics is appropriate for patients who are less ill. Even when the diagnosis of pyelonephritis is based upon failure of a short course of oral therapy, prolonged oral therapy (2–6 weeks) with a wide variety of antibiotics can eradicate infection.[4,7] The optimal duration of therapy remains unknown, and recommendations vary from 14 days to several months. Two studies showed no difference in relapse rates between patients treated for 2 weeks vs. those treated for 6 weeks.[4] Irrespective of the chosen duration of therapy, high relapse and reinfection rates require that patients receive long-term microbiologic and clinical follow-up. Urine cultures should be performed for several months after cessation of therapy. Positive cultures following appropriate treatment are an indication for re-treatment and evaluation for anatomic lesions (ultrasound, intravenous pyelogram, cystoscopy, etc.).

KEY FEATURES

Definition
Infection of upper urinary tract—includes renal parenchyma. Almost always associated with lower tract disease (UTI)

Pathophysiology
Ascending infection (urethra to bladder to ureter to kidney); "complicating" factors include obstruction, indwelling catheters
- Congenital anomalies
- Enlarged prostate
- Bladder lesions
- Extrinsic lesions (tumors)

Complications: sepsis, renal papillary necrosis, perinephric abscess, renal dysfunction, renal failure (rarely)

Epidemiology
- UTI most common in women
- Pregnant women especially susceptible (including complications)
- Men usually have underlying causes
- Other high-risk groups: diabetics, elderly, infants, chronically ill

Microbiology
- Enteric gram negative bacilli (E. coli, Klebsiella, Proteus, Enterobacter, Pseudomonas)
- Others: staphylococci, group D streptococci (especially enterococci)
- Chlamydia, genital mycoplasms (? role in upper tract disease)

Diagnosis
- UTI: dysuria, frequency, urgency, suprapubic tenderness
- Pyelonephritis: add the following—fever, chills, nausea, vomiting, costovertebral angle pain/tenderness
- All correlate poorly with presence of or extent of disease

- Urine Gram's stain, blood, and urine cultures important
- Microbiologic diagnosis and clinical follow-up essential

Treatment
- Inpatient vs. outpatient therapy depends on clinical state, risk group
- Fluid therapy important
- Antibiotics: ampicillin with or without aminoglycosides, or trimethoprim/sulfamethoxazole good empiric therapy, but many other agents are acceptable. Once cultures are available, physician can switch to another agent if necessary
- Duration: at least 2 weeks; up to 6 weeks if necessary
- Follow-up: repeat cultures essential up to 2 years later because of very high relapse and reinfection rates

REFERENCES

1. Roberts JA: Pathogenesis of pyelonephritis. J Urol 129:1102–1106, 1983.

    This review article summarizes experimental data about route of infection, bacterial virulence factors, reflux, and host immune responses, and includes 70 references in the field.

2. Braude AL: Current concepts of pyelonephritis. Medicine 52:257–264, 1973.

    Although this review was written 10 years before the first reference, it discusses much of the earlier experimental data that have contributed to this field and includes 49 references.

3. Vivaldi E, Cotran R, Zangwill DP, Kass EH: Ascending infection as a mechanism in pathogenesis of experimental nonobstructive pyelonephritis. Proc Soc Exp Biol Med 102:242–244, 1959.

    This is one of the original papers showing experimentally that pyelonephritis could occur by an ascending route. The laboratory from which this paper was published (Dr. Kass') was one of the frontrunners in defining UTIs and exploring pathogenesis.

4. Andriole VT: Current concepts of urinary tract infections. Semin Infect Dis 3:89–130, 1980.

    More comprehensive than the previously cited reviews, this excellent review of selected topics covers a wide range of relevant areas, with emphasis on those areas that are still controversial and on topics where more research work needs to be done. This paper lists 213 references.

5. Schecter H, Leonard CD, Scribner BH: Chronic pyelonephritis as a cause of renal failure in dialysis candidates. JAMA 216:514–517, 1971.

    One of many clinical series showing that chronic pyelonephritis in the absence of an underlying structural defect was a rare cause of end-stage chronic renal failure. This retrospective analysis of the histories of 173 dialysis patients identified 13% in whom chronic pyelonephritis was the primary cause of renal failure, but all of these patients had structural defects.

6. Hellebusch AA: Renal papillary necrosis. A urological emergency. JAMA 210:1098–1100, 1969.

    A short description of this entity with four case reports including photographs of salient radiologic findings.

7. Kaye D, Santoro J: Urinary tract infections. In Mandell GL, Douglas RG, Bennett JE (eds): Principles and Practice of Infectious Diseases. New York, John Wiley and Sons, 1979, pp 537–570.

An excellent chapter on the entire spectrum of UTIs with review of current under-standing of pathophysiology and emphasis on clinical information. This chapter also in-cludes 216 references.

8. Thornton GF, Andriole VT: Bacteriuria during indwelling catheter drainage. JAMA 214:339–342, 1970.
   One of multiple clinical studies emphasizing the high risk of UTI in patients requiring prolonged indwelling catheter drainage and demonstrating efficacy of closed sterile drain-age systems in limiting this complication.

9. Abraham E, Brenner BE, Simon RR: Cystitis and pyelonephritis. Ann Emerg Med 12:228–234, 1983.
   Another review with emphasis on clinical information with particular emphasis on diagnosis and treatment. This paper includes 94 references.

10. Little PJ, Wardener HE: Acute pyelonephritis. Incidence of reinfection in 100 patients. Lancet 2:1277–1278, 1966.
    One of the early clinical articles showing the high rate of recurrence in these patients despite appropriate treatment and emphasizing this particular problem in pregnant women.

11. McCabe WR, Jackson GG: Treatment of pyelonephritis. Bacterial and host factors in success or failure among 252 patients. N Engl J Med 272:1037–1044, 1965.
    Extensive microbiologic investigation, analysis of host factors, and 3-year follow-up of patients treated for chronic pyelonephritis, with the intent of identifying factors that influenced treatment outcome. About two thirds of patients had relapse; causes for the majority of relapses could not be found.

12. Mundt KA, Polk BF: Identification of site of urinary tract infections by antibody-coated bacteria assay. Lancet 4:1172–1175, 1979.
    Review of published literature about the antibody-coated bacteria assay for deter-mining site of UTI involvement, with the goal of determining its usefulness. The authors calculate sensitivity, specificity, and predictive value from published data, and conclude that this assay has no present role in management of patients.

13. Komaroff AL, Pass TM, McCue JD, Cohen AB, Hendricks TM, Friedland G: Management strategies for urinary and vaginal infections. Arch Intern Med 138:1069–1073, 1978.
    Clinical data were accumulated on 821 women coming to a primary care setting complaining of UTI symptoms. Predictive values of various symptoms and laboratory findings were calculated, and a nomogram for appropriate diagnostic management was proposed.

14. Rice PA, Vayo HE, Libman H: Sexually transmitted diseases. In Noble J (ed): Textbook of General Medicine and Primary Care. Boston/Toronto, Little, Brown, 1987, pp 1730–1742.
    A detailed summary of urethritis and cystitis in female and male patients.

Pelvic Inflammatory Disease

Rochelle L. Epstein, M.D.

Pelvic inflammatory disease (PID) is the general name for infections of the female upper genital tract. The disease is also called salpingo-oophoritis, since although infection primarily involves the uterus and fallopian tubes, extension to surrounding peritoneum to involve the ovaries and neighboring structures is common. The mortality rate in PID is low; however, the disease has major clinical significance because of important medical and social consequences of infection.

Over the past 15 years, the incidence of PID has risen sharply in the United States, parallel to an increase that has been observed in the frequency of all sexually transmitted diseases. It has been estimated that PID accounts for 2.0–2.5 million outpatient visits per year, and enough hospital days to keep six 400-bed hospitals full at all times. The major medical sequelae of PID, including involuntary infertility, ectopic pregnancy, and chronic pelvic pain, have had major impact on the lives of women who have experienced even a single episode of this infection. Twenty to 30% of involuntary infertility in the United States is due to fallopian tube obstruction, which in most cases has resulted from prior pelvic infection. The incidence of ectopic pregnancy is seven times higher in women who have had an episode of PID than in those who have not. Chronic pelvic pain syndromes occur in 18% of patients who have had PID, compared with 6% in the general female population, and often result in major surgical procedures and major disruptions of personal lifestyles.

PID is generally an ascending infection resulting from penetration of organisms from the vagina and cervix into the normally sterile uterus and fallopian tubes. Exceptions to this rule are rare (e.g., tuberculous salpingitis results from hematogenous spread; secondary PID results from local spread from an infectious origin outside of the genital tract). PID can result from two major exogenous sources: (1) venereal infections, such as gonorrhea; or (2) iatrogenic causes, such as intrauterine devices (IUD) or medical procedures (e.g., hysterosalpingogram). The causes of nonsurgical endogenous PID, infections caused by pathogenic organisms that are normal members of the vaginal flora, are still poorly understood. PID can be caused by a variety of organisms other than *Neisseria gonorrhoeae*, including many common aerobic and anaerobic bacteria, *Mycoplasma hominis, Ureaplasma urealyticum*, and *Chlamydia trachomatis*. Up to 50% of cases are polymicrobial infections. *Mycobacterium tuberculosis* causes PID rarely. Patients with IUDs are especially prone to serious infections, especially with group A beta hemolytic streptococci and Actinomyces species. The incidence of gonococcal PID varies, depending upon the population studied, but has been estimated to be between 45% and 80% of cases. This form of the disease tends to occur in younger patients and is more likely to be the cause when the illness represents the first episode of the disease for the patient.

Despite many studies that have demonstrated disparities in case diagnosis when based upon clinical observations compared with laparoscopic findings, clinical evaluation by history and findings on physical examination remains the most practical method of diagnosis for most patients. The usual diagnostic criteria include some combination of (1) clinical symptoms: fever, lower abdominal pain, abdominal tenderness; (2) findings on pelvic examination: cervical motion tenderness, adnexal tenderness, pelvic mass and/or induration; and (3) laboratory findings: leukocytosis, elevated erythrocyte sedimentation rate (ESR), Gram's stain of cervical material positive for gonococcus. Patients can present with a wide spectrum of severity of clinical illness, from mild abdominal pain to severe systemic toxicity. The disease can be present in the absence of any single finding or laboratory result listed in this article. It is therefore essential for the physician to consider this diagnosis in all sexually active women. A pelvic examination should be performed on any woman with abdominal or pelvic complaints. Differential diagnosis must include other pelvic and abdominal processes that could have similar presentation, e.g., ectopic pregnancy, endometriosis, corpus luteum hemorrhage, ovarian tumors, mesenteric adenitis, inflammatory bowel disease, and appendicitis. Common characteristics of PID to consider include the following:

1. Pain associated with PID is usually bilateral and constant (can be more severe on one side or the other).
2. Vaginal discharge is extremely common.
3. Dysuria occurs in 20% of cases.
4. Abnormal menstrual bleeding occurs in 35–40% of patients (especially common in gonococcal PID).
5. Twenty-five per cent of patients have nausea, vomiting, or anorexia.

A Gram's stain of cervical material should always be performed. The demonstration of gram negative *intracellular* diplococci correlates with a positive culture for *N. gonorrhoeae* in over 90% of cases (high specificity). Unfortunately, the sensitivity of this test is much lower: only 48–71% of patients with positive cultures have had a positive Gram's stain. The rate of transmission of gonorrhea to sexual partners is extremely high. Thus, all sexual contacts of patients with gonococcal PID should receive appropriate antibiotic treatment.

Special tests are sometimes necessary for diagnosis of complicated cases. These include (1) culdocentesis: should be performed if ectopic pregnancy is a serious consideration; (2) pelvic ultrasound: especially useful for diagnosis of ovarian cysts or abscesses; and (3) laparoscopy: currently reserved for patients who fail to improve with antibiotic therapy, or any patient in whom the diagnosis is in doubt. Surgical exploration may be required for patients who present with signs of an acute abdomen or pelvic mass.

Treatment of this infection depends in part upon the severity of clinical illness. Antimicrobial treatment is directed primarily at *N. gonorrhoeae*, *C. trachomatis*, and anaerobic species. Table 1 lists the Centers for Disease Control (CDC) recommended antibiotic regimens for ambulatory and hospitalized patients.[8] Outpatient treatment is acceptable if the patient is able to take oral medications and does not have findings suggestive of pelvic mass or acute abdomen, and if good follow-up care is available. More severely ill patients may require hospitalization for intravenous medication and supportive care, or for further diagnostic evaluation.

KEY FEATURES

PID is *common;* there are three major sequelae: infertility, ectopic pregnancy, and chronic pelvic pain.

Exogenous sources: sexually transmitted or iatrogenic (IUDs or procedures); *endogenous* sources: vaginal flora or local spread.

Most infections are *mixed* (more than a single organism) and often

Table 1.   TREATMENT REGIMENS FOR PELVIC INFLAMMATORY DISEASE

Ambulatory Treatment

Cefoxitin 2.0 gm IM, or amoxicillin 3.0 gm PO, or ampicillin 3.5 gm PO, or aqueous procaine penicillin G 4.8 million U IM at 2 sites or ceftriaxone 250 mg IM (all once only)

plus

Probenecid 1.0 gm PO (once only; not given with ceftriaxone)

plus

Doxycycline 100 mg PO bid (or tetracycline 500 mg PO qid) for 10–14 days

Inpatient Treatment

Doxycycline 100 mg IV q12h plus cefoxitin 2.0 gm IV q6–8h for at least 4 days and at least 48 hours after defervescence, with doxycycline 100 mg PO bid thereafter to conclude 10–14 days of therapy

or

Clindamycin 600 mg IV q6–8h plus gentamicin/tobramycin 2.0 mg/kg IV followed by 1.5 mg/kg IV q8h (if renal function is normal) for at least 4 days and at least 48 hours after defervescence, followed by clindamycin 450 mg PO q6–8h to conclude 10–14 days of therapy

Adapted from 1985 STD treatment guidelines. Morbid Mortal Weekly Rep 34(suppl): 92S–94S, 1985.

include both aerobic and anaerobic organisms. Common pathogens include *Neisseria gonorrhoeae, Chlamydia trachomatis, Mycoplasma hominis, Ureaplasma urealyticum,* and other common aerobic and anaerobic bacteria.

Clinical findings include the following:
1. Usual symptoms: fever, lower abdominal pain, abdominal tenderness
2. Other common symptoms: vaginal discharge, dysuria, abnormal menstrual bleeding, nausea, vomiting, anorexia
3. Pelvic examination: cervical motion tenderness, adnexal tenderness, pelvic mass and/or induration
4. Laboratory: leukocytosis, elevated ESR, positive Gram's stain of cervical material for gonococcus (intracellular gram negative diplococci)

Differential diagnosis: Ectopic pregnancy, endometriosis, corpus luteum hemorrhage, ovarian tumors, mesenteric adenitis, inflammatory bowel disease, appendicitis

Treatment: Antibiotics (see Table 1), supportive care

BIBLIOGRAPHY

1. Polk BF, Branch WT: Salpingitis. *In* Branch WT Jr: Office Practice of Medicine. Philadelphia, WB Saunders Co, 1982, pp 450–455.
   An excellent and concise, clinically oriented review of salpingitis, including a comprehensive bibliography for further reference.

2. Eisenbach DA: Polymicrobial etiology of acute pelvic inflammatory disease. N Engl J Med 293:166–171, 1975.
   A carefully performed microbiologic study demonstrating the vast number of aerobic and anaerobic organisms associated with this disease.

3. Jacobson L, Westrom L: Objectivized diagnosis of acute pelvic inflammatory disease. Diagnostic and prognostic value of routine laparoscopy. Am J Obstet Gynecol 105:1088–1098, 1969.
   This Swedish study examined the relationship (and discrepancies) between history and physical examination vs. laparoscopy for diagnosis.

4. Sweet RL, Mills J, Hadley KW, et al: Use of laparoscopy to determine the microbiologic etiology of acute salpingitis. Am J Obstet Gynecol 134:68–74, 1979.
   This smaller American study of laparoscopy also showed some discrepancies between laparoscopic findings and the clinical presentation.

5. Westrom L: Effect of acute pelvic inflammatory disease on fertility. Am J Obstet Gynecol 122:707–713, 1975.
   This study examined the relationship between PID and infertility.

6. Centers for Disease Control (CDC): Treatment guidelines. Morbid Mortal Weekly Rep 34 (suppl.):92S–94S, 1985.
   Extensive treatment guidelines with concise rationales for most sexually transmitted diseases.

7. Rice PA, Vayo HE, Libman H: Sexually transmitted disease. *In* Noble J (ed). Textbook of General Medicine and Primary Care. Boston/Toronto, Little, Brown, 1987, pp 1734–1739.

A current review of the entire area of sexually transmitted diseases, including PID, with extensive bibliography.

8. Treatment of sexually transmitted diseases. Med Letter Drugs Therapeut 30:5–10, 1988.
   Treatment recommendations advocating inclusion of cefoxitin or ceftriaxone and dox-ycycline in primary treatment regimens for PID, predicated on increasing prevalence of penicillin-resistant Neisseria gonorrhoeae *and emergence of tetracycline-resistant strains.*

Malaria

David Schwartz, M.D.
Brant L. Viner, M.D.

With as many as 300 million worldwide cases per year, malaria continues to be one of the leading medical concerns in temperate and tropical countries.[1] The abandonment of mosquito control programs combined with the antimalarial resistance of *Plasmodium falciparum* has led to a resurgence of this disease throughout the world. Owing to increased world travel, immigration, and military activity, malaria remains the most common acute febrile illness imported into the United States.[2] As a rule, malaria in the United States is imported in over 95% of cases and occurs predominantly (over 75%) in foreigners.[2] Exceptions include congenital malaria, blood transfusion–associated malaria,[3] and malaria resulting from shared needles among drug addicts. With over 1100 cases occurring annually in the United States,[2] U.S. physicians must be capable of recognizing and treating patients with this disease.

As with most parasitic infections, a cursory review of the life cycle will aid in understanding the clinical picture as well as the therapeutic options. The plasmodium goes through both a sexual (sporogony) and an asexual (schizogony) stage. Both stages require a parasitic relationship with a host organism—Anopheles mosquitos for the sexual stage and humans for the asexual stage. The sexual phase begins when a suitable Anopheles mosquito ingests mature gametocytes in a blood meal taken from an infected human host. These gametocytes mate, forming an oocyte, which develops in the stomach lining of the mosquito. Once mature, the oocyte releases several hundred sporozoites, which migrate to the salivary glands, remaining dormant until they are injected into a susceptible human host—thus initiating the asexual stage. The sporozoites are rapidly (within 30 minutes) cleared from the circulation and individually infect hepatocytes. These sporozoites may remain dormant or may grow and divide, releasing several thousand merozoites into the circulation. Once released, the merozoites infect red blood cells and can be identified as a ring-shaped trophozoite within a RBC. The trophozoite then develops and divides, forming a mature schizont (RBC packed with merozoites). The schizont ruptures and the merozoites penetrate fresh RBCs, thereby initiating a new generation of parasites. After several generations some merozoites will develop into sexually differentiated gametocytes. When these gametocytes are ingested by an Anopheles mosquito, the malarial life cycle is completed.

There are several distinctions among species of plamodia (*falciparum, vivax, malariae,* and *ovale*), but clinically, the only important distinction is between *P. falciparum* and the others.[4] Falciparum malaria, unlike the other types, is often chloroquine resistant and can result in death in the absence of underlying diseases. Additionally, falciparum infections should be viewed as a medical emergency because they are capable of killing their host within 24 hours of the onset of symptoms. The characteristics that allow for this excess mortality in falciparum infections include the following:

1. *P. falciparum* infects all red blood cells, whereas the other species infect either old or young red blood cells.
2. *P. falciparum* causes a much higher level of parasitemia (40–500,000 organisms/ml vs. 10–30,000 organisms/ml). This overwhelming parasitemia is associated with marked hemolysis with resultant complications.
3. *P. falciparum* causes the infected RBC to become sticky and adhere to the capillary endothelium. This sludging is associated with diffuse and focal ischemic changes throughout the body.
4. *P. falciparum* is the only form resistant to conventional antimalarials.

Thus, recognition of the falciparum infection is crucial and may be life saving.

Morphologic and clinical features that distinguish falciparum infection from the others include the following:

1. Falciparum infections are usually manifested while an individual is in an endemic region or within 2 months of leaving such a region. The reason for this is that *P. falciparum* is unable to remain dormant in hepatocytes.
2. Clinically, all patients with malaria may have fevers, myalgias, headache, mild anemia, and splenomegaly, but severe hemolytic anemia, CNS changes, acute renal failure, and massive hemoglobinuria are usually seen only in *P. falciparum* infections. The fever curve is not reliable in distinguishing subtypes of malaria.
3. Morphologically, falciparum infection will demonstrate only ring forms within RBCs and banana-shaped gametocytes, whereas the other species will have ameboid-appearing trophozoites and mature schizonts in addition to their ring and gamete forms. An additional subtle point is that

the ring forms of *P. falciparum* are hair-like and more than one ring form may infect the same RBC, whereas ring forms in the other species are coarse and usually have only one ring form per RBC.

These points should help one distinguish between falciparum and other Plasmodium infections, but when in doubt one should obtain the proper smears and treat empirically for falciparum infection.

Once the diagnosis is considered, a few simple steps should be taken before initiating therapy. Blood specimens for the thin and thick smears are best obtained from finger sticks because samples from capillary blood will demonstrate a much higher parasite load. If *P. falciparum* is not of clinical concern (person outside endemic region for more than 2 months, mild febrile illness, and minimal parasitemia with suspected trophozoites or schizonts on smear), one should be certain of the diagnosis prior to initiating therapy because urgent therapy is not necessary. Lastly, if *P. falciparum* infection is suspected, a detailed travel and transfusion history should be elicited to determine if the infected host could have been exposed to chloroquine resistant organisms.[1,5]

Once the diagnosis and resistant patterns have been determined, treatment[6] of malarial infection is quite straightforward and is outlined in the key features section. For all uncomplicated attacks of malarial infections in which chloroquine resistant *P. falciparum* is not an issue, chloroquine phosphate by mouth is the drug of choice. If the patient is unable to take oral medications, IV quinine dihydrochloride or IM chloroquine hydrochloride is preferred. In *P. vivax* and *P. ovale* infections, a 2-week course of primaquine phosphate must be given to eradicate the hepatic phase of the infection. Because *P. falciparum* does not have a prolonged hepatic phase, treatment with primaquine is not necessary. In attacks that are due to chloroquine resistant *P. falciparum*, all patients should be hospitalized and treated with IV quinine dihydrochloride and either PO Fansidar (pyrimethamine plus sulfadoxine) or PO tetracycline. There is evidence that steroids are detrimental in the treatment of the CNS complications of *P. falciparum* infections,[7] and at this point, only vigorous supportive care can be recommended.

A discussion of malaria would not be complete without a note concerning chemoprophylaxis. For those individuals visiting areas without chloroquine resistant organisms, a weekly dose of chloroquine (300 mg base PO) should be administered 1 week prior to travel and continuing for 6 weeks after returning to the United States. During the final 2 weeks of therapy, patients who have spent prolonged periods in areas endemic for *P. vivax* or *P. ovale* may be given primaquine (15 mg base PO qd) to eradicate the hepatic phase of the infection. Most patients traveling through chloroquine resistant regions should be given three Fansidar tablets to be taken as a single dose in the event of a febrile illness *if medical care is not readily available.* Patients traveling to areas endemic for chloroquine and Fansidar resistant *P. falciparum* (Thailand, Kampuchea, Burma), may be candidates for prophylaxis with doxycycline (100 mg PO qd) beginning 1–2 days prior to travel and continued for 4 weeks after return.

With the exception of chloroquine, antimalarial agents should be used cautiously in patients who are pregnant or who suffer from G6PD deficiency. Information on prevention of malaria in travelers is now available 24 hours a day from the CDC (404-639-1610).

KEY FEATURES

PATHOPHYSIOLOGIC DISTINCTIONS

Organism	RBCs Infected	Level of Parasitemia
P. falciparum	All	20–2000 k/ml
Others	Young or old	6–50 k/ml

CLINICAL DISTINCTIONS

Organism	Incubation Period (Bite to Symptoms)	Symptomatology	Morphology
P. falciparum	9–14 days	Fevers, headache, focal and diffuse CNS changes, severe acute renal failure with hemoglobinuria Myocarditis Massive, tender splenomegaly	Rings: hair-like with multiple forms per RBC Gametocytes: banana shaped Ameboid trophozoites and schizonts not seen
Others	Weeks to years	Fevers, headache, myalgias, anemia Splenomegaly	Rings: coarse with single organism per RBC Ameboid trophozoites and mature schizonts present Gametocytes: round or oval appearing

DRUG THERAPY

Infection	Drug	Adult Dose
All except chloroquine resistant *P. falciparum*		
Oral	Chloroquine phosphate	600 mg base PO, then 300 mg base PO in 6 hours, then 300 mg base PO qd × 2 days
Parenteral	Quinine dihydrochloride	600 mg in 300 cc NS IV over 2 to 4 hours q8h until patient able to take oral medications
	or	
	Chloroquine HCl	200 mg base IM q6h (painful; may cause abscesses)
Then for eradication of relapse (*P. vivax* and *P. ovale* only)		
	Primaquine phosphate	15 mg base PO qd × 14 days or 45 mg base PO q week × 8 weeks
Chloroquine resistant *P. falciparum*		
Oral	Quinine sulfate	650 mg PO tid × 3 to 10 days
	plus	
	Tetracycline HCl	250 mg PO qid × 7 to 10 days
	and/or	
	Pyrimethamine	25 mg PO bid × 3 days
	plus	
	Sulfadiazine	500 mg PO qid × 5 days
Parenteral	Quinine dihydrochloride	As above
	or	
	Quinidine gluconate	Investigational drug for this condition. Monitor ECG in ICU setting. Call CDC for protocol (daytime 404-488-4046; nights, weekends, holidays 404-639-2888)

REFERENCES

1. Wyler DJ: Malaria—resurgence, resistance and research. N Engl J Med 308:875, 1983.
   A complete review of prevalence, world trends, resistance patterns, and problems in control. In addition, it provides a complete biomedical discussion reviewing the factors that prevent the development of a vaccine.

2. Centers for Disease Control: Malaria Surveillance Annual Summary 1982: Issued November 1983.
   Summary statistics for malaria in the United States.

3. Guerrero IC, Weniger BC, Schultz MG: Transfusion malaria in the United States, 1972–1981. Ann Intern Med 99:221, 1983.
   Report of 26 cases of transfusion-associated malarial infections in the United States. Only one case was due to P. ovale, while the rest were evenly split among P. falciparum, P. vivax, and P. malariae. A recommendation is made that potential donors be deferred for 3 years after an unexplained febrile illness occurs 1 year after exposure to malaria.

4. Fitzgerald FT: Malaria: A modern dilemma. West J Med 136:220, 1982.
   A general review of the prevalence, clinical manifestations, diagnostic methods, and therapeutic interventions.

5. Centers for Disease Control: Recommendations for the prevention of malaria in travelers. MMWR 37:277, 1988.
6. Drugs for parasitic infections. Medical Letter 30:15, 1988.
   Outlines the medical therapy for malarial infections and prophylactic measures for exposed individuals.

7. Warrell DA, Looareesuwan S, Warrell MJ et al: Dexamethasone proves deleterious in cerebral malaria: A double-blind trial in 100 comatose patients. N Engl J Med 306:313, 1982.

Human Immunodeficiency Virus Infection

Howard Libman, M.D.

BACKGROUND

Human immunodeficiency virus (HIV), previously known as human T-lymphotropic virus type III/lymphadenopathy-associated virus (HTLV-III/LAV), is the cause of the acquired immune deficiency syndrome (AIDS) and AIDS-related complex (ARC).[1-4] AIDS was first recognized as a clinical problem in the United States at the end of the last decade as physicians in New York and California became aware of an unusual assortment of serious infections and malignancies in male homosexuals and bisexuals. Soon thereafter, a similar problem was noted among intravenous drug abusers in the same geographic areas. An intensive epidemiologic review by the Centers for Disease Control (CDC) strongly suggested that this outbreak, characterized by impaired cellular immunity, represented a new clinical syndrome. Attempts to identify an immunosuppressive infectious agent were finally successful in 1984, when Gallo isolated a new retrovirus from the lymphocytes of affected patients.[5] HIV is now known to cause dysfunction and lysis of helper T lymphocytes, significantly impairing both cellular and humoral immunity. The virus also has the ability to infect neurons and other cell lines.

EPIDEMIOLOGY

HIV infection is epidemic in certain populations.[6-8] It is estimated that at least 1.5 million people in the United States are infected with the virus and that a majority of these will develop ARC or AIDS. Between June 1981 and March 1988, 55,315 patients with AIDS had been reported to the CDC; more than 250,000 cases are anticipated by 1991. HIV is transmitted primarily by means of sexual contact with an infected individual or parenteral exposure to infectious body fluids. Specific risk factors associated with AIDS include homosexuality/bisexuality (present in 73% of patients), intravenous drug abuse (24%), and having received blood product transfusion(s) (3%). Others at risk for AIDS include heterosexual contacts of persons already infected (3%) and children of infected women (1%); 3% of patients have no identifiable risk factor.

CLINICAL MANIFESTATIONS

Primary HIV infection may be asymptomatic or characterized by a viral syndrome with aseptic meningitis that lasts 2–3 weeks.[9] Within 6 months of initial infection, antibody to the virus is detectable in the serum. The patient may remain clinically well for a prolonged period of time, or, after several months to years, ARC or AIDS may develop. ARC, described mainly in homosexual and bisexual males, is manifested by the gradual onset of fever, night sweats, fatigue, anorexia, weight loss, diarrhea, and persistent generalized lymphadenopathy. Thrush, shingles, other skin infections, and refractory dermatitis have also been reported. On physical examination, the patient appears chronically ill and, in addition to lymphadenopathy, may have hepatosplenomegaly. Mild anemia, leukopenia with absolute lymphopenia, hypoalbuminemia, hypergammaglobulinemia, impaired delayed hypersensitivity, and a low T lymphocyte helper-suppressor ratio are usual laboratory findings. The HIV antibody test is positive in over 90% of cases.

AIDS, which often evolves in a manner similar to ARC, is characterized by opportunistic infection or neoplasm, profound wasting, or encephalopathy. The majority of infected patients have *Pneumocystis carinii* pneumonia, presenting with dyspnea, a nonproductive cough, and frequently an unremarkable lung examination. Chest roentgenogram shows a diffuse interstitial pattern, and diagnosis is generally made by bronchoscopy with lavage.[10] A wide variety of other opportunistic infections have been described as well (Table 1); recurrent bacterial pneumonias may also occur.[11] Kaposi's sarcoma, previously known as a rare localized soft tissue tumor with a benign clinical course, is the most common neoplasm reported in patients with AIDS.[12] Physical examination reveals violaceous nodular lesions of the skin that spread rapidly, disseminating cutaneously and viscerally. Diagnosis is suspected clinically and confirmed by biopsy. Undifferentiated non-Hodgkin's lymphoma and primary lymphoma of the central nervous system also occur with increased frequency in AIDS. Other clinical abnormalities, including a variety of neurologic syndromes,[13,14] chronic renal failure/nephrotic syn-

Table 1.   INDICATOR DISEASES FOR THE DIAGNOSIS OF AIDS

Positive HIV Test Necessary	HIV Test Results Not Necessary
Bacterial infections, multiple or recurrent (child <13 years)	Candidiasis of esophagus or bronchopulmonary tract‡
Coccidioidomycosis, disseminated	Cryptococcosis, extrapulmonary
HIV encephalopathy*	Cryptosporidiosis, chronic
HIV wasting syndrome*	Cytomegalovirus infection, disseminated‡
Histoplasmosis, disseminated	Herpes simplex, chronic mucocutaneous or visceral
Isosporiasis, chronic	
Kaposi's sarcoma	Kaposi's sarcoma†‡
Lymphoma of the brain, primary	Lymphoma of the brain, primary†
Lymphoma, undifferentiated non-Hodgkin's	Lymphoid interstitial pneumonitis (child <13 years)‡
Salmonella septicemia, recurrent	
Tuberculosis, extrapulmonary	Mycobacterial disease, atypical/disseminated‡
	Pneumocystis pneumonia‡
	Progressive multifocal leukoencephalopathy
	Toxoplasmosis of the brain‡

*Diagnosis of exclusion.
†In patient less than 60 years old.
‡Positive HIV antibody test necessary if diagnosis is made presumptively (see reference 18).

drome,[15] bone marrow suppression, autoimmune phenomena, and ophthalmic disorders,[16] have also been described. Anemia, leukopenia, thrombocytopenia, abnormal renal and hepatic function tests, proteinuria, and immunologic abnormalities similar to those in ARC are often present. Serum antibody to HIV is almost always detectable.

DIAGNOSIS

ARC is a clinical syndrome that has not been precisely defined. It is an illness of greater than 3 months' duration characterized by constitutional symptoms and generalized lymphadenopathy not attributable to other causes. A diagnostic evaluation should be performed on all patients with suspected ARC to exclude other possibilities (e.g., secondary syphilis, cytomegalovirus infection, hepatitis B, and Hodgkin's disease).[17] Specific case criteria for AIDS were established by the CDC in 1983 and have recently been revised to take into account the availability of HIV antibody testing[18] (Table 1).

An HIV antibody test[19] is considered positive if the enzyme-linked immunosorbent assay (ELISA) is positive on a repeated basis and this is confirmed by the more specific Western blot assay. Although serologic testing has proved useful in the routine screening of blood products, its clinical utility is limited to those instances in which patient management might be affected. It is important to realize that (1) screening asymptomatic populations at low risk for HIV infection will result in a high false positive rate; (2) testing high-risk populations with nonspecific complaints may confuse, rather than clarify, the clinical situation; (3) serologic evidence of HIV infection is not required to diagnose ARC and is not always necessary to diagnose AIDS; (4) the natural history of HIV infection is uncertain, and treatment remains problematic; and (5) test results have the potential for psychological harm and to be used in a discriminatory manner. The US Public Health Service has recently published specific recommendations regarding the use of HIV antibody testing.[20]

PROGNOSIS

The natural history of infection with HIV is still unclear.[21-25] Whereas some asymptomatic seropositive patients (approximately 25% over five years) have developed ARC, and others (10%) AIDS, the remainder are clinically well but have evidence of immunologic dysfunction. Once ARC has evolved, there is generally little or no clinical improvement, and at least 10% of patients with ARC develop AIDS. The cumulative probability of survival with AIDS is 48.8% at one year and 15.2% at five years. Patients with Kaposi's sarcoma alone have the best prognosis, whereas those with opportunistic infection other than *P. carinii* pneumonia have the worst. Other factors affecting mortality include the age, sex, and race or ethnicity of the patient, and the route of acquisition of the virus.

MANAGEMENT

The care of patients with HIV infection requires a multidisciplinary approach, involving the primary care physician, appropriate subspecialty consultants, neurologist, psychiatrist, and social worker. Psychiatric support of those afflicted and their significant others is essential because of the anxiety, depression, neurologic impairment, and social isolation that often accompany HIV infection.[26] Asymptomatic patients who are seropositive should be provided a regular opportunity by their health care provider to verbalize their feelings, ask questions, and discuss any physical complaints they might have.

Management of patients with ARC is mainly supportive. Therapy with oral nystatin suspension or clotrimazole troches is usually effective for thrush; refractory cases necessitate oral administration of ketoconazole. Care of patients with AIDS involves the treatment, when possible, of opportunistic disease processes[27,28] (Table 2). *P. carinii* pneumonia[29-31] often responds to trimethoprim-sulfamethoxazole (TMP-SMZ), although drug toxicity and relapse following cessation of therapy are common. Treatment is generally continued for 3 weeks. Pentamidine is as effective as TMP-SMZ and, in patients with AIDS, probably no more toxic. Aerosolized pentamidine administered on an intermittent basis appears to hold the greatest promise for

Table 2.   **TREATMENT OF OPPORTUNISTIC INFECTIONS ASSOCIATED WITH AIDS***

Infection	Treatment/Dosage	Toxicity
Candidiasis, oral	Nystatin suspension 500,000 U PO qid	Gastrointestinal intolerance
	or	
	Clotrimazole troche 10 mg PO qid	Gastrointestinal intolerance
	or	
	Ketoconazole† 200–400 mg/day PO	Gastrointestinal intolerance, hepatotoxicity, gynecomastia, impotence
Cryptococcal meningitis	Amphotericin B‡ 0.5 mg/kg/day IV	Fever, altered mental status, nephrotoxicity, pancytopenia, hypokalemia, hypomagnesemia
Cytomegalovirus infection	Ganciclovir (investigational)	Leukopenia
Herpes simplex infection, mucocutaneous	Acyclovir 5 mg/kg IV q8h *or* 200–400 mg PO five times/ day	Phlebitis, altered mental status, nephrotoxicity, hepatotoxicity
Herpes zoster infection, disseminated	Acyclovir 10 mg/kg IV q8h	Same as for herpes simplex
P. carinii pneumonia	Trimethoprim-sulfamethoxazole 20 mg/kg/day TMP; 100 mg/ kg/day SMZ PO or IV *or* Pentamidine 4 mg/kg/day IV	Fever, rash, leukopenia, hepatotoxicity
Leukopenia, hypoglycemia, hyperglycemia, nephrotoxicity, hepatotoxicity
Toxoplasmosis	Sulfadiazine and pyrimethamine: 100 mg/kg/day PO and 25–50 mg/day PO (with folinic acid)	Fever, rash, hemolytic anemia, pancytopenia

*There is no demonstrated effective therapy for cryptosporidiosis[40] or *Mycobacterium avium* complex infection.[41] Treatment of syphilis may require modification in patients with concomitant HIV infection.[42]

†Drug of choice for esophageal involvement.

‡Alternatively, may be used at a reduced dose in conjunction with flucytosine.

prophylaxis against recurrent infection. Acyclovir is useful in the treatment of mucocutaneous herpes simplex and disseminated herpes zoster infections. Ganciclovir, an investigational agent, appears beneficial in patients with cytomegalovirus infection.[32] However, leukopenia is a frequent side effect, and relapse is common upon dicontinuation of the drug. Cryptococcal meningitis is treated with amphotericin B, sometimes in conjunction with flucytosine,[33] and toxoplasmosis of the brain is managed with sulfadiazine and pyrimethamine;[34] long-term maintenance therapy is necessary to prevent recurrence of both diseases. Palliative chemotherapy and radiation therapy have been useful in the treatment of Kaposi's sarcoma.

Clinical trials are underway to assess a variety of antiviral and immune-modulating agents that may be effective against HIV. Azidothymidine (AZT) is the only drug thus far that has been shown to be of clinical benefit. In a double-blind, placebo-controlled trial[35] involving 282 patients with AIDS (manifested by *P. carinii* pneumonia) or ARC followed for a median of four months, 19 in the placebo group and only 1 in the treatment group died. Toxicity of the agent includes leukopenia, macrocytic anemia, gastrointestinal intolerance, and altered mental status. Whether the drug will prove useful over a longer period of time and in other populations with HIV infection is currently being studied. Prototype vaccine preparations are in the early stages of clinical investigation.

PREVENTION

Despite public fears to the contrary, HIV infection is rather difficult to transmit. Casual contact, even when prolonged, does not place one at increased risk for infection.[36] Patients should be counseled to avoid promiscuous sexual activity, especially with members of high-risk populations; use a condom during sexual intercourse; and not share razors, toothbrushes, needles, or other objects that could be contaminated with blood.[37] Seroconversion has been described in individuals following percutaneous (risk <1% per occurrence) or mucous membrane exposure to body fluids of infected patients, but health care workers as a whole appear to be at low risk for occupational acquisition of HIV infection.[38] Universal precautions are strongly recommended in dealing with blood and other body fluids of *all* patients regardless of whether specific risk factors have been identified.[39]

KEY FEATURES

Human immodeficiency virus (HIV) is the pathogen responsible for acquired immune deficiency syndrome (AIDS) and AIDS-related complex (ARC).

The organism causes dysfunction and lysis of helper T lymphocytes, significantly impairing cellular and humoral immunity, and has the ability to infect neurons and other cell lines.

It is estimated that 1.5 million people in the United States are infected with HIV and that a majority of these will develop ARC or AIDS. HIV is transmitted almost exclusively by means of sexual contact with an infected individual or by parenteral exposure to infectious body fluids.

ARC is a clinical syndrome manifested by fever, night sweats, fatigue, anorexia, weight loss, diarrhea, and persistent generalized lymphadenopathy. It is a diagnosis of exclusion that does not require HIV antibody testing.

AIDS is characterized by the development of opportunistic infection or neoplasm, profound wasting, or encephalopathy. Specific case criteria for AIDS have been established by the CDC and were recently revised to take into account the availability of HIV antibody testing (Table 1).

The natural history of infection with HIV is still unclear. Over 50% of patients with AIDS are dead within one year of diagnosis, and nearly 85% within five years.

The care of patients with HIV infection is best provided by means of a multidisciplinary approach, involving the primary care physician, appropriate subspecialty consultants, neurologist, psychiatrist, and social worker.

Management of the patient with ARC requires excluding other causes of generalized lymphadenopathy and careful clinical reassessment on a regular basis. Management of the patient with AIDS involves treatment, when possible, of opportunistic disease processes, including infections (Table 2).

Azidothymidine (AZT) is the only antiviral drug thus far that has been shown to be of benefit in the treatment of HIV infection. Clinical trials are underway to assess the efficacy of other antiviral and immune-modulating agents.

Casual contact, even when prolonged, does not place one at increased risk for HIV infection. Practical recommendations aimed at modifying high-risk behaviors may slow transmission of the virus. These include avoiding promiscuous sexual activity, using a condom during sexual intercourse, and not sharing objects that could be contaminated with blood.

Health care workers as a whole appear to be at low risk for occupational acquisition of HIV infection. Universal precautions should be used in dealing with blood and other body fluids of *all* patients.

REFERENCES

1. Fauci AS, Macher AM, Longo DL, et al: Acquired immunodeficiency syndrome: Epidemiologic, clinical, immunologic, and therapeutic considerations. Ann Intern Med *100*:92–106, 1984.
2. Fauci AS, Masur H, Gelmann EP, Markham PD, Hahn BH, Lane HC: The acquired immunodeficiency sydrome: An update. Ann Intern Med *102*:800-813, 1985.
3. Bowen DL, Lane HC, Fauci AS: Immunopathogenesis of the acquired immunodeficiency syndrome. Ann Intern Med *103*:704–709, 1985.
4. Landesman SH, Ginzburg HM, Weiss SH: The AIDS epidemic. N Engl J Med *312*:521–525, 1985.
   Review articles on the basic laboratory and clinical aspects of human immunodeficiency virus infection.

5. Gallo RC, Salahuddin SZ, Popovic M, et al: Frequent detection and isolation of cytopathic retroviruses (HTLV-III) from patients with AIDS and at risk for AIDS. Science *224*:500–503, 1984.

Peripheral blood lympocytes from 47 of 97 patients with AIDS or "pre-AIDS" were found to express and release a new T-lymphotropic retrovirus (named HTLV-III) when grown in cell culture. Control group lymphocytes did not produce the virus.

6. Burke DS, Brundage JF, Herbold JR, et al: Human immunodeficiency virus infections among civilian applicants for United States military service, October 1985 to March 1986: Demographic factors associated with seropositivity. N Engl J Med 317:131–136, 1987.
   The mean prevalence of HIV infection in applicants for military serve was 1.50 per 1000. Older age, black race, male sex, and residence in an urban area were significant independent predictors of a positive HIV antibody test.

7. Centers for Disease Control: Human immunodeficiency virus infection in the United States: A review of current knowledge. MMWR 36(suppl 6S):1–48, 1987.
   Summary of CDC epidemiologic data.

8. Friedland GH, Klein RS: Transmission of the human immunodeficiency virus. N Engl J Med 317:1125–1135, 1987.
   Accumulated data strongly support the conclusion that transmission of HIV occurs only through blood, sexual activity, and perinatal events.

9. Ho DD, Sarngadharan MG, Resnick L, Veronese FD, Rota TR, Hirsch MS: Primary human T-lymphotropic virus type III infection. Ann Intern Med 103:880–883, 1985.
   Description of case reports.

10. Broaddus C, Dake MD, Stulbarg MS, et al: Bronchoalveolar lavage and transbronchial biopsy for the diagnosis of pulmonary infections in the acquired immunodeficiency syndrome. Ann Intern Med 102:747–752, 1985.
    For the diagnosis of P. carinii pneumonia, the sensitivity of bronchoalveolar lavage alone was 89%; transbronchial biopsy, 97%; and both precedures combined, 100%.

11. Polsky B, Gold JWM, Whimbey E, et al: Bacterial pneumonia in patients with acquired immunodeficiency syndrome. Ann Intern Med 104:38–41, 1986.
    Eighteen episodes of community-acquired bacterial pneumonia in 13 patients with AIDS are reported.

12. Friedman-Kien AE, Laubenstein LJ, Rubinstein P, et al: Disseminated Kaposi's sarcoma in homosexual men. Ann Intern Med 96:693–700, 1982.
    Early report of an uncommon sarcoma behaving in an atypical fashion in patients with acquired immunodeficiency.

13. Levy RM, Bredesen DE, Rosenblum ML: Neurological manifestations of the acquired immunodeficiency syndrome (AIDS): Experience at UCSF and review of the literature. J Neurosurg 62:475–495, 1985.
    The most common neurologic complications encountered in 315 patients with AIDS or ARC included toxoplasmosis (103 cases), subacute encephalitis (54), cranial or peripheral nerve complications (51), cryptococcosis (41), aseptic meningitis (21), primary CNS lymphoma (15), and metastatic lymphoma (12).

14. Gabuzda DH, Hirsch MS: Neurologic manifestations of infection with human immunodeficiency virus: Clinical features and pathogenesis. Ann Intern Med 107:383–391, 1987.
    Clinical review. Subacute encephalitis caused by HIV infection is the most frequent cause of neurologic dysfunction in AIDS, resulting in cognitive, motor, and behavioral abnormalities. Pathologic evidence of this disease is found in 90% of patients at autopsy.

15. Rao TKS, Friedman EA, Nicastri AD: The types of renal disease in the acquired immunodeficiency syndrome. N Engl J Med 316:1062–1068, 1987.
    Ten per cent of patients with AIDS had renal dysfunction, with a majority showing

evidence of nephropathy characterized by massive proteinuria and/or azotemia. Survival for more than 6 months was rare in those with chronic disease.

16. Palestine AG, Rodrigues MM, Macher AM, et al: Ophthalmic involvement in acquired immunodeficiency syndrome. Ophthalmology 91:1092–1099, 1984.
    Clinical review. Ocular findings were of four major categories: cytomegalovirus (CMV) retinitis, cotton-wool spots, conjunctival Kaposi's sarcoma, and neuro-ophthalmic motility abnormalities. CMV retinitis was an important cause of visual loss.

17. Libman H: Generalized lymphadenopathy. J Gen Intern Med 2:48–58, 1987.
    Review article. ARC is a clinical syndrome of exclusion with an extensive differential diagnosis. Laboratory testing and consideration of lymph node biopsy are recommended.

18. Centers for Disease Control: Revision of the CDC surveillance case definition for acquired immunodeficiency syndrome. MMWR 36(suppl. 1S):1–15, 1987.
    Revised CDC criteria incorporating the HIV antibody status of the patient.

19. Steckelberg JM, Cockerill FR, III: Serologic testing for human immunodeficiency virus antibodies. Mayo Clinic Proc 63:373–380, 1988.
    Description of available methods of testing and their sensitivities, specificities, and predictive values.

20. Centers for Disease Control: Public health service guidelines for counseling and antibody testing to prevent HIV infection and AIDS. MMWR 36:509–515, 1987.
    Broad recommendations are offered based upon public health and epidemiologic concerns.

21. Centers for Disease Control: Update: Acquired immunodeficiency syndrome in the San Francisco cohort study, 1978–1985. MMWR 34:573–575, 1985.

22. Francis DP, Jaffe HW, Fultz PN, Getchell JP, McDougal JS, Feorino PM: The natural history of infection with the lymphadenopathy-associated virus human T-lymphotropic virus type III. Ann Intern Med 103:719–722, 1985.

23. Melbye M, Biggar RJ, Ebbesen P, et al: Long-term seropositivity for human T-lymphotropic virus type III in homosexual men without the acquired immunodeficiency syndrome: Development of immunologic and clinical abnormalities. Ann Intern Med 104:496–500, 1986.

24. Goedert JJ, Biggar RJ, Weiss SH, et al: Three-year incidence of AIDS in five cohorts of HTLV-III–infected risk group members. Science 231:992–995, 1986.

25. Rothenberg R, Woelfel M, Stoneburner R, Milberg J, Parker R, Truman B: Survival with the acquired immunodeficiency syndrome: Experience with 5833 cases in New York City. N Engl J Med 317:1297–1302, 1987.
    Articles addressing the prognosis of asymptomatic carriage of HIV, ARC, and AIDS.

26. Holland JC, Tross S: The psychosocial and neuropsychiatric sequelae of the acquired immunodeficiency syndrome and related disorders. Ann Intern Med 103:760–764, 1985.
    Psychologic problems associated with HIV infection are common and often multifactorial in origin. Management guidelines are proposed.

27. Grant IH, Armstrong D: Management of infectious complications in acquired immunodeficiency syndrome. Am J Med 81(suppl 1A):59–72, 1986.

28. Kaplan LD, Wofsy CB, Volberding PA: Treatment of patients with acquired immunodeficiency syndrome and associated manifestations. JAMA 257:1367–1374, 1987.
    Reviews of the current management of opportunistic diseases associated with AIDS.

29. Treatment of Pneumocystis carinii pneumonia. Med Letter 29:103–104, 1987.

30. Gordin FM, Simon GL, Wofsy CB, Mills J: Adverse reactions to trimethoprim-sulfameth-

oxazole in patients with the acquired immunodeficiency syndrome. Ann Intern Med 100:495–499, 1984.
31. Wharton JM, Coleman DL, Wofsy CB, et al: Trimethoprim-sulfamethoxazole or pentamidine for Pneumocystis carinii pneumonia in the acquired immunodeficiency syndrome: A prospective randomized trial. Ann Intern Med 105:37–44, 1986.
    Articles addressing the therapeutic options for pneumocystis pneumonia.

32. Laskin OL, Cederberg DM, Mills J, et al: Ganciclovir for the treatment and suppression of serious infections caused by cytomegalovirus. Am J Med 83:201–207, 1987.
    Eighty-seven per cent of patients with retinitis had improvement or stabilization of their disease so long as therapy was continued.

33. Zuger A, Louie E, Holzman RS, Simberkoff MS, Rahal JJ: Cryptococcal disease in patients with the acquired immunodeficiency syndrome: Diagnostic features and outcome of treatment. Ann Intern Med 104:234–240, 1986.
    Cerebrospinal fluid antigen and culture, and serum antigen were the most sensitive diagnostic tests. Although patients often responded favorably to amphotericin B, relapsing infection occurred if therapy was stopped.

34. Leport C, Raffi F, Matheron S, et al: Treatment of central nervous system toxoplasmosis with pyrimethamine/sulfadiazine combination in 35 patients with the acquired immunodeficiency syndrome: Efficacy of long-term continuous therapy. Am J Med 84:94–100, 1988.
    Thirty-one of 35 patients showed evidence of clinical improvement during the first two months of therapy. Side effects, including hematologic toxicity and rash, were common but rarely necessitated discontinuation of the agents. Long-term continuous therapy was necessary to prevent relapse.

35. Fischl MA, Richman DD, Grieco MH, et al: The efficacy of azidothymidine (AZT) in the treatment of patients with AIDS and AIDS-related complex: A double-blind, placebo-controlled trial. N Engl J Med 317:185–191, 1987.
    AZT decreased mortality and the frequency of opportunistic infections in subgroups of patients with AIDS or ARC over 8–24 weeks of observation.

36. Friedland GH, Saltzman BR, Rogers MF, et al: Lack of transmission of HTLV-III/LAV infection to household contacts of patients with AIDS or AIDS-related complex with oral candidiasis. N Engl J Med 314:344–349, 1986.
    Only 1 of 101 nonsexual household contacts of patients with AIDS had evidence of HIV infection, and this case had probably been acquired perinatally.

37. Centers for Disease Control: Additional recommendations to reduce sexual and drug abuse–related transmission of human T-lymphotropic virus type III/lymphadenopathy-associated virus. MMWR 35:152–155, 1986.
    Practical recommendations to reduce the spread of HIV infection.

38. Centers for Disease Control: Update: Acquired immunodeficiency syndrome and human immunodeficiency virus infection among health-care workers. MMWR 37:229–239, 1988.
    There have been 15 documented cases of seroconversion in health care workers without reported nonoccupational risk factors for HIV infection. Needlestick injuries have been more frequent than contamination of mucous membranes or intact skin.

39. Centers for Disease Control: Recommendations for prevention of HIV transmission in health-care settings. MMWR 36(suppl 2S):1–18, 1987.
    Detailed recommendations for health care workers.

40. Pitlik SD, Fainstein V, Garza D, et al: Human cryptosporidiosis: Spectrum of disease. Arch Intern Med 143:2269–2275, 1983.
    Diarrheal illness may occur in immunocompetent, as well as immunocompromised,

hosts. In the former group, the disease is self-limited; in the latter, it is protracted, associated with malabsorption syndrome, and often results in death.

41. Centers for Disease Control: Diagnosis and management of mycobacterial infection and disease in persons wtih human immunodeficiency virus infection. Ann Intern Med 106:254–256, 1987.

   A purified protein derivative (PPD) skin test is recommended for all patients with HIV infection. In those with active tuberculosis, initial therapy should consist of three drugs, and treatment may need to be continued longer than the standard duration of 9 months. There are no definitive data on the efficacy of the treatment of infection caused by M. avium complex.

42. Tramont EC: Syphilis in the AIDS era (editorial). N Engl J Med 316:1600–1601, 1987.

   Neurosyphilis has developed in an accelerated fashion in some patients with HIV infection appropriately treated for early syphilis, and current treatment protocols may be inadequate. Syphilis serologic studies are recommended in all patients with HIV infection.

SECTION 6
NEPHROLOGY

Metabolic Acidosis

Claire Fritsche, M.D.

Metabolic acidosis results from (1) retention, overproduction, or exogenous addition of organic or inorganic acids to the body fluids; or (2) loss of HCO_3^- from the body. Acidemia is corrected with the buffers hemoglobin, phosphates, proteins, or bone, or through alveolar hyperventilation. Respiratory compensation is rapid and reaches steady state at 24 hours. The kidney compensates for acidosis by excreting increased NH_4^+ and titratable acids. Severe acidosis results in decreased vascular resistance, ventricular depression and irritability with hypotension, pulmonary edema, ventricular fibrillation, and tissue hypoxia. Compensatory signs include Kussmaul's respiration and, in chronic acidosis, osteopenia. Plasma pH, pCO_2, and HCO_3^- are low, and plasma K^+ is normal or high even with K^+ deficits. The anion gap is normal or high $[Na^+ - (Cl^- + HCO_3^-) = 8 - 12$ mEq/L = normal gap]. The unmeasured anions consist of phosphate, proteins, sulfate and organic acids. Metabolic acidosis is categorized as anion gap or non–anion gap.

INCREASED ANION GAP ACIDOSIS

Four conditions are included in anion gap acidosis: renal failure, ketoacidosis, lactic acidosis, and acidosis from drugs and toxins.

Renal Failure

Normally, metabolism produces fixed acids at a rate of 70–100 mEq/day. In renal failure, the kidneys cannot excrete the daily load of sulfate, phosphate, and organic anions. Plasma HCO_3^- falls by <2 mEq/L/day. If replacement with >100 mEq $NaHCO_3$/day is required, another cause for acidosis should be sought.[3]

Ketoacidosis

Ketoacidosis occurs in alcoholism, diabetes, or starvation. Routine screening for ketones with Acetest or Ketostix detects only acetoacetic acid and not β-OH butyric acid. However, patients with poor tissue oxygenation or alcoholic ketosis have high β-OH butyrate to acetoacetate ratios. *Alcoholic ketosis* occurs in patients with prolonged ethanol intake, decreased food intake, and vomiting. The acidosis responds rapidly to abstinence, intravenous glucose, and saline, rarely requiring $NaHCO_3$. Likewise, alkali therapy is not recommended in *diabetic ketosis* unless the serum HCO_3^- is <10 mEq/L and should be stopped when the serum HCO_3^- reaches 15 mEq/L. When diabetic ketosis is treated (insulin, fluids, electrolytes), organic acid production ceases and metabolism of partially oxidized substances results in HCO_3^- accumulation. This, along with improved renal function, returns HCO_3^- to normal. Overcorrection with alkali results in hypokalemia and a mixed metabolic alkalosis and respiratory alkalosis.[3] *Starvation* causes mild ketoacidosis requiring no alkali therapy.

Lactic Acidosis

Lactic acidosis (lactate >4 mEq/L, pH <7.25) occurs when normal production of lactate (60 mEq/hour) is exceeded or ineffectively utilized. Causes are divided into type A (tissue hypoxia) and type B. Tissue hypoxia results from cardiovascular collapse, asphyxia, carbon monoxide or cyanogen poisoning, respiratory failure, severe anemia, or congestive heart failure. The multiple causes for type B include neoplasia; liver failure (especially with hypoglycemia); convulsions; inborn errors of metabolism; diabetes mellitus; and ingestion of phenformin, ethanol, methanol, ethylene glycol, and salicylates. Patients with short gut syndrome develop D-lactic acidosis.[22] Clinical laboratories routinely measure L-lactate, not D-lactate. Treatment starts with correction of the cause. In type A, measures include improvement of perfusion, oxygenation, and correction of volume depletion. If patients are volume expanded with high peripheral resistance, vasodilators such as nitroprusside may be beneficial. In types A and B, $NaHCO_3$ is given when plasma HCO_3^- is <10 mEq/L and pH is <7.20. The deficit is calculated as follows:

(40% body weight in kg) × (normal HCO_3^- [mEq/L]

$$- \text{ measured } HCO_3^-).$$

To prevent overshoot and central respiratory alkalosis, half of the calculated deficit is given, arterial blood gas determinations repeated, and HCO_3^- corrected to 15–18 mEq/L. Treatment problems include hypernatremia, hyperosmolality, and volume overload. Treatment with dichloroacetate, which enhances activity of pyruvate dehydrogenase, has improved acidosis but not survival.[10] The mortality rate of patients with lactic acidosis is 80% despite therapy.

Acidosis from Drugs and Toxins

Chronic paraldehyde ingestion results in severe acidosis, intoxication, confusion, nausea, and pungent breath odor. The lactate level is elevated, and plasma ketones are falsely positive. The minimum lethal blood level of paraldehyde is 50 mg/dl.[1] Treatment requires correction of hypotension and acidosis.

In adults, salicylate toxicity usually presents as a simple respiratory alkalosis or as combined respiratory alkalosis and metabolic acidosis with hyperventilation, nausea, tinnitus, stupor, coma, and convulsions. Noncardiac pulmonary edema occurs in the older adult smoker who chronically ingests salicylates.[15] Metabolic acidosis, ketosis, depressed uric acid concentration, and coagulopathy are common.

Methanol poisonings (paints, varnishes, paint remover, windshield cleaners) result in a high anion gap, profound acidosis with measured osmolality significantly greater than calculated osmolality. Methanol is not harmful, but its metabolites, formaldehyde and formic acid, lead to overproduction of organic acids, including lactic and keto-acids. Patients present 12–48 hours after ingestion with drunkenness, nausea, vomiting, pancreatitis, seizures, blurred vision, retinal edema, optic atrophy, blindness, and coma. One hundred milliliters of methanol or blood levels >100 mg/dl are lethal.[2] Immediate treatment includes $NaHCO_3$ (to correct acidosis) and ethanol (to inhibit methanol metabolism).

Ethylene glycol (antifreeze) poisoning results in high anion gap acidosis with measured plasma osmolality higher than calculated osmolality. Ethylene glycol is not harmful, but its metabolites, oxalic and other organic acids and lactic acid, contribute to toxicity. Symptoms and signs within a few hours include drunkenness, seizures, coma, hypertension, myopathy, cardiac failure, pulmonary edema, and acute oliguric renal failure with oxalate crystalluria and hypocalcemia. The lethal dose is 100 ml.[14] Ethylene glycol serum levels should be measured, but therapy must be started immediately. Treatment is the same as for methanol: $NaHCO_3$, ethanol, and hemodialysis. In addition, if the patient is not in oliguric renal failure, diuresis should be maintained with fluid replacement and osmotic (mannitol) and loop (furosemide [Lasix]) diuretics. (For details, see section 10, Selected Toxicologic Emergencies.)

NORMAL ANION GAP ACIDOSIS

Hyperchloremic metabolic acidosis is categorized under (1) GI, (2) renal, and (3) miscellaneous causes. Loss of HCO_3^- from the GI tract is associated with diarrhea, small bowel or pancreatic drainage, external fistulae, ureterosigmoidostomies, and obstructed ileal conduits. Treatment includes correction of the underlying problem and $NaHCO_3$ as needed.

Renal causes of non–anion gap acidosis include carbonic anhydrase inhibitor intoxication, renal tubular acidosis (RTA), and chronic renal failure. Proximal (type 2) RTA, a defect in proximal tubular HCO_3^- transport, is associated with hyperphosphaturia, aminoaciduria, glycosuria, hyperuricuria, hypouricemia, hypokalemia, and hypophosphatemia. Nephrocalcinosis, renal stones, and bone disease are rare. To enhance proximal HCO_3^- reabsorption, moderate salt restriction and mild diuretics (thiazide, amiloride) are recommended.[20,21]

In classic type I distal RTA, the distal nephron cannot maintain a significant H^+ gradient. Even with severe acidosis, the urinary pH remains above 6. Low or normal serum K^+, hypercalciuria, nephrocalcinosis, renal stones, and bone disease are associated. Treatment includes K^+ replacement and 1–2 mEq/kg/day of $NaHCO_3$ or citrate solution.[20,21]

Type 4 RTA is a complex disorder associated with one or several renal abnormalities. These include aldosterone resistance, hyporenin-hypoaldosteronism, decreased distal nephron H^+ secretion, decreased NH_3 production, or generalized distal nephron tubular defects.[23] Features include hyperkalemia, plasma $HCO_3^- > 15$ mEq/L, and urinary pHs that can fall below 5.5. Diabetes mellitus, interstitial nephritis, and obstructive uropathy are associated. Besides correction of volume depletion if present , or correction of the underlying illness, initial therapy is designed to treat the hyperkalemia because acidosis is mild.[18,19] When K^+ cannot be controlled, sodium polystyrene sulfonate (Kayexalate) or loop diuretics (if the patient is volume expanded) can be used. Fludrocortisone (0.1–0.5 mg/day) may be used, but high doses may be required and diuretics are necessary to correct the attendant volume overload. $NaHCO_3$ is given if acidosis is not corrected with control of K^+.

Early chronic renal failure leads to a non–anion gap acidosis as a result of nephron loss leading to decreased titratable acid and NH_4^+ in urine. Alkali therapy is used.

Finally, hyperalimentation leads to hyperchloremic metabolic acidosis when amino acid cations are infused in excess of organic anions. Increasing the organic anion concentration (e.g., acetate) and decreasing Cl^- correct the acidosis.

KEY FEATURES

TREATMENT OF METABOLIC ACIDOSIS

Increased Anion Gap
Renal Failure
Treatment: less than 100 mEq $NaHCO_3$/day

Ketoacidosis
$NaHCO_3$ only if plasma HCO_3^- <10 mEq/L. Correct to 15 mEq/L
Lactic Acidosis
Correct cause
$NaHCO_3$ if plasma HCO_3^- <10 mEq/L. Correct to 15 mEq/L
HCO_3^- deficit = (40% body weight in kg) × (normal HCO_3^- [mEq/L]
   − measured HCO_3^-)
Hemodialysis
Peritoneal dialysis
Drugs, Toxins
Paraldehyde
  Alkali, volume correction
Salicylate
  Alkaline diuresis
  Hemodialysis if renal insufficiency or salicylate levels >80 mg/dl
Methanol
  Alkali
  Folate 50–70 mg IV every 4 hours for 24 hours
  Ethanol 0.6 gm/kg loading dose; then 5–10 gm/hour
  Hemodialysis if methanol >50 mg/dl, lethal ingestion, visual im-
    pairment
  Ethanol infusion during dialysis: 66 mg/kg/hour for nondrinkers;
    154 mg/kg/hour for drinkers
Ethylene glycol
  Treatment: as in methanol overdose
Normal Anion Gap
Gastrointestinal Tract
Treatment: underlying cause and alkali
Renal
Proximal type 2 RTA
  Thiazide, amiloride, moderate salt restriction
  Children 3–13 mEq sodium and/or potassium bicarbonate solution/
    kg/day
Type 1 distal RTA
  1–2 mEq $NaHCO_3$/kg/day
Type 4 distal RTA
  High Na^+, low K^+ diet if patient tolerant of volume expansion
  Kayexalate
  Fludrocortisone (0.1–.5 mg/day)
  $NaHCO_3$
  Loop diuretics
Early chronic renal failure
  Alkali

REFERENCES

1. Cohen JJ, Kassirer JP: Metabolic acidosis. In Cohen JJ, Kassirer JP: Acid-Base. Boston, Little, Brown, 1982, pp 121–225.
2. Rose BD: Metabolic acidosis. In Rose BD: Clinical Physiology of Acid Base and Electrolyte Disorders. New York, McGraw-Hill, 1977, pp 323–353.
3. Schrier RW: Pathogenesis and management of metabolic acidosis and alkalosis. In Schrier RW (ed): Renal and Electrolyte Disorders, 2nd ed. Boston, Little, Brown, 1980, pp 115–158.

These three references all give a concise physiologic and practical approach to metabolic acidosis.

4. Narins R, et al: Diagnostic strategies in disorders of fluid, electrolyte and acid-base homeostasis. Am J Med 72:496–520, 1982.
5. Narins R, Emmett M: Simple and mixed acid-base disorders: A practical approach. Medicine 59:161–185, 1980.
6. Bia M, Thier S: Mixed acid-base disturbances: A clinical approach. Med Clin North Am 65:547–561, 1981.
7. Tannen RL: Ammonia and acid-base homeostasis. Med Clin North Am 67:781, 1983.
   References 4–7 are excellent discussions of the basics in acid-base physiology and address the problems of mixed disturbances.

8. Fraley D, et al: Stimulation of lactate production by administration of bicarbonate in a patient with a solid neoplasm and lactic acidosis. N Engl J Med 303(19):1100–1102, 1980.
   Pitfalls of treatment in specialized cases.

9. Fields A, et al: Chronic lactic acidosis in a patient with cancer. Cancer 47:2026–2029, 1981.
10. Starpoole PW, et al: Treatment of lactic acidosis with dichloroacetate. N Engl J Med 309–96, 1983.
    Outlines treatment with dichloroacetate in 11 patients; 6 had improved acidosis, but only 1 survived.

11. Kriesberg RA: Lactic homeostasis and lactic acidosis. Ann Intern Med 92:227–237, 1980.
12. Madias NE: Lactic acidosis. Kidney Int 29:752–774, 1986.
13. Kriesberg RA: Pathogenesis and management of lactic acidosis. Ann Rev Med 35:181–193, 1984.
    References 11–13 are good reviews of the pathophysiology and current treatment of lactic acidosis.

14. CPC—Case 38—1979. N Engl J Med 301:650–657, 1979.
    Excellent review by Dr. Norman Levinsky of the toxic ingestions causing metabolic acidosis, concentrating on differentiation of ethylene glycol from methanol.

15. Heffner G, Sahn S: Salicylate induced pulmonary edema. Ann Intern Med 95:405–409, 1981.
16. Hill G: Salicylate intoxication. N Engl J Med 288:1110–1113, 1973.
    Review of the physiologic abnormalities and appropriate treatment.

17. Gonda A, et al: Hemodialysis for methanol intoxication. Am J Med 64:749, 1978.
18. Knochel J: The syndrome of hyporeninemic hypoaldosteronism. Ann Rev Med 30:145–153, 1979.
19. Battle D, et al: Hyperkalemic distal renal tubular acidosis associated with obstructive uropathy. N Engl J Med 304:373–380, 1981.
    Earliest recognition of this entity with explanation of cause.

20. Battle D, Arruda J: Renal tubular acidosis syndromes. Min Electrol Metab 5:83–99, 1981.
21. Battle D: Renal tubular acidosis. Med Clin North Am 67:859–878, 1983.
    References 20 and 21 are quite similar, but the last especially is a good review with comparison charts.

22. Dahlquist N, et al: D-lactic acidosis and encephalopathy after jejunoileostomy: Response to overfeeding and to fasting in humans. Mayo Clinic Proc 59:141–145, 1984.
    Good bibliography for this unusual syndrome.

23. Battle DC: Segmental characterization of defects in collecting tubule acidification. Kidney Int 30:546–554, 1986.
    Excellent basic physiologic description of H+ secretion.

Metabolic Alkalosis

Claire Fritsche, M.D.

Metabolic alkalosis is divided into two phases: initiation and maintenance. Initiation occurs in three ways: (1) H^+ loss from extracellular fluid (ECF), (2) HCO_3^- addition to ECF, or (3) loss[7] of fluid containing Cl^-. The first, H^+ loss, can be from several sources. GI loss of HCl through nasogastric suction or vomiting results in rising plasma HCO_3^-. Renal loss from mineralocorticoid excess results when H^+ secretion is directly stimulated in the distal nephron. Ion shifts across fluid compartments may initiate metabolic alkalosis. With major K^+ deficits, K^+ moves into ECF from cells to maintain the ratio of intracellular and extracellular K^+. To maintain neutrality, H^+ from carbonic acid enters cells and HCO_3^- remains in ECF. The second mode of initiation, through net addition of HCO_3^- or its precursors (lactate, citrate, acetate) to ECF, results when these compounds are administered in amounts greater than the daily acid production. Finally, alkalemia is initiated when ECF volume contraction around a constant HCO_3^- space leads to an increased HCO_3^- concentration.

Alkalemia is transient when usual restorative measures are available.[5] Immediate buffering of body fluids by addition of H^+ (from phosphate, proteins, and lactic acid) to ECF titrates surplus HCO_3^-. Respiratory compensation through alveolar hypoventilation causing pCO_2 to rise (not >55 mmHg) and pH to fall is limited by hypoxemia. The kidney ultimately excretes the excess HCO_3^- and returns the pH to normal.

Contravening factors may result in the maintenance of alkalosis, a phase that is classified as Cl^- responsive, Cl^- resistant, or miscellaneous. Patients with Cl^- responsive alkalosis have urinary Cl^- <10 mmol/L and are commonly volume depleted.[4] Decreased ECF results in enhanced electroneutral proximal Na^+ reabsorption. The amount of Cl^- available for reabsorption is limited because of previous losses from the GI or urinary tracts. Therefore, Na^+-H^+ exchange occurs with net HCO_3^- reabsorption perpetuating the alkalosis. In the distal nephron, there is increased H^+ secretion with HCO_3^- generation that also tends to maintain the alkalosis. This increase may be aldosterone dependent. Limited availability of Cl^- in the distal nephron also perpetuates alkaloses because HCO_3^- is secreted in exchange for Cl^- at this site.[17] Cl^- responsive alkalosis may result from vomiting, nasogastric suction, diarrhea, villous adenoma, and diuretic therapy. Posthypercapneic alkalosis is also Cl⁻ responsive. Chronic hypercapnia increases Cl⁻ and H⁺ excretion and HCO_3^- reabsorption. Correcting hypercapnia usually results in retention of Cl⁻ and excretion of HCO_3^- unless patients are on low Na⁺ diets or have decreased intravascular volume. Then, proximal Na⁺ reabsorption is enhanced with maintenance of alkalemia as described.

Patients with Cl⁻ resistant alkalosis have urinary Cl⁻ >10 mmol/L and have excess mineralocorticoids.[4] Na⁺ is avidly reabsorbed distally and H⁺ is secreted. Cl⁻ availability is unimportant. This classification of alkalosis includes Cushing's syndrome, Bartter's syndrome, hyperaldosteronism, and ingestion of licorice containing glycyrrhizic acid. Patients with severe K⁺ depletion (K⁺ <2 mEq/L) have urinary Cl⁻ >20 mmol/L, without excess mineralocorticoid activity, and have alkalemias improved only with correction of the K⁺ deficit.[3]

Those patients who do not fit into the Cl⁻ resistant or responsive category have exogenous sources of alkali (excessive $NaHCO_3$, nonreabsorbable antacids, massive transfusions of blood with citrate anticoagulant or of Plasmanate* with acetate) and limited ability to excrete HCO_3^- (e.g., renal insufficiency). Glucose ingestion after starvation, hypoparathyroidism, and non–parathormone-induced hypercalcemia are included in the miscellaneous category for maintenance of alkalosis.

Clinical features stem from volume depletion or hypokalemia (orthostasis, weakness, muscle cramps). Arrhythmias associated with digoxin are more common. Paresthesias and carpopedal spasm occur in moderate alkalosis; seizures and arrhythmias are seen in severe alkalosis. Compensatory hypoventilation in patients with underlying lung disease may require correction of alkalosis to improve declining ventilatory function. Treatment is based on the cause. Underlying problems should be corrected (e.g., discontinuing nasogastric suction, halting Cl⁻ diarrhea, reducing diuretics, etc.). Cimetidine is given to raise gastric pH when nasogastric suction must be continued. Volume and Cl⁻ are restored with NaCl and KCl in the Cl⁻ sensitive group. In severe K⁺ depletion, K⁺ is replaced before ECF deficits are corrected. Mineralocorticoid excesses are treated specifically or their effects blocked by spironolactone or amiloride in the Cl⁻ resistant group.

When usual corrective measures fail, alternative treatment exists. Tidal volume and respiratory rate can be decreased as an immediate measure to lower the pH of mechanically ventilated patients (maintaining oxygenation). In congestive heart failure, ascites, nephrotic syndrome, renal failure, or severe alkalosis (pH >7.6), acetazolamide, acid therapy, or dialysis can be used. Acetazolamide (250 mg bid–tid, by the oral or intravenous route),[2,3]

---

*Trademark for a commercial preparation of human plasma protein fraction.

a carbonic anhydrase inhibitor and proximal diuretic, increases renal HCO_3^-, K^+, and Na^+ excretion (urine pH >7). Serum pH must be monitored because inhibition of carbonic anhydrase in the lung could block CO_2 expiration. Acid is administered when acetazolamide is ineffective or when patients develop seizures, arrhythmias, or serum pH >7.6, not easily correctable by routine measures. The amount of acid is at least equal to the HCO_3^- excess. HCO_3^- excess = (40% total body weight in kg) × (plasma HCO_3^- [mEq/L] − desired or normal HCO_3^-). Acid need may be underestimated if causes for alkalosis are ongoing. HCl is administered over 8–24 hours as a 0.1–0.15 N solution in 5% dextrose in water [(40% body weight in kg) × (measured plasma HCO_3^- [mEq/L] − desired HCO_3) = mEq H^+ required] and must be infused through a central vein.[7,9,10] Severe mediastinitis has resulted from central catheters penetrating the vessel wall. Although HCl is corrosive, a Swedish group administered 0.15 N HCl peripherally, buffered in an amino acid solution and infused with a fat emulsion.[8] NH_4Cl (metabolized in the liver to HCl, NH_3, and then to urea) can be given in a peripheral vein or orally. Twenty milligrams of NH_4Cl/ml, which is approximately equal to 350 mEq/L of H^+ ion, can be given intravenously at a maximal rate of 500 ml/hour.[1] More rapid administration leads to CNS toxicity. NH_4Cl is contraindicated in liver or renal disease because of accumulation of NH_3 and urea. Three hundred milliliters of 10% arginine monohydrochloride supplies 150 mEq of H^+ and can be given over an hour if necessary.[1] However, because the arginine cation displaces K^+ from cells, dangerous hyperkalemia can result, especially in patients with abnormal renal function. Finally, high-Cl, low-acetate bath dialysis is used in patients in renal failure and for those who cannot tolerate fluid loading.

KEY FEATURES

METABOLIC ALKALOSIS

Cl⁻ Responsive
Causes: vomiting, nasogastric suction, Cl⁻ diarrhea, villous adenomas, diuretic therapy, posthypercapnia
Features: volume depletion, urinary Cl⁻ <10 mmol/L
Treatment: correct underlying problem, cimetidine, volume + Cl⁻ restoration
Cl⁻ Resistant
Causes: Cushing's syndrome, Bartter's syndrome, hyperaldosteronism, licorice, severe K^+ depletion
Features: volume repletion, urinary Cl⁻ >10 mmol/L
Treatment: correct underlying cause; spironolactone, amiloride

Miscellaneous
 Causes: excessive $NaHCO_3$, massive transfusion of blood and Plasmanate, hypoparathyroidism, glucose after starvation
Alternative Treatment for Refractory Alkalosis
1. Decrease tidal volume, respiratory rate of ventilated patient
2. Acetazolamide (250 mg bid–tid PO or IV)
3. Acid needed = HCO_3^- excess = (40% total body weight in kg) × (plasma HCO_3^- − desired HCO_3^-); HCl (0.15N in 5% dextrose in water over 8–24 hours) in central line

REFERENCES

1. Cohen JJ, Kassirer JP: Metabolic alkalosis. In Cohen JJ, Kassirer JP: Acid-Base. Boston, Little, Brown, 1982, pp 227–306.
2. Harrington JT: Metabolic alkalosis. Kidney Int 26:88–97, 1984.
3. Schrier RW: Pathogenesis and management of metabolic acidosis and alkalosis. In Schrier RW (ed): Renal and Electrolyte Disorders, 2nd ed. Boston, Little, Brown, 1980, pp 115–158.
    References 1–3 all give a concise physiologic and practical approach to metabolic alkalosis.

4. Narins R, et al: Diagnostic strategies in disorders of fluid, electrolyte and acid-base homeostasis. Am J Med 72:496–520, 1982.
5. Narins R, Emmett M: Simple and mixed acid-base disorders: A practical approach. Medicine 59:161–185, 1980.
6. Bia M, Thier S: Mixed acid-base disturbances: A clinical approach. Med Clin North Am 65:347–361, 1981.
    References 4–6 are excellent discussions in acid-base physiology and address problems of mixed disturbances.

7. Kurtzman N: Metabolic alkalosis. Kidney 9:27–32, 1976.
    Quick review of initiation, maintenance, and treatment.

8. Knutsen OH: New method for administration of hydrochloric acid in metabolic alkalosis. Lancet 1:953–956, 1983.
    Method of peripheral administration of HCl with amino acids and fat emulsion reviewed in two patients.

9. Williams SE: Hydrogen ion infusion for treating severe metabolic alkalosis. Br Med J 1:1189, 1976.
    Method for calculating H^+ deficit is given.

10. Harken A, et al: Hydrochloric acid in correction of metabolic alkalosis. Arch Surg 110:819–812, 1975.
    Method for preparing HCl and calculating dose necessary is given.

11. Danilewitz M, et al: Ranitidine suppression of gastric hypersecretion resistant to cimetidine. N Engl J Med 306:20–22, 1982.
12. Barton C, et al: Cimetidine in the management of metabolic acidosis induced by nasogastric drainage. Arch Surg 114:70–74, 1979.
    References 11 and 12 discuss the use of H_2 blockers in treatment of metabolic alkalosis.

13. Madias N, Levey A: Metabolic alkalosis due to absorption of "nonabsorbable" antacids. Am J Med 74:155–158, 1983.

14. Madias N, et al: Increased anion gap in metabolic alkalosis. N Engl J Med 300:1421–1423, 1979.
    Added interpretation of the anion gap.
15. Brater D, Morrelli H: Systemic alkalosis and digitalis related arrhythmias. Acta Med Scand (Suppl)647:79–85, 1981.
16. Bear R, et al: Effect of metabolic alkalosis on respiratory function in patients with chronic obstructive lung disease. CMA Journal 117:900–903, 1977.
    Authors present eight patients with chronic obstructive pulmonary disease and metabolic alkalosis and conclude a benefit from correction of alkalosis.
17. Borkan S, et al: Renal response to metabolic alkalosis induced by isovolemic hemofiltration in the dog. Kidney Int 32:322–328, 1987.
    Presents evidence supporting importance of Cl⁻ in correction of alkalosis.

Respiratory Acid-Base Disorders

Claire Fritsche, M.D.

RESPIRATORY ACIDOSIS

Diminished effective alveolar ventilation leads to inadequate excretion of metabolically produced CO_2. From the Henderson-Hasselbalch equation,

$$pH = 6.1 + \log \frac{[HCO_3^-]}{.03\ pCO_2}$$; as pCO_2 rises, pH falls, resulting in respiratory

acidosis. Immediate defense against acidosis is provided by the intracellular buffers, hemoglobin, phosphates, protein, and lactate. Renal compensation occurs in 12–24 hours with increased H^+ secretion.[5] Because more Na^+ is reabsorbed in exchange for H^+, Cl^- excretion is increased. In acute respiratory acidosis, only immediate buffering is available, causing HCO_3^- to increase by 3–4 mEq/L.[5] Acute respiratory acidosis may be caused by neuromuscular abnormalities (e.g., Guillain-Barré syndrome, myasthenia gravis, brain stem or spinal cord abnormalities), drug overdose, flail chest, airway obstruction, pneumonia, smoke inhalation, pulmonary edema, and pulmonary emboli. Patients manifest signs and symptoms of respiratory failure, including headache, fatigue, altered mental status, tremor, somnolence, coma, blurred vision, and papilledema. The pH and pO_2 are decreased, pCO_2 is elevated, HCO_3^- is elevated (not greater than 30 mEq/L),[6] and plasma Cl^- is normal. In chronic respiratory acidosis, in addition to buffering, renal compensation is in effect. Causes include neuromuscular disorders (e.g., amyotrophic lateral sclerosis (ALS), pickwickian syndrome, polio, diaphragmatic paralysis), sedation, kyphoscoliosis, severe pulmonary interstitial fibrosis, and, most often, chronic obstructive pulmonary disease (COPD).

Clinical features are associated with the underlying disease, and cor pulmonale may coexist. Laboratory abnormalities include increased pCO_2 and HCO_3^-, decreased plasma Cl^- and pH (but not less than 7.20),[5] and a normal anion gap. Respiratory failure must be treated and volume overload avoided. If artificial ventilation is used, care should be taken to lower pCO_2 slowly (especially in patients with underlying chronic respiratory acidosis), or CNS alkalosis may result, leading to seizures and coma.[7]

RESPIRATORY ALKALOSIS

When alveolar ventilation increases, pulmonary excretion exceeds production of CO_2. From the equation $pH = 6.1 + \log \dfrac{[HCO_3^-]}{.03\ pCO_2}$, as pCO_2 falls, pH rises and respiratory alkalosis results. Immediate defense against alkalosis occurs when H^+ is released from intracellular buffers, consuming HCO_3^-. Lactic acid and other organic acid production increases. HCO_3^- may fall to 15 mEq/L but usually is not below 18 mEq/L.[5] Renal compensation occurs more slowly with reduced net acid excretion, reduced generation of HCO_3^-, and decreased NH_4^+ excretion. Na^+ and K^+ excretion increases over the first 24–48 hours but then returns to normal.[5] Respiratory alkalosis may be caused by CNS abnormalities (e.g., head trauma, CNS tumor, or hemorrhage), hypoxemia (e.g., congestive heart failure, pulmonary emboli, pulmonary disorders, altitude), anxiety, fever, thyrotoxicosis, salicylism, hepatic insufficiency, sepsis, and problematic artificial ventilation. There are no specific features associated with chronic alkalosis, but acute respiratory alkalosis may result in lightheadedness, perioral and extremity paresthesias, carpopedal spasm, muscle cramps, tinnitus, hyperactive reflexes, tetany, seizures, and cardiac arrhythmias.[1] In most circumstances, treatment is limited to correction of the underlying disorder. Symptomatic patients with psychogenic hyperventilation should rebreathe into a paper bag. Artificially ventilated patients who are overbreathing may require sedation or treatment with paralyzing agents to control respiratory rate. Decreasing minute ventilation, increasing dead space, or adding 3% carbon dioxide[3] are alternative treatments of respirator-induced alkalosis.

KEY FEATURES

RESPIRATORY ACIDOSIS AND RESPIRATORY ALKALOSIS

Respiratory Acidosis

Acute

Causes: neuromuscular (Guillain-Barré syndrome, myasthenia gravis, brain stem or spinal cord abnormalities), drug overdose, flail chest, airway obstruction, pneumonia, smoke inhalation, pulmonary edema, pulmonary emboli

Chronic

Causes: neuromuscular (ALS, pickwickian syndrome, polio, diaphragmatic paralysis), sedation, kyphoscoliosis, severe pulmonary interstitial fibrosis, COPD

Treatment: artificial ventilation with special care to correct acidosis *slowly*, especially in chronic acidosis

Respiratory Alkalosis

Causes: CNS (head trauma, CNS tremors, bleeds), hypoxemia, anxiety, fever, thyrotoxicosis, salicylism, hepatic insufficiency, gram negative sepsis, artificial ventilation

Treatment includes the following:

1. Correct cause
2. Rebreathe into paper bag
3. Ventilator: decrease minute ventilation, increase dead space, 3% CO_2, sedation with or without pancuronium bromide (Pavulon) for agitation

REFERENCES

1. Cohen JJ, Kassirer JP: Respiratory acidosis; respiratory alkalosis (Chaps 10 and 11). *In* Cohen JJ, Kassirer JP: Acid-Base. Boston, Little, Brown, 1982, pp 307–376.
2. Rose BD: Respiratory acidosis; respiratory alkalosis (Chaps 19 and 20). *In* Rose BD: Clinical Physiology of Acid-Base and Electrolyte Disorders. New York, McGraw-Hill, 1977, pp 354–376.
3. Schrier, RW: Pathogenesis and management of respiratory and mixed acid-base disorders. *In* Schrier RW (ed): Renal and Electrolyte Disorders, 2nd ed. Boston, Little, Brown, 1980, pp 159–182.

    References 1–3 give a concise physiologic and practical approach to respiratory acidosis and alkalosis.

4. Narins R, et al: Diagnostic strategies in disorders of fluid, electrolyte amd acid-base homeostasis. Am J Med 72:496–520, 1982.
5. Narins R, Emmett M: Simple and mixed acid-base disorders: A practical approach. Medicine 59:161–185, 1980.
6. Bia M, Thier S: Mixed acid-base disturbances: A clinical approach. Med Clin North Am 65:347–361, 1981.

    References 4–6 are excellent discussions in acid-base physiology and address problems of mixed disturbances.

7. Arieff A, et al: Intracellular pH of brain: Alterations in acute respiratory acidosis and alkalosis. Am J Physiol 230:804–812, 1976.

    Dog study to show ranges of cellular pH in the brain during wide fluctuations in pCO₂.

Acute Renal Failure

David Bernard, M.D.

Acute renal failure refers to the sudden onset of renal insufficiency resulting in rapidly progressive azotemia (a rise in the BUN of 10–20 mg%/day and creatinine of 0.5–2.0 mg%/day). Although oliguria, the daily passage of under 400 ml of urine, has been considered a cardinal sign of acute renal failure, nonoliguric forms are present in about half of cases.[1] Because urea originates from the catabolism of protein, the level of BUN will rise much faster when acute renal failure is associated with a hypercatabolic state, such as burns or sepsis; on the other hand, because the major source of creatinine in the blood is muscle, the serum creatinine will rise at a rate greater than 2 mg%/day only when acute renal failure is associated with rhabdomyolysis, but not simply from hypercatabolism.[2] Approximately 50% of acute renal failure occurs in association with surgery or trauma, 30% in a medical setting or related to nephrotoxins, and the balance in association with pregnancy.

It is useful to classify the causes of acute renal failure into pre-renal causes, in which there is inadequate renal perfusion from hypovolemia or poor cardiac output; post-renal causes, in which there is urinary obstruction; and renal causes, which encompass all the intrinsic renal parenchymal diseases. In pre- and post-renal disorders, specific therapy is often available and curative and these must be excluded first. Of the many renal parenchymal causes, so-called acute nonspecific renal failure or acute tubular necrosis (ATN) is responsible in 75% of cases. Four major factors are thought to be important in the pathogenesis of ATN.[4] Renal ischemia is probably the most common cause and develops as an extension of pre-renal failure when reversal of deficits of blood volume or cardiac output can no longer restore renal function to normal. Release of the heme pigments hemoglobin and myoglobin into the circulation may cause ATN. Nontraumatic rhabdomyolysis is common, often not recognized, and may be seen in association with seizures, vigorous exercise, prolonged coma, viral myositis, and drug abuse.[2,3] Nephrotoxins, especially drugs and radiographic contrast media,[6] are an increasingly common cause. Pregnancy and obstetric-related circumstances such as postpartum hemorrhage and septic abortion make up the balance.

In evaluating a patient with acute renal failure, one must first identify any reversible causes, such as circulatory failure (pre-renal factors), or obstruction (post-renal). In many cases, the cause of renal failure can be determined from the history and clinical features. Special emphasis must be placed on drug exposure or occupational and environmental nephrotoxins. The physical examination should include assessment of fluid balance and cardiac function, and should always include rectal and pelvic examinations to assess the possibility of obstruction. Other features are helpful in establishing the differential diagnosis, as follows:

The *urine sediment*: In ATN, a diagnostic sediment is seen in about 80% of cases and consists of large numbers of deeply pigmented ("muddy brown"), coarsely granular casts and large numbers of renal tubular epithelial cells free and in casts. In pre-renal and post-renal failure, the sediment is usually benign. In specific forms of renal parenchymal disease, such as acute glomerulonephritis or interstitial nephritis, urine sediment may offer clues to the underlying pathology.

The *urine composition* is frequently useful in separating pre-renal from intrinsic renal failure, although no consistent pattern is present in obstruction.[7] The urine sodium concentration on a random urine specimen is usually low in pre-renal failure (less than 10 mEq/L) and high in ATN (greater than 25 mEq/L). Urine osmolality and specific gravity tend to be high in pre-renal causes (ratio of urine to plasma greater than 1.5) and low in ATN (ratio less than 1.1). The "renal failure index" (the urinary sodium concentration divided by urine to plasma creatinine ratio) or the fractional excretion of sodium (clearance of sodium divided by clearance of creatinine) is low in pre-renal failure (less than 1) and high (over 4) in renal failure. In nonoliguric forms of ATN, the urine features are not always so typical and the urine sodium concentration may be less than 25 mEq/L in some cases.[7] *Radiologic studies* are used predominantly to rule out obstruction. For this purpose, ultrasonography is most useful, although if a high degree of suspicion of urinary obstruction is present, retrograde or anterograde ureteric catheterization should be performed even if the ultrasound does not suggest obstruction. Occasionally, in cases in which it is felt that specific treatment may be available for acute renal failure, such as in cases of rapidly progressive glomerulonephritis, a renal biopsy may be needed to establish the diagnosis.

The management of acute renal failure should be considered under two headings—prevention and treatment of the established case. Because ATN usually occurs in a predictable clinical setting, anticipation of the disease is the key to prevention. Prompt and adequate replacement of fluid and blood losses in surgical, burn, and trauma patients may prevent post-ischemic ATN, whereas the incidence of ATN in the medical setting can be reduced by effective management of cardiac and septic shock, the avoidance of potential nephrotoxic drugs, and dose modifications for elderly or compromised patients. The value of mannitol or potent diuretics in preventing acute renal failure is more controversial.[8] Some authorities advocate their use to maintain high urine flow rates of 2–4 L/day for 2–3 days after events known to be associated with a high incidence of ATN. These include severe muscle crushing injuries, mismatched blood transfusions, intravascular hemolysis, and acute hyperuricemia.[8] In an oliguric patient, once reversible factors have been excluded or dealt with, an adequate volume of fluid should be given to establish a state of positive fluid balance; saline or colloid solutions may be used. If such therapy does not lead to an increase in urine output in an oliguric patient, a single large dose of mannitol (up to 25 gm) or furosemide (200–400 mg) can be given.[8] If urine flow rate does not increase following the initial doses of these agents, repeated high doses of diuretic should not be given, but rather therapy for established ATN should be instituted. Such management can be considered under the following discussion:

Restrict intake of all substances normally excreted by the kidney: This includes fluids (300–400 ml/day plus an amount for urine volume and any extrarenal losses should be allowed); sodium and potassium, which are given to replace obvious losses only; and drugs normally excreted by the kidney.

Supply adequate nutrition: Initially, protein intake is restricted to 20–40 gm/day (of high biologic value protein) to limit the rate of rise of BUN, and 100 gm of carbohydrate is given to slow protein catabolism. However, this diet will induce a state of negative nitrogen balance and cannot be continued for long. As soon as the patient is stable, usually once dialysis is commenced, a relatively normal diet supplying adequate calories and essential amino acids should be started. If the patient cannot ingest food by mouth, parenteral nutrition should be started promptly. Some studies have suggested that aggressive feeding of acute renal failure patients, supplying adequate calories and essential amino acids, may improve the overall prognosis and enhance the rate of recovery of renal function.[9]

The biochemical abnormalities of renal failure must be monitored carefully: Hyperkalemia and acidosis rarely need treatment on their own, generally being corrected when dialysis is begun for other reasons. Occasionally infusions of glucose and ion exchange resins are needed to control hyperkalemia before dialysis is commenced, and sodium bicarbonate treatment may be necessary if the serum bicarbonate concentration falls below 16 mEq/L.

Prevent infection: Because infection is the most common cause of death in acute renal failure, every effort should be made to reduce the risk of nosocomial infection.

Dialysis treatment: is used more frequently and earlier today than previously. Although patients without complications can be managed well by conservative measures, routine periodic dialysis simplifies therapy, makes the patient feel better, and allows liberalization of diet and fluid restrictions. Specific indications for dialysis include the following:

1. Any uremic sign or symptom (e.g. mental confusion, GI upset, peri-carditis, bleeding)
2. A BUN over 100–150 mg% or creatinine of over 10–12 mg%, or a rapidly rising BUN (over 25–30 mg%/day)
3. Hyperkalemia uncontrolled by conventional means
4. Severe acidosis uncontrolled by conventional means
5. Significant fluid overload

Peritoneal dialysis is usually the first form of therapy begun, and most patients can be managed quite adequately by this means. It is effective and easy to perform, has the advantage of avoiding heparinization in the bleeding patient, and allows dialysis to be accomplished in the hypotensive patient in whom blood flows for hemodialysis may be inadequate. However, because peritoneal dialysis is inefficient and requires immobilization, hemodialysis is generally started as soon as it is evident that oliguria will not resolve promptly, or immediately in hypercatabolic patients.

Despite these measures, the prognosis for recovery from acute renal failure remains poor, about half the patients failing to recover. Death is usually from complications of the underlying disease rather than from renal failure itself.

KEY FEATURES

In typical cases of acute renal failure, BUN rises by 10–20 mg%/day creatinine by 0.5–2.0 mg%/day.

In hypercatabolic forms of acute renal failure, BUN rises at 25–30 mg%/day; in rhabdomyolysis, creatinine rises at over 2 mg%/day.

Always exclude pre-renal and post-renal causes:
- Careful history and physical to include assessment of fluid status
- A benign urine sediment favors pre-renal or post-renal factors
- A low spot urine sodium concentration or low fractional sodium excretion favors pre-renal causes
- If there is high suspicion of obstruction, perform pyelogram even if ultrasound is normal
  Prevent ATN by:
- Prompt restoration of fluid losses
- Rapid treatment of shock
- Judicious use of nephrotoxic drugs
- Prophylactic diuretics in patients suffering muscle crushing injuries, incompatible blood transfusions, and acute hyperuricemia
  Once oliguric renal failure is established:
- Vigorously and adequately replace fluids (colloid and saline); administer until fluid balance is clearly positive.
- If oliguria persists, give single dose of mannitol (25 gm) or furosemide (200–400 mg)

If urine flow increases, continue to monitor renal function

If oliguria persists, treat for established renal failure:

1. Restrict intake of all substances needing renal excretion (fluids, sodium, potassium, drugs)
2. Supply adequate nutrition
3. Treat biochemical complications (acidosis and hyperkalemia)
4. Prevent infection (aseptic techniques)
5. Begin dialysis (usually peritoneally first), generally before uremia manifests. Certainly, if:
   a. Any uremic sign or symptom develops
   b. BUN over 100–150 mg% or rising fast; creatinine over 10–12 mg%
   c. Acidosis not easily treatable medically
   d. Hyperkalemia not easily treatable medically
   e. Severe fluid overload present

REFERENCES

1. Anderson RJ, et al: Nonoliguric acute renal failure. New Engl J Med 296:1134, 1977.
   A prospective study of the incidence, causes, and outcome of nonoliguric acute renal failure. Of 92 patients studied, 54 were found to be nonoliguric throughout the course of the disease. Morbidity and mortality were lower in this group than in the oliguric cases. It should be emphasized, however, that this is the only study reporting a lower mortality rate in nonoliguric ATN. At least 12 other studies have failed to confirm this finding.

2. Grossman RA, et al: Nontraumatic rhabdomyolysis and acute renal failure. New Engl J Med 291:807, 1974.
   The clinical and biochemical features of acute renal failure from nontraumatic rhabdomyolysis are described. The disease is highly suggested by the findings of a triad of urine dipstick-positive for blood, pigmented granular casts in the urine sediment in the absence of red blood cells, and marked elevation of serum creatinine phosphokinase level. In addition, an unusually rapid increase in serum levels of creatinine, potassium, and phosphate is noted, and serum calcium concentration is often low early in the course of the disease.

3. Gabow PA, Kaehny WD, Kelleher SP: The spectrum of rhabdomyolysis. Medicine 61:141, 1982.
   The causes, clinical features, and prognosis of rhabdomyolysis-related acute renal failure are presented and contrasted with cases of rhabdomyolysis in which normal renal function was preserved.

4. Rasmussen HH, Ibels LS: Acute renal failure. Multivariate analysis of causes and risk factors. Am J Med 73:211, 1982.
   An analysis of the risk factors for the development of acute renal failure in 143 patients with the disease. About half the patients had more than one risk factor, with hypotension, excessive aminoglycoside exposure, and dehydration being the most important insults.

5. Henrich WL, Blachley JD: Acute renal failure with prostaglandin inhibition. Semin Nephrol 1:57, 1981.
   The pathophysiology of acute renal failure from nonsteroidal anti-inflammatory agents is reviewed, and the patients prone to this complication are outlined. Patients with cirrhosis, congestive heart failure, nephrotic syndrome, and volume depletion (secondary to conditions such as diuretic therapy and gastrointestinal fluid loss) are at especially high risk.

Although all anti-inflammatory agents seem likely to be able to produce this condition, sulindac may not because it appears not to inhibit renal prostaglandin production.

6. Harkonen S, Kjellstrand C: Contrast nephropathy. Am J Nephrol 1:69, 1981.
    A detailed review emphasizing the particular risk of this entity in patients with pre-existing renal insufficiency and in patients with diabetes mellitus. Type I diabetics with severe renal disease have an over 90% incidence of nephrotoxicity, with as many as half sustaining permanent renal damage. Hypertension, old age, and peripheral vascular disease may increase the risk in susceptible patients. In multiple myeloma, the risk of renal failure from radiographic contrast media is quite low if the patients are well hydrated and have normal renal function.

7. Miller TR, et al: Urinary diagnostic indices in acute renal failure. A prospective study. Ann Intern Med 89:47, 1978.
    Renal failure patients could be separated into pre-renal and ATN categories from the findings of the urinary chemical composition and concentration. Post-renal cases were not reliably categorized, seeming to appear like pre-renal cases when the renal failure was mild and like ATN once renal insufficiency was more advanced.

8. Levinsky NG, Bernard DB, Johnston PA: Mannitol and loop diuretics in acute renal failure. In Brenner BM, Lazarus JM (eds): Acute Renal Failure. Philadelphia, WB Saunders Co, 1983, pp 712–722.
    An extensive literature review on the value of diuretic therapy in preventing and treating acute renal failure. Guidelines are offered as to when and how these agents should be used and to whom they should be given.

9. Abel RM, et al: Improved survival from acute renal failure after treatment with intravenous essential L-amino acids and glucose. N Engl J Med 288:695, 1973.
    The authors compared the effects of hyperalimentation with glucose and amino acids versus glucose alone in patients with acute renal failure. The group given amino acids had a lower morbidity rate, recovered renal function more rapidly, and had a lower mortality.

10. Kaplan AA, Longnecker RE, Folkert VW: Continuous arteriovenous hemofiltration. A report of six months experience. Ann Intern Med 100:358, 1984.
    The authors describe the technique of continuous hemofiltration and review their results in 15 patients. The procedure was found to be a convenient and safe method for achieving continuous fluid, electrolyte, and acid-base control in patients with acute renal failure.

Hypernatremia and Hyponatremia

Wilfred Lieberthal, M.D.

The water content of the body (50–60% of total body weight) is distributed between the intracellular (ICF) and the extracellular (ECF) compartments: two thirds of total body water is within cells, whereas one third is extracellular. Cell membranes are freely permeable to water, which moves between cells and interstitial tissue to maintain osmotic equivalence between these two compartments. A fall in ECF osmolality (hypotonicity) results in a shift of water into cells, whereas hypertonicity results in a movement of water out of cells into the extracellular fluid (ECF). Serum osmolality is normally maintained between 280 and 300 mOsm/kg of water.

Sodium, with its associated anions, accounts for more than 90% of the osmolality of the ECF and is the primary determinant of the effective osmolality (tonicity) of the ECF compartment. Therefore, with few exceptions, changes in the concentration of sodium in plasma reflect proportional alterations in plasma tonicity. Normal serum sodium concentration ranges between 135 and 145 mEq/L. The clinical consequences of hyponatremia and hypernatremia are largely due to the associated changes in tonicity and the resultant shifts of water into and out of cells. The serum sodium concentration provides no information about the total amount of sodium in body fluid, since it reflects only the relative proportions of sodium and water in the ECF. Thus, the presence of hyponatremia or hypernatremia indicates that factors controlling body fluid *osmolality* are abnormal; either may be associated with a normal, decreased, or increased total body sodium.

The serum osmolality and therefore the sodium concentration is maintained within a remarkable narrow range despite wide variations in dietary sodium and fluid intake. If an individual is deprived of water, plasma osmolality will rise as a result of continued insensible and urinary losses of water. An increase in plasma osmolality above 280 mOsm/kg (or a serum sodium concentration of 135 mEq/L) stimulates the release of antidiuretic hormone (ADH) from the posterior pituitary. ADH enhances water reabsorption from the collecting ducts of the kidney and the excretion of a concentrated urine, thus limiting free water loss. Renal water retention will continue until the individual drinks water. Thirst is usually stimulated above a serum osmolality of 300 mOsm/kg (serum sodium level of 145 mEq). Increased water intake results in a fall in plasma osmolality that both inhibits the thirst mechanism and reduces ADH release. When the serum osmolality falls below 280 mOsm/kg of water, ADH secretion ceases and a maximally dilute urine is excreted until the serum osmolality rises into the normal range. The release of ADH may be stimulated by factors other than plasma osmolality, such as marked volume depletion, pain, anxiety, and a variety of drugs.[1] These factors may result in renal water retention despite a normal or reduced serum osmolality.

HYPONATREMIA

Causes

There are two situations in which hyponatremia does not reflect the presence of hypo-osmolality and requires no treatment. Pseudohyponatremia (or factitious hyponatremia) refers to situations in which the clinical laboratory provides a falsely low measure of serum sodium concentration. This occurs in the presence of severe hyperlipidemia or hyperproteinemia. In this situation, plasma osmolality is normal. Hyperglycemia results in hyponatremia in the presence of a plasma osmolality that is actually *increased*. Intracellular water enters the ECF by osmosis and dilutes out the plasma sodium. (Plasma sodium will decrease about 1.7–2.0 mEq/L for every increase of 100 mg/dl in plasma glucose above normal.)

Once pseudohyponatremia and hyperglycemia have been excluded, one can assume hyponatremia indicates the presence of hypotonicity. The next step in the clinical evaluation is an assessment of the extracellular volume status of the patient. Management of a hyponatremic state is facilitated by determining whether the patient has an associated increased total body sodium (with edema), a decreased total body sodium (and hypovolemia), or an apparently normal extracellular volume status.[4]

Clinical Features

The signs and symptoms of hyponatremia are predominantly neuropsychiatric and range from lethargy and confusion to grand mal seizures and coma.[2,3] The severity of the symptoms depends on the degree of hyponatremia and the rate at which the serum sodium concentration is lowered; acute hyponatremia has a significantly higher morbidity and mortality rate than chronic hyponatremia. In general, signs and symptoms of hyponatremia do not occur until the serum sodium level falls below 120 mEq/L, and most patients with the severest manifestations (coma, seizures) have a serum sodium concentration below 110–115 mEq/L.

Hyponatremia Associated with Extracellular Volume Depletion

This situation arises in patients who have lost both salt and water and have ready access to water. If a volume-depleted person is allowed to drink water freely, hyponatremia will develop because severe hypovolemia stimulates both thirst and ADH secretion and impairs renal water excretion.[4]

Diagnosis. Clinical signs of ECF depletion are usually present, i.e., poor skin turgor, dry mucous membranes, absence of sweating, and postural hypotension.

Treatment. All that is usually required to correct hyponatremia associated with hypovolemia is the intravenous administration of appropriate amounts of isotonic saline. As soon as extracellular volume is restored to normal, ADH will be suppressed and the kidney will excrete a maximally dilute urine. The serum sodium concentration will rise rapidly to the normal range.

Hyponatremia Associated with Expansion of Extracellular Volume

In patients with edema that is due to cardiac failure, cirrhosis, or nephrotic syndrome, the ingestion of large amounts of water will lead to hyponatremia. Although total body sodium is markedly increased in these patients, "effective" circulating blood volume is reduced. The kidneys respond to this apparent hypovolemia in a manner similar to the response associated with true or absolute hypovolemia. These mechanisms prevent appropriate urine dilution and lead to water retention. Hyponatremia in association with edema may also occur in patients with advanced renal failure who have unrestricted water intake. The defect in water excretion in these patients is a result of severe reduction in the glomerular filtration rate, which limits the formation and hence the excretion of free water.

Diagnosis. This category of hyponatremia is easy to recognize clinically because the patient has obvious edema.

Therapy. In the edematous hyponatremic patient, both sodium and water intake should be limited. Unless oliguria is present, restriction of water intake to less than 1000 ml/day will result in a gradual correction of the serum sodium concentration over a number of days.

The need for rapid correction of the serum sodium concentration in edematous patients who are manifesting marked symptoms and signs of hypotonicity presents a difficult management problem. The use of loop diuretics (furosemide and ethacrynic acid) followed by replacement of sodium losses with hypertonic saline is usually effective but requires careful monitoring. In patients with advanced renal failure, hemodialysis may be the most appropriate intervention.

Hyponatremia Associated with Normal Extracellular Volume

Many clinical conditions are associated with euvolemic hyponatremia, such as the following:

1. Water intoxication may result from an abnormally large oral intake of water (psychogenic water drinking) or from the excessive parenteral administration of hypotonic fluid. Acute water intoxication is a particularly dangerous cause of hyponatremia, because it results in a rapid fall in serum osmolality. In these patients, life-threatening complications

such as seizures and coma may develop at serum sodium concentrations above 120 mEq/L.

2. Endocrinopathies, particularly hypoadrenalism and hypothyroidism, are important but unusual causes of hyponatremia. The mechanisms responsible for the abnormality in water secretion in these conditions have not been clarified.

3. Diuretic use may result in hyponatremia in patients who are not significantly volume depleted. This typically occurs in patients who have been on thiazide diuretics for prolonged periods and are severely potassium depleted. Discontinuation of the diuretic and correction of the potassium deficit will usually correct the hyponatremia.[5]

4. The syndrome of inappropriate secretion of ADH (SIADH) involves a sustained or intermittent elevation of the plasma level of ADH that cannot be ascribed to any physiologic stimulus, osmotic or nonosmotic.[6] SIADH occurs in a variety of circumstances, which may be classified into three main groups: (1) malignant tumors that produce ADH or substances with ADH-like activity (oat cell carcinoma of the lung, cancer of the prostate), (2) diseases of the CNS (tumors, trauma, infection, stroke), and (3) certain drugs (chlorpropamide, tolbutamide, clofibrate, vincristine, opiates, carbamazepine) that may stimulate ADH release or potentiate its renal tubular action or both.[7] SIADH is a diagnosis of exclusion, which can only be made once other conditions known to affect water excretion (renal, adrenal, and thyroid disease; hypovolemia and edematous states) have been excluded.

Treatment. In patients who are asymptomatic or who have only mild symptoms of hyponatremia, water restriction is usually all that is required. Reversible factors contributing to the hyponatremia should be sought. If the patient is unable or unwilling to restrict water intake, the use of a drug that antagonizes the renal action of ADH should be considered. Demeclocycline (300–600 mg qid) is usually effective.[8]

In patients who manifest neurologic signs of hypotonicity or who have severe hyponatremia (sodium below 110 mEq/L), rapid elevation of the serum sodium concentration is indicated. This is achieved by the infusion of hypertonic saline as a 3% (510 mEq/L) or a 5% (853 mEq/L) solution. Hypertonic saline should be given in amounts necessary to raise the serum sodium to a safe level (120–125 mEq/L). The approximate sodium deficit (in mEq) is calculated as follows:

$$\text{(Desired serum sodium concentration}$$

$$- \text{ measured serum sodium concentration)} \times (0.6)$$

$$\times \text{ (total body weight [kg])}$$

The rate at which the serum sodium level should be raised is controversial,[9] since there is evidence that brain damage can result if the serum sodium concentration is raised too slowly or too rapidly. However, available evidence suggests that a rate of 1 mEq/L/hr is effective and safe.

There is uniform agreement that elevation of the sodium level into the normal range is both unnecessary and dangerous.

HYPERNATREMIA

Hypernatremia always indicates hypertonicity of body fluids. Because hypertonicity is normally a potent stimulus to thirst, hypernatremia occurs in patients who are unable to respond to thirst by ingesting water (usually very ill or comatose patients or infants). For this reason, hypernatremia is encountered far less commonly than hyponatremia.

Causes

Hypernatremia may result from loss of hypotonic fluid, from loss of pure water, or from gain of sodium.[10]

Hypernatremia is most commonly associated with losses of hypotonic fluid from the gastrointestinal tract, skin, or kidneys. Severe gastroenteritis may result in hypernatremia, most commonly in infants. Excessive loss of hypotonic fluid may also occur from the skin as a result of profuse sweating. An osmotic diuresis (as a result of hyperglycemia or administration of mannitol) results in loss of hypotonic urine.

Losses of pure water occur far less commonly than losses of hypotonic fluid. Increased insensible losses of water may occur from the skin (during fever) or from the lungs (during hyperventilation). Renal losses of water result from abnormalities in the concentrating mechanism, owing either to a deficiency of ADH (central diabetes insipidus) or to a renal resistance to the action of ADH (nephrogenic diabetes insipidus).

The administration of inappropriate amounts of hypertonic saline (during the treatment of hyponatremia) or of sodium bicarbonate (during cardiopulmonary resuscitation or metabolic acidosis) is the most frequent cause of salt intoxication in adult clinical practice.

Therapy

If the hypernatremic patient is severely volume depleted, initial therapy involves correction of the sodium deficit because hypovolemia is more life threatening than hypernatremia. This is best achieved by the administration of isotonic saline. Only once ECF volume has been restored should hypotonic fluid be given to correct the hypernatremia.

In the hypernatremic patient who has lost hypotonic fluid, hypotonic saline solution (half-normal or quarter-normal saline) should be used to correct the hypernatremia. The use of tap water (administered orally) or 5% dextrose in water (administered intravenously) should be limited to the less common situation in which loss of pure water has occurred.

The amount of water needed to correct hypernatremia to a serum sodium concentration of 140 mEq/L may be approximated by the following formula:

$$\text{Normal total body water (TBW)(L)} = 0.6 \times \text{normal body weight (kg)}$$

$$\text{Current TBW} = \frac{140 \times \text{normal TBW}}{\text{measured } Na^+ \text{ concentration}}$$

$$\text{Body water deficit} = \text{normal TBW} - \text{current TBW}$$

Rapid correction of hypernatremia is unnecessary and may result in cerebral edema, with further neurologic deterioration.[10] Half the calculated water deficit should be replaced over the first 12–24 hours and the rest over the following 24–48 hours.

KEY FEATURES

A. *Hyponatremia*
1. In all cases of hyponatremia, search for reversible factors (drugs, endocrine diseases, volume depletion).
2. Water restriction (1000 ml/day) is effective in all cases of hyponatremia, but correction of serum sodium concentration occurs slowly over several days.
3. Rapid correction of hyponatremia with hypertonic saline is indicated only when CNS impairment is present or when hyponatremia is profound (110 mEq/L).
4. When administering hypertonic saline:
   a. Do not aim for a normal serum sodium concentration but for a sodium level between 120 and 125 mEq/L.
   b. Monitor patient for signs of volume overload.
   c. In edematous patients (especially those with congestive heart failure), hypertonic saline is hazardous and should be used with potent diuretics.
   d. In patients with severe renal failure, use of hypertonic saline is not recommended. Dialysis is the safest and most effective treatment.
B. *Hypernatremia*
1. Correction of hypernatremia must be *gradual*. Give only half the water deficit in the first 12–24 hours and the rest over the next 24–48 hours. Monitor serum sodium level frequently.
2. Use hypotonic saline as replacement in most cases.

3. Use dextrose in water (IV) or tap water (orally) only if losses of pure water have occurred.
4. Use normal saline in patients with associated signs of severe intravascular volume depletion. Give saline until the patient is hemodynamically stable, and then give hypotonic fluids until hypernatremia is corrected.

REFERENCES

1. Schrier RW, Berl T: Nonosmolar factors affecting renal water excretion. N Engl J Med 292:81, 141, 1975.
   Excellent review of multiple nonosmolar factors that can stimulate ADH and thereby lead to hyponatremia.

2. Arieff H, Llach F, Massry SG: Neurological manifestations and morbidity of hyponatremia. Medicine 55:121, 1976.
   Describes the clinical manifestations of hyponatremia and correlates mortality with degree of brain swelling.

3. Arieff AI, Guisado R: Effects on the central nervous system of hypernatremic and hyponatremic states. Kidney Int 10:104–116, 1976.
   Discusses CNS manifestations and management of hypernatremia and hyponatremia.

4. Defronzo RA, Thier SO: Pathophysiologic approach to hyponatremia. Arch Intern Med 140:897–902, 1980.
   Review of hyponatremia stressing value of classifying causes according to state of extracellular volume.

5. Fichman MP, Vorherr H, Kleeman CR, Telfer N: Diuretic induced hyponatremia. Ann Intern Med. 75:853–863, 1971.
   A description of 25 nonedematous patients who developed hyponatremia associated with severe potassium depletion. Hyponatremia is corrected with discontinuation of diuretic and potassium replacement.

6. Martinez-Maldonado M: Inappropriate antidiuretic hormone secretion of unknown origin. Kidney Int 17:554, 1980.
   Discusses causes and management of SIADH.

7. Moses AM, Miller M: Drug-induced dilutional hyponatremia. N Engl J Med 291:1234–1238, 1974.
   Review of the important drugs capable of producing water retention hyponatremia.

8. Forrest JM, Cox M, Hang C, Morrison G, Bia M, Singer I: Superiority of demeclocycline over lithium in the treatment of the chronic syndrome of inappropriate antidiuretic hormone. N Engl J Med 298:173, 1978.
9. Narins RG: Editorial. Therapy of hyponatremia. Does haste make waste? New Engl J Med 314:1573–1575, 1986.
10. Feig PU, McCurdy DK: The hypertonic state. N Engl J Med 297:1444, 1977.
    Discusses CNS manifestations and management of hypernatremia and hyponatremia.

Hyperkalemia and Hypokalemia

Wilfred Lieberthal, M.D.

Potassium is predominantly an intracellular cation. Only 2% (60 mEq) of total body potassium (approx. 4200 mEq) is situated in the extracellular space. However, the concentration of potassium in extracellular fluid (ECF) plays a vital role in the function of cardiac and skeletal muscle and is normally maintained within a narrow range (3.8–5.0 mEq/L). The serum concentration of potassium may be perturbed either by alterations in total body potassium balance or by shifts of potassium between the intracellular and extracellular compartments.

The kidney, by regulating urinary excretion of potassium, is the major determinant of total body potassium balance. Extrarenal losses from stool and skin amount to less than 5–10% of the ingested load of potassium (approximately 50–150 mEq/day). Urinary potassium is derived predominantly from the secretion of potassium into renal tubular fluid by the distal nephron because potassium filtered at the glomerulus is almost entirely reabsorbed by the proximal renal tubule. The major factors that increase renal tubular secretion and thereby enhance renal excretion of potassium are (1) elevated aldosterone activity, (2) systemic alkalosis, and (3) increased volume flow or sodium delivery through the distal nephron. Conversely, renal excretion of potassium is limited by renal failure (reduced glomerular filtration rate) and by factors that decrease distal renal tubular potassium secretion (aldosterone deficiency, systemic acidosis, and reduced volume flow through the distal nephron).[1]

The serum potassium concentration is also affected by factors that alter the distribution of potassium between the intracellular and extracellular compartments. Alterations in acid-base balance have an important effect on the distribution of potassium.[2] Systemic acidosis results in the movement of potassium out of cells, whereas systemic alkalosis promotes cellular uptake of potassium. Insulin, aldosterone, and catecholamines (via beta receptor stimulation) also increase cellular uptake of potassium and play a role in the immediate defense against hyperkalemia following an external potassium load.[3,4]

HYPERKALEMIA

Causes

Pseudohyperkalemia, or artifactual hyperkalemia, requires no treatment. It is most commonly due to hemolysis of the blood sample or prolonged tourniquet placement. Also, in blood dyscrasias associated with extreme thrombocytosis (greater than 700,000/mm³) or leukocytosis (greater than 50,000/mm³) release of potassium from these elements during clotting may result in an apparently high serum potassium level. In these situations, potassium measured in an anticoagulated (plasma) sample is normal.

Transcellular shifts of potassium from intracellular to extracellular space occur in states of metabolic or respiratory acidosis and in diseases associated with massive cellular destruction (rhabdomyolysis, hemolysis, or tumor lysis). Deficiencies of insulin or aldosterone as well as beta adrenergic blockade may contribute to hyperkalemia by impairing cellular uptake of potassium.[3,4] High potassium intake alone, in the absence of a renal excretory defect, rarely results in hyperkalemia. However, in all cases of hyperkalemia exogenous sources of potassium must be identified and discontinued. Suspect substances include foods with high potassium content, potassium-containing salt substitutes, stored blood, and large doses of potassium penicillin (1.7 mEq/million U).

Reduced renal excretion of potassium is present in the majority of cases of chronic hyperkalemia and is an important complication of severe acute and chronic renal failure. However, impairment of distal renal tubular secretion of potassium may result in hyperkalemia even when renal function is normal or only mildly reduced. Reduced renal tubular secretion may be due to a deficiency of aldosterone (Addison's disease, hyporeninemic hypoaldosteronism,[5,6] and drugs such as nonsteroidal anti-inflammatory agents and angiotensin-converting enzyme inhibitors[7]) or to the use of potassium-sparing diuretics such as triamterene, spironolactone, or amiloride. These drugs should be used with caution, if at all, in patients with a serum creatinine concentration above 2.5–3.0 mg%. Renal tubular secretion of potassium is also decreased by factors that reduce sodium delivery to the distal nephron—typically, extracellular volume depletion.

Clinical Manifestations

The most important manifestation of hyperkalemia is its effect on cardiac function. Hyperkalemia makes the heart increasingly refractory to excitation. ECG changes provide a useful guide to the severity of the hyperkalemia. The ECG manifestations progress from peaking of the T waves (usually seen at serum potassium concentrations above 6.5 mEq/L); to prolongation of the P-R interval, loss of P waves, and widening of the QRS complex (at serum potassium levels above 7.5 mEq/L); and finally to a sine wave and cardiac asystole (potassium above 8.5 mEq/L). It must be emphasized, however, that the correlation between potassium levels and ECG change is only approximate. Severe cardiac toxicity may be seen at lower levels of serum potassium, especially if the potassium level rises very rapidly or if other electrolyte abnormalities that enhance the neuromuscular effects of hyperkalemia (hypocalcemia, hyponatremia, acidosis) are present. Thus, in assessing the severity of hyperkalemia both the serum potassium level and the ECG must be taken into account (see Key Features).

Treatment

Several interventions are available to treat hyperkalemia. The effects of hyperkalemia on cardiac muscle can be directly antagonized by the intravenous administration of calcium. Calcium gluconate (10 ml of a 10% solution) may be administered intravenously over 2 minutes. This is best done with ECG monitoring. If the cardiac abnormalities persist or recur, this dose of calcium gluconate may be repeated twice at 5-minute intervals. Calcium should be used with caution in digitalized patients. Calcium infusion is indicated only when major ECG abnormalities are present. The ameliorating effect of calcium on cardiac toxicity is transient (approximately 1 hour), so that other procedures must be instituted to reduce the serum potassium level once the immediate danger of cardiac toxicity has been averted.

Potassium can be driven into cells by the intravenous administration of glucose as well as sodium bicarbonate. Both these forms of treatment work within 20–30 minutes and last 4–6 hours. This treatment is indicated in all patients with a serum potassium concentration above 6.5 mEq/L and in patients with any ECG abnormality of hyperkalemia.

Glucose may be given as an intravenous bolus of 25–50 gm (50–100 ml of 50% dextrose) together with 5–10 U of regular insulin. The rapid alkalinization of the ECF with 1–2 ampules of sodium bicarbonate (given intravenously over 10–20 minutes) is a useful adjunct to glucose infusion and is particularly valuable when metabolic acidosis is present. (This mode of treatment can be simplified by using a "cocktail" consisting of 1 L of 10% glucose containing 20 U regular insulin and two ampules of sodium bicarbonate. Half a liter is given over the first half hour and the rest over the next 2–3 hours.)

Potassium can be removed from the body by increasing potassium loss from the GI tract. This is done by the administration of sodium polystyrene sulfonate (Kayexalate and others), a cation exchange resin that exchanges sodium for potassium. Kayexalate can be given orally or rectally. When it is given orally (as 25–50 gm in 20–30 ml of 70% sorbitol), the onset of action is 2–6 hours. This dose can be repeated three to five times per day. Rectal administration (as 50 gm in 100 ml of sorbitol or 5% dextrose in water) has an effect within 30–90 minutes and is indicated if a rapid onset of action is required or if oral administration is contraindicated. The enema must be retained for 30–60 minutes to be maximally effective and can be repeated hourly as necessary.

An exchange resin is indicated as the sole form of treatment in cases of mild hyperkalemia (serum potassium level 5.5–6.5 mEq/L, no ECG abnormalities) and together with the more rapidly acting modes of therapy in moderate and severe hyperkalemia.

Dialysis is another effective means of removing potassium but is indicated only when the more conservative modes of therapy are ineffective or contraindicated.

Finally, in all cases of hyperkalemia, reversible factors that may be contributing to this problem (e.g., volume depletion, drugs, hypoaldosteronism) must be sought and treated, or eliminated.

HYPOKALEMIA

Causes

Hypokalemia associated with normal total body potassium occurs in situations associated with a shift of potassium from the ECF into cells. This is most commonly seen during respiratory or metabolic alkalosis or following insulin administration. The treatment of diabetic ketoacidosis may result in precipitous falls in serum potassium concentration as a result of cellular uptake of potassium as metabolic acidosis and insulin deficiency are simultaneously corrected.[8] Treatment of megaloblastic anemia with vitamin B_{12} is a rare cause of hypokalemia and results from the rapid uptake of potassium by newly formed red blood cells.

Hypokalemia associated with potassium deficiency is usually the result of inappropriate loss of potassium from the body. Decreased intake alone rarely results in significant hypokalemia.

Losses of potassium from the gastrointestinal tract may result from diarrhea, laxative abuse, enteric fistulae, and rarely from a villous adenoma (a colonic tumor that secretes potassium-rich fluid). Because the potassium content of gastric juice is low, the hypokalemia associated with vomiting and nasogastric section is largely the result of the associated metabolic alkalosis that causes increased urinary losses of potassium.

Loss of potassium from the skin is an unusual cause of hypokalemia but may occur during profuse sweating or in patients with extensive burns.

Increased renal excretion of potassium occurs in a number of widely diverse clinical situations.[9] It is diagnostically useful to separate these causes according to whether hypertension is present or absent.

Renal loss of potassium associated with normal blood pressure may result from multiple causes. Diuretic-induced hypokalemia is seen primarily in patients given diuretics to treat edema states such as congestive heart failure, cirrhosis, or the nephrotic syndrome. Hypokalemia occurs far less commonly in nonedematous patients given diuretics, e.g., for hypertension.[10] Increased urinary losses of potassium are also a feature of metabolic or respiratory alkalosis. Renal tubular acidosis, magnesium deficiency, and Bartter's syndrome are less common causes of renal potassium wasting.

In a hypertensive individual with hypokalemia, either spontaneous or diuretic induced, certain secondary causes of hypertension must be excluded. Renal wasting of potassium in association with hypertension is usually the result of elevated levels of aldosterone, which may be primary (as in primary hyperaldosteronism) or secondary to high levels of circulating renin (as in renal artery stenosis and malignant hypertension).

Clinical Manifestations

Skeletal muscle involvement produces weakness, paralysis, hyporeflexia, and, rarely, flaccid paralysis (usually serum potassium levels below 2 mEq/L). Cardiac manifestations include the typical ECG changes (flattening and inversion of T waves, prominent U waves, and depressed S-T segments) as well as tachydysrhythmias and an increased sensitivity to digitalis.

Diagnosis

The urinary potassium concentration may be helpful in distinguishing between renal causes (in which urinary potassium is high—greater than 20 mEq/L) and non-renal causes (in which renal conservation results in low urinary potassium concentrations, usually less than 20 mEq/L).

Most causes of hypokalemia are associated with metabolic alkalosis. The combination of hypokalemia and metabolic acidosis is usually due to one of two abnormalities: renal tubular acidosis or, more commonly, gastrointestinal fluid losses.

Treatment

The correction of hypokalemia should always be undertaken with caution. Rapid potassium replacement is seldom necessary and may cause transient hyperkalemia.

The magnitude of the potassium deficit can be estimated when the serum potassium concentration is in the range of 2–4 mEq/L. Within this range, a fall in serum potassium of 1 mEq/L is associated with a total deficit of 150–200 mEq of potassium. Below 2 mEq/L, the deficit usually exceeds 400 mEq but cannot be more accurately estimated.

Oral potassium replacement is usually effective and is preferred over intravenous treatment in most cases. In patients with metabolic alkalosis, it is generally advisable to replace potassium deficits with potassium chloride. Potassium chloride solutions are effective and inexpensive but have an unpleasant taste and may cause epigastric distress. If gastrointestinal symptoms are a problem, potassium can be given as a tablet (KCl in a wax matrix) or as potassium gluconate, both of which are better tolerated. In patients with hypokalemia and metabolic acidosis, both deficits can be simultaneously corrected with potassium citrate or potassium bicarbonate.

Intravenous potassium is indicated only in patients who cannot take oral potassium or who have severe hypokalemia with cardiac arrhythmias or skeletal muscle paralysis. Parenteral potassium preparations are highly concentrated and must be diluted before administration; the concentration of administered potassium should not exceed 40 mEq/L. The rate of infusion depends upon the urgency of the situation, but it should never exceed 30–40 mEq/hour.

In patients on long-term diuretic therapy, the routine administration of potassium salts is not recommended. Potassium should be administered prophylactically to patients receiving diuretics who have edema; are receiving digitalis preparations; have severe liver disease, because of the risk of hypokalemia precipitating hepatic encephalopathy; or have underlying cardiac disease or a serum potassium level <3.0 mEq/L.[11] In other patients receiving regular diuretic therapy, serum potassium levels should be monitored and potassium supplement given only to those whose serum potassium concentration falls to below normal range.

KEY FEATURES

HYPERKALEMIA

Forms of Treatment Available
A. Antagonize cardiac effects
 1. 10% calcium gluconate (10–30 ml)
B. Drive K^+ into cells
 1. Glucose 25–50 gm as 50% glucose (50–100 ml) with 5–10 U regular insulin IV
 2. Sodium bicarbonate 1–2 ampules (44–88 mEq) over 10–20 minutes IV
C. Remove K from body

1. Cation exchange resin
   a. Orally: 25–50 gm in 20–30 ml 70% sorbitol 2–3 times/day
   b. Rectally: 50 gm in 100 ml D5W retained for 30–60 minutes
2. Dialysis
   a. Peritoneal removes approximately 15 mEq/hour
   b. Hemodialysis removes >50 mEq/hour

Use Both Plasma (K+) and ECG Changes to Guide Treatment

ECG		Plasma K+ (mEq/L)	Treatment
Normal	*and*	5.5–6.5	Exchange resin
Peaked T waves	*and/or*	6.5–7.5	Glucose and insulin and/or bicarbonate plus Kayexalate
Absent P wave; broad QRS; sine wave		At any level	Calcium infusion; plus glucose, insulin, and/or bicarbonate; plus Kayexalate

HYPOKALEMIA

A. Estimate total body deficit

Plasma K+ (mEq/L)	Deficit (mEq)
3.0–4.0	100–200
2.0–3.0	200–400
<2.0	≥400

B. Use oral replacement wherever possible —generally not more than 200 mEq/day
   1. Potassium chloride usually (10% solution contains 1.3 mEq/ml)
   2. Potassium citrate if acidosis is present (contains 1 mEq/ml)
C. Consider intravenous administration if
   1. Patient cannot take oral preparations
   2. Serum potassium <2 mEq/L
   3. Muscle paralysis (especially respiratory)
   4. Cardiac arrhythmias, digitalis toxicity
D. Guidelines to IV therapy
   1. Rate: seldom requires >10 mEq/hour, not >30–40 mEq/hour
   2. Concentration: not >40 mEq/L

REFERENCES

1. Cohen JJ: Disorders of potassium balance. Hosp Pract *14*:119, 1979.
   Review of disorders of potassium balance with good discussion of pathophysiology.

2. Adrogue HJ, Madias NE: Changes in plasma potassium concentration during acute acid base disturbances. Am J Med *71*:456, 1981.
3. Rose RM, Silva P, Young JB, Lansberg L, Brown RS, Rowe JW, Epstein FH: Adrenergic modulation of extrarenal potassium disposal. N Engl J Med *302*:431, 1980.
   The increase in serum potassium concentration following an intravenous load of potassium was studied in nine normal volunteers. Adrenergic blockade with propranolol augmented the rise in serum potassium and prolonged the elevation without decreasing urinary potassium excretion. The authors suggest that in patients with impaired potassium disposal, beta adrenergic blockade may increase the risk of hyperkalemia.

4. Cox M, Sterns RH, Singer I: The defense against hyperkalemia: The role of insulin and aldosterone. N Engl J Med 299:525, 1978.

   Review of the part played by insulin and aldosterone in regulating internal potassium balance.

5. Vaamonde CA, Perez G, Oster SR: Syndromes of aldosterone deficiency. Min Electr Metab 5:121–134, 1981.
6. DeFranzo RA: Hyperkalemia and hyporeninemic hypoaldosteronism. Kidney Int 17:118–134, 1980.
7. Ponce PS, Jennings AE, Madias NE, Harrington JT: Drug induced hyperkalemia. Medicine 64:357–370, 1985.

   Review of the mechanisms by which drugs cause hyperkalemia.

8. Beigelman PM: Potassium in severe diabetic ketoacidosis. Am J Med 54:419–420, 1973.
9. Kliger AS, Hayslett JP: Disorders of potassium balance. *In* Brenner BM, Stein JH (eds): Acid-Base and Potassium Homeostasis. Contemporary Issues in Nephrology 2. New York, Churchill-Livingstone, 1978, pp 168–204.

   A review of the disorders of potassium homeostasis with a thorough discussion of the causes of hypokalemia.

10. Kassirer JP, Harrington JT: Diuretics and potassium metabolism: A reassessment of the need, effectiveness, and safety of potassium therapy. Kidney Int 11:505, 1977.
11. Tannen RL: Diuretic-induced hypokalemia. Kidney Int 28:988–1000, 1985.

   A careful assessment of the risks and benefits of potassium replacement therapy in patients on diuretics.

Hematuria

Beldon A. Idelson, M.D.

Although rarely constituting a medical emergency, hematuria (gross or microscopic) should be considered as a sign of serious urinary tract disease or a manifestation of a systemic disease. The bleeding may be coming from the kidney or from any part of the urinary excretory system from the renal pelvis to the distal urethra. Most patients with hematuria will have some signs or symptoms pointing to a site of bleeding in the urinary tract or to the presence of some associated systemic disease; however, the remaining 20% will be totally asymptomatic. The cause of the bleeding will ultimately be identifiable in over 90% of cases.

In about 65% of patients, a bleeding site will be identified in the lower urinary tract or ureters. The bladder itself will be the source in about 35%, and nearly half of these patients will turn out to have a bladder neoplasm. Of patients presenting with *gross* hematuria, about 15–20% will turn out to have a neoplasm in the urinary tract.[1] Thus, the finding of hematuria, either gross or microscopic, is a significant finding that demands prompt investigation.

The first step in evaluation is to confirm that the red color of the urine is indeed due to red blood cells. Red urine in the absence of red cells and with a negative dipstick may be caused by a number of dyes in food and drugs (Table 1); on the other hand, red or brown urine without red blood cells but with a positive dipstick is caused by hemoglobinuria or myoglobinuria. After these causes are excluded, a systematic search for the bleeding site can be pursued. [1-3]

With gross hematuria, a description of the pattern can give helpful information. [1] Total hematuria (bleeding throughout voiding) is indicative of bleeding from the ureter or kidney but may be seen with severe bladder hemorrhage as well; initial hematuria (bleeding only at the beginning of voiding) generally suggests urethral bleeding beyond the bladder neck; terminal hematuria (bleeding at the end of voiding) is indicative of posterior urethral or bladder neck bleeding. Blood-stained undergarments with clear urine indicate distal urethral bleeding.

Gross hematuria in a male over the age of 60 is most likely caused by benign prostatic hypertrophy (BPH). Such patients usually present with symptoms of bladder neck outlet obstruction, e.g., hesitancy, poor stream, and dribbling. Although rectal examination will confirm the diagnosis, further evaluation by cystoscopy will reveal a bladder tumor as the actual cause of bleeding in a significant minority of patients.

The history of renal or ureteral colic is characteristic; calculi are responsible for hematuria in approximately 20% of patients.

The family history of sickle cell disease should lead to the search for sickle hemoglobin in a young black patient with painful or asymptomatic, microscopic or gross hematuria. Sickle cell screening should be performed in all young black patients with hematuria. Sickle trait or disease is the cause of gross hematuria in about one third of black patients; hematuria is the most

Table 1.   COMMON CAUSES OF RED-BROWN URINE IN ABSENCE OF
RED BLOOD CELLS

With *positive* dipstick for hemoglobin
  Hemoglobin, myoglobin
With *negative* dipstick for hemoglobin
  Anthocyanin pigment (beets and berries)
  Red-colored candies
  Vegetable dyes in food coloring
  Porphyrins
  Phenazopyridine hydrochloride (pyridium)
  Phenothiazines
  Senna (cathartics, rhubarb, cascara)
  Phenolphthalein (in alkaline urine)

common presentation of sickle trait. The bleeding generally stops in a few days but recurs in approximately 50% of cases.[4]

A history of fevers, skin rash, or arthralgias suggests a systemic disease. Easy bruising or abnormal bleeding should raise the possibility of coagulopathy or ingestion of an anticoagulant drug. A recent upper respiratory infection should raise the question of acute glomerulonephritis. The importance of a complete history and systems review cannot be overestimated in the initial evaluation of patients with hematuria.[4]

Careful physical examination may yield signs of a systemic disease or bleeding diathesis. Fluid overload and hypertension in a young, previously well patient may suggest acute glomerulonephritis. Murmurs, joint swelling, skin lesions, fever, and so forth should suggest systemic lupus erythematosus (SLE), bacterial endocarditis (BE), or vasculitis. Abdominal examination may detect polycystic kidneys.

Careful urinalysis is often extremely valuable in pinpointing the cause of bleeding. RBC casts point to glomerular diseases, whereas hematuria with WBCs and bacteria indicates infection at some level. Red and white blood cells without bacteria may be seen in nephrolithiasis, tumors, papillary necrosis, or adjacent sequestered infection. Phase contrast microscopy should be performed next. Dysmorphic RBCs, even in the absence of RBC casts, points strongly to a glomerular origin of the hematuria.[5]

Laboratory studies should be guided by the early clinical information. Symptoms of cystitis should lead to a urine culture. Multisystem involvement should indicate antinuclear antibody (ANA) serum complement, etc. Every patient should have serum creatinine determined as a measure of overall renal function. Next, an intravenous pyelogram (IVP) should be performed. This will show stones, particularly radiolucent stones, and the size and symmetry of the two kidneys. Polycystic kidney disease or mass lesions will often be evident. Filling defects as a result of tumor, sloughed papillae, or blood clot may be demonstrated by IVP. Chronic papillary necrosis, tuberculosis, and medullary sponge kidney have distinctive findings that may be seen on IVP.

Further evaluation depends on the IVP. The finding of a mass lesion should lead to a CT scan or ultrasound.[6] A lucent defect in the renal pelvis should lead to a search for lower urinary tract disease by cystoscopy; the likelihood of a bladder neoplasm in this setting is around 15%. If a detailed history, thorough physical examination, and coagulation screen are normal, and the IVP, ultrasound, and cystoscopy are likewise negative, the major causes of hematuria remaining are glomerular diseases. An arteriovenous malformation may be discovered by arteriography, but many are too small to be visualized. Bladder infestation with *Schistosoma haematobium* should be considered in appropriate populations.

Recurrent gross hematuria without other manifestations of systemic

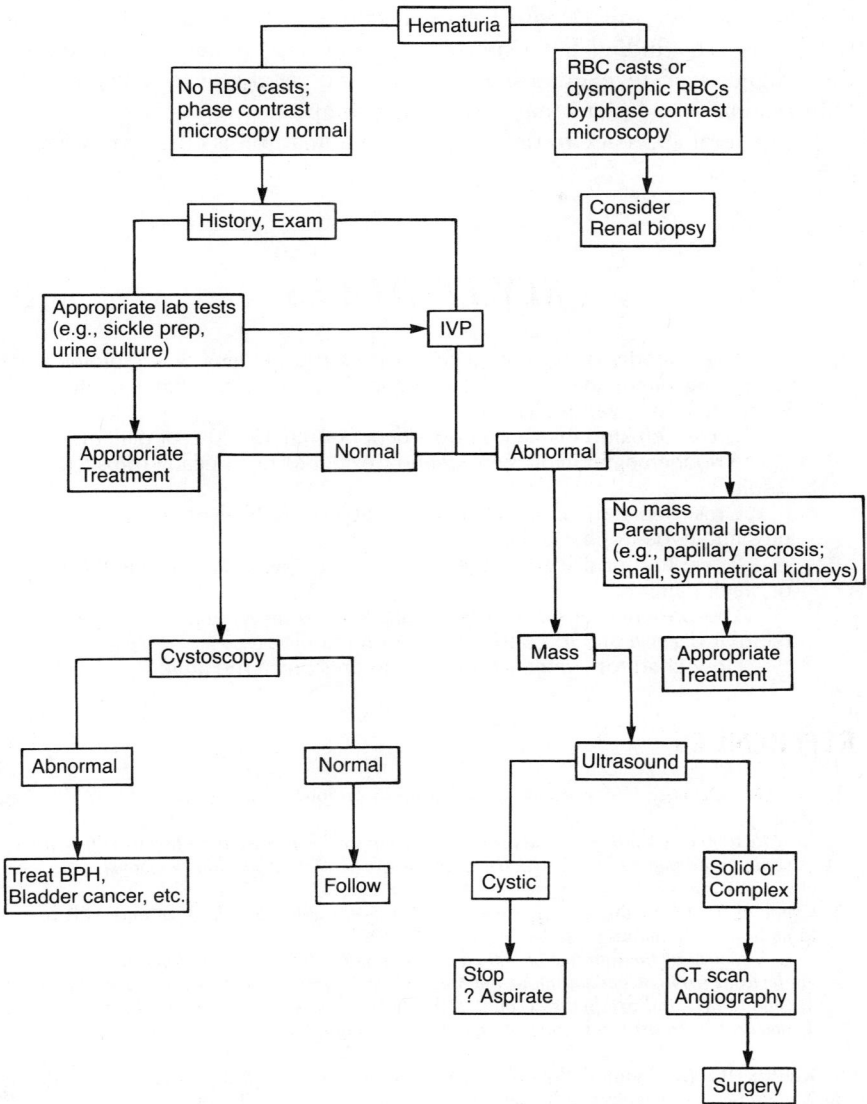

Figure 1. Evaluation of a patient with hematuria. BPH = benign prostatic hypertrophy.

disease and usually occurring immediately after an upper respiratory infection suggests Berger's disease.[4] A renal biopsy may be useful to establish the diagnosis by finding deposition of IgA in the mesangium; in such patients, the prognosis of developing hypertension and renal failure is about 20%. Other glomerular lesions may be found by biopsy as well.

A general approach to the patient with hematuria is outlined in Figure 1.

KEY FEATURES

The majority of patients with hematuria have signs or symptoms suggesting either the site of bleeding within the urinary tract or the presence of a systemic disease.

Gross hematuria is caused by a neoplasm in 15–20% of patients.

A nonhemoglobin pigment is simply excluded by a negative dipstick result.

Gross hematuria in a male over age 60 is most likely due to benign prostatic hypertrophy (BPH).

Sickle trait or disease is the cause of gross hematuria in one third of black patients.

The presence of RBC casts should lead to an evaluation for glomerular disease and to consideration of renal biopsy.

Flow chart for evaluation of hematuria is given in Figure 1.

REFERENCES

1. Lee LW, Davis E: Gross urinary hemorrhage: A symptom, not a disease. JAMA 153:782, 1953.
   In 1000 consecutive patients who underwent urologic evaluation for gross hematuria, 22% had malignancy of the urinary tract, whereas 8% had no cause demonstrated.

2. Greene LF, O'Shaughnessy EJ, Hendricks ED: Study of five hundred patients with asymptomatic microhematuria. JAMA 161:610–613, 1956.
   A review of the findings of 500 consecutive patients with microscopic hematuria who underwent urologic evaluation at the Mayo Clinic. Asymptomatic benign prostatic hypertrophy (BPH) and urethritis accounted for 45% of cases. In contrast to findings in gross hematuria, urinary tract cancer was detected in only 2%.

3. Kudish HG: Determining the cause of hematuria. Postgrad Med J 58:118–122, 1975.
4. Abuelo G: The diagnosis of hematuria. Arch Intern Med 143:967–970, 1983.
   A comprehensive review of causes of hematuria and evaluation.

5. Fairly KF, Birch DF: Hematuria: A simplified method for identifying glomerular bleeding. Kidney Int 21:105–108, 1982.
6. Gatenby RA: Diagnostic evaluation of a renal mass. Semin Oncol 10:401–412, 1983.
   Excellent review of the diagnostic modalities available and critical evaluation of their specificity and sensitivity. A comprehensive algorithm for work-up of a renal mass is presented.

Nephrolithiasis

David Bernard, M.D.

Nephrolithiasis, the formation of stones in the upper tract of the kidneys, is one of the most common of all renal diseases. It has been estimated that 1 in 1000 people in the United States is hospitalized for this condition each year, while the overall prevalence of kidney stones of all types is 3–5 per 1000 of an unselected American population.[1] Until fairly recently, the pathogenesis of most kidney stones was not well understood, so that prevention, the key factor in the treatment of this condition, was inadequate. Today, as the cause of stones is better appreciated, efficient methods for reducing new stone formation are now available for many patients.[2,3] Indeed, in over 90% of cases, a metabolic derangement predisposing the patient to kidney stones can be demonstrated.

Kidney stones are composed of one or more of the following four major constituents: calcium, either as phosphate or as oxalate; uric acid; cystine, found exclusively in patients with cystinuria; and struvite (triple phosphate stone; infection stone), found in association with recurrent urinary tract infection by urea-splitting organisms. Over 70% of all stones contain calcium, as pure calcium oxalate, as pure calcium phosphate, or as a mixture of oxalate and phosphate.[3]

Kidney stones may be associated with several clinical syndromes.[1,4,5] They are frequently *asymptomatic*, being discovered at the time radiographs are taken for some other reason; they may produce *hematuria* (gross or microscopic); and they may predispose the patient to *urinary tract infections* or produce *pyuria*. Also, when a stone breaks loose from the calyx and drops into the ureter, *renal colic* results. This last, most dramatic clinical manifestation of kidney stone disease arises from impaction of the stone in the ureter. The outstanding symptom of an attack of colic is excruciating pain, the site of which depends on where the stone lodges. When the site is high in the proximal ureter, pain is felt in the upper abdominal quadrant on that side or in the flank; if the stone moves lower down into the ureter, the pain radiates from the flank and lower ribs downward and forward to the pelvis and inguinal ligament; if the stone impacts in the distal part of the ureter, pain is felt in the lower abdomen and may radiate into the groin and testicle or labia. Stones impacting near the junction of ureter and bladder may, in addition to causing pain, mimic cystitis and produce urinary urgency and frequency.

The management of kidney stones should be discussed in three categories: the acute attack, the early and late complications of the condition, and the dietary and drug therapy aimed at preventing recurrent stone formation. In approaching the patient with an acute attack of abdominal pain thought to be due to renal colic, the first step is to confirm the diagnosis. This may sometimes be done with confidence from the patient's history (previous similar attacks, knowledge about the presence of stones, a typical history of pain radiation into the groin) or from the physical examination and urinalysis revealing hematuria. However, frequently, a radiologic study is required. Although a kidney, ureter, and bladder (KUB) radiograph will reveal a radiodense stone (calcium containing, struvite, or cystine), a uric acid stone, which is radiolucent, will not be seen. By far, the most useful diagnostic early investigation to perform in a patient suspected of suffering from acute renal colic is an intravenous pyelogram (IVP). This examination should be performed as soon as possible after the diagnosis is entertained, directly from the emergency room if possible, because not only will it offer diagnostic confirmation of the condition but it also will direct future therapy by demonstrating the size of the stone, the site of stone impaction, and whether the obstruction to urine flow is partial or complete.

Initial treatment requires intensive supportive measures: adequate analgesia and sedation are needed to alleviate the extreme pain, and intravenous fluids are usually necessary because nausea and vomiting are common. Antibiotics are indicated in the presence of fever.[5,6] Beyond these general measures, further management will depend on the characteristics of the stone itself, as defined by the IVP. Once it is known how large the stone is and where it has impacted, a judgment must be made as to the likelihood of its passing spontaneously—treatment will then depend on this prediction. For example, treatment will be conservative and expectant if it is judged likely that the stone will pass spontaneously and the patient's vital signs are stable, even in the presence of fever and presumed urosepsis;[6] on the other hand, early surgical removal may be planned if spontaneous passage is thought unlikely; and all grades of possibilities are present between these two extremes. Most stones pass spontaneously and therapy with hydration and analgesia is all that is necessary, particularly when the stone is small and impacted low down in the ureter.[5,6] On the other hand, larger stones, particularly if they impact high up, are less likely to pass on their own and will usually need early surgical removal. Studies have shown that stones 10 mm or more in size rarely pass spontaneously and usually need surgical extraction.[5] Two additional factors determine the urgency with which a stone should be removed—the clinical condition of the patient and the degree of urinary obstruction. If conservative therapy is failing to control symptoms or if hemodynamics are deteriorating, the stone should be removed even if it is small and low down. In these cases, it may be possible to extract calculus with a "basket" through the bladder so as to avoid formal ureterolithotomy. The degree of obstruction is critically important in determining how long it is safe to maintain an expectant approach. In the presence of complete obstruction, even if the patient is comfortable, no more than 4 or 5 days should be allowed to elapse before removing the stone surgically. On the other hand, if the obstruction to the urinary tract is only partial and the patient is comfortable and free of urinary infection, the stone can be left *in situ* for several weeks or months while waiting for it to pass without any fear that renal damage will occur.[5]

Once it is decided to remove the stone, several options are available. The open surgical treatment of stones has largely disappeared. The advent of endourologic procedures (percutaneous nephrolithotomy) and of extracorporeal shock wave lithotripsy permits effective removal of over 90% of renal stones. The former technique makes use of stone extraction via flexible nephroscopes placed percutaneously into the collecting system. The procedure is performed under local anesthesia and permits shorter hospitalization and quicker recovery than an open surgical procedure. Extracorporeal shock wave lithotripsy is a noninvasive technique that uses hydraulic shock waves focused on the stones to pulverize and break them up. The stone fragments then pass spontaneously. This promising new technology is not yet widely available. Stones in the lower one third of the ureter are removed by basket extraction via the bladder.

The presence of stones in the kidney or their passage through the urinary tract may result in other problems requiring specific management. For example, at the time of an acute attack of renal colic, obstruction of a solitary kidney may lead to acute renal failure, whereas associated urinary tract infection or bacteremia would need to be treated.[6] Later complications include stricture formation in the ureter or urethra and recurrent urinary tract infections.

Perhaps the most important aspect of the management of renal stones is to prevent recurrent stone formation. This would, of course, avoid all the complications outlined above. In the majority of cases (over 90%) recurrent stone formation can be eliminated or markedly reduced. This requires elucidating the causative factors in each case and utilizing dietary and drug methods to correct them. Although a detailed history and physical examination are important in identifying a stone and its cause, laboratory studies are usually more important. Blood levels of calcium, uric acid, electrolytes, and parathyroid hormone are measured; 24-hour urine excretion rates of calcium, uric acid, citrate, and oxalate are calculated (and cystine in suspicious, familial cases); and any stone removed is subjected to crystallographic analysis. Each metabolic derangement has its own specific therapy and most are gratifyingly successful.

KEY FEATURES

A. Over 70% of all kidney stones contain calcium, and of these, a clearly definable metabolic abnormality responsible for stone formation can be detected in 90% of cases.
B. Clinical consequences of kidney stones include the following:
   1. They may be asymptomatic
   2. They may cause hematuria
   3. They may predispose the patient to recurrent urinary tract infection
   4. They may produce acute renal colic
C. Treatment of the acute attack:
   1. Analgesia and sedation
   2. Antibiotics in the presence of fever
   3. Intravenous fluids
   4. Obtain intravenous pyelogram (IVP) early to assess the *size* of stone, *site* of impaction, and degree of urinary *obstruction*
      a. If small and low in ureter, treat conservatively
      b. If large (over 10 mm) and high, plan early removal
      c. If obstruction complete, remove within 5 days
D. Always send any stone passed or removed for full chemical analysis
E. If stone removal is preferred, generally use nonsurgical techniques (endourologic technology and extracorporeal shock wave lithotripsy)
F. Treat stone complications:
   1. Acute renal failure
   2. Strictures
   3. Urinary infection (often recurrent)
G. Prevent recurrent stone formation
   1. Identify stone constituents
   2. Measure serum calcium, uric acid, electrolytes, and parathyroid hormone
   3. Measure 24-hour urine calcium, uric acid, citrate, oxalate, cystine
   4. Each type of stone has its own specific prevention approach

REFERENCES AND SUGGESTED READINGS

1. Malek RS: Renal lithiasis: A practical approach. J Urol 118:893, 1977.
   A good overview of the incidence, clinical features, and causes of kidney stones.

2. Coe FL: Prevention of kidney stones. Am J Med 71:514, 1981.
   A brief but excellent review of this topic. Dr. Coe emphasizes that although not all the factors responsible for stone formation are known, recurrent stone disease is now

preventable in most cases. A concise approach to the clinical evaluation of the patient with kidney stones is offered.

3. Coe FL: Treated and untreated recurrent calcium nephrolithiasis in patients with idiopathic hypercalciuria, hyperuricosuria or no metabolic disorder. Ann Intern Med 87:404, 1977.

    An important paper that presents a review of the underlying metabolic defects and response to treatment in 202 patients with recurrent calcium oxalate kidney stones. Thiazides were given for idiopathic hypercalciuria, allopurinol for hyperuricosuria, and both agents for those patients with no discernible metabolic abnormality. A dramatic reduction in new stone formation was achieved with this approach.

4. Millman S, et al: Pathogenesis and clinical course of mixed calcium oxalate and uric acid nephrolithiasis. Kidney Int 22:366, 1982.

    Stone-forming patients with idiopathic hypercalciuria, hyperuricosuria, or both were studied in relation to clinical course, the physicochemical factors in the urine promoting stone formation, and response to therapy. Pure uric acid stone formers developed the most stones per year, pure calcium oxalate stone formers the least, with the mixed calcium oxalate and uric acid group being intermediate. Differences were also noted among the various types in relation to complications (lowest in pure uric acid stones) and need for surgical treatment (lowest in mixed calicum oxalate and uric acid group). Response of stones to treatment aimed at reducing the metabolic defect was excellent.

5. Elliot JJ: Calcium oxalate urinary calculi: Clinical and chemical aspects. Medicine 62:36, 1983.

    The clinical features of stone disease in 117 patients with calcium oxalate calculi are presented, including the age distribution (under 25 years to over 75 years), mode of clinical presentation (most frequently the spontaneous passage of a ureteral stone), ratio of spontaneous stone passage to surgical extraction (2:1 in patients under 55 and 1:1 in older patients), and the time taken before spontaneous passage occurred (under 4 days to 6 months). In the absence of urinary obstruction, two patients with stones were followed without intervention for 6 months. Endoscopic manipulation was performed if the stone was near the ureterovesical junction or was obstructing but not moving. The largest stone removed successfully via endoscopy was 8 mm in length, whereas all stones 10 mm or more needed formal surgical removal. Recurrence was low in patients treated for their first stone attack (4% over 10 years) but high in patients when several stones had previously been passed (15–30% over 9 years).

6. Klein LA, Koyle M, Berg NS: The emergency management of patients with ureteral calculi and fever. J Urol 129:938, 1983.

    Although a conservative approach with hydration and analgesia is the accepted initial management of patients with acute ureteral obstruction by calculus, in the presence of fever, many physicians consider emergency drainage to be indicated for fear of gram negative bacteremia developing. This paper argues that such an aggressive approach is unnecessary. The authors treated 14 patients with ureteral calculi and fever (as high as 103° F in some cases) with antibiotics, fluids, and careful monitoring and avoided early surgery, which can in any case be difficult and complicated. In 11 cases, no surgical intervention was ever needed, and all patients recovered fully, supporting a careful monitoring approach as correct initial management in all cases with renal colic.

7. Chaussy C, et al: First clinical experience with extracorporeally induced destruction of kidney stones by shock waves. J Urol 127:417, 1982.

    A fairly new technique for stone removal based on the use of high-energy shock waves to pulverize the stone and crush it into fragments small enough to be passed spontaneously. An underwater condenser is used, which emits a spark causing explosive evaporation of surrounding water and shock waves that can be focused onto a kidney stone. The technique successfully eliminated 54 of 59 stones from the renal pelvis but 0 of 2 from the ureter; in only 15% of cases was colic observed during passage of the fragments.

8. Pak CYC, et al: A simple test for the diagnosis of absorptive, resorptive and renal hypercalciurias. N Engl J Med 292:497, 1975.

This widely quoted paper claimed to offer a way in which the various causes of hypercalciuria could be separated. Unfortunately, significant overlapping of the various types occurs and because initial treatment is in any case probably similar for all forms of idiopathic hypercalciuria, efforts at classifying the patients seem not worthwhile.

9. Bordier P, et al: On the pathogenesis of so-called idiopathic hypercalciuria. Am J Med 63:398, 1977.

The causes of hypercalciuria in a group of 47 patients were classified on the basis of the urinary calcium excretion following a week of low calcium intake (400 mg/24 hours), the serum parathyroid levels, and the response to thiazide and vitamin D therapy. In patients with predominantly gastrointestinal hyperabsorption of calcium, urinary calcium concentration became normal on the reduced intake diet. Two other subcategories were identified: patients with primary renal tubular leak of calcium and patients in whom the primary defect appeared to be renal tubular leak of phosphate. The latter would produce hypophosphatemia, which stimulates the synthesis of 1,25-dihydroxyvitamin D_3, which promotes enhanced calcium absorption from the gut.

10. Pak CYC, et al: Evidence justifying a high fluid intake in treatment of nephrolithiasis. Ann Intern Med 93:36, 1980.

In vitro or in vivo dilution of urine from stone formers was shown to reduce the propensity for the crystallization of calcium salts significantly. This is the first study to offer a sound scientific reason for encouraging patients with stones to ingest large fluid volumes.

11. Smith LH, Hofman AF: Acquired hyperoxaluria, urolithiasis, and intestinal disease: A new digestive disorder? Gastroenterology 66:1257, 1974.

Hyperoxaluria with calcium oxalate nephrolithiasis in patients who have disease or absence of the small bowel was first described in 1969. This paper reviews the mechanism involved (malabsorbed fatty acids precipitating with gut calcium, leaving dietary oxalate in solution and free to be absorbed) and discusses the therapeutic approach.

12. Vargas AD, Bragin SD, Mendez R: Staghorn calculus: Its clinical presentation, complications and management. J Urol 127:860, 1982.

The high incidence of complications in this condition is emphasized in this study of 95 patients with staghorn calculi. Only 1% of cases had silent stones, clinical complications occurred in 53% of patients, and only 51% of kidneys were considered to be undamaged. The authors conclude that complete surgical removal of the calculus and medical adjunctive therapy should be performed early in the course of the disease to prevent the development of complications and renal damage.

13. Griffith DP: Infection-induced renal calculi. Kidney Int 21:422, 1982.

A good review of this problem that makes a plea for earlier and more vigorous surgical therapy for these patients. The advantages and disadvantages of acetohydroxamic acid is presented, the point being made that the drug may play its most important role in preventing new stone growth in patients with resistant urinary infection with urea-splitting organisms who have reasonably good renal function and slight or absent obstruction to urine flow. It is unlikely to be effective in dissolving existing large staghorn stones.

Uremia

Beldon A. Idelson, M.D.

There are many causes of progressive renal function loss leading to end-stage renal disease. Patients will have remarkably few symptoms and only minor laboratory abnormalities except for elevated BUN and serum creatinine levels until more than 70% of kidney function has been lost. Thus, early renal failure is characterized by elevated serum creatinine and BUN without other significant biochemical abnormalities. Only in far advanced renal failure do plasma potassium and phosphate concentrations rise, acidosis develop, and sodium balance become positive. The syndrome of uremia results from the combined loss of excretory, regulatory, and endocrine functions of the kidney. Acute and generally reversible problems may supervene at any time in the azotemic patient.

MANAGEMENT OF ACUTE PROBLEMS IN CHRONIC RENAL FAILURE

General Measures

It is important to recognize and correct reversible causes of deterioration in patients with stable chronic renal failure.

The major correctable causes of worsening of renal failure are given in Table 1. Hypovolemia is especially important to identify and treat because it is common, often subtle, but usually not difficult to correct. Post-renal urinary tract obstruction may be due to prostatism, stones, or bladder dysfunction; obstruction is best evaluated by ultrasound examination. Nephrotoxins, including medications, are an important cause of worsening. Con-

Table 1.   REVERSIBLE CAUSES OF WORSENING RENAL FAILURE

Hypovolemia
Obstruction
Nephrotoxins
Hypertension
Infection
Congestive heart failure
Hypercalcemia

gestive heart failure with a fall in cardiac output and poorly controlled hypertension are important reversible causes of sudden worsening of chronic renal failure.

As renal failure becomes more severe, and remediable causes of deterioration are excluded, manifestations of the uremic state must be treated, and diet is modified to manage nitrogen balance and regulate electrolyte and water intake. A carefully planned conservative regimen should be begun when the glomerular filtration rate (GFR) falls below 25 ml/minute regardless of the presence of symptoms.

In the patient with chronic renal failure, dialysis is generally begun arbitrarily when the creatinine clearance falls to a level of 5–7 ml/minute. However, in many instances, acute problems supervene and mandate earlier institution of either peritoneal dialysis or hemodialysis on an urgent and occasionally emergent basis. Generally agreed upon criteria for the initiation of dialysis include (1) early symptoms of uremia—usually neurologic or gastrointestinal, (2) pericarditis, (3) intractable volume overload, (4) hyperkalemia, (5) peripheral neuropathy, and (6) problems in hemostasis. Dialysis is often necessary on an urgent basis to prepare the chronic renal failure patient for surgery. An unrelated but life-saving role for hemodialysis or hemoperfusion arises in the setting of certain intoxications, especially those involving salicylates, methanol, ethylene glycol, and theophylline preparations.

The complications of emergent peritoneal dialysis include peritonitis, hemorrhage, bowel perforation, and occasionally respiratory compromise as a result of the expansion of intra-abdominal volume. The complications of hemodialysis are more numerous and are listed in Table 2.

Table 2.   MEDICAL COMPLICATIONS OF HEMODIALYSIS

A. Psychological	F. Metabolic and Endocrine
B. Neurologic	1. Hyperlipidemia
1. Dysequilibrium syndrome	2. Hypothyroidism and goiter
2. Subdural hematoma	3. Infertility and sexual dysfunction
3. Dialysis dementia	G. Renal osteodystrophy
C. Cardiovascular	H. Vascular access problems
1. Pericarditis	1. Infection
2. Accelerated atherosclerosis	2. "Steal" syndrome
3. Infective endocarditis	3. Aneurysm and thrombosis
4. Congestive heart failure	I. Mechanical problems
D. Gastrointestinal	1. Air embolism
1. Hepatitis	2. Hyperthermia
2. Refractory ascites	3. Errors in dialysate composition
E. Hematologic	J. Miscellaneous
1. Anemia	1. Pyrexial reactions
2. Hypersplenism	2. Muscle cramps
	3. Leukopenia

Data from Lazarus JM: Kidney Int 18:783–796, 1980.

Specific Problems and Interventions

Sodium. Sodium balance is maintained until very late in the course of chronic renal failure, explaining the absence of edema in most of these patients.[1,2] There is a lower limit of sodium excretion, and thus severely curtailed intake will lead to volume depletion. Patients with chronic renal failure are especially prone to volume depletion with intensive diuretic administration or gastrointestinal fluid losses. A sodium intake of 50–100 mEq daily (3–6 gm of salt) is reasonable. Occasionally patients will have gross sodium wasting and must receive 150–200 mEq sodium/day.

Water. Urinary concentration and dilution are severely impaired in CRF, and the urine is essentially isotonic. The volume of daily fluid intake should be approximately 500–700 ml above urine output.

Potassium. Potassium balance and plasma potassium concentration are preserved until very late, owing to increased renal tubular excretion and an enhancement of intestinal potassium excretion.[1,2] Acute deterioration of chronic renal failure, acidosis, hemolysis, dietary indiscretion, or hypercatabolism often underlie hyperkalemia. Potassium-sparing diuretics (spironolactone, amiloride, or triamterene) should be used with caution if at all. Potassium intake should be restricted to 2 gm (50 mEq)/day. (See Article 6–6, Hyperkalemia and Hypokalemia, for further comments on the management of hyperkalemia.) Hypokalemia is uncommon in chronic renal failure but may be due to poor intake, gastrointestinal losses, or overzealous administration of cation exchange resins.

Metabolic Acidosis. Metabolic acidosis is common when the GFR falls below 25 ml/minute. It may be seen earlier in patients with tubulointerstitial disease. Generally, metabolic acidosis is well tolerated and not treated unless the serum bicarbonate concentration falls below 16–18 mEq/L. Sodium bicarbonate in a dose of 30–60 mEq/day (2.0–5.0 gm) will maintain the plasma bicarbonate level close to 20 mEq/L in most patients.[1,2]

Uric Acid. Although hyperuricemia up to 10 mg/dl is common, articular gout is infrequent. The presence of gout in chronic renal failure should suggest the possibility of lead nephropathy, amyloidosis, or polycystic kidney disease. Colchicine or nonsteroidal anti-inflammatory agents may be used in the usual doses. Routine use of allopurinol to lower the serum acid concentration is not necessary.

Cardiovascular

Pericarditis. This is a late sign of chronic renal failure and is best managed by beginning dialysis. Nonsteroidal anti-inflammatory agents control fever and chest pain but do not alter the course. The patient should be watched carefully for tamponade, which may be treated by pericardiocentesis with or without instillation of intrapericardial steroids.[8]

Myocardial Complications. Cardiac hypertrophy frequently occurs as a result of anemia and chronic salt and water excess.[8] Congestive heart failure may be present. Hyperkalemia or, less commonly, disorders of calcium balance may produce clinically important arrhythmias. Occasionally, cardiac enlargement without hypertension, profound anemia, or volume overload is seen. This may be a specific uremic cardiomyopathy and is characterized by increased end-systolic and end-diastolic ventricular volume, hypokinesia of the myocardium, and decreased ejection fraction. This is best managed by beginning regular dialysis.

Hypertension. This is usually related to volume overload and is managed by sodium restriction with or without diuretics. It may be necessary to add other antihypertensive agents (methyldopa, clonidine, or hydralazine). Beta blocking agents and angiotensin converting enzyme inhibitors are useful in some instances.

Neurologic. Strokes of all types are common and may cause death in as many as 30% of dialysis patients under the age of 50. Seizures may occur in terminal chronic renal failure and are due to uremic encephalopathy, hypertensive encephalopathy, metabolic alkalosis from vomiting, or water intoxication with hyponatremia. Uremic encephalopathy is best managed by dialysis. Peripheral neuropathy with sensory symptoms of paresthesias is common. Autonomic neuropathy is also common and may contribute to postural hypotension and impotence.[9]

Other. Chronic renal failure is associated with myriad derangements of other homeostatic mechanisms and organ system function.[3–7,9,11] These changes are for the most part chronic and progressive but may, on occasion, manifest acutely. Striking elevations in VLDL and triglycerides are often recorded.[3] With phosphate retention in late stages of disease, hyperphosphatemia and hypocalcemia may ensue, requiring treatment with phosphate-binding antacids and/or vitamin D preparations.[4–5] Anemia seldom requires specific attention beyond correction of other causes, but the bleeding diathesis resulting from uremic platelet dysfunction may warrant emergent dialysis.[6] Gastrointestinal symptoms are early manifestations of uremia and suggest the need for initiation of dialysis; pancreatitis may occur in the setting of uremia and confuse this issue.[7]

KEY FEATURES

Patients with chronic renal failure are generally asymptomatic and have few biochemical abnormalities (other than azotemia) until over 70% of renal function has been lost.

The most common correctable cause of sudden deterioration of chronic renal failure is hypovolemia.

Most patients cannot maximally conserve sodium and easily become volume depleted in the face of reduced salt intake and/or seemingly trivial losses.

Hyperkalemia is unusual, and when it occurs it is generally caused by dietary indiscretion, acute acidosis, hypercatabolism, hemolysis, or the use of potassium-sparing diuretics.

Metabolic acidosis is usually asymptomatic and mild; treatment with $NaHCO_3$ is given when the serum bicarbonate concentration is under 16–18 mEq/L.

Serum phosphate concentration should be maintained below 5 mg/dl by the use of aluminum hydroxide antacids.

Prompt institution of dialysis should be effected when early signs of uremia are evident.

Dialysis is mandatory when pericarditis, neuropathy, or progressive volume overload occurs.

REFERENCES AND SUGGESTED READINGS

1. Mitch WE, Wilcox CS: Disorders of body fluids, sodium and potassium in chronic renal failure. Am J Med 72:536–550, 1982.
2. Morrison G, Murray TG: Electrolyte, acid-base and fluid homeostasis in chronic renal failure. Med Clin North Am 65:429–447, 1981.
3. Haas LB, Wahl PW, Sherrard DJ: A longitudinal study of lipid abnormalities in renal failure. Nephron 33:145–149, 1983.
4. Coburn JW, Llach F: Renal osteodystrophy and maintenance dialysis in replacement of renal function by dialysis. In Drukker W, Parsons FM, Maher JF (eds): Replacement of Renal Function by Dialysis. Boston, Martinus Nijhoff Publishers, 1983, pp 679–711.
5. Massry SG, Ritz E: The pathogenesis of secondary hyperparathyroidism of renal failure. Is there a controversy? Arch Intern Med 138:853–856, 1978.
6. Fried W: Hematologic abnormalities in chronic renal failure. Semin Nephrol 1:176–187, 1981.

    A thorough review of the mechanisms and available therapies, particularly the anemia of renal failure.

7. Zelnick EB, Goyal RK: Gastrointestinal manifestations of chronic renal failure. Semin Nephrol 1:124–136, 1981.
8. Compty CM, Shapiro FL: Cardiac complications of regular dialysis therapy in replacement of renal function by dialysis. In Drukker W, Parsons FM, Maher JF (eds): Replacement of Renal Function by Dialysis. Boston, Martinus Nijhoff Publishers, 1983, pp 595–610.
9. Reese GN, Appel SH: Neurologic complications of renal failure. Semin Nephrol 1:137–150, 1981.

    An excellent presentation of neurologic manifestations in untreated uremia and dialysis and after transplantation.

10. Lazarus JM: Complications of hemodialysis: An overview. Kidney Int 18:783–796, 1980.

    This is a comprehensive examination of the complications of hemodialysis as they relate to (1) the consequences of the procedure itself, and (2) the results of incompletely treated uremia.

11. Emmanouel DS, Lindheimer MD, Katz AI: Endocrine abnormalities in chronic renal failure: Pathogenetic principles and clinical implications. Semin Nephrol 1:151–175, 1981.

    This discussion and review centers mainly around the three most clinically apparent disorders: thyroid dysfunction, sexual and reproductive abnormalities, and abnormal glu-cose metabolism. There is a superb introduction, outlining the general mechanisms by which endocrinopathies may arise in uremia.

SECTION 7
NEUROLOGY

Transient Ischemic Attacks

Fereydoun Shahrokhi, M.D.
Barbara A. McQuinn, M.D.
Robert A. Witzburg, M.D.

Transient ischemic attack (TIA) is defined as an episode of focal neurologic dysfunction that is due to cerebral ischemia with complete resolution within 24 hours. In most patients, TIA symptoms last less than 1 hour. The interruption of cerebral blood flow responsible for TIA may, of course, lead to persistent neurologic deficit; therefore, prompt attention is necessary for all patients with TIA.

Atherosclerosis of the cervicocranial arterial trunks is the most common cause of TIA. Atherosclerosis most frequently occurs in the area of the carotid bifurcation or in the course of the basilar artery, but the middle cerebral arteries, the vertebral arteries, and the subclavian arteries may also be affected. The advancing atherothrombotic process may lead to hemodynamically significant narrowing, occlusion, and/or distal embolism. Emboli may consist of platelets, plaque deposits, or fibrin accumulations.[1] Simultaneous involvement of multiple territories or proximal and distal stenosis in the same arterial system may further complicate both diagnosis and treatment. Local hemodynamic changes cannot be considered in isolation but must be viewed in the context of overall cerebral circulation. The three major collateral systems are the circle of Willis, the external-internal carotid connections through the ophthalmic artery, and the corticomeningeal small vessels. Potential contributions of other factors, such as increased blood viscosity, decreased cardiac output, arterial hypotension, anemia, and hypoxemia, must be considered.

Short-lived (10–30 minute) TIAs are thought to result from cerebrovascular atherothrombosis, resulting in either low-flow states or artery-to-artery embolism. Less frequently, cardiogenic embolism may cause TIAs.[2-4] The latter is usually associated with the sudden onset of neurologic deficits in multiple arterial territories, with symptoms lasting several hours. Other causes of TIA include transient hypotension, cardiac arrhythmia, hemiplegic migraine, clinical fluctuation during the course of lacunar stroke, sickle cell disease, hypercoagulable states, polycythemia, vasculitis, metabolic disturbance, and subdural hematoma.

TIAs can be distinguished from stroke only during the recovery stage. They may occur in any vascular territory and may cause stroke syndromes related to the particular vessels or borderzone areas involved. The incidence of stroke in TIA patients is reported to be 5–6% per year and is unrelated to the number of preceding TIAs, which may vary from one to several hundred. It is thought that the stroke risk is higher in patients with crescendo TIA as well as within the first few weeks following a TIA. However, TIA is also a marker for cardiovascular disease, and more than 50% of TIA patients die of heart disease rather than of cerebrovascular causes.[5]

Transient monocular blindness (amaurosis fugax), a TIA of the ophthalmic artery, is described by many patients as a swift, painless spread of a shade over one eye with a subsequent gradual clearing. Other patients describe this as a rapid global blurring or a segmental visual loss in one eye. Although amaurosis fugax is frequently a harbinger of stroke, the attacks themselves are rarely associated with a simultaneous hemiparesis. Carotid TIAs produce a contralateral hemiparesis and/or sensory loss, usually in the territory of the middle cerebral artery. Vertebrobasilar (brain stem) TIAs may be associated with paralysis or numbness of one or both sides of the body as well as with diplopia, dysarthria, dizziness, bilateral facial numbness, and ataxia.

The differential diagnosis of TIA includes migraine phenomena, atypical or sensory seizures, labyrinthine vertigo, syncope, nonspecific dizziness, and hyperventilation syndrome. Migraine "accompaniments," the transient and usually benign neurologic phenomena that may precede headache or occur even in the absence of headache, may mimic TIA.[6] The presence of scintillating visual phenomena, the slow evolution of symptoms, and the subsequent throbbing headache are helpful clues. In migraine, the clinical deficits spread gradually and in an orderly fashion. The progression usually occurs over a period of 5–30 minutes and may involve more than one arterial territory. A positive personal or family history of migraine, an early age at onset of symptoms, and a history of similar episodes in the past suggest a diagnosis of migraine.

Sensory seizures may also be difficult to distinguish from TIA. As in complicated migraine, these patients experience a progression of subjective symptoms, often without regard to vascular territory. The time course of the symptom march is much shorter in seizure than in migraine, lasting less than a minute. Distinguishing features may include similar episodes associated with motor seizures, confusion, aura or loss of consciousness, epileptiform discharges on EEG, or a positive clinical response to anticonvulsant therapy.

The rotary sensation, or true vertigo, of peripheral vestibular (labyrinthine) dysfunction must be differentiated from a somewhat less distinct vertigo or dizziness that is due to vertebrobasilar TIA. In patients with acute vertigo, associated signs or symptoms of cranial nerve, sensory, or motor dysfunction implicate posterior circulation ischemia. The presence of progressive hearing loss, tinnitus in one ear, or positional exacerbation of symptoms or nystagmus may suggest peripheral vestibular disease. Hyperventilation causes paresthesias in the hands and around the mouth, as well as a sense of floating dizziness and faintness. The symptoms may accompany excitement, anxiety, or depression, but the hyperventilation itself is usually not noticed by the patient. The syndrome usually occurs in younger patients and rarely presents a serious problem in differential diagnosis. The symptoms can be reproduced in the examining room with less than 3 minutes of hyperventilation.

Syncope of cardiac or other causes is due to an abrupt reduction in the cerebral perfusion pressure while the patient is in the upright posture. Cerebral perfusion and alertness are restored when the patient falls and becomes horizontal. Loss of muscle tone leading to the fall thus provides a valuable compensatory measure to protect the brain from prolonged ischemia. The cranial nerve, motor, and sensory symptoms related to posterior circulation TIA are absent in patients with syncope.

The proper evaluation of a patient with TIA includes attention to known risk factors for cerebrovascular disease, as enumerated previously. As in the evaluation of stroke, each patient should have an ECG, routine hematologic and chemical studies, head CT scan, and, if relevant, echocardiography, sedimentation rate, and noninvasive carotid studies. If surgical intervention is contemplated, the definitive preoperative study is still arteriography, although digital subtraction angiography (DSA) may ultimately replace conventional arteriography. Other imaging techniques, such as positron emission tomography (PET) scan and magnetic resonance imaging (MRI), may become useful in the evaluation of regional brain tissue viability. CT scan is essential to demonstrate existing infarcts or, less frequently, other pathology that may mimic TIA. The important diagnosis of exclusion is usually subdural hematoma.

The currently available noninvasive vascular studies include oculoplethysmography (OPG), Doppler ultrasound, beta mode ultrasound, and phonoangiography. OPG measures the blood pressure in the central retinal artery, providing an indirect estimate of perfusion pressure in the internal carotid artery. Doppler ultrasound estimates stenosis by measuring the velocity of the moving red blood cell column. Directional Doppler ultrasound may detect reversal of flow in the supraorbital and other superficial branches of the internal carotid artery. This reversal of flow is due to retrograde filling from the ipsilateral superficial temporal artery. Beta mode (real time) scanning, another ultrasound study, images the static vessel walls and may show stenosis or large ulcerated plaques in the common and/or internal carotid arteries. Such a battery of noninvasive studies may provide substantial information about the state of the arterial wall and of the blood flow in the cervical carotid arteries. Unfortunately, clear direction in the application of such information to treatment of an individual patient is lacking at this time.

TREATMENT

The treatment of a patient with TIA is largely aimed at the prevention of recurrent episodes, as well as aborting progression to completed stroke. Although currently available therapy may be effective in the symptomatic therapy of TIA, the actual prevention of stroke remains an elusive goal. Available treatment modalities include antiplatelet agents, anticoagulants, and arterial surgery. Only aspirin therapy has been shown unequivocally to reduce the subsequent risk of stroke.[7-11] Surgery for patients with vertebrobasilar TIA remains experimental; therefore, except for those at a few centers, clinicians managing patients with vertebrobasilar ischemia must choose between antiplatelet therapy and anticoagulant therapy. Given the ongoing controversy in this area, it is clear that each individual patient must be managed as a unique clinical problem, rather than by a "cookbook" approach. In the future, as clinical studies are refined by classifying TIA patients into pathophysiologic subgroups, it may be possible to demonstrate superior efficacy or safety for a given treatment.

Surgical procedures for prevention of cerebral infarction have included carotid endarterectomy and external-internal carotid bypass. A well-controlled multicenter trial showed no benefit from the bypass for patients with middle cerebral artery TIA that is due to intracranial occlusive disease.[25] When the most severe stenosis is in the surgically accessible cervical portion of the carotid artery, endarterectomy is considered. Controversy regarding the indications and risk:benefit ratio for carotid endarterectomy is unresolved.[26-29] Significant reduction of the blood pressure distal to the carotid artery stenosis occurs with 70–75% stenosis.[1,18] Additional factors that may contribute to the impairment of cerebral perfusion include inadequacy of the circle of Willis or other collateral systems. Unless the combined mortality/morbidity of vascular surgery and angiography is less than 3%, a more conservative, nonoperative approach is appropriate.[20] Restenosis at the operative site is unusual, occurring in only 3.6% of the patients over 2 years.[21] Cervical carotid endarterectomy is currently advised for patients with appropriate carotid system TIA and hemodynamically significant stenosis (greater than 50%). The presence of ulcerated plaques larger than 5 mm constitutes a less well-accepted indication for surgical intervention. End-arterectomy for asymptomatic carotid stenosis is not recommended.[22-24]

Carotid endarterectomy is an effective modality for the symptom of TIA. However, it has not been clearly established that carotid endarterectomy actually reduces the risk of subsequent infarction in the territory of the operated vessel. Therefore, it is vital that patients be selected with an effort to minimize operative morbidity and mortality for a procedure of potential but not unequivocal benefit in the prevention of stroke.[26] An occasional patient may be referred for surgical intervention on the basis of serious contraindications for treatment with aspirin or anticoagulants.

Platelet aggregation in the early stage of clotting is thought to be an important step in the pathogenesis of TIA and stroke. In the Canadian Cooperative Study, aspirin therapy produced a 31% reduction in the risk of stroke or death in patients with TIA.[8] This effect was much less dramatic in women than in men. Currently, a lower dose of aspirin is advocated by some investigators, but no large-scale trials have evaluated doses less than 1000 mg of aspirin per day.[9] Dipyridamole (Persantine), a phosphodiesterase inhibitor, has been much less effective than aspirin, and although it is frequently added to aspirin therapy, there are no data to support its use. Antiplatelet therapy appears to be less effective in TIA of the posterior circulation and is of no value in the prevention of cardiac emboli. We presently recommend aspirin in the dose of 650 mg twice daily, as used in the Canadian Study.

The use of anticoagulant therapy in the secondary prevention of TIA and stroke remains controversial. Full-dose anticoagulation with heparin followed by coumarin is thought by some investigators to offer benefits that justify the risk of hemorrhage.[10-14] However, no large-scale randomized trial convincingly supports this contention in patients with atherothrombotic or cerebrovascular disease.[30] Indeed, there is some evidence suggesting an increased risk of infarction and death in these patients.[12] Despite this, it is relatively common practice to begin treatment of patients with recent onset TIA in the carotid distribution with intravenous heparin followed by coumarin if surgery is not chosen.[15,16] Although firm data are lacking, more support exists for the use of anticoagulants for the patient with stroke in evolution.[12] In patients with cardiogenic embolism, anticoagulation is appropriate.[11,17]

KEY FEATURES

TIA is defined as an episode of transient focal neurologic dysfunction, completely resolving in less than 24 hours, as a result of cerebral ischemia. TIAs result from the same conditions responsible for stroke, most commonly cerebral atherosclerosis or cardiogenic embolism.

The differential diagnosis of TIA includes complicated migraine, atypical seizure, vertigo, syncope, orthostatic hypotension, and hyperventilation syndrome. Detailed history is most helpful in differentiating these disorders.

Potential modes of therapy include antiplatelet medication, anticoagulants, and carotid endarterectomy. Antiplatelet therapy (650 mg aspirin twice daily) is clearly beneficial in men and may be helpful in women. Other therapies are controversial, and management must be individualized carefully.

REFERENCES

1. Kistler JP, et al: Therapy of ischemic vascular disease due to atherosclerosis. Part I: N Engl J Med *311*:27–34, 1984. Part II: N Engl J Med *311*:100–105, 1984.

    A good review of the pathophysiology and management of cerebral ischemic events is presented. The discussion includes that of treatment options for patients with carotid TIA and/or minor completed stroke, as well as the more difficult problems of symptomatic carotid bruits, small-vessel occlusive disease, or vertebrobasilar system atherosclerosis.

2. Dyken ML, et al: Risk factors in stroke. Stroke *15*:1105–1111, 1984.

    An analysis of environmental, genetic, medical, and other conditions that may predispose an individual to stroke is given. Hypertension, diabetes, cardiac disease, and prior TIAs were identified as potentially treatable risk factors for CVA.

3. Easton J, Sherman DG: Management of cerebral embolism of cardiac origin. Stroke *11*(5):433–442, 1980.

    The authors review the data concerning cardiac conditions associated with embolic stroke. Systemic embolus is reported in 10–20% of patients with rheumatic heart disease, 5–12% of patients with recent myocardial infarction (MI), and 10–20% of patients with nonrheumatic atrial fibrillation (AF). Anticoagulation was felt to reduce the embolic recurrence rate to 10–25% of its natural incidence, depending on the condition studied. Recommendations for immediate anticoagulation in cardiac cerebral embolism are made. The authors suggest a 3-month period of anticoagulation for post-MI patients and a treatable period of several weeks following cardioversion for AF patients. For patients with a noncorrectable cardiac lesion, indefinite anticoagulation was suggested.

4. Barnett HJM: Cardiac causes of cerebral ischemia. *In* Toole JF (ed): Cerebral Vascular Disorders. New York, Raven Press, 1984, pp 168–197.

    A brief but excellent review of the cardiac causes of cerebral ischemia.

5. Muuronen A, Kaste M: Outcome of 314 patients with transient ischemic attacks. Stroke *13*:24–31, 1982.

    The results of follow-up (mean 7.8 years) of 314 consecutive cases of TIA treated between 1967 and 1976 are presented. As of 1979, 4.8% of patients suffered a CVA, whereas 12.7% suffered a myocardial infarction. The presence of hypertension correlated inversely with survival at 10 years.

6. Bartleson JD: Transient and persistent neurological manifestations of migraine. Stroke *15*(2):383–386, 1984.

    A review of the clinical symptoms of complicated migraine (i.e., migraine with associated ischemic symptomatology). Prophylactic treatment with beta blocking medications and the infrequent but unfortunate occurrence of stroke as sequela to migraine are some of the topics covered in this informative discussion.

7. Canadian Cooperative Study Group: A randomized trial of aspirin and sulfinpyrazone in threatened stroke. N Engl J Med 299:53–59, 1978.
   This report is one of the original prospective trials of antiplatelet agents in cerebral ischemia.

8. Hersch J: Progress review: The relationship between dose of aspirin, side-effects, and antithrombotic effectiveness. Stroke 1:1–4, 1985.
   The controversy surrounding the determination of the optimal antithrombotic dosage of aspirin is reviewed. No convincing evidence was found for superior effectiveness of any single dose; however, the author notes that the lower frequency of side effects as well as theoretical considerations support the use of a low-dose regimen.

9. Millikan CH, McDowell FH: Treatment of transient ischemic attacks. Stroke 9:299–308, 1978.
   It is suggested that the beneficial effects of anticoagulants override their risk of hemorrhage.

10. Olsson JE, et al: Anticoagulant versus antiplatelet therapy as prophylactic against infarction in transient ischemic attacks. Stroke 11:4–9, 1980.
    This randomized study comparing antiplatelet agents to anticoagulants suggested that the latter are more effective in preventing stroke after TIA or minor stroke, although they carry a greater risk of bleeding.

11. Sherman DG, et al: Cerebral embolism. ACCP-NHLBI National Conference on Antithrombotic Therapy. Chest 89:82S–98S, 1986.
    This section composes a part of an extensive review of antithrombotic therapy. Evidence supporting therapy is presented at various levels of certainty. All sections are well referenced.

12. Sage J, Van Uitert RL: Risk of recurrent stroke in patients with atrial fibrillation and nonvalvular heart disease. Stroke 14(4):537–540, 1983.
    A study of 140 patients with nonvalvular atrial fibrillation and subsequent CVA revealed a stroke recurrence rate of 20% per year over the following nine years. None of the patients received anticoagulants. The recurrence rate was independent of the presence of chronic vs. intermittent atrial fibrillation.

13. Weksler B, Lewin M: Anticoagulation in cerebral ischemia. Stroke 14(5):658–663, 1983.
    This review article details the controversy surrounding the use of antiplatelet vs. anticoagulant therapy for stroke prevention. Historical review of published reports suggests that the outcomes of both modes of therapy are roughly equivalent.

14. Shields RW, et al: Anticoagulant-related hemorrhage in acute cerebral embolism. Stroke 15(3):426–437, 1984.
    Five cases of hemorrhage into CT-proven, originally nonhemorrhagic infarcts were reviewed. Two patients were over-anticoagulated. All five patients had quite extensive middle cerebral artery infarcts. The report underscores the risk of too-early or excessive anticoagulation in patients with large infarcts.

15. Irino T et al: Sanguineous cerebrospinal fluid in recanalized cerebral infarction. Stroke 8:22, 1981.
    About one in three embolic cerebral infarctions shows CSF evidence of hemorrhagic transformation, mostly within the first several days.

16. Whisnant JP, et al: Carotid and vertebral basilar transient ischemic attacks: Effects of anticoagulants, hypertension and cardiac disorders on survival and stroke occurrence: A population study. Ann Neurol 3:107–115, 1978.
    Patients treated with anticoagulants had no significant difference in survival from

untreated patients. Hemorrhagic complications were more likely to occur in patients on long-term (>1 year) anticoagulation and in those over 65 years of age.

17. Sandok BA, et al: Guidelines for the management of transient ischemic attacks. Mayo Clinic Proc 53:665, 1978.
    The study suggests that long-term treatment with anticoagulants after 2–4 months following stroke has diminished benefits and an increased risk of hemorrhage.

18. Wolf P, et al: Duration of atrial fibrillation and imminence of stroke: The Framingham Study. Stroke 14(5):664–667, 1983.
    Nonrheumatic atrial fibrillation (AF) was found to increase the risk of CVA fivefold as determined by 30-year follow-up in the prospective Framingham study. Stroke recurrence within 6 months of the initial event was over twice as common (47% vs. 20%) in stroke accompanied by AF. In patients with AF and rheumatic heart disease, the probability of stroke was found to be increased by 17-fold.

19. Toole JF: Surgical management of transient ischemic attacks. In Toole JF (ed): Cerebral Vascular Disorders. New York, Raven Press, 1984, Chap 8.
    A succinct review of the subject and the rationale for surgical management.

20. Fields WS, et al: Joint study of extracranial arterial occlusion. V. Progress report of prognosis following surgery or non-surgical treatment for transient cerebral ischemic attacks and cervical artery lesions. JAMA 211:1995–2003, 1970.

21. Mohr JP: Transient ischemic attacks and the prevention of strokes. N Engl J Med 299:93–95, 1978.
    It is suggested that the combined morbidity of angiography and surgery should be less than 3%. Otherwise, surgery would be more dangerous than no treatment, over the short-term period.

22. Cossman D, et al: Early re-stenosis after carotid endarterectomy. Arch Surg 113:275–278, 1978.
    The rate of recurrent stenosis at a previously operated endarterectomy site was found to be 3.6% over a 2-year period.

23. Yatsu FM, Fields WS: Asymptomatic carotid bruit: Stenosis or ulceration, a conservative approach. Arch Neurol 42:383–385, 1985.
    This review of the literature suggests that the incidence of cerebral events in patients with asymptomatic carotid bruits is doubled. However, the risk of TIA or stroke within the appropriate (ipsilateral) carotid territory was little higher than in the general population, at 0.1–0.4% per year. Therefore, the authors conclude that bruits may simply be markers for atherosclerotic disease and suggest conservative management unless warning TIAs or greater than 80% stenosis develops.

24. Quinones-Baldrich WJ, Moore WS: Asymptomatic carotid stenosis: Rationale for management. Arch Neurol 42:378–382, 1985.
    The risk of a stroke in patients with asymptomatic carotid bruit was considered to be 1–2% per year. It was concluded that prophylactic endarterectomy may be helpful in patients with stenosis exceeding 70% by angiogram but only if performed in centers where the perioperative morbidity and mortality averages less than 2%.

25. The EC/IC Bypass Study Group: Failure of extracranial-intracranial arterial bypass to reduce the risk of ischemic stroke. New Engl J Med 313:1191–1200, 1985.
    A large, prospective trial comparing extracranial-intracranial arterial bypass to non-surgical treatment for carotid-distribution TIA. No benefit was demonstrated for the surgical group, despite relatively low morbidity related to the procedure itself.

26. Barnett HJM, Plum F, Walton JN: Carotid endarterectomy—an expression of concern. Stroke 15:941–943, 1984.

   Concern was expressed over reports that the average morbidity and mortality from endarterectomy in the United States may approach 10%—over three times higher than the 2.9% "allowable" combined risk of arteriography and operation calculated from co-operative study data regarding the natural history of carotid disease. The authors counsel physicians practicing in institutions with higher than acceptable surgical complication rates to discontinue referral of patients for surgery.

27. Patterson RH: Can carotid endarterectomy be justified? Yes. Arch Neurol 44:651–652, 1987.
28. Jonas S: Can carotid endarterectomy be justified? No. Arch Neurol 44:652–654, 1987.
29. Hachinski V: Carotid endarterectomy (editorial). Arch Neurol 44:654, 1987.

   References 27–29 compose a three-part opinion piece highlighting the controversy regarding carotid endarterectomy.

30. Kieth DS, et al: Heparin therapy for recent transient focal cerebral ischemia. Mayo Clin Proc 62:1101–1106, 1987.

   Retrospective, population-based study of stroke-free individuals who were examined within 30 days of their first TIA during the period 1955–1979. Of the 289 patients so identified, 102 (35%) received heparin therapy. There were no differences in survival, survival free of stroke, or survival free of TIA attributable to heparin. Hemorrhagic complications occurred at a rate of 3.2/100 person-days of therapy.

Stroke

Fereydoun Shahrokhi, M.D.
Barbara A. McQuinn, M.D.
Robert A. Witzburg, M.D.

Stroke is defined as the sudden onset of a neurologic deficit that is due to a vascular lesion and lasts more than 24 hours. It is this abruptness of the neurologic deterioration that distinguishes stroke from other diseases associated with focal central nervous system dysfunction. Stroke is caused by either of two mechanisms: hemorrhagic destruction or ischemic infarction of brain tissue. Included among hemorrhagic strokes are primary intracerebral hemorrhages, usually resulting from hypertensive vascular disease.

ISCHEMIC STROKE

Diagnosis and Management

The blood supply of the brain is provided by two carotid arteries and two vertebral arteries. The vertebral arteries join on the anterior surface of the brain stem to form the common trunk of the basilar artery. The symptoms and signs of the various strokes are determined by the involved arteries. The following summarizes the more common ischemic cerebrovascular syndromes according to their respective territories:

I. Infarction in the major arterial territories:
   A. Internal carotid territory ("anterior circulation"): The carotid circulation supplies most of the cerebral hemispheric circulation, with the exception of the posterior (occipital) portion and the thalamus.
   B. Vertebrobasilar territory ("posterior circulation"): This territory supports the occipital and medial temporal lobes, the thalamus, the brain stem, and the cerebellum.
II. Infarction in the borderzone (watershed) territories: The zones between the neighboring arterial branches of the system just cited.
III. Small, deep, penetrating arteriolar territories: Occlusion of these arteries results in well-circumscribed lacunar infarcts in the deep subcortical structures (basil ganglian, the white matter, and the brain stem).
IV. Subcortical arteriosclerotic encephalopathy (Binswanger's disease): This entity consists of gradual or stepwise ischemic deterioration of the white matter diffusely in the periventricular areas over 2 years and is commonly associated with dementia.

The most common cause of ischemic stroke is atherosclerosis of the major cervical and intracranial arteries with local narrowing or occlusion or distal embolization.[1,2] Emboli originating in the heart also cause stroke. Patients with atrial fibrillation, recent myocardial infarction, valvular heart disease, mitral valve prolapse, atrial myxoma, and bacterial endocarditis are at risk for embolic stroke.[2-5] Abrupt onset of neurologic deficits within several seconds (usually less than 1 minute) is common in embolic stroke. A slower, progressive, or stuttering onset, over minutes, hours, or days, is usually seen in thrombotic or lacunar stroke but may rarely also result from recurrence or fragmentation of cardiac emboli.[11] Hemiparesis upon awakening in the morning is very common with thrombotic process. Many atherosclerotic infarctions are preceded by similar but transient deficits, i.e., transient ischemic attacks (see Transient Ischemic Attacks). The symptoms and signs of these attacks disappear within 24 hours. Established ("completed") infarctions may still show rapid clinical improvement within the first several weeks, though subsequent recovery is slower and may continue for up to 1 year. Apparently 6% of cardiac strokes are hemorrhagic at presentation, whereas such hemorrhage is rare in thrombotic stroke.[18] Other, less common causes of stroke include hemiplegic migraine, vasculitis, septic arteritis, lupus erythematosus, fibromuscular dysplasia, hypercoagulable states, hemoglobi-

nopathy, erythrocytosis, hyperviscosity syndrome, and thrombotic thrombocytopenic purpura. Traumatic or, less commonly, spontaneous carotid
dissection may also result in stroke.[6,7] Borderzone infarcts are caused by a
sudden uncompensated drop in cerebral perfusion pressure. Cardiac arrhythmias, general anesthesia, overzealous use of antihypertensive medications, and cardiac arrest are some of the common causes. Lacunar infarcts
are thought to be caused by the lipohyalinosis in the walls of the small
perforating arteries and are seen only in hypertensive patients.[8] Heart failure, low pO_2, severe anemia, hypokalemia, and alcohol intoxication have
also been associated with increased risk of stroke.[7,23,24]

Clinical Presentations

Anterior Circulation

Middle cerebral artery (MCA) infarction is the most common stroke
syndrome. This artery supplies the lateral aspects of the hemispheres, including sensory and motor cortices, along with the language association
centers on the dominant (usually left) side and the nondominant cortex
involved in spatial appreciation, speech prosody, and certain aspects of mood
and affect. A typical left MCA infarct causes a right-sided weakness in the
face and arm and, to a lesser degree, in the leg. Sensory loss may include
a mild dulling of pinprick on the right, with relatively more severe loss of
fine proprioception and two-point discrimination in the same areas. In addition, language impairment (aphasia) is common. An infarct of the anterior
portion of the MCA territory ("superior division") would be expected to
produce an expressive aphasia and predominantly motor signs; that affecting
the posterior MCA territory ("inferior division") may produce receptive aphasia and predominantly sensory loss.

Deep lethargy is unusual at the onset of an uncomplicated MCA infarct.
However, the gradual development of edema in the infarcted area over
several hours to a few days may lead to lethargy, particularly in a large
stroke. The presence of deep obtundation at stroke onset suggests the presence of intracerebral hemorrhage, brain stem infarct, massive internal carotid
territory infarct, the additive effect of pre-existing CVAs, or superimposed
infectious or metabolic disorders.

Occlusion of the internal carotid artery (ICA) is associated with the
symptoms of MCA infarct, as well as additional deficits from anterior cerebral
artery infarction. In rare patients, the posterior cerebral artery originates
from the internal carotid, and thus occlusion of the latter may cause massive
infarction of an entire hemisphere. ICA infarction causes paralysis affecting
the leg to the same degree as that of the face and arm. The frontal lobes are

affected, and behavioral disturbances may follow. In addition, lethargy is often present as a result of the immense size of the infarction. There may be an ipsilateral Horner's syndrome from the stretching of the ascending ocular sympathetic rami within the carotid sheath.

Posterior Circulation

The vertebrobasilar system supplies the brain stem, cerebellum, occipital cortex, and thalamus. Therefore, arterial occlusion in this system results in a variety of clinical syndromes, depending on the area in which it occurs.

Occlusion of the basilar artery, depending on its level and the efficiency of the collateral circulation, may cause a variable degree of paralysis in all four extremities, sensory loss, variable ocular palsies, paralysis of conjugate gaze, difficulty in swallowing, dysarthria, mutism, or impairment of consciousness ranging from drowsiness to deep coma.

Locked-in syndrome, a result of pontine infarction, is associated with a mute, quadriparetic state. However, the patient's alertness is preserved and the patient may be able to communicate via eye movement or blinking. The locked-in syndrome is often associated with other signs of pontine stroke, including "ocular bobbing" (spontaneous vertical eye movements); corneal reflex loss; and constricted, sluggishly reactive pupils. Locked-in syndrome can also be seen in central pontine myelinolysis, which by some accounts follows the medical management of serum sodium disturbance.

Occlusion of either the posterior inferior cerebellar artery or a vertebral artery causes the lateral medullary (Wallenberg's) syndrome, in which pin and temperature sensation is diminished on the ipsilateral face and on the contralateral body. In addition, ipsilateral ataxia and Horner's syndrome occur, along with vertigo, hoarseness, and nystagmus. Motor weakness is usually not seen.

Borderzone (Watershed) Infarction

Bilateral borderzone infarction is caused by a sudden loss of cerebral perfusion pressure and may be evident following cardiac arrest or severe hypotension of any origin. A common clinical accompaniment of borderzone infarction is the "man in the barrel syndrome," in which greater weakness occurs in the hips and shoulders than in the hands and feet. Dementia and/ or transcortical aphasias may accompany borderzone stroke. Unilateral watershed infarction may occur in the borderzone between any two or among three arterial territories. Most frequently, the borderzone between the middle and posterior cerebral arteries is involved. Less commonly, borderzone stroke may be seen in the brain stem or cerebellum.

Lacunar Infarction

Lacunar infarcts are small (0.5–1.5 cm) ischemic lesions in the deep white matter, basal ganglia, brain stem, or cerebellum. They are named for their well-circumscribed, "lake-like" appearance on both CT and pathologic examination and are believed to reflect occlusive disease in the tiny, deep perforating arteries. Hypertension is considered the major risk factor for lacunar stroke. Although such infarcts are often clinically silent, numerous lacunar stroke syndromes have been described. The most common of these are pure motor stroke, pure sensory stroke, clumsy-hand dysarthria syndrome, and ataxia with ipsilateral hemiparesis. The occurrence of multiple lacunar strokes in one individual is common and may cause dementia.

Management and Prognosis

Treatment of stroke in the acute phase includes bed rest plus administration of O_2 during the first few days, to decrease metabolic demand and protect vulnerable surrounding brain areas. Medical problems contributing to decreased cerebral oxygenation should be treated aggressively. Arterial blood pressure often transiently rises at the time of ischemic stroke and usually returns to baseline in a few hours or days. It is safer not to treat this "compensatory" hypertension unless the blood pressure is extremely high. The course of ischemic stroke remains unpredictable for about 24 hours in those strokes related to the anterior circulation, and for about 1 week in brain stem strokes. Immobilization of patients for longer than a few days is unnecessary, and physical therapy should soon be instituted to prevent deep vein thrombosis, pulmonary embolism, pneumonitis, bed sores, and urinary tract infections.

Depending on the circumstances, a search may be undertaken for treatable sources of recurrent cerebral ischemic events. The useful tests may include ECG; echocardiogram; sedimentation rate; and, in some cases, noninvasive carotid studies, arterial or venous digital subtraction angiography, or, in selected instances, arteriography.

The use of anticoagulant therapy (heparin followed by warfarin) remains controversial. There is no evidence supporting the use of immediate anticoagulation to modify the course of completed thrombotic stroke, and there is some suggestion in the literature that such therapy may be dangerous.[18,25] At the present time, support for the use of anticoagulants is available only for patients with embolic stroke. In such cases, the risk of recurrent cerebral embolism is 12–15% in the first two weeks and there is no safe interval immediately following the index event. That is, the risk is approximately 1% per day, beginning with the first day. However, several trials have demonstrated the safety of anticoagulation in these patients, and in appropriately selected cases treatment should be started without delay.[18-22] Most authors consider it prudent to wait 24–48 hours after embolic stroke, demonstrate the absence of hemorrhage by head CT, and then initiate heparin therapy. Contraindications to treatment include uncontrolled hypertension, advanced age, massive infarction, and the presence of intracerebral or subarachnoid hemorrhage, in addition to the usual cautions for the use of these drugs. The proper duration of treatment is frequently ill defined, but it is determined by the standard of therapy for the underlying lesion rather than by the stroke syndrome.

Platelet aggregation is thought to be an important underlying factor in patients with carotid thromboembolism. Thus, antiplatelet medication is often administered to prevent recurrent ischemic events.[10,11] Aspirin in doses ranging from 40 mg to 1500 mg/day with or without dipyridamole (Persantine) 50–75 mg tid is commonly prescribed, although proof of treatment efficacy is lacking. Other treatments, including fibrinolysis, pentoxifylline, naloxone, calcium channel blockade, and prostacycline, are still considered investigational.[26] The cerebral vasodilators are considered ineffective or even harmful, as they may exaggerate local cerebral hypoperfusion by creating steal syndromes. The role of endarterectomy and of surgical bypass in cerebral atherosclerotic diseases is discussed in the article on transient ischemic attacks.

The prognosis of stroke is much worse, and the mortality rate is significantly higher, when a depressed level of consciousness develops. The permanent loss of the ability to walk is also associated with a shortened life expectancy. Because of concomitant atherosclerotic cardiovascular disease, stroke patients are at increased risk of death from heart disease.[12,13] In fact, stroke patients who survive their event are more likely to die of subsequent myocardial infarction than from recurrent stroke.[14] For this reason, the recognition and treatment of cardiac disorders, hypertension, and other systemic illnesses become especially crucial in the post-stroke period. The prognosis for rehabilitation is related to the type as well as to the degree of neurologic dysfunction produced by a stroke. In general, patients with prominent unilateral neglect and denial of illness (nondominant hemispheric stroke) and those with severe receptive aphasia, lethargy, ataxia, or chronic behavioral disorders following stroke are poor rehabilitation candidates.

INTRACEREBRAL HEMORRHAGE

Primary intracerebral hemorrhage accounts for 10–20% of all strokes. The most common causes include hypertensive vascular disease, ruptured aneurysm or arteriovenous malformation, and overzealous anticoagulation therapy. Blood dyscrasias, hemorrhagic transformation of an ischemic infarct, cortical vein thrombosis, bleeding into tumors, amphetamine or cocaine abuse, and cerebral amyloid angiopathy have also been associated with hemorrhagic stroke.[14] Traumatic intracranial hemorrhage may at times be confused with a primary spontaneous event.

The most common type of spontaneous intracranial bleeding is hypertensive intracerebral hemorrhage.[14] This occurs most often in the putamen, but it also occurs in the thalamus, pons, deep white matter, and cerebellum. The underlying pathology is thought to be lipohyalinosis and necrosis of small penetrating arterioles, i.e., the same general process that is felt to be responsible for lacunar infarction. Formation of microaneurysms (of Charcot-Bouchard) may precede the arteriolar rupture.

The symptoms of intracerebral hemorrhage may include lethargy, headache, and nuchal rigidity. However, it is important to note that neck stiffness is found only when there is both leakage of blood into the subarachnoid space and preservation of a level of consciousness sufficient to allow appreciation of pain. An immediate and definitive diagnosis of intracerebral hemorrhage is best made by CT scan. In putamenal and thalamic hemorrhage, the symptoms usually evolve over a few minutes. In addition to headache and rapid deterioration of consciousness, contralateral hemiparesis is frequently present. Large pontine hemorrhages may lead to coma and quadriparesis in a matter of minutes. Lobar cerebral hemorrhages[15] also cause lethargy, stiff neck, and contralateral hemiparesis. In addition, there may be earache and contralateral superior quadrantanopia with temporal lobe hematoma; ipsilateral temporoparietal pain and contralateral sensory loss with parietal lobe hemorrhage; and, finally, ipsilateral eye pain with contralateral hemianopia in occipital lobe hematoma.

Cerebellar hemorrhage deserves special attention. The extra-axial location of these hematomas in relation to vital centers of the brain stem, along with their relatively slower clinical evolution, usually makes surgical treatment possible. The symptoms of cerebellar hematoma, in addition to gradually progressive lethargy, may include an ipsilateral peripheral facial paresis, sixth nerve palsy, and limb ataxia, as well as dysarthria, truncal ataxia, skewed eye deviation, deviation of the eyes to the opposite side, and vertical ocular bobbing. Again, CT scan gives an immediate and definitive diagnosis. Surgical decompression of the hematoma may be life saving when the lethargy resulting from distortion of the brain stem is severe or progressive. Ventriculoperitoneal shunt is effective when a significant hydrocephalus has resulted from compression of the fourth ventricle by the hematoma.

Large intracerebral hemorrhages have a high mortality rate.[16] The single most important sign of poor prognosis is progressive deterioration of the level of consciousness, usually owing to increased intracranial pressure. This event calls for immediate cranial CT scan and consideration of surgical decompression. Relative contraindications for surgical evacuation include a history of bleeding disorder, involvement of deep subcortical structures by the hematoma, or hematoma in close proximity to vital language or brain stem centers. Ventriculoperitoneal (VP) shunting may be helpful if significant hydrocephalus has resulted. The danger of unwittingly performing surgery on a patient with cerebral amyloid angiopathy must also be counted among the risks of operation. Although this slowly progressive vascular disease often manifests with multiple spontaneous intracerebral bleeds, it may present with a single large hematoma.[17] Decompressive surgery is hazardous in such patients, owing to the risk of severe intraoperative hemorrhage from the friable arterial vessels.

The medical management of increased intracranial pressure from intracerebral hemorrhage includes hyperventilation, fluid restriction, intravenous corticosteroids, and head elevation at about 30 degrees. Intravenous hyperosmolar agents such as mannitol may be useful as a temporizing method for transiently reducing intracranial pressure in neurologically unstable patients awaiting surgery. The correction of coagulopathy and control of hypertension should not be overlooked.

KEY FEATURES

A. Definition of stroke: Sudden onset of neurologic deficit that lasts more than 24 hours and is due to vascular disease
B. Stroke types
   1. Ischemic-thrombotic
   2. Hemorrhagic
   3. Intracerebral hemorrhage
C. Patient evaluation
   1. History of cardiovascular disease, trauma, drug abuse
   2. Serial neurologic examinations
   3. Cardiovascular evaluation
   4. CT scan: emergency procedure if embolic stroke or intracerebral hemorrhage is suspected
D. Treatment: In general, supportive
   1. Embolic stroke: consider immediate anticoagulation (controversial: see text)
   2. Intracerebral hemorrhage: consider surgical evaluation and/or decompression with shunt
E. Prognosis: Massive infarction, prolonged alteration of consciousness, extensive brain stem dysfunction signify a poor prognosis

REFERENCES

1. Ressin MS, et al: Mechanisms of acute carotid stroke. Ann Neurol 6:245–252, 1979.
    Sixty-four patients with acute stroke and arteriographically documented tight (2 mm)

stenosis or occlusion of the ipsilateral carotid artery were studied. Forty-two patients (66%) had angiographic evidence of intracranial embolization distal to the involved cervical carotid artery. These patients were less likely to have suffered from previous TIAs and were more likely to present with moderate to severe neurologic deficit at stroke onset than were patients with no radiologic evidence of embolus.

2. Easton J, Sherman DG: Management of cerebral embolism of cardiac origin. Stroke 11(5):433–442, 1980.

   The authors review the data concerning cardiac conditions associated with embolic stroke. Systemic embolus is reported in 10–20% of patients with rheumatic heart disease, 5–12% of patients with recent myocardial infarction (MI), and 10–20% of patients with nonrheumatic atrial fibrillation (AF). Anticoagulation was felt to reduce the embolic recurrence rate to 10–25% of its natural incidence, depending on the condition studied. Recommendations for immediate anticoagulation in cardiac cerebral embolism are made. The authors suggest a 3-month period of anticoagulation for post-MI patients and a treatment period of several weeks following cardioversion for AF patients. For patients with a noncorrectable cardiac lesion, indefinite anticoagulation was suggested.

3. Sage J, Van Uitert RL: Risk of recurrent stroke in patients with atrial fibrillation and nonvalvular heart disease. Stroke 14(4):537–540, 1983.

   A study of 140 patients with nonvalvular atrial fibrillation and subsequent CVA revealed a stroke recurrence rate of 20% per year over the following 9 years. None of the patients received anticoagulants. The recurrence rate was independent of the presence of chronic vs. intermittent atrial fibrillation.

4. Wolf P, et al: Duration of atrial fibrillation and imminence of stroke: The Framingham study. Stroke 14(5):664–667, 1983.

   Nonrheumatic atrial fibrillation (AF) was found to increase the risk of CVA fivefold as determined by 30-year follow-up in the prospective Framingham study. Stroke recurrence within 6 months of the initial event was over twice as common (47% vs. 20%) in stroke accompanied by AF. In patients with AF and rheumatic heart disease, the probability of stroke was found to be increased by 17-fold.

5. Boughner DR, Barnett HJM: The enigma of the risk of stroke in mitral valve prolapse. Stroke 16:175–177, 1985.

   Patients with mitral valve prolapse (MVP), a common condition with a 5–7% incidence in the adult population, rarely develop cerebral symptoms. However, a disproportionately higher percentage of young stroke patients have MVP. This editorial reviews current progress in the identification of which MVP patients are at risk for stroke. Current evidence is discussed that suggests that the concurrent myxomatous degeneration of cardiac valves besides the mitral increases the risk of stroke.

6. Bartleson JD: Transient and persistent neurological manifestation of migraine. Stroke 15(2):383–386, 1984.

   The article is a handy review of the clinical symptoms of complicated migraine (i.e., migraine with associated ischemic symptomatology). Prophylactic treatment with beta blocking medications and the infrequent but unfortunate occurrence of strokes as sequelae to migraine are some of the topics covered in this informative discussion.

7. Irey NS, et al: Oral contraceptives and stroke in young women: A clinicopathologic correlation. Neurology 28:1216–1219, 1978.

   Postmortem studies on three young women with oral contraceptive–associated CVA disclosed pathologic internal thickening in the cerebral vasculature. Similar systemic vascular changes had been previously described in association with exogenous steroid use.

8. Fisher CM: Lacunar strokes: A review. Neurology 32:871–876, 1982.

   Over 20 discrete clinical syndromes resulting from lacunar infarctions are described in detail. The author also comments on the declining incidence of the lacunar state (a progressive, well-characterized neurologic deterioration associated with recurrent lacunar CVA) and a lacunar stroke in general, and relates this to trends toward early diagnosis and treatment of hypertension.

9. Hillbom M, Kaste M: Ethanol intoxication: A risk factor of ischemic brain infarction. Stroke 14(5):694–699, 1983.

In 100 consecutive patients with radiographically verified ischemic CVA, ethanol intoxication in the preceding 24 hours was found to be 4–7 times as common in men and 6–15 times as common in women than in the age-matched general population. Alcohol intoxication was concluded to be a significant risk factor for cerebral infarction. The risk was felt to be highest in middle-aged women and in young men.

10. Grolta JC, et al: Does platelet antiaggregant therapy lessen the severity of stroke? Neurology 35:632–636, 1985.

Four large studies of platelet antiaggregant drugs in cerebral ischemia are reviewed. In three of the four studies, a trend toward less severe recurrent ischemic events in the treated versus the control group was noted. The authors acknowledge that other factors contributing to stroke severity (patient age, location of lesion, presumed stroke mechanism, etc.) were not specifically reviewed and controlled in this study.

11. Kistler JP, et al: Therapy of ischemic vascular disease due to atherothrombosis. Part I: N Engl J Med 311:27–34, 1984. Part II: N Engl J Med 311:100–105, 1984.

A good review of the pathophysiology and management of cerebral ischemic events is presented. The discussion includes that of treatment options for patients with carotid TIA and/or minor completed stroke, as well as the more difficult problems of asymptomatic carotid bruits, small vessel occlusive disease, or vertebrobasilar system atherosclerosis.

12. Heyman A, et al: Risk of stroke in asymptomatic persons with cervical carotid bruits. N Engl J Med 302:838–841, 1980.

A community survey of 1620 persons over age 45 without prior history of neurologic disease revealed 72 people (4.4%) with cervical carotid bruits. Greater age, female sex, and the presence of hypertension were associated with a high frequency of bruits. Correction for age and blood pressure revealed, during a 6-year follow-up period, a sevenfold higher risk of stroke in men but not in women with cervical bruits. However, the stroke commonly did not occur ipsilateral to the bruit, and the frequency of death from subsequent heart disease was higher than that from stroke. The authors conclude that cervical bruits simply serve as markers for generalized atherosclerosis.

13. Muuronen A, Kaste M: Outcome of 314 patients with transient ischemic attacks. Stroke 13:24–31, 1982.

The results of follow-up (mean 7.8 years) of 314 consecutive cases of TIA treated between 1967 and 1976 are presented. As of 1979, 4.8% of patients suffered a CVA, whereas 12.7% suffered a myocardial infarction. The presence of hypertension correlated inversely with survival at 10 years.

14. Ojemann RG, Heros RC: Spontaneous brain hemorrhage. Stroke 14:468–475, 1983.

The pathophysiology, diagnostic evaluation, and medical vs. surgical treatment options in intracerebral hemorrhage are discussed. The article offers clinical descriptions of intracerebral hematoma by location and by etiology and is quite a useful and informative review of the subject.

15. Ropper AH, Davis KR: Lobar cerebral hemorrhages: Acute clinical syndromes in 26 cases. Ann Neurol 8:141–147, 1980.

The acute clinical and radiologic findings in 26 patients with intrahemispheric cerebral hemorrhage are described. Eight of the 26 patients had chronic hypertension, 2 had arteriovenous malformations, 1 had metastatic tumor, and 2 had bleeding tendencies as a result of anticoagulation therapy. The pathology responsible for the remaining hemorrhages was undetermined.

16. Helwig-Larsen S, et al: Prognosis for patients treated conservatively for spontaneous intracerebral hematoma. Stroke 15(6):1045–1048, 1984.
    In a Danish study of 53 cases with medically managed intracerebral hemorrhage, 30% of patients were found to have recovered fully at 4½ years, with normal neurologic examinations. Thirteen per cent had minor CNS sequelae, and 17% had debilitating deficits. Twenty-seven per cent of patients died at the time of the acute event, and 7 additional patients died during the follow-up period. Ninety per cent of patients with hematomas larger than 50 ml in size died acutely, whereas only 10% of those with smaller hematomas died.

17. Cosgrove GR, et al: Cerebral amyloid angiopathy. Neurology 35:625–631, 1985.
    The clinical findings in a series of 24 autopsy-proven cases of cerebral amyloid angiopathy are discussed. Two thirds of the patients presented with spontaneous intracerebral hemorrhage. The other common clinical accompaniment was dementia. Hemorrhages that were multiple, frontoparietal or parieto-occipital in location, and superficial or ruptured into the ventricles were found to be suggestive of the disorder, especially in demented patients.

18. Sherman DG, et al: Cerebral embolism. ACCP-NHLBI National Conference on Antithrombotic Therapy. Chest 89:82S–98S, 1986.
    This section composes a part of an extensive review of antithrombotic therapy. Evidence supporting therapy is presented at various levels of certainty. All sections are well referenced.

19. Koller RB: Recurrent embolic cerebral infarction and anticoagulation. Neurology 32:283–285, 1982.
    A retrospective review of the hospital course of 44 patients with embolic stroke. Eleven patients suffered recurrent cerebral embolism, three of whom died as a result. There were two recurrences within the first 48 hours. Seventeen embolic infarctions in fifteen patients were managed with anticoagulant therapy (thirteen heparin, four warfarin). There were no complications of therapy, and no patient suffered hemorrhage into the infarcted area.

20. Cerebral Embolism Study Group: Immediate anticoagulation of embolic stroke: A randomized trial. Stroke 14:668–676, 1983.
    A multicenter prospective trial of immediate vs. delayed (14 days) anticoagulation of patients with cardiogenic embolic brain infarction. Of all patients not receiving sodium warfarin (Coumadin) at the time of the index stroke, only 2 of 56 (4%) had hemorrhagic infarction. Follow-up CT scan in 40 patients showed late hemorrhage in 2 additional patients. All 4 hemorrhagic infarctions occurred in nonanticoagulated patients with large strokes. There were no major complications among 24 patients who were immediately heparinized after embolic stroke. A trend toward reduction of early recurrent embolic stroke was seen.

21. Ramirez-Lasserpas M, Quinones MR: Heparin therapy for stroke: Hemorrhagic complications and risk factors for intracerebral hemorrhage. Neurology 34:114–117, 1984.
    A combined retrospective and prospective study of 510 patients treated with continuous infusion heparin for acute cerebral infarction, reversible ischemic neurologic deficit, or transient ischemic attack. Overall, hemorrhage occurred in 16 (3.1%) patients, 3 of whom (0.6%) had CNS bleeding. Risk factors included abnormal CT scan, multiple infarcts, known source of embolus, severe neurologic deficit, and presence of cerebral infarction.

22. Furlan AJ, et al: Hemorrhage and anticoagulation after nonseptic embolic brain infarction. Neurology 32:280–282, 1982.
    Among 54 consecutive patients presenting with embolic stroke, CT scan demonstrated

hemorrhage in only 2%. No secondary hemorrhage occurred among 25 patients immediately anticoagulated, and no recurrent emboli occurred once adequate anticoagulation was achieved. Among the 20 patients who had persistent sources of emboli but were not anticoagulated, 5 (25%) suffered recurrent cerebral embolism 1–7 days after the initial event.

23. Gill JS, Zekula AV, Shipley MJ, et al: Stroke and alcohol consumption. N Engl J Med 315:1041–1046, 1986.

    A retrospective, case-control study of 230 stroke patients evaluating the relative risk of stroke in nondrinkers, light drinkers, and heavy drinkers. Among men, light drinkers were at lowest risk for stroke and heavy drinkers (consuming more than 300 gm weekly) had a fourfold increase in risk compared with nondrinkers. The number of women in this study who drank heavily was too small to demonstrate a change in risk. The study relies on patient report of recent alcohol consumption as the primary measure of intake.

24. Khaw KT, Barrett-Connor E: Dietary potassium and stroke-associated mortality. N Engl J Med 316:235–240, 1987.

    This study evaluates the relationship between potassium intake and stroke-associated mortality in a population-based cohort of 859 men and women (aged 50–79 years) in Southern California. At 12 years, 24 stroke-associated deaths had occurred. Men in the lowest tertile of potassium intake had a relative risk of 2.8 compared with the remainder of the group. For women, the relative risk was 4.8. This effect was independent of known cardiovascular risk factors as well as other dietary variables.

25. Duke RJ, et al: Intravenous heparin for the prevention of stroke progressive in acute partial stable stroke: A randomized controlled trial. AIM 105:825–828, 1986.

    A prospective, double-blind, placebo-controlled trial involving 225 patients with acute partial, stable thrombotic stroke. Patients in the treatment group received continuous infusion heparin for 7 days. No neurologic differences between treatment and control groups were identified at 7 days, 3 months, or 1 year, although a greater number of deaths occurred in the heparin group 3–12 months after treatment.

26. Gelmers HJ, et al: A controlled trial of nimodipine in acute ischemic stroke. N Engl J Med 318:203–207, 1988.

    A prospective, double-blind, randomized, placebo-controlled trial of nimodipine, a calcium channel blocker, in the first 4 weeks following acute ischemic stroke. During the treatment period, mortality from all causes was reduced in the nimodipine group (8.6% vs. 20.4%). In addition, a better neurologic outcome was evident in the treatment group at 6 months' follow-up examination. The therapeutic effect appeared to be limited to men.

27. Meyer FB, et al: Focal cerebral ischemia: Pathophysiologic mechanisms and rationale for future avenues of treatment. Mayo Clin Proc 62:35–55, 1987.

    An excellent, state-of-the-art review of pathophysiology of stroke syndromes and discussion of therapeutic modalities on the horizon.

Headache, Part I: A Clinical Approach

Nagagopal Venna, M.D.

When a patient is seen for the chief symptom of headache, the diagnosis usually is a benign disorder such as tension headache or migraine, but the differential diagnosis includes life-threatening conditions such as subarachnoid hemorrhage or brain tumor. Thus, the clinician must evaluate each patient with care.

PATHOGENESIS OF HEADACHE

Intracranial lesions, with or without increased intracranial pressure, cause headaches by displacement, traction, and irritation of the pain-sensitive basal dura, walls of venous sinuses, and trunks of the major arteries at the base of the brain. The parenchyma of the brain itself is insensitive. A ball-valve mechanism of obstruction to CSF outflow causes the headache of third ventricle cyst. Dilatation of the external carotid artery is implicated in headaches of migraine, transient cerebral ischemic attacks, and febrile-toxic states. A specific inflammation of external carotid artery branches underlies the headache and jaw claudication of giant cell arteritis. Excessive contraction of the muscles of the scalp, neck, and jaws seems to be involved in tension headaches and temporomandibular joint (TMJ) dysfunction.

Patterns of referral of pain are important to recognize. Pain arising in the posterior fossa may be referred to the forehead because the tentorium is innervated by the trigeminal nerve. Also, a posterior fossa mass can cause pain and stiffness of the neck by irritation of the second and third cervical roots. Pain from the upper cervical spine may be referred to the forehead and temples. Lesions in the pituitary fossa and sphenoid sinus may cause pain over the vertex or frontotemporal areas. Pain from the eye, paranasal sinuses, and teeth is frequently referred to the forehead and temples. Indeed, the source of headache may be as remote as an abdominal pheochromocytoma.

DIAGNOSTIC APPROACH TO HEADACHE

Despite the bewildering diversity of possible causes, a systematic and broad-based clinical approach usually leads to the diagnosis. A narrow focus may result in inappropriate referrals as well as inaccurate diagnosis and treatment, as exemplified by futile dental extractions for trigeminal neuralgia, ineffective remedies for cluster headache misconstrued as "sinus headache," or misdiagnosis of an intracranial lesion as tension headache. It is careful history and physical examination that solve the diagnostic problem in most cases of headache; rarely do laboratory tests prove to be vital.

Severity of headache does not correlate with seriousness of the etiology: cluster and migraine headaches can be excruciating while the headache of brain tumor or sentinel subarachnoid hemorrhage may be only moderately painful. Headache accompanied by regional symptoms is not necessarily due to regional pathology: headache with a red eye or nasal stuffiness is characteristic of cluster headache and mimics glaucoma, iritis or allergic rhinitis. Recent onset or a notable alteration in the pattern of chronic headaches should be viewed with caution: a life-long sufferer of migraine is not immune to rupture of cerebral aneurysm.

History

With practice, the history can be rapidly surveyed to elicit key features of onset, location, spread, quality, severity, duration, and aggravating and relieving factors. The sickening, throbbing hemicranial pain of migraine, the boring fronto-orbital pain of cluster headache, the peculiar burning pain over the temple in giant cell arteritis, and the constant sensation of pressure and tight band around the head of tension headache are readily recognizable. In evaluating a new headache, the rapidity of onset is important. Subarachnoid hemorrhage has a sharp onset, whereas the headache of migraine or meningitis, though equally severe, evolves over many minutes or hours. Mechanical features of headache include coughing, straining, bending, standing, and lying down. Such movements may aggravate ongoing headaches of migraine and sinusitis, but when headache is induced or relieved by these maneuvers, intracranial mass lesion or obstruction to CSF outflow should be suspected. For example, headache of third ventricle colloid cyst is brought on by lying down and is relieved by holding the head down between the knees. Post–lumbar puncture headache is largely limited to erect position. Cough may precipitate severe pain in some pituitary tumors, though bursting headache, occurring only in a bout of cough, may be benign. However, the lack of mechanical characteristics is not helpful. Headache that occurs recurrently in sexual intercourse may be due to a benign orgasmic cephalalgia, but if the first episode is severe it may be necessary to consider intracranial hemorrhage. The effects of foods and drugs provide clues to cases of "hot dog" or "ice cream" headache. Migraine may be exacerbated by nitroglycerin, reserpine, or theophylline; cluster headaches may be aggravated by alcohol. Headache that awakens the patient from sound sleep is frequently due to hemorrhage or other intracranial mass lesions. The exception is a cluster headache that often awakens the patient with clockwork regularity a few hours after falling asleep. This is different from headache present on awakening in the morning, as in tension headache, migraine, frontal sinusitis, and severe diastolic hypertension. Headache of ethmoidal and frontal sinusitis is worse in the morning, whereas that of maxillary and sphenoid sinusitis worsens as the day passes because of position-dependent drainage patterns.

Clues to the etiology of headache often lie in the phenomena that accompany the episode and may indicate dysfunction of eyes, sinuses, teeth, TMJ, cervical spine, or jaws. Fronto-orbital headache associated with tearing and redness of the eye and nasal stuffiness characterizes cluster headache. Jaw claudication strongly suggests temporal arteritis. Neurologic symptoms may include changes in behavior; level of consciousness; and motor, sensory, visual, auditory, and language functions. The tempo of the evolution and regression of the phenomena is critical: scintillating scotomata that enlarge and regress over 20–30 minutes are pathognomonic of classic migraine. Temporal headache with amaurosis fugax in an elderly person suggests giant cell arteritis, although carotid atherosclerotic transient ischemic attacks, glaucoma, or retinal detachment can mimic this. New onset frontal headache with diplopia raises the specter of enlarging posterior communicating artery aneurysm, but painful third cranial nerve palsies also occur in diabetes, ophthalmoplegic migraine, and temporal arteritis. Headache with seizures suggests arteriovenous malformations or other brain lesions. Episodic headache accompanied by systemic symptoms such as anxiety, pallor, palpitations, tremor, or perspiration suggests pheochromocytoma; severe episodes of migraine may cause prostration and transient polyuria, vomiting, or diarrhea. Certain headaches are associated with telltale behaviors. Patients with a typical migraine prefer to lie down in a dark, quiet room and try to fall asleep, whereas a cluster headache patient paces the floor.

In patients with recurring headaches, interval history of regional, neurologic, psychiatric, and systemic symptoms may indicate whether the headache is a benign syndrome like migraine or a symptom of an ongoing process. Headache is a common feature of depression and anxiety, so that emotional changes must be appraised. Patients' concerns about the nature of the headache should be explored.

Headache of recent onset is potentially serious, whereas headache on and off for years is likely to be benign. Recent substantial change in the pattern of long-standing headache or its accompaniments, though not necessarily ominous, should be evaluated carefully. The influence of life stresses may be apparent in migraine that appears at puberty; tends to be worsened by oral contraceptives, pregnancy, or hypertension; and tends to fade after menopause. A striking feature of cluster headaches is their recurrence in clusters of 1–3 months with asymptomatic intervals of months to years, whereas tension headaches may be constant for months.

Physical Examination

This discussion of the physical examination focuses on patients without obvious signs like obtundation or hemiparesis. Initial evaluations include a thorough general physical examination. Regional examination includes the orbits, sinuses, teeth and gums, oropharynx, calvaria, and scalp. Superficial temporal and facial arteries are palpated for pulse, thickening, and tenderness. The TMJ is examined for tenderness, pain on movement, spasm, and crepitation. The cervical spine is checked for mobility and tenderness. Auscultation over orbits, skull, mastoid process, and neck may reveal bruit of intracranial arteriovenous malformation or carotid occlusive disease.

Comprehensive neurologic examination, including mental state and gait, is performed. Optic fundi are scrutinized for papilledema, if necessary, after dilating the pupils in stable situations. Lack of papilledema does not rule out intracranial mass lesion. Mapping of visual fields by finger or a 4-mm pinhead may provide the only sign in headaches caused by pituitary tumors, as patients are often unaware of even dense defects.

Tests of Intracranial Lesions

Skull radiographs are underutilized in the investigation of headache. A lateral view of the skull may reveal changes in the sella not seen on usual CT scans in pituitary tumors. Frontal views of the sinuses that include ethmoid and sphenoid sinuses should be obtained. CT scan has made investigation of headache patients safer and easier, but it is normal in most of the common headache syndromes. Noncontrast study in acute lesions and contrast study in recurrent chronic headache give the best yields. The scan is sensitive for intracranial hemorrhage, including subdural hematoma, tumor, arteriovenous malformation, and other focal lesions. However, there are important pitfalls: the sellar region is a notorious blind spot, so that lateral skull views, polytomograms, and special CT scan views of the sella are essential. Certain lesions such as isodense subacute subdural hematoma, especially when bilateral, may not be obvious on CT scan or may be misinterpreted as pseudotumor cerebri. If contrast material is not used, lesions isodense with brain, such as cysts of the third ventricle, pituitary tumors, some arteriovenous malformations and angiomas, as well as certain primary and metastatic tumors, may be missed. Artifact from bone may obscure cerebellopontine angle mass lesions. In 10% of patients with subarachnoid hemorrhage, CT scan is negative. The CT scan may be useful in detecting infection of paranasal sinuses, especially sphenoid and ethmoid sinuses, even when radiographs are negative. The magnetic resonance imaging (MRI) scan is now the test of choice for lesions in the pituitary and posterior fossa, as it is devoid of bone artifact.

The proper timing for performance of lumbar puncture (LP) is a vexing question in acute headaches, and critical delays occur awaiting a "rule-out" CT scan in cases of acute bacterial meningitis. In such a patient, spinal fluid analysis takes precedence, even if the patient is obtunded, as long as there is no evidence of herniation. In subarachnoid hemorrhage, with negative CT scan only spinal tap will establish the diagnosis.

Cerebral angiography is needed in selected cases, such as the patient with acute headache and third cranial nerve palsy as a result of an enlarging posterior communicating artery aneurysm. EEG has a limited role in the rare instances of seizures manifested predominantly by episodic headache, though this occurs usually in association with neurologic symptoms. When giant cell arteritis is suspected, an urgent erythrocyte sedimentation rate (ESR) determination and temporal artery biopsy are indicated. Migraine syndrome occurring in patients with multiple system dysfunction should raise suspicion of systemic lupus erythematosus, and appropriate immunologic tests must be performed.

KEY FEATURES

Etiologic diagnosis is the critical first step in managing a patient with headache.

Important headache characteristics include location; quality; intensity; aggravating, relieving, or precipitating factors; and timing.

Headache accompaniments include regional, neurologic, systemic, and behavioral manifestations.

Physical examination:

1. General: BP, cardiovascular, skin.

2. Regional: scalp; calvaria; eyes; sinuses; teeth; throat; TMJ; superficial temporal and facial arterial pulses; orbital, cranial, and cervical bruits.

3. Neurologic: mental status, visual acuity and fields, afferent pupillary defect, optic disks.

4. Psychiatric: depression, confusion.

Laboratory evaluation is usually unhelpful. ESR should be obtained for suspected temporal arteritis.

Tests for intracranial disease: skull radiographs, CT scan, MRI scan, cerebral angiography, cervical spine radiographs.
Special studies include temporal artery biopsy, lumbar puncture.

Headache, Part II: Management of Common Headache Syndrome

Nagagopal Venna, M.D.

MIGRAINE

Migraine is a common cause of chronic recurrent headaches with protean neurologic accompaniments. Despite intense research, its etiology remains elusive.

Features Common to All Subtypes of Migraine

The Migraine Diathesis. A family history of migraine occurs in 60% of patients, and there is a female preponderance of 3:1. Onset is usually in childhood, adolescence, or young adulthood, but it may occur at any age. It is often preceded in childhood by motion sickness, cyclical vomiting, or recurrent abdominal pain. Hormonal upheavals of puberty, pregnancy, oral contraceptive use, menstruation, or menopause exacerbate, precipitate, or occasionally ameliorate migraine. Association has been described between migraine and mitral valve prolapse, Raynaud's phenomenon, Prinzmetal's angina, left-handedness, and polycystic ovary disease. Certain foods; head trauma; hypertension; vasoactive drugs like nitroglycerin, reserpine, hydralazine, prazosin, and theophylline; and alcohol may aggravate the headache. The episodes of migraine often change over the years: common migraine may become classic, neurologic accompaniments may occur without headache, and the attacks tend to fade in later life. Episodic migraine may become more continuous when combined with tension headache.

Headache is only a part of a wider clinical disturbance with a 1–2 day prodrome of irritability, euphoria, increased energy, or depression. Perception of sounds, sights, and smells becomes keener, and there may be fluid retention and increase in appetite or craving for certain foods. The headache may evolve over many minutes to an hour or so but rarely is explosive. It does not awaken the patient from sleep but may occur on awakening. It is predominantly hemicranial, often becoming bilateral, and when hemicranial it may switch sides in different attacks. It is usually throbbing but can be steady and lasts from a few hours to a few days. Nausea, anorexia, and vomiting are common. There may be tenderness or even swelling over the temple at the height of an attack. Typically, the patient prefers to lie down in a quiet, darkened room, trying to sleep off the headache. The headache may be followed by exhaustion, depression or euphoria, and polyuria.

Subtypes of Migraine

Common Migraine. This is by far the most common type, has the attributes enumerated previously, and lacks visual or other focal neurologic disturbances.

Classic Migraine. Though the most spectacular, it constitutes only 15% of all forms of migraine. The episodes begin abruptly with visual hallucinations in the form of scintillating scotomata, zigzag lines, bright spots, circles, and stars, sometimes resembling colorful fireworks. A pathognomonic but not invariable feature is the build-up and movement of these hallucinations from the center of vision to the periphery. As scintillations regress, hemianopia or total blindness may appear in their wake. Throbbing headache sets in as vision returns to normal along with the usual accompaniment of migraine. The visual aura distinguishes this subtype.

Complicated Migraine. Complicated migraine refers to migraine in association with neurologic disturbances other than those of classic type. The headache is preceded, accompanied, or followed by hemiplegia, hand-face-mouth paresthesias, unilateral ophthalmoplegia, uniocular visual loss, or symptoms of brain stem dysfunction (hemiplegic, cheiro-oral, ophthalmoplegic, retinal, and basilar artery migraine, respectively). The deficits usually resolve in minutes to hours, but they may persist for several days and recur in subsequent attacks.

Diagnosis

Diagnosis is clinical, as there are no confirmatory tests. Migraine in the family, onset in early life, association with childhood motion sickness, cyclical vomiting, recurrent abdominal pain, and major alterations of headache patterns by endocrine milestones and vasoactive drugs provide supportive evidence. In the individual episode, the symptoms surrounding the headache, such as nausea, vomiting, photophobia, sonophobia, autonomic alterations, and mood and vegetative disturbances, are suggestive. When focal neurologic disturbances occur, their build-up over 20–30 minutes is pathognomonic but not always present. Unilateral headache that switches sides or alternating neurologic disturbances in different episodes support migraine, though consistent occurrence on the same side does not refute the diagnosis.

Laboratory evaluation is indicated in the first episodes of complicated migraine, especially in the absence of characteristic crescendo, with persistence of focal deficits, abnormal interval neurologic examination, or unexpected change in the character of headache or in the presence of systemic illness. Migraine-like syndrome occurs in systemic lupus erythematosus, and appropriate tests may be helpful. CT scan with contrast enhancement is needed to rule out arteriovenous malformation. In the first attack of ophthalmoplegic migraine, cerebral angiogram may be indicated to rule out saccular aneurysm. EEG rarely reveals seizures mimicking migraine or may identify migraine with epileptiform discharge, a syndrome frequently responsive to anticonvulsant therapy. When migraine headache is explosive, lumbar puncture and CT scan rule out subarachnoid hemorrhage.

Treatment

Abortive treatment is tailored to the frequency and severity of the headache (Table 1). Mild episodes respond to aspirin, acetaminophen, or other nonsteroidal anti-inflammatory drugs. Ergotamine is time honored and effective for more severe attacks when administered early in the episode. Status migrainosus, an occasional complication with incapacitating headache

Table 1.   TREATMENT OF MIGRAINE

Abortive Treatment
Mild attacks:
  Aspirin 300–600 mg
  Combinations such as Fiorinal (aspirin, caffeine, butalbital)
Moderate to severe attacks:
  Oral ergotamine tartrate (e.g.: Ergomar, Gynergen); ergotamine combined with caffeine and sedatives, such as Cafergot, Wigraine, Migralam, etc.
  Suppositories when nausea, vomiting occur; 2 mg early in the attack, repeat in ½ hour if needed
  Maximum dosage: 65 mg of ergotamine per attack; 10 mg/week
Status migrainosus:
  Hospitalize patient in a quiet, dark room
  Discontinue ergotamine
  IV fluids as needed
  Analgesia with narcotics plus an antiemetic
  Sedatives (oral benzodiazepines)
  Some intractable cases respond to prednisone 60 mg/day for a week

Prophylactic Therapy
Propranolol: 20 mg tid, increased gradually up to 80 mg tid; most patients need about 120 mg/day. If responsive, long-acting, once-a-day form may be conveniently used
Amitriptyline: start with 25 mg at night—increase up to 150 mg/day, in divided doses
Methysergide: start with 2 mg/day, increase to 2 mg tid. Not more than 4 months of continuous therapy, but can be resumed after 1-month drug holiday.
Calcium channel blockers: until more experience is accrued, reserved for resistant cases
Verapamil: 60 mg qid
Nifedipine: 10 mg bid–qid

lasting more than 3 days, is managed by hospitalization in a quiet environment, withdrawal of ergot preparations, judicious use of narcotic analgesics and anti-inflammatory drugs, antiemetics and sedation, and intravenous hydration as needed. Precipitating factors, which are often psychological stresses, should be dealt with. Intractable cases may respond to a short course of prednisone.

Prophylactic therapy alleviates frequent migraine (>2–3/month). The various drugs seem to be about equally effective; the choice in a particular patient depends on the presence of contraindications to the drugs and on previous response to other drugs. Propranolol is now widely and successfully used for prophylaxis. Amitriptyline, a well-tolerated tricyclic antidepressant, is effective with or without associated tension headache or depression. Methysergide, though effective, is reserved for resistant cases because of occasional side effects of retroperitoneal and cardiac valvular fibrosis. It should not be given more than 4 months continuously but can be resumed after a drug holiday of 1 month. Calcium channel blockers are the latest addition to the prophylactic armamentarium and may benefit both classic and common migraine.

CLUSTER HEADACHE

Cluster headache is a distinctive syndrome, but pathogenesis and etiology are obscure. Males outnumber females by 5:1, and most patients are 20–40 years of age. The episodes of steady, boring headache occur abruptly, centered over the eye and temple and are often excruciatingly intense. Characteristic accompaniments are tearing and bloodshot eye, stuffy nose, sweaty and flushed face, and sometimes a transient Horner's syndrome, all ipsilateral to the headache. The pain lasts about an hour and may recur a few times a day. Some patients are awakened by the headache with clockwork precision a few hours after falling asleep. The patient paces the floor in the grip of pain. There is no nausea or vomiting, nor do neurologic deficits occur. Characteristically, a series of headaches occur in clusters lasting up to 1–3 months followed by headache-free periods of months to years. Physical examination during headache reveals injection of the ipsilateral eye and sometimes Horner's syndrome. Interval examination is normal, but some patients may have deep nasolabial folds, prominent furrows on the forehead and across the chin, and facial telangiectasia.

The nature of cluster headache, its regional accompaniments, and its temporal pattern are diagnostic. The uninitiated often mistake it for eye, dental, or sinus disease, leading to misdirected therapy. However, it is important to rule out iridocyclitis, dental abscess, or acute sinusitis in the first attacks. There are no confirmatory laboratory tests.

Effective abortive treatment is provided by intramuscular ergotamine or dihydroergotamine or inhalation of 100% oxygen, but prophylactic therapy is needed for the duration of the cluster. Avoidance of cigarettes and alcohol is important. Ergotamine and methysergide in the younger patient; prednisone in refractory cases, often combined with ergotamine; and lithium carbonate in patients over 40 years as well as propranolol and calcium channel blockers are effective agents (Table 2).

TENSION HEADACHE

Tension headache, undoubtedly, is one of the most common forms of headache and is frequently seen in conjunction with migraine ("mixed headaches"). The distinction between common migraine and tension headache is often blurred, but tension headache is a recognizable clinical syndrome. The pain is suboccipital with radiation to the neck, vertex, and forehead. It is usually described as a constant, dull pressure or a heaviness over the head; or a tight, squeezing band around the head. Pain may fluctuate but persist for days, weeks, or months, intensified by emotional stress. Physical examination is negative except for areas of tenderness over the occiput and posterior aspect of the neck. The overlap with migraine is suggested in patients who experience nausea and vomiting or throbbing exacerbations against a background of constant pain. Depression, anxiety, and other emotional stresses as well as regional disorders such as cervical spondylosis and TMJ disease should be looked for.

Some patients respond to counseling and simple analgesics. Narcotics are to be avoided. Antidepressant drugs may be beneficial whether or not depression is present. Amitriptyline in doses starting at 25 mg at bedtime and gradually increased up to 150 mg/day is useful. In mixed tension-migraine headaches, propranolol may be effective. A compassionate, supportive attitude is essential.

Table 2.   TREATMENT OF CLUSTER HEADACHE

Abortive Treatment
Ergotamine tartrate: 1–2 mg IM, repeat in 1 hour if necessary; not more than 6 mg/week
or
Dihydroergotamine mesylate: 2 mg IM (DHE-45), repeat in 1 hour if needed; not more than 6 mg/day
or
100% oxygen: 10 L/minute for 10 minutes
Prophylactic Treatment (for the duration of cluster)
Ergotamine tartrate: if headaches occur only at night, 2 mg at bedtime; for more frequent headache, 1 mg bid or tid
Propranolol: as for migraine
Methysergide: as for migraine
Lithium carbonate: for patients over the age 40 years; 300 mg 2–4 times a day; careful blood level follow-up
Prednisone: for intractable cases; 40–60 mg/day for a week, tapered over 3 weeks

POST-TRAUMATIC HEADACHES

Persistent headache after blunt head trauma is common. The spectrum extends from an unrelenting headache lasting weeks to the fluctuating benign headache of post-concussion syndrome. An unusual subtype, dysautonomic cephalgia, has recently been defined.

Post-traumatic headache may be due to intracranial hematoma. A subdural hematoma is the most common cause in this group and accumulates over several weeks. In older patients, a chronic subdural hematoma may evolve over months after even trivial injury. Rarely, a subacute epidural or delayed intracerebral hematoma may be responsible.

The patient typically returns after the head trauma with unrelenting headache, often aggravated by changes in position of head and body, cough or straining, and accompanied by vomiting. Headache may awaken the patient. Fluctuating depression of consciousness, gait disturbance, behavioral change, seizures, or focal neurologic symptoms are highly suspicious. Neurologic examination may be quite normal or show drowsiness, papilledema, ataxia, Babinski's responses, mild hemiparesis, or an akinetic mute state. Lethargy is usually more prominent than focal signs.

Persistent headache after head injury should be thoroughly evaluated. The "mechanical features" of headache and neurologic disturbances should be viewed with concern. The CT scan will identify subdural, epidural, or rare intracerebral hematomas. One must be careful not to miss an isodense subdural hematoma, which is most likely to occur 3–6 weeks after trauma. When it is unilateral, such a collection shows itself by lateral displacement of the brain. It is axiomatic that "lateralized mass effect without a mass is subacute subdural hematoma until proved otherwise." A pitfall in CT diagnosis is the occurrence of bilateral isodense subdural hematomas—without displacement of the midline. A scan with loss of definition of cortical sulci and slit-like ventricles suggesting "pseudotumor cerebri" in this context should be suspected to be subdural hematomas. Contrast-enhanced CT scan and radiotracer brain scans may help delineate these better, but rarely angiography may be needed. These are eminently treatable by surgical evacuation.

Headache of Post-concussion Syndrome

The headache of post-concussion syndrome is the most common type of chronic post-traumatic headache. The pain is part of a polysymptomatic syndrome of postural dizziness; impairment of concentration and attention; and changes in behavior such as irritability, depression, decreased libido, and insomnia. The headache is generalized, steady or throbbing, mild or moderate in severity, often clearly aggravated by anxiety or work needing concentration. It improves over weeks or months and is not accompanied by depression of consciousness or other neurologic symptoms. Physical examination is normal. Diagnosis is clinical, but in the early post-traumatic period or if there is doubt, a head CT scan is recommended.

Reassurance about the benign natural course of the disease is an essential part of management, along with periodic follow-up clinical examinations. Simple analgesics are recommended and narcotics avoided. Antidepressants such as amitriptyline are sometimes helpful in the more refractory cases.

Post-traumatic Vascular Headaches

Headaches with the characteristics of migraine may occur after head trauma. In persons with migraine diathesis, the trauma may trigger recurrent migraine. These patients respond to usual prophylactic therapy with propranolol or antidepressant drugs.

Post-traumatic Dysautonomic Cephalgia

This subtype is probably more common than realized and follows injury to the anterior neck, though head trauma is frequently associated. Injury to the sympathetic network surrounding the carotid artery is implicated. The pain is hemicranial and is associated with ipsilateral facial hyperhidrosis and pupillary dilation, followed by transient partial Horner's syndrome. Propranolol is useful in this self-limited disorder.

GIANT CELL ARTERITIS

Headache is a presenting feature of giant cell arteritis (GCA). Early identification of this disorder is vital so that visual loss and other less common neurologic sequelae can be prevented by corticosteroid therapy. GCA usually appears subacutely in persons over the age of 55 years. The headache may be quite specific, located mainly over the temple, spreading to face, jaw, occiput, and vertex. It is constant, boring, and can be excruciating, often with a curious burning quality and with throbbing or lancing exacerbations. Pain tends to worsen at night; on exposure to cold; and on contact with the scalp while brushing the hair, laying the head on a pillow, or wearing eyeglasses. However, the headache may be nonspecific or resemble other headache syndromes, particularly vascular or tension headache.

Regional headache accompaniments are characteristic. An almost pathognomonic feature is jaw claudication on chewing or talking. Amaurosis fugax is ominous, presaging unilateral or bilateral blindness. Blanching or pain of the tongue is rare. Systemic accompaniments take the form of polymyalgia rheumatica with malaise, weight loss, anorexia, depression, fever, and body aches and pains. Temporal arteries may be tender and nonpulsatile but are occasionally normal. Tender nodules are sometimes felt over the temporal and occipital areas. In severe cases, there may be scalp or tongue necrosis.

In case of any persistent headache of new onset and of a few days' to a few months' duration, appearing in an individual over the age of 55, GCA must be considered. Headache may be nonspecific, and in biopsy-proved cases the temporal arteries can be clinically normal. Important clues are provided by regional and systemic accompaniments of the headache. The erythrocyte sedimentation rate (ESR) should be obtained urgently and is usually markedly elevated (>100 mm). However, if vision is threatened, steroid therapy should be initiated pending further tests, and a normal ESR does not rule out the disorder. The diagnosis is confirmed by temporal artery biopsy. Large segments (4–6 cm) of artery should be obtained so that false negative findings as a result of skipped lesions can be avoided. If findings are negative, biopsy of an asymptomatic contralateral temporal artery may establish the diagnosis.

There is a 50% risk of visual loss, often bilateral, in the first few months of symptoms. Steroid therapy should be promptly initiated in doses of 60–80 mg of prednisone a day. If vision is threatened, hydrocortisone may be given intravenously followed by oral prednisone. Most patients need therapy for at least a year. Longer-term therapy is dictated by ESR and clinical activity.

HEADACHE FROM INTRACRANIAL MASS LESION AND/OR RAISED INTRACRANIAL PRESSURE

The fear of brain tumor looms large in the minds of patient and physician with regard to new onset headaches. Headache is indeed a cardinal symptom of brain tumor, and identical headaches occur with other mass lesions such as subdural hematoma or brain abscess. Masses in the posterior fossa are especially likely to present with headache as an early and prominent symptom. The headaches may occur with or without increase in intracranial pressure; conversely, raised intracranial pressure and headaches may occur without mass lesions, as in pseudotumor cerebri. On the other hand, headache may be absent in many such patients.

The qualities of the headache may be nondescript, but its temporal profile is more suggestive. In most cases, the headache is of new onset and of a few weeks' to a few months' duration. Exceptionally, with slow-growing tumors such as pituitary adenomas, patients experience headache for a few years. The headaches are persistent and gradually increase in severity, but in pseudotumor cerebri they may be quite intermittent and may remit spontaneously. Diurnal fluctuation in severity is common, the headache being worse in the morning and improving as the day goes on. Headache may awaken the patient from sleep. Mechanical features in which headaches are markedly aggravated or precipitated by change in position of head and body, coughing, and straining are prominent with masses in or close to the lateral, third, and fourth ventricles and the aqueduct or in the region of the foramen magnum. The pain is a dull ache but may have a throbbing "vascular headache" quality. It is usually mild to moderate in intensity but can be excruciating. The "vascular" quality is particularly typical of pseudotumor cerebri and in fact may respond to propranolol. In supratentorial lesions, unilateral headache is usually on the side of the mass. In posterior fossa lesions, the pain is characteristically over the occiput and posterior aspect of neck but may be referred to the supraorbital area. Sellar and perisellar lesions cause bifrontal or vertex pain. Regional accompaniments of headache are notable in posterior fossa lesions and consist of neck stiffness and head tilt. Neurologic accompaniments are obviously important and may involve motor, sensory, coordination, gait, and continence functions as well as symptoms referable to cranial nerve dysfunction. Diplopia and obscuration of vision are symptoms of increased intracranial pressure. Obscurations are characterized by momentary and abrupt graying-out of vision in one or both eyes in association with papilledema. More subtle accompaniments are in the form of personality changes—the history from family and friends is important. An unusual symptom complex occurs in patients with third ventricle cysts and other midline mass lesions in which the paroxysms of headaches are associated with sudden brief loss of consciousness or sudden loss of muscle tone causing drop attacks.

Neurologic abnormalities may be readily evident or may be quite subtle and uncovered only by careful examination. Unilateral anosmia may be the clue to a subfrontal meningioma. Bitemporal visual field impairment often exists without the patient being aware of it. Afferent pupillary defect (Marcus Gunn's pupil) may be the only sign of compression of the anterior visual pathway. Lesions in the region of aqueduct such as pinealoma may be quite silent other than headache, but the clinical syndrome, consisting of decreased upgaze, small pupils and lid retraction, provides the clue. Temporal lobe mass may be suggested by upper quadrantic visual field defect ("pie in the sky defect"). Masses in the midline of the cerebellum cause severe difficulty with gait, but relatively little abnormality might be found when the patient is examined in bed. Elementary neurologic examination may be entirely normal in some lesions of the frontal and medial temporal lobes, but careful documentation of behavior and mental state will lead to the diagnosis.

The need for laboratory investigation of intracranial mass lesion is determined by a combination of factors in the history and physical examination. The presence of neurologic symptoms other than those characteristic of migraine and/or abnormal neurologic signs, including personality and behavioral change are serious indications. Headache of recent onset that is persistent or progressive and that cannot be diagnosed as a specific headache syndrome should be worked up further despite normal clinical neurologic examination. The specific tests, CT scan of brain, EEG, angiography, have been outlined previously.

KEY FEATURES

MIGRAINE
Diagnosis
Diagnosis is based on clinical analysis of history and normal physical examination.

There are no diagnostic laboratory abnormalities.

The migraine episode is characterized by a constellation of focal neurologic, autonomic, gastrointestinal, and behavioral accompaniments.

Long-term history reveals influence of endocrine milestones, vasoactive drugs, and age.

Migraine diathesis, in the family and in childhood (motion sickness, cyclical vomiting, recurrent benign abdominal pain), provides supportive evidence.

Laboratory Investigation
May be necessary to rule out disorders that mimic migraine and is indicated in the first episodes of complicated migraine and in migraine with systemic illness, abrupt change in character, or explosive onset of headache.

ESR, ANA: Migraine syndrome may occur in patients with systemic lupus erythematosus (SLE); these tests may be helpful.

CT scan with contrast: Helps rule out intracranial vascular malformations (headaches and visual disturbances always affecting same side) and a giant aneurysm (simulates ophthalmoplegic migraine).

EEG: Useful in the rare instance of cephalgia as an ictal manifestation. Migraine patients often have dysrhythmic abnormalities.

Lumbar puncture: To rule out subarachnoid hemorrhage when headaches appear explosively.

Cerebral angiography: May be needed in the first episode of ophthalmoplegic or retinal migraine to rule out carotid aneurysm.

Treatment
Abortive treatment: Tailored to severity and frequency of headaches. Aspirin, other nonsteroidal anti-inflammatory drugs, and ergotamine.

Prophylaxis
Indicated for severe frequent headaches (>3/month)

Choice of drug depends on associated medical problems, side effects, and contraindications. Propranolol, methysergide, amitriptyline, calcium channel blockers.

CLUSTER HEADACHE

Diagnosis
1. Clinical picture is distinctive
2. Predominance in young men
3. Headache accompanied by ipsilateral conjunctival injection, eye tearing, nasal stuffiness, transient Horner's syndrome
4. Prominent creases on face
5. Clustering of headaches. Nocturnal periodicity. In initial episodes, rule out iritis, acute glaucoma, dental abscess, sinusitis

Abortive Treatment
1. IM ergotamine or dihydroergotamine
2. Inhalation of 100% oxygen 10 L/minute for 10 minutes

Prophylactic Treatment
1. Necessary for the duration of cluster
2. Ergotamine
3. Propranolol
4. Lithium carbonate indicated in patients >40 years and in chronic cluster
5. Prednisone: Short courses for intractable headache

TENSION HEADACHE

Diagnosis
1. Diagnosis is clinical; overlaps common migraine
2. Nonepisodic, pressure or band-like pain
3. Normal clinical examination
4. Look for depression, anxiety, regional dysfunction such as temporomandibular joint disease

Treatment
1. Supportive rapport with patient
2. Non-narcotic analgesics
3. Amitriptyline
4. Biofeedback
5. Treat aggravating regional disturbances such as cervical spondylosis

POST-TRAUMATIC HEADACHES

Headache from Intracranial Mass Lesion
Diagnosis: Persistent or worsening headache, alteration of consciousness, focal neurologic symptoms, behavioral changes, "mechanical" qualities to headache should arouse suspicion.

CT scan: sensitive test. Beware of pitfall of isodense lesions such as subacute subdural hematoma. "Hypernormal scan," a scan read as pseudotumor cerebri, is suspicious of bilateral isodense subdural hematomas.

Radionuclide brain scan is helpful in isodense subdural hematoma;

cerebral angiography occasionally needed in such cases, especially if bilateral.

Headache of Post-concussion Syndrome

Diagnosis is based on clinical examination. Headache as part of multisymptomatic syndrome. No alteration of consciousness or no abnormal neurologic symptoms or signs.

Treatment: reassurance, amitriptyline, follow-up.

Post-traumatic Migraine

Diagnosis by history and normal physical examination. Responds to propranolol prophylaxis.

Post-traumatic Dysautonomic Cephalgia

Diagnosis is based on recurrent headaches, accompanied by hemifacial hyperhidrosis and pupillary dilation after anterior neck injury.

Treatment: Propranolol; self-limited course.

GIANT CELL ARTERITIS (GCA)

Headache is the presenting symptom. High degree of suspicion is essential to diagnose this condition before devastating blindness occurs. The following features of headache should suggest GCA: new onset in elderly person, duration of days to a few months. Typical headaches are centered over temporal area, being burning and constant with throbbing or lancing exacerbations. Exacerbations occur at night, by cold, by contact with scalp.

Headache may be entirely nonspecific.

Headache accompaniments include: jaw claudication, unilateral or bilateral visual impairment, polymyalgia rheumatica.

Physical signs strongly suggestive of GCA include tender, nonpulsatile temporal arteries. Tender nodules over temporal, occipital areas may be seen.

Biopsy-proven GCA may have clinically normal temporal arteries.

Laboratory Abnormalities

ESR >100 mm is the rule, but nearly 30% may be normal.

Temporal artery biopsy is diagnostic.

If one side is negative, asymptomatic side may be positive.

Differential Diagnosis

Carotid aneurysm, ophthalmoplegic migraine.

Treatment

Corticosteroids should be started before vision is affected. When clinical suspicion is strong, steroids should be started urgently, pending biopsy.

HEADACHE OF INTRACRANIAL MASS LESIONS

History

The headaches are often nondescript, resembling tension or vascular headaches. Temporal profile of short duration, persistence, and progressive course is much more important.

"Mechanical features," positional variations, diurnal fluctuation, awakening from sleep by headache, obscurations of vision, and diplopia are suggestive.

Paroxysms of headache with brief loss of consciousness or drop attacks are suggestive of mass lesions in or close to ventricular cavities.

Physical Examination

Abnormalities may be subtle.

Anosmia, field defects, afferent pupillary defect, gait disturbance, personality and behavioral abnormalities should be sought in patients with apparently normal examination.

Laboratory Investigation

Required when headaches are accompanied by neurologic symptoms (other than those typical of migraine) and/or signs.

Even when clinical neurologic examination is normal, investigation is indicated in cases in which headache is of new onset and progressive and is not explicable as a well-defined headache disease such as migraine. MRI scan is superior to CT scan in detecting lesions in the posterior fossa and pituitary region.

BIBLIOGRAPHY

1. Lance JW: Neurological progress: Headache. Ann Neurol 10:1–10, 1981.

   Good concise review of etiology, pathogenesis, and treatment of migraine, cluster, and tension headaches with brief review of temporal arteritis, carotodynia, trigeminal neuralgia, the novel neck-tongue syndrome, cough, and coital headaches. About 90 references.

Migraine

2. Saper JR: State of the art: Migraine. Part I: Classification and pathogenesis. Part II: Treatment. JAMA 239:2380–2383, 2480–2484, 1978.

   A comprehensive review of all aspects of migraine.

3. Bickerstaff ER: Basilar artery migraine. Lancet 1:15–17, 1961.

   The paper delineates a distinctive subtype of migraine, based on a study of 34 patients. It occurs in adolescent girls with a family history of migraine. The premonitory phase consists of visual impairment; vertigo; ataxia; dysarthria; and numbness of face, tongue, and body. As these fade, a throbbing headache sets in.

4. Carroll D: Retinal migraine. Headache 10:9–13, 1970.

   This paper describes a rare variant in the group of recurrent episodes of transient monocular visual loss without headache. Sometimes permanent field defects remain.

5. Brandt KD, Lessel S: Migrainous phenomenon in systemic lupus erythematosus. Arthritis Rheumat 21:7–16, 1978.

   This paper describes migraine-like episodes with visual hallucinations in 11 patients with SLE. The headaches correlated with disease flare-ups and responded to steroid therapy better than to conventional antimigraine medications.

6. Mayer JS, Hardenberg J: Clinical effectiveness of calcium entry blockers in prophylactic treatment of migraine and cluster headaches. Headache 23:266–272, 1983.
    Thirteen patients with classic migraine, fourteen with common migraine, and eight with cluster headaches were treated with calcium channel blockers in a double-blind, cross-over study. Nimodipine, verapamil, and nifedipine were all effective, but nimodipine was the most effective and had the fewest side effects.

7. Glista CG, Mellinger JR, Rooces ED: Familial hemiplegic migraine. Mayo Clinic Proc 50:307, 1975.
    Describes ten members of one family with hemiplegic migraine. In each person, the attacks were stereotyped and only one had persistent hemiparesis. Propranolol decreased frequency and severity of attacks.

8. Friedman AP, Haarter H, Merritt HH: Ophthalmoplegic migraine. Trans Am Neurol Assn 86:169, 1961.
    Episodes start with headache. After the headache is established, ipsilateral ocular palsy evolves, most commonly affecting the third cranial nerve and possibly including the pupil. The paresis may last for a few days to a few months. Angiography ruled out other explanations.

9. Dorfman LJ, Marshall WH, Enzmann ER: Cerebral infarction and migraine—clinical and radiological correlation. Neurology 29:317–322, 1979.
    Four young adults with migraine had CT scan evidence of cerebral infarction, two with persistent neurologic deficits, one without symptoms, and one with transient deficits.

10. Fisher CM: Late-life migraine accompaniments: Further experience. Stroke 17:1033–1042, 1986.
    This report of 85 patients is an addition to Fisher's previous report on 120 similar patients. It highlights the occurrence of migraine phenomena in the older patients, and the need to consider migraine as a cause of transient cerebral ischemia in this group. Headache is present in half of the patients. Episodes last 15–25 minutes with a build-up of scintillations and hemiparesthesias. Cerebral angiograms are normal. Episodes tend to recur over 5–10 years and run a benign course without permanent residual deficit.

Cluster Headache

11. Kudrow L: Cluster headache: Diagnosis and management. Headache 19:142–150, 1979.
    An excellent review of clinical features, subtypes, pathogenesis, and treatment of this syndrome, with 51 references. Good tables highlighting clinical features and treatment are provided.

12. Price RW, Posner JB: Chronic paroxysmal hemicrania. A disabling headache syndrome responding to indomethacin. Ann Neurol 3:183–184, 1978.
    The individual headache episodes are identical to cluster headache but recur daily for years. Response to indomethacin is striking.

13. Lance JE, Curran DA: Treatment of chronic tension headache. Lancet 1:1236–1239, 1964.
    This study documents the efficacy of amitriptyline in chronic tension headache, with over 50% good response, becoming more than 80% in patients of 60 years of age.

14. Diamond S: Depression and headache. Headache 23:122–126, 1983.
    This article is a good review of depression presenting as headache. It emphasizes the prevalence of this condition, the "tension headache" quality, and the need to probe into

the history to elicit the masked depression. Reviews the good response to tricyclic anti-depressants.

15. Vijayan N: A new post-traumatic headache syndrome: Clinical and therapeutic observation. Headache 17:19–22, 1977.

    Article describes seven patients with episodic frontotemporal headache accompanied by transient ipsilateral facial sweating and dilation of pupils. Patients had anterior neck injuries. Partial damage of sympathetic nerves in the neck is the postulated mechanism. Patients responded to propranolol but not to ergotamine.

16. Goodman BW: Review: Temporal arteritis. Am J Med 67:839–852, 1979.

    A masterly review of all aspects of giant cell arteritis, including the pitfalls in diagnosis and a review of treatment (165 references).

17. Lance JW: Headaches related to sexual activity. J Neurol Neurosurg Psychiat 39:1226–1236, 1976.

    Article describes this condition under recognized benign syndrome of recurrent tension-like headaches occurring during sexual excitement or vascular-type headache during orgasm occurring without evidence of structural lesion and a benign course. Only 2 of the 21 patients had mild neurologic symptoms associated with headaches.

Aneurysmal Subarachnoid Hemorrhage

Joe I. Ordia, M.D.

Spontaneous subarachnoid hemorrhage (SAH) is nontraumatic bleeding that occurs primarily within the subarachnoid space. The incidence in the United States is about 11 per 100,000 population. Of the estimated 26,000 cases seen annually, 80% are due to a ruptured berry aneurysm.[1] Hypertension atherosclerosis, ruptured arteriovenous malformation (AVM), coagulopathy, and bleeding into a tumor account for most of the others. After age 20 years, aneurysms are more prevalent than AVMs, with a peak incidence in the fifth and sixth decades. There is a slight female preponderance. Histologically, these aneurysms involve defects in the media (absence of the internal elastic lamina) and degeneration of the intima.

When a spontaneous SAH occurs, a definitive diagnosis may not be immediately apparent, but a ruptured aneurysm must be assumed until proved otherwise. The condition is characterized by an explosive headache of sudden onset. However, the severe headache may be preceded by milder "sentinel headaches" caused by small "warning leaks."[2] The headache may be accompanied by nausea and vomiting, loss of consciousness, lethargy, or photophobia. Seizure is the presenting feature in 5% of cases. An occasional patient presents in an acute confusional state without complaining of head-ache. Ptosis and diplopia occur from direct compression of the oculomotor nerve. Nuchal rigidity, low-grade fever, and other signs of meningeal irritation are common. Hemiparesis, facial palsy, and aphasia may be present. Subhyaloid hemorrhages are characteristic findings on funduscopy; papilledema may occur 12–24 hours later. Some patients have ECG changes (Q waves, elevated ST segment, inverted T waves) suggestive of a myocardial infarction, but these are usually transient. The level of consciousness is the single most important prognostic sign, and it is the basis of all the grading systems.[3–5] The World Federation of Neurological Surgeons (WFNS) has proposed a new scale[5] based on the Glasgow Coma Scale (GCS). The Botterell classification is frequently used and is summarized as follows:

Grade 1: Conscious, with or without signs of subarachnoid blood
Grade 2: Drowsy, without significant deficit
Grade 3: Drowsy and confused or with minimal deficit
Grade 4: Deteriorating with major neurologic deficit
Grade 5: Moribund, with vegetative disturbance and extensor rigidity

Patients 50 years or older or who have an associated major medical problem are dropped an additional grade. Grade 4 and 5 patients are rarely candidates for aneurysm surgery. They may, however, undergo evacuation of intracerebral hematoma or ventriculostomy or CSF shunting for relief of hydrocephalus.

Computed tomography (CT) can establish the diagnosis of SAH in about 90% of cases and is the initial test of choice. The amount of subarachnoid blood on CT is of value in predicting the severity of vasospasm.[6] CT scan is useful to recognize hydrocephalus, intracerebral hematoma, cerebral infarction, and cerebral edema.

Lumbar puncture (LP) may be hazardous if there is an intracranial hematoma or a ventricular obstruction. It is to be avoided in such cases because of the risk of transtentorial herniation. In cases in which there are no such contraindications, this author favors at least an initial LP. If a rebleed is suspected, the baseline RBC count is used for comparison. In patients with symptomatic communicating hydrocephalus, serial LPs to reduce CSF pressure may be extremely helpful.

Ruptured aneurysms are notorious for high mortality rates. About one third of the victims die before they reach the hospital. Results of early surgical obliteration reported in earlier series were dismal. In a series of 228 patients, Graf reported a 44.5% mortality rate among patients operated upon within 14 days and a 23.2% death rate in those operated upon after 2 weeks.[7] The recently insulted brain is swollen, tight, fragile, and difficult to retract. Vasospasm impairs cerebral perfusion. There is, however, an increasing role for early aneurysm surgery (i.e., within 3 days of the SAH), particularly in grades 1 and 2 patients.[8,9]

The frequently inevitable delay of operation is fraught with the risks of recurrent hemorrhage and vasospasm. The highest frequency of rebleeding is during the first 2 weeks, reaching a peak during the fifth to ninth day. In the Cooperative Aneurysm Study (CAS), 23.7% of patients treated with bed rest alone hemorrhaged during this peak period.[10] Such bleeding carries a mortality rate of 85.5%. After 6 weeks, the rate of secondary hemorrhage is about 3% per year. Vasospasm is thought to be due to the release of vasoactive breakdown products of subarachnoid blood. Serotonin, norepinephrine, oxy-hemoglobin, prostaglandins, and thromboxane have all been implicated. The clinical syndrome of delayed ischemic deficit (DID)[11] rarely develops before the third day, but reaches a peak around day 8.

During the first 2 weeks following an SAH, medical therapy is directed at prevention of rebleeding and vasospasm. The principles involved are regulated bed rest,[10] antihypertensive therapy, and antifibrinolytic therapy. Strict bed rest is enforced. The head of the bed is elevated 15–30 degrees. Turning is allowed so as to avoid decubitus ulcers. The vital signs; level of consciousness; and verbal, motor, and pupillary responses are checked frequently. Taking of rectal temperatures is avoided. The lighting is subdued. Radio and television are not allowed, and visitors are limited to close relatives. A soft diet is ordered. Grade 4 and 5 patients may require tube feeding. Stool softeners (Colace, Metamucil) help to regulate bowel movements. Fluid and electrolyte balance is maintained. Airway and oxygenation are closely monitored. All patients receive seizure prophylaxis, and headaches are treated with analgesics. Intractable headaches that are due to communicating hydrocephalus may respond to LP. The agitated patient is mildly sedated with phenobarbital, chloral hydrate, or librium. Elastic stockings or pneumatic compression boots are utilized, and passive range of motion exercises are performed to reduce thromboembolic complications. Antihypertensive therapy reduces systolic thrust on the fragile wall of the aneurysm. The goal is normotension with blood pressure at levels adequate for cerebral perfusion. Hypotension must be avoided because it predisposes the patient to infarction. The systolic pressure is kept between 110 and 160 mmHg.

Subarachnoid blood activates the conversion of plasminogen to plasmin, an active fibrinolysin. This lyses the clot that seals the site of aneurysmal leak. Epsilon-aminocaproic acid (EACA or Amicar) blocks the conversion of inactive plasminogen to plasmin.[12] A daily dosage of 24–36 gm dissolved in 500 ml of 5% dextrose in water is given as a constant intravenous infusion. Absorption via the oral route (2.0–2.5 gm q2h) is variable, and diarrhea is common. In the Cooperative Aneurysm Study, patients receiving EACA had a 10% incidence of rebleeding in the first 2 weeks, compared with 22.6% in patients randomized to bed rest alone.[13] Some centers in Europe use the highly potent amino-methyl-cyclohexane carboxylic acid or tranexamic acid (AMCHA). Antifibrinolytic therapy increases the risk of thromboembolism and is contraindicated in pregnancy. Restlessness, psychosis, and increased incidence of hydrocephalus have been reported with antifibrinolysins. The protective effect of antifibrinolytic therapy is neutralized by the increased mortality from ischemic complications.[14]

Cerebral vasospasm presents the ultimate in therapeutic difficulty. Although kanamycin and reserpine deplete the amount of circulating serotonin, they have not proved to be effective against vasospasm and are no longer used. Nimodipine and other calcium channel blockers are potent cerebral vasodilators.[15] They are the subject of ongoing investigations, and they may provide effective therapy for cerebral vasospasm.[16] Until a direct treatment is available, our current efforts are directed at ameliorating its effect on the brain. Intravascular volume expansion is achieved with colloid or blood to improve cerebral perfusion. Hemodilution may enhance oxygen delivery. The systolic pressure is kept between 140 and 160 mmHg (up to 200 mmHg if the aneurysm has been successfully clipped) with phenylephrine or dopamine. If the CT scan shows cerebral swelling or edema, steroids (dexamethazone) are administered.

After 2 weeks, grade 1, 2, and 3 patients undergo complete cerebral angiography. Those without significant vasospasm undergo surgery. Advances in microsurgical techniques have remarkably improved the results of intracranial operations. Clipping is the procedure of choice. Other strategies include obliteration of the neck with a ligature, wrapping with muscle, encasement in self-hardening plastics, and carotid ligation. Angiography is repeated after another 2 weeks if surgery was further delayed because of vasospasm, and also in patients in whom the source of hemorrhage was not apparent on the initial study. Spasm, thrombosis, and edema may preclude angiographic visualization of an aneurysm. Grade 4 and 5 patients are rarely candidates for aneurysm surgery. The regulated bed rest and antifibrinolytic therapy are discontinued 3 weeks after the last hemorrhage.

KEY FEATURES

Spontaneous subarachnoid hemorrhage (SAH) is frequently the result of a ruptured aneurysm. About a third of the patients die before they can be hospitalized. Half of those admitted soon after the hemorrhage die during the hospitalization, primarily from rebleeding, cerebral vasospasm, and infarction. Attempts to forestall these devastating events by early surgery have met with only limited success.

Diagnostic steps include a high degree of clinical suspicion, CT scan of the brain, LP in selected cases, and cerebral angiography.

Surgical outcome is better if surgery is delayed for about 2 weeks to allow the swollen brain to relax and the peak period of rebleed and vasospasm to pass.

Medical management during this period is aimed at preventing recurrent bleeding and vasospasm. The cardinal aspects of treatment are as follows:

1. Regulated bed rest
2. Antihypertensive therapy
3. Antifibrinolytic therapy

There are promising results with new calcium channel blockers in the management of vasospasm.

REFERENCES

1. Kurtzke JF: Epidemiology of cerebrovascular disease. Joint Council CVD, Survey Report, Rochester, MN, Whiting Press, 1980.
   Incidence of SAH: 11 per 100,000 population.

2. LeBlanc R: The minor leak preceding subarachnoid hemorrhage. J Neurosurg 66:35–39, 1987.
   Thirty-nine per cent of patients with aneurysmal SAH had a preceding "warning leak."

3. Botterell EH, Longheed WM, Scott JW, Vandeweter SL: Hypothermia and interruption of carotid, or carotid and vertebral, circulation in the surgical management of intracranial aneurysms. J Neurosurg 13:1–42, 1956.
   A neurologic grading system for patients with SAH is described.

4. Nibbelink DW, Forner JC, Henderson WG: Intracranial aneurysms and subarachnoid hemorrhage—report on a randomized treatment study. Stroke 8:202–218, 1977.
   Cooperative Aneurysm Study Neurological Status Scale is given as follows:
   Grade 1: Symptom free
   Grade 2: Minor symptoms (headaches, meningeal irritation, diplopia)
   Grade 3: Major neurologic deficit, but fully responsive
   Grade 4: Impaired state of alertness but capable of protective or other adaptive responses to noxious stimuli
   Grade 5: Poorly responsive but with stable vital signs
   Grade 6: No response to address or shaking, non-adaptive response to noxious stimuli, and progressive instability of vital signs

5. Drake C: Report of World Federation of Neurological Surgeons Committee on a Universal Subarachnoid Hemorrhage Grading Scale. J Neurosurg 68:985–986, 1988.
   Proposed WFNS SAH scale is as follows:

WFNS Grade	GCS Score	Motor Deficit
I	15	Absent
II	14–13	Absent
III	14–13	Present
IV	12–7	Present or absent
V	6–3	Present or absent

6. Fisher CM, Kistler JP, Davis JM: Relation of cerebral vasospasms to subarachnoid hemorrhage visualized by computerized tomographic scanning. Neurosurgery 6:1–4, 1980.
   The amount of blood in the basal cisterns is predictive of vasospasm.

7. Graf CJ, Nibbelink DW: Cooperative study of intracranial aneurysms and subarachnoid hemorrhage: Report on a neurosurgical treatment and study: III. Intracranial Surgery. Stroke 5:557–601, 1974.

   Two hundred twenty-eight patients with aneurysms on the anterior portion of the circle of Willis were operated upon at different times. Mortality in those operated on within 14 days from the last SAH was 44.5%; after 14 days, 23.2%.

8. Hunt WE, Miller CA: The results of early operation for aneurysm. Clin Neurosurg 24:208–215, 1976.

   Early intervention is justified in a small percentage of cases with aneurysmal hemorrhage.

9. Flamm ES: The timing of aneurysm surgery 1985. Clin Neurosurg 33:145–158, 1986.

   Early surgery may improve the overall outcome.

10. Nibbelink DW, Turner JC, Henderson WG: Intracranial aneurysms and subarachnoid hemorrhage—report on a randomized treatment study. IV-A. Regulated bed rest. Stroke 8:202–221, 1977.

    Aneurysm patients randomized to 3 weeks of regulated bed rest without surgery had a dismal mortality rate of 55.1% during the mean follow-up interval of 6.5 years.

11. Fisher CM, Roberson GH, Ojemann RG: Cerebral vasospasm with ruptured saccular aneurysm—the clinical manifestations. Neurosurgery 1:245–248, 1977.

    The features of delayed ischemic deficit are described.

12. Nibbelink DW, Jacobson CD: Plasminogen depletion during administration of epsilon-aminocaproic acid. Thromb Diathes Haemorrh (Stuttg) 29:598–602, 1973.

    EACA inhibits the production of plasminogen and blocks its conversion to plasmin.

13. Adams HP Jr, Nibbelink DW, Torner JC, Sahs AL: Antifibrinolytic therapy in patients with aneurysmal subarachnoid hemorrhage. A report of the Cooperative Aneurysm Study. Arch Neurol 38:25–29, 1981.

    EACA lowers the incidence of rebleeding during the first 2 weeks following aneurysmal rupture.

14. Vermeulen M, Lindsay KW, Murray GD, et al.: Antifibrinolytic treatment in subarachnoid hemorrhage. N Engl J Med 311:432–437, 1984.

    Overall mortality is not affected by antifibrinolytic therapy.

15. Allen GS, Ahn HS, Preziosi TJ, et al: Cerebral arterial spasm—A controlled trial of Nimodipine in patients with subarachnoid hemorrhage. N Engl J Med 308:619–524, 1983.

    Nimodipine, a calcium channel blocker, produced beneficial effect. Only 1 patient died among the 56 patients in the treatment group. Eight patients out of 56 receiving placebo died.

16. Petruk KC, West M, Mohr G, et al: Nimodipine treatment in poor-grade aneurysm patients. Results of a multicenter double-blind placebo-controlled trial. J Neurosurg 68:505–517, 1988.

    Nimodipine reduces the effect of vasospasm and improves outcome in poor-grade patients with SAH.

Myasthenia Gravis

Jonathan Newmark, M.D.
Nagagopal Venna, M.D.

Though myasthenia gravis (MG) is a rare disease with an incidence of 1 in 20,000, patients may periodically require urgent attention for life-threatening but reversible paralytic crises that punctuate the chronic course of the disease. The initial diagnosis is often missed for a long time because clinical signs may be inconspicuous or atypical.

It is now established that MG is an autoimmune disease with antibodies targeted at the acetylcholine receptors on the postsynaptic membrane of skeletal neuromuscular junctions. However, the factors that incite the immune attack are not known except for the rare cases associated with D-penicillamine. The clinical hallmark of MG is weakness, worsened by exertion and improved by rest. Extraocular muscles are affected early, causing fluctuating ptosis and diplopia. Similar weakness often spreads to muscles of the face, jaw, palate, pharynx, tongue, neck, and extremities and in severe cases to diaphragm and intercostal muscles causing respiratory failure. The weakness can be remarkably asymmetrical, presenting, for example, as unilateral ptosis. Painless weakness can be brought out by exercise of specific muscles; ptosis may be readily evoked by sustained upgaze without blinking. Sparing of pupillary reflexes despite extraocular paresis is a characteristic finding. Even with prominent symptoms, objective weakness may be difficult to demonstrate. Tendon and superficial reflexes, sensation, and cerebellar function are unaffected.

More than 30 drugs are known to cause myasthenic symptoms. The physician should review the drug history of any patient in whom the diagnosis of MG is considered. A high degree of suspicion is essential for diagnosis, but confirmation is straightforward in most patients. A battery of tests that reflect different aspects of the disease should be performed to support the clinical diagnosis. The tests are also important to refute the diagnosis in patients with congenital ptosis, neurasthenia, masked depression, and other vague fluctuating symptoms incorrectly labeled myasthenic so that inappropriate and toxic treatment is avoided. The intravenous edrophonium (Tensilon) test should be done first: it can be performed simply and safely, results are immediate, and the test is positive in 90% of cases. Edrophonium reverses myasthenia by increasing acetylcholine availability at neuromuscular synapses by inhibiting cholinesterase. An intravenous line is established, and the heart rate is monitored to recognize the occasional bradycardia that may occur. Atropine 1 mg is kept ready to reverse bradycardia and/or intestinal cramps, both of which are usually trivial and transient reactions to the drug. A baseline of strength is established for the index muscles most affected or most readily testable, such as eyelids or orbicularis oculi. Forced vital capacity can be equally well tested and may be more easily quantitated. A placebo of 1 ml normal saline is injected first. Next, 0.2 cc (2 mg) of Tensilon is injected IV as a test dose. If there are no untoward effects, a further 8 mg is injected in one minute. Reversal of weakness is usually instantaneous and frequently dramatic, but lasts only about 10 minutes.

Electromyographic (EMG) examination reveals pathognomonic fatigability of neuromuscular transmission on repetitive nerve stimulation in 90% of patients when distal, proximal, and cranial muscles are sampled together. The recently developed single-fiber EMG is helpful in difficult cases. Antibodies to acetylcholine receptor protein (>5 U) are detectable in about 90% of patients and may be a valuable diagnostic aid because false positive tests are rare. Because 10% of patients with MG harbor a thymoma, chest radiograph and CT scan of the mediastinum should be obtained.

The paraneoplastic Eaton-Lambert syndrome resembles myasthenia gravis more in its name (myasthenic syndrome) than in its clinical features. The weakness is in proximal girdle muscles, but bulbar and extraocular movements are spread and EMG shows a transient increment of strength on repetitive stimulation and enhancement after brief exercise of affected muscles. There is little or no improvement with edrophonium.

Patients on maintenance therapy for MG often present with bulbar and respiratory failure that evolves with treacherous swiftness; intercurrent infection, surgery, pregnancy, aminoglycoside antibiotics, excess of anticholinesterase drugs, and abrupt withdrawal or reduction and sometimes initiation of treatment with high doses of corticosteroids may precipitate the crises but they are often spontaneous. Rarely, myasthenic crisis may be the presenting feature of myasthenia gravis. In the presence of respiratory compromise, urgent endotracheal intubation and ventilation take precedence over attempts to differentiate myasthenic crisis from cholinergic crisis. Even after the respiratory status is stabilized, this distinction may not be clear. A patient may in fact suffer simultaneously from both cholinergic excess and myasthenic weakness. For instance, some patients noticing deteriorating strength take increasing amounts of anticholinesterase drugs, so that when they arrive in crisis they show miosis and excessive secretions in the upper respiratory tract, fasciculations, and abdominal cramps, indicating cholinergic excess as well as myasthenic weakness. An edrophonium test should be performed only after the respiratory state is secure and may sometimes distinguish myasthenic crisis from acute cholinergic crisis. It is best, in any case, to withdraw cholinesterase inhibitors for several days and resume them, if needed, in smaller doses. Plasmapheresis is a useful adjunct in myasthenic crisis where it is readily available, and it may decrease the duration of the severe phase requiring intensive care. Acute, severe cases must be distinguished from Guillain-Barré syndrome, botulism, potassium-related myopathies, and acute polymyositis. With modern intensive care, crisis should represent a transient, manageable complication, rather than a fatal event.

MAINTENANCE TREATMENT

The long-term management of patients with MG is best carried out by physicians with expertise in this disease. The clinical spectrum of the disease is wide, ranging from the purely ocular form to fulminating generalized disease, although most patients experience a long course with intermittent exacerbations. Anticholinesterase drugs may suffice in symptomatic treatment of patients with mild disease. Pyridostigmine (Mestinon) is commonly used in doses of 60 mg every 3–6 hours. A long-acting preparation can be given at night. Thymectomy is indicated in most adult patients with generalized myasthenia of more than a year's duration. It is, of course, required in all patients with thymomas. Thymectomy may affect a fundamental immune pathology in MG and may produce a permanent remission in nearly 40% of patients. Adrenal corticosteroids offer another major modality of treatment of MG, to which about 80% of patients respond. Patients who are not candidates for thymectomy or who have not improved after thymectomy, and patients with generalized or oculobulbar disease who are not satisfactorily controlled by anticholinesterase drugs are appropriate candidates for steroid therapy. A commonly used method is to start prednisone at a high dose of 100 mg daily for a month, tapering to alternate-day dose very slowly. Another method is to start with a low dose of 20–30 mg/day and gradually build up the dose to 80–100 mg/day and then reach a maintenance level. The latter method produces a slower improvement but avoids the occasional worsening of MG in the first few weeks of high-dose therapy. Azathioprine is a cytotoxic immunosuppressive drug that is useful in patients who do not respond to steroids or those in whom steroids cause unacceptable side effects.

The initial enthusiasm for plasmapheresis has waned. It has become clear that plasmapheresis does not produce lasting benefit, but it is a useful adjunct in critical relapses.

Many patients with severe MG need to be on multiple modalities of therapy. For instance, a patient after thymectomy may still need to be maintained on corticosteroids and anticholinesterases at least for a few years, supplemented by plasmapheresis during exacerbations.

KEY FEATURES

Myasthenia gravis (MG) is an autoimmune disorder mediated by antibodies against postsynaptic acetylcholine receptors at skeletal neuromuscular junctions.

Clinical Characteristics
1. Weakness of muscles increased by exercise and improved by rest
2. Predilection for extraocular muscles while sparing pupils
3. Frequent involvement of facial-cervical-bulbar and limb muscles
4. Occurrence of paralytic crises with respiratory failure

Diagnostic Tests
1. IV edrophonium (Tensilon)
2. EMG with repetitive nerve stimulation
3. Single-fiber electromyography
4. Acetylcholine receptor antibodies in serum
5. Radiography and CT scan of chest for detection of thymoma

Treatment
Symptomatic Treatment
A. Myasthenic Crisis
    1. Intubation and ventilation
    2. Edrophonium (Tensilon) test to help differentiate myasthenic from cholinergic crises
    3. Treatment of precipitating factors
    4. Plasmapheresis
    5. Readjustments of maintenance drugs
B. Maintenance
    1. Anticholinesterase drugs (pyridostigmine)

Specific Treatment
1. Thymectomy in most patients
2. Adrenal corticosteroids
3. Azathioprine
4. Plasmapheresis
5. Combination of modalities just cited for severe cases

REFERENCES

1. Seybold ME: Myasthenia gravis. JAMA 250:2516, 1983.
   A good general review of all aspects of MG, including controversies in management.

2. Drachman DB: Myasthenia gravis. N Engl J Med 298:139, 298 (2 parts), 1978.
   Good review of pathophysiology by the author who elucidated many aspects of it; has clinicophysiologic correlation. Useful flow charts for choices among treatment modalities are given.

3. Perlo VP, Arnason B, Poskanzer D, et al: The role of thymectomy in the treatment of myasthenia gravis. Ann NY Acad Sci 183:308–315, 1971.
   A review of 267 patients from Massachusetts General and Mt. Sinai Hospitals who

underwent thymectomy for MG without thymoma. Seventy-six patients achieved improvement or remissions: 50% had done so by 2½ years, and 26% required more than 5 years. All age groups and both sexes responded. Remissions were permanent in all but one patient.

4. McQuillen MP, Leone MG: A treatment carol: Thymectomy revisited. Neurology 27:1103–1106, 1977.

   The authors compare five large series of patients with MG treated by thymectomy with five large series of medically treated patients from various medical centers and show the lack of evidence that thymectomy is superior in inducing remissions. Authors point out the need for randomized controlled trials to establish the role of thymectomy.

5. Pascuzzi RM, Coslett HB, Johns TR: Long-term corticosteroid treatment of myasthenia gravis: Report of 116 patients. Ann Neurol 15:291, 1984.

   A good study of the experience of long-term treatment of 116 patients with a mean follow-up of 3–8 years, ages 8–82 years. Twenty-seven per cent of patients achieved remission, 52% had marked improvement, and 14% had moderate improvement, within 3 weeks in most. The median time for maximal improvement was 6 months. Ten patients experienced severe exacerbations requiring assisted ventilation, all with 2 weeks of therapy. The maximal improvement was maintained for the duration of follow-up. Although patients noted on/off phenomenon on alternate-day therapy, this eventually disappeared.

6. Hertel G, Merteaus HG, Reuther P, Ricker K: The treatment of myasthenia gravis with azathioprine. In Dan PC (ed): Plasmapheresis and Immunosuppression of Myasthenia Gravis. Boston, Houghton-Mifflin, 1975, pp 315–318.

   The largest series to date of 250 patients treated with 150–200 mg of azathioprine a day for as long as 15 years. Onset of improvement occurred gradually over 2–12 months. Transient exacerbations sometimes seen with a steroid therapy did not occur. Side effects were minor.

7. Newsom-David J, et al: Long-term effects of repeated plasma exchange in myasthenia gravis. Lancet 1:464–468, 1979.

   Study of six patients treated with plasmapheresis. Concludes that the therapy is effective in the short term but that it provided no cumulative long-term benefit.

8. Argov Z, Mastaglia FL: Disorders of neuromuscular transmission caused by drugs. N Engl J Med 301:409–413, 1979.

   Article lists an alarming number of drugs that have been shown to cause myasthenic symptoms, with brief discussion of pathophysiology.

9. Rowland LP: Controversies in the treatment of myasthenia gravis. J Neurol Neurosurg Psychiat 43:654–659, 1980.

   This is a masterly systematic review addressing specific dilemmas facing the clinician. There is a critical assessment of limitation of the Tensilon test in distinguishing cholinergic from myasthenic crisis. Anticholinesterase drugs, corticosteroids, thymectomy, azathioprine, and plasmapheresis are all critically examined and put in perspective. There is a sobering table of 30 unanswered questions in the treatment of MG!

10. Tindall RSA, Rollins JA, Phillips JA, et al: Preliminary results of a double-blind, randomized, placebo-controlled trial of cyclosporine in myasthenia gravis. N Engl J Med 316:719–724, 1987.

    This report adds another form of immunotherapy for patients with myasthenia gravis. Twenty patients with generalized MG of recent onset not controlled by acetylcholine-esterases were randomly assigned to cyclosporine or placebo. Over a treatment period of 1 year, clinical improvement and decline in acetylcholine receptor antibodies were better than in the placebo group. If these findings are confirmed in further trials, cyclosporine would be a useful adjunct to the treatment of MG, especially for patients unable to tolerate steroids.

Dizziness and Vertigo: Part I

Nagagopal Venna, M.D.

Dizziness, a common and often disabling symptom, often elicits a less than enthusiastic response from the physician because of its reputation as a symptom for which satisfactory explanation is rarely uncovered. This in turn leads to a sense of desperation and abandonment in the patient. However, with the application of a systematic clinical method and the use of selected laboratory tests and consultation, accurate diagnosis can be reached in many instances, providing the basis for rational management.

CLINICAL APPROACH

Careful and focused history and physical examination are indispensable. At first, it should be determined whether the patient's dizziness is vertigo or not. Vertigo is a hallucination of rotation or, less commonly, linear displacement of the body or of the environment. Out of the amorphous array of sensations described as dizziness, vertigo crystallizes the problem as vestibular derangement. The patient is asked to describe nonrotatory sensations without using the word "dizziness." Patients usually describe their feeling as lightheadedness, wooziness, drunkenness, faintness, imbalance, or anxiety. These are less specific than vertigo and need a broader-based approach because their mechanisms range from postural hypotension to hyperventilation. Presyncope should be identified when patients describe episodes of dizziness, lightheadedness, or faintness, occurring over a period of a few minutes and sometimes associated with graying of vision, perspiration, and pallor. Such spells indicate cardiac or vasovagal dysfunction or postural hypotension. A caveat is that patients with vestibular disease sometimes present with ill-defined giddiness rather than with vertigo. Provocative factors for dizziness are probed next. A key feature is the effect of changes in head and body position. Benign and central positional vertigo syndromes are defined by their specific induction by head turning, looking up, or turning to one side. Dizziness of postural hypotension occurs on standing, especially after prolonged rest. Many patients with constant dizziness experience worsening by postural change, but this feature is not diagnostically critical. Vertigo provoked by Valsalva's maneuver suggests craniocervical junction abnormality, whereas dizziness brought on by hyperventilation indicates psychogenic mechanisms. Vertigo provoked by coughing and sneezing occurs in perilymphatic fistula. Dizziness without external provocation may be due to disorders like cardiac arrhythmias and vertebrobasilar ischemia migraine.

Dizziness Accompaniments: Regional

Certain symptoms linked to vertigo—oscillopsia (i.e., illusion of to-and-fro movement of the environment), nausea, vomiting, and prostration—are not diagnostically helpful. The clue to the cause of dizziness often lies in its regional accompaniments. Ear symptoms of fullness, tinnitus, and decreased hearing characterize Ménière's disease. Deafness, hemifacial paresthesias, and facial paresis typify cerebellopontine angle (CPA) lesions such as acoustic neuroma. Limb ataxia with or without gait ataxia is the hallmark of cerebellar dysfunction, whereas brain stem disease produces dizziness accompanied by dysarthria, diplopia, bilateral facial or limb paresthesias, weakness, and drop attacks. Epileptic dizziness may be accompanied by absences and automatisms. Dizziness with headache and visual aura suggests migraine, whereas perioral and digital paresthesias suggest hyperventilation syndrome.

Constructing the temporal profile of the symptoms facilitates differential diagnosis. A monophasic illness with acute persistent dizziness suggests vestibular neuronitis, whereas chronic recurrent episodic dizziness represents benign positional vertigo. Chronic nonepisodic dizziness is usually part of a psychogenic or multisensory disorder.

Physical Examination

The general physical examination should focus on cardiac disease in the form of arrhythmias, valvular disease, and hypertension. Blood pressure is determined in supine and upright postures. Dizziness-provoking tests are key steps in the diagnosis. The *Nylen-Bárány maneuver* is the basis of defining peripheral and central positional vertigo syndromes. After explanation, the patient is seated at the edge of the examining table and the head is quickly lowered to 45 degrees from the body and turned 45 degrees to one side. In this head-hanging position, induced vertigo and nystagmus are observed and characterized. The test is repeated after return to sitting position with the head hanging and turned to the other side. Critical features to note are severity of vertigo, latency, direction, duration, and fatigability of nystagmus on repeated testing. Electronystagmography is not a substitute for this bedside test. Valsalva's maneuver and a few minutes of hyperventilation are other provocative tests and become significant when the patient's symptoms are reproduced. In patients with vertigo after head trauma or barotrauma, the fistula test may identify oval/round window rupture, a potentially curable cause of vertigo. To perform the test, the tragus of the ear is firmly and quickly pressed into the ear canal. Better still, the external canal pressure is increased by pneumatic otoscope. When the fistula test is positive, a bout of vertigo and nystagmus is induced.

Careful neurologic examination is necessary. Attention is paid to inspection of the ear; hearing acuity; Rinne's and Weber's tests; corneal reflexes; facial weakness; and limb, trunk, and gait ataxia. In a patient with acute vertigo, inability to stand or walk may be the only clue to cerebellar infarction or hemorrhage. Absence of corneal reflex on the deaf side is a telltale sign of acoustic neuroma. An assessment is made of the patient's overall behavior, mood, and thought content, looking for clues for psychiatric illness.

Laboratory Examination

Numerous laboratory tests are available, but they must be selected on the basis of the clinical picture. Inappropriate tests often obscure the correct diagnosis. The vestibular system can be tested by electronystagmography (ENG) and caloric testing. ENG is especially useful to detect and characterize clinically inapparent nystagmus, as in some cases of positional vertigo, Ménière's disease, or vestibular neuronitis, after the acute illness has subsided. For technical reasons, positional nystagmus evident clinically may not be recorded by ENG. Regional pathology is studied by audiometry, which characterizes fluctuating sensorineural deafness in Ménière's disease and steadily progressive deafness in acoustic neuroma, and helps distinguish conductive deafness from nerve deafness. The auditory pathways are physiologically tested by brain stem auditory evoked response (BAER), which is sensitive for acoustic neuroma and brain stem diseases like multiple sclerosis.

Anatomy of the petrous bone, cerebellar pontine angle area, cerebellum, and brain stem can now be elegantly and noninvasively studied by CT scanning. In acute vertigo, noncontrast study is appropriate so that cerebellar infarction or hemorrhage can be detected. When cerebellar stroke is suspected but the immediate scan is negative, it is critical to repeat the test in a few days. In recurrent or chronic cases, a contrast scan gives a better yield for tumors in the posterior fossa. Acoustic neuroma is often isodense with brain and, unless large, may be missed on a plain study. In cases of recurrent dizziness that are due to temporal lobe seizure, electroencephalogram (EEG) is the key to diagnosis. Serologic tests for syphilis are performed in Ménière's syndrome because both acquired and congenital syphilis may produce it. Erythrocyte sedimentation rate (ESR) and antinuclear antibody (ANA) may be needed in the rare cases of arteritis involving the labyrinthine artery presenting with acute vertigo and deafness. Consultations with an otolaryngologist and cardiologist and neurologist or psychiatrist are obtained based on thorough initial evaluation. In elderly patients with chronic imbalance, it is wise to rule out hypothyroidism by thyroid function tests.

KEY FEATURES

Systematic, focused history and examination are critical for diagnosis.

Determine if dizziness means vertigo, which implies vestibular dysfunction.

Identify presyncope, because it is always cardiovascular in its etiology.

Determine if dizziness is spontaneous or provoked.

Determine regional *dizziness accompaniments* referable to derangement in specific systems:

- Auditory
- Cerebellar pontine angle structures
- Cerebellum
- Brain stem
- Cerebral hemispheres (seizure phenomena)
- Widespread cerebral disturbances (migraine, presyncope)

Determine the psychiatric history as appropriate.

Determine the temporal profile.

Physical examination is as follows:

A. General examination

B. Regional examination
   1. Auditory: Hearing acuity, Rinne's and Weber's tests
   2. Neurologic: Corneal reflexes, facial strength, cerebellar/brain stem function

C. Dizziness-provoking tests
   1. Nylen-Bárány positional testing
   2. Fistula test
   3. Valsalva's maneuver
   4. Hyperventilation

D. Psychiatric assessment

The laboratory evaluation is tailored to the clinical setting. The following tests may be used:

   1. Electronystagmography (ENG)
   2. Caloric tests
   3. Audiometry
   4. CT scan of posterior fossa

Dizziness and Vertigo: Part II

Nagagopal Venna, M.D.

The etiologic diagnosis of dizziness syndromes is facilitated by subdivision into three groups, based on temporal profile.

GROUP A: ACUTE MONOPHASIC PERSISTENT VERTIGO

Patients present with acute prolonged vertigo lasting hours to days. The clinical setting and selected laboratory tests enable diagnosis in most instances.

Vestibular Neuronitis. This occurs most often in the third and the fourth decades with acute vertigo, unaccompanied by auditory or neurologic symptoms and often preceded by recent upper respiratory infection, measles, infectious mononucleosis, or similar illness in the family. Physical examination shows spontaneous unidirectional nystagmus away from the affected ear while hearing, and neurologic functions are normal. Audiometry confirms lack of cochlear dysfunction, but caloric tests show vestibular paresis. A similar illness plus peripheral facial paralysis and vesicles on the external ear indicates herpes zoster oticus (Ramsay Hunt syndrome). Signs of brain stem dysfunction (internuclear ophthalmoplegia, optic neuritis) may indicate that the illness is part of multiple sclerosis. The course is benign with spontaneous resolution in 4–6 weeks, although positional vertigo may persist for 6 months. Recurrences are rare, and treatment is symptomatic.

Ménière's Disease. The first attack of Ménière's disease may simulate vestibular neuronitis closely. Although it is typically accompanied by auditory symptoms, these may be absent in the early attacks. Onset in middle or late life and further course clarify the diagnosis.

Brain Stem–Cerebellar Infarction and Cerebellar Hemorrhage. Cerebellar infarction or hemorrhage and brain stem infarction in the territories of posterior inferior, anterior inferior, and superior cerebellar arteries (PICA, AICA, and SCA, respectively) present with acute vertigo and ataxia. The principal clue is the clinical setting—an elderly person with hypertension, diabetes, or heart disease. In cerebellar stroke there is nystagmus, usually to the side of the lesion, and ipsilateral limb ataxia. In midline lesions, the only accompanying finding may be inability to walk. CT is sensitive to hemorrhage, but infarction is easily missed because of bone artifact or because the scan is performed too early. The PICA, AICA, and SCA occlusions are diagnosed by the unique constellation of neurologic signs accompanying the vertigo and nystagmus, and CT scan is usually normal. Small cerebellar strokes are liable to be misdiagnosed as vestibular neuronitis or Ménière's disease; thus, a high degree of suspicion should be maintained in older patients with cardiovascular disease.

GROUP B: CHRONIC RECURRENT EPISODIC DIZZINESS

These patients present with episodic vertigo of minutes to hours punctuated by asymptomatic periods and recurring over months to years.

Benign Positional Vertigo (BPV). This common cause of recurrent vertigo is frequently missed. The bouts of vertigo last less than a minute and are provoked specifically by movements of the head, as in suddenly turning the head to one side, rolling over on the side in bed, and looking up to reach overhead. There are no neurologic or auditory accompaniments. The Nylen-Bárány test usually establishes the diagnosis by inducing a characteristic prominent positional vertigo accompanied by nystagmus. In the head-hanging lateral position, undirectional rotatory-upbeat nystagmus appears after 10–15 seconds and away from the undermost ear. Nystagmus is transient despite maintaining the head position and fatigues on repeated testing. The rest of the examination is normal. Diagnosis is clinical, but caution is needed because positional vertigo and nystagmus can be due to lesions in the posterior fossa (acoustic neuroma, cerebellar metastases, or multiple sclerosis). In this central positional vertigo, nystagmus appears without a latency in head-hanging position and lasts as long as the position is maintained; the direction of nystagmus changes in different head positions, and there may be downbeat nystagmus. It does not fatigue with repeated testing, and dizziness is mild.

Audiometry is normal whereas caloric tests show vestibular paresis in a third of cases and electronystagmography (ENG) is helpful when nystagmus is not clinically apparent. Further tests are not usually indicated but clinical follow-up is needed.

BPV often occurs as an idiopathic illness in the elderly. It also commonly follows blunt head trauma and rarely follows an attack of vestibular neuronitis. Prognosis is good, with spontaneous resolution in months. Physical therapy is sometimes helpful in symptomatic treatment.

Ménière's Disease. Recurrent episodic vertigo in the fourth to sixth decade is the hallmark of Ménière's disease. The episodes begin abruptly, last several hours to a day, and are accompanied by unilateral fullness in the ear, tinnitus, and transient hearing impairment. However, early episodes may be monosymptomatic. With repeated episodes, deafness progresses. Examination in the acute phase may reveal nystagmus away from the affected ear, sensorineural deafness, and normal neurologic function. Characteristically, hearing improves as the attack subsides. Audiogram demonstrates a sensorineural hearing loss that is most marked for low frequencies and that fluctuates on repeated testing. ENG may reveal nystagmus not clinically apparent. Caloric tests show vestibular paresis. Brain stem auditory evoked responses (BAER) are normal. ENT consultation is essential because several otologic diseases resemble Ménière's disease. A contrast-enhanced CT scan of the posterior fossa is indicated to rule out cerebellar pontine angle tumor. Because syphilitic labyrinthitis can cause Ménière's syndrome, serologic tests for syphilis are indicated. Treatment is symptomatic.

Perilymphatic Fistula. This eminently treatable cause of vertigo provoked by position, cough, and sneezing occurs as an unusual sequela to blunt head trauma or barotrauma causing rupture of the oval and/or round window. Fistula test is usually positive but diagnosis is confirmed by exploring the middle ear.

Vertebrobasilar Transient Ischemic Attacks. Vertebrobasilar occlusive disease can cause recurrent vertigo, lasting about 15 minutes and characteristically accompanied by dysarthria, diplopia, bilateral paresthesias, and drop attacks. Interval examination is normal except for evidence of cardiovascular disease. The diagnosis is clinical. Though vertigo may occur alone early on, sooner or later other symptoms of brain stem dysfunction appear with vertigo. Thus, recurrent episodes of monosymptomatic vertigo should make this diagnosis suspect.

Epileptic Vertigo. In this treatable condition, dizzy spells last a few seconds and may be accompanied by head and eye turning or brief nystagmus, nausea, tinnitus, anxiety, and contralateral paresthesias. The EEG is crucial, showing an epileptic focus in the temporal lobe or parietal association cortex. CT scan may be abnormal as well.

Cerebellar Pontine Angle Tumor. Most cerebellar pontine angle tumors present with progressive unilateral deafness and chronic dysequilibrium, but rarely recurrent vertigo may occur.

Hyperventilation. Discrete attacks of dizziness are a prominent manifestation of conditions associated with hyperventilation. Patients describe vague lightheadedness, or wooziness without nausea, vomiting, or hearing aberration, often accompanied by tingling around the lips, fingers, and toes. Patients tend to be chronically incapacitated by dizziness and may be fearful of developing symptoms in public. Physical examination is normal except for reproduction of symptoms by hyperventilation. Caloric tests may elicit histrionic or bizarre responses rather than vestibular paresis. When the patient reports vertigo, the eyes may be seen to converge, strongly indicating a psychogenic basis.

Postural Hypotension–Cardiac Arrhythmias. Postural hypotension produces recurrent faintness in an upright position and is particularly notable after prolonged bed rest. The diagnosis is easily established once it is considered. Intermittent cardiac arrhythmias and heart block are common causes of spontaneous recurrent dizziness or presyncope. Clinical cardiac examination and Holter's monitoring help confirm the diagnosis.

Alcohol-Related Vertigo. Alcohol ingestion is an important cause of positional nystagmus, sometimes associated with positional vertigo. The nystagmus usually resolves in about 12 hours after a single drink. Thus, in cases of positional vertigo, the state of alcohol intoxication must be known to interpret test results properly.

Migraine and Benign Paroxysmal Vertigo. Migraine is an underrecognized cause of recurrent dizziness or vertigo in young people. It may occur as part of a widespread migraine syndrome or with vertigo as the predominant manifestation. Diagnosis is clinical, based on a personal and family history of migraine and motion sickness and on normal clinical examination. Prophylactic treatment with propranolol or pizotifen is often effective.

GROUP C: CHRONIC NONEPISODIC DIZZINESS

This large group consists of patients with more or less constant nonvertiginous dizziness accompanied by lightheadedness, a sense of imbalance, or fear of falling.

Psychogenic Dizziness. Constant dizziness is a common presenting symptom of psychological distress. Typically, patients seem to be incapacitated by the vague dizziness. Physical examination is normal, though in some patients hyperventilation provokes the symptoms. Caloric tests and audiograms are normal or produce bizarre responses. Psychiatric evaluation reveals hysteria, depression, thought disorder, or anxiety states.

Multisensory Dizziness. This is especially common in the elderly. There is a history of chronic vague dizziness and gait imbalance with or without postural fluctuation. Examination shows no nystagmus, and provocative tests are negative. However, general examination reveals multiple sensory deficits: an elderly diabetic patient with decreased vision that is due to cataracts, decreased proprioception as a result of peripheral neuropathies, and postural hypotension secondary to autonomic neuropathy is a typical example. The diagnosis is clinical. Myxedema is an important treatable cause of these symptoms that is sometimes associated with hearing impairment.

Cerebellar Pontine Angle Tumor. About 50% of patients with acoustic neuroma complain of chronic gait instability, which they may call dizziness. Frequently patients are unaware of deafness. Physical examination reveals unilateral nerve deafness and in advanced cases decreased corneal reflex and limb ataxia. Caloric tests show vestibular paresis, audiogram confirms nerve deafness, and the BAER test shows retrocochlear abnormality. Contrast-enhanced CT scan of the cerebellar pontine angle area, sometimes with tomograms of the internal auditory meatus, will establish the diagnosis.

KEY FEATURES

DIZZINESS AND VERTIGO

Acute Monophasic Persistent Vertigo
Vestibular neuronitis
Ménière's disease
Cerebellar infarction or hemorrhage
Brain stem infarction

Chronic Recurrent Episodic Dizziness
Benign positional vertigo
Ménière's disease
Vertebrobasilar transient ischemic attacks
Migraine
Hyperventilation
Epileptic vertigo
Presyncope

Chronic Nonepisodic Dizziness
Psychogenic
Multisensory deficits
Cerebellar pontine angle tumor

BIBLIOGRAPHY

1. Drachman DA, Hart CW: An approach to the dizzy patient. Neurology 22:323–334, 1972.
    This important paper outlines a systematic clinical and laboratory system that led to a satisfactory diagnosis in most patients referred for dizziness. The diagnostic breakdown reflects general experience. Causes of dizziness in 104 patients are listed (%):
    Peripheral vestibular disease: 38
    Hyperventilation syndromes and other psychiatric syndromes: 32
    Multiple sensory deficits: 13
    Brain stem vascular disease: 5
    Other neurologic disorders: 4
    Cardiovascular diseases: 4
    Multiple sclerosis: 2
    Visual disorders: 2
    Endocrine disorders: 1
    Uncertain diagnosis: 9

2. Tower HMA: Clinical algorithms: Dizziness and vertigo. Br Med J 288:1739–1743, 1984.

This is a useful algorithmic approach to dizziness and vertigo, giving a broad overview in a flow-sheet form.

3. Leherer JF, Rubin RC, Poole DC, et al: Perilymphatic fistula—a definitive and curable cause of vertigo following head trauma. Western J Med *141*:57–60, 1984.

    These 33 patients with perilymphatic fistula from rupture of oval and/or round windows after blunt head trauma had persistent vertigo, sometimes with unilateral deafness, and positive fistula test. Middle ear exploration and closure of fistula with tissue graft led to resolution of vertigo in 32 patients. In 12 of 20 patients with deafness, hearing improved. The authors recommend surgical intervention after a minimum of 3 months of symptoms to allow for patients with spontaneous resolution, and earlier intervention in patients with hearing loss. This condition should be considered in persistent vertigo after head trauma and otolaryngologic consultation obtained.

4. Huang CY, Yu YL: Small cerebellar strokes may mimic labyrinthine lesions. J Neurol Neurosurg Psychiat *48*:263–265, 1985.

    This paper shows that small infarctions or hemorrhage in the cerebellum can present with a clinical syndrome simulating acute peripheral vestibular lesions—abrupt onset of vertigo, nausea, ataxia, and unidirectional nystagmus. Headache, obtundation, and brain stem signs associated with larger lesions were absent in 6 out of 39 cases. CT scan was crucial to diagnosis. Thus, the diagnosis of vestibular neuronitis or first episode of Ménière's disease in an older patient with hypertensive and cardiovascular disease should not be accepted without ruling out cerebellar stroke.

Benign Positional Vertigo

5. Brandt T, Daroff RB: Physical therapy for benign paroxysmal positional vertigo. Arch Otolaryngol *16*:484–485, 1980.

    A regimen of positional exercises relieved BPV in 66 of 67 patients within 2 weeks. The patient sits with eyes closed and tilts the body bilaterally so that the side of the head lies on the bed until evoked vertigo subsides. The patient returns to an upright posture for 30 seconds and assumes a head-down position to the other side for 30 seconds. The sequence is repeated until no vertigo is experienced. The maneuver is repeated every 3 hours when awake until 3 consecutive vertigo-free days are achieved.

6. Gacek RR: Singular neurectomy update. Ann Otol Rhinol Laryngol *91*:469–473, 1982.

    Ninety-six surgical sections of the posterior ampullary nerve were reviewed by middle ear approach for persistent BPV. Ninety-one per cent of patients were relieved of vertigo, and 7% had sensorineural hearing loss as a complication. In the rare patients in whom disabling BPV persists beyond 1 year, singular nerve section is an effective and safe procedure in the hands of experts.

7. Carthorne T, Hinchcliffe R: Positional nystagmus of the central type as evidence of subtentorial metastases. Brain *84*:415–426, 1961.

    Six patients with cerebellar metastases presented with recent onset of vertigo and imbalance, some with positional vertigo. In all patients, "central" positional nystagmus appeared as soon as the head-hanging position was held; the nystagmus was not fatigued by repeated testing, and vertigo was mild. It is essential that if the characteristics of nystagmus do not fit those of BPV, posterior fossa lesions should be ruled out.

Epileptic Vertigo

8. Kogeorgos J, Scott DF, Swash M: Epileptic dizziness. Br Med J *282*:687–689, 1981.

    Thirty patients with temporal lobe seizures presented with dizzy spells. The episodes occurred without provocation and lasted a few seconds; many of the patients had vertigo and nausea. About 50% had episodes of absences, anxiety, and automatisms, usually independent of dizzy spells. EEG was crucial to the diagnosis. Response to anticonvulsants was good. This paper emphasizes the importance of considering temporal lobe epilepsy in patients with brief spontaneous episodic vertigo otherwise likely to be misdiagnosed as psychogenic.

Ménière's Disease

9. Dickins JRE, Graham SS: Ménière's disease 1978–1982. Am J Otol 5:137–155, 1983.
   This is a good review of diagnostic pathophysiologic, medical, surgical, and therapeutic aspects of Ménière's disease, emphasizing the areas of continued controversy (250 references).

Migraine and Vertigo

10. Behan PO, Carlin J: Benign recurrent vertigo. *In* Rose FC (ed): Advances in Migraine Research and Therapy. New York, Raven Press, 1982, pp 49–55.
    Thirty-two young patients, mostly women, had vertigo lasting hours to days and recurring over months to years. Nine patients had transient tinnitus, and two had transient decrease in hearing; 30% had headaches, and 50% experienced scintillations or scotomata. Some patients had a personal history of common or classic migraine, a family history identical to that of patients with recurrent vertigo in childhood, and in one case subsequent development of classic migraine. The clinical and laboratory evaluations were normal except for ENG findings of positional or spontaneous nystagmus. Most patients responded well to prophylaxis with pizotifen or propranolol, both established medications for migraine. The authors feel that this form of vertigo is an unrecognized variant of migraine.

Positional Vertigo

11. Janetta PJ, Moller MB, Moller AR: Disabling positional vertigo. N Engl J Med 310:1700–1705, 1984.
    Nine patients had a new syndrome characterized by chronic continuous disabling vertigo/imbalance in the upright position. Five patients had tinnitus. In seven, it was spontaneous, and in two it followed head trauma. BAER in eight patients indicated eighth cranial nerve dysfunction. Because medical therapy was unsuccessful, these patients underwent exploration of the posterior fossa and were found to have compression of the vestibular and/or cochlear nerves at the brain stem. There, nerves were decompressed by interposing soft plastic felt between vessels and nerves. All patients were relieved of vertigo in a follow-up of 5 months to 11 years.
    This report points to vascular compression of nerve roots in the rare cases of vertigo. This surgery should be undertaken only after a thorough evaluation and by surgeons with special expertise.

12. Aschan G, Bergstedt M: Positional alcoholic nystagmus in man following repeated alcohol doses. Acta Otolaryngol (suppl) 330:15, 1975.
    This paper describes the effects of alcohol ingestion on positional vertigo and nystagmus within 30 minutes of drinking moderate amounts of alcohol. Positional nystagmus appears often with vertigo. The nystagmus is right beating with the right lateral position and left beating in the left lateral position, reaching its maximum about 2 hours later. At 4 hours, the direction of nystagmus reverses and eventually subsides in 12 hours.

Acute Inflammatory Polyradiculoneuropathy: The Guillain-Barré Syndrome

Jeremy D. Schmahmann, M.D., Ch.B.
Nagagopal Venna, M.D.

Acute inflammatory polyradiculoneuropathy is a segmental demyelinating disease affecting many levels of the peripheral nervous system. Described clinically by Landry in 1859 and elaborated upon by Guillain, Barré, and Strohl in 1917, it has become known as the Guillain-Barré syndrome (GBS).[1,2] Although the cause remains under investigation, the pathogenesis appears to be an immune-mediated attack by humoral antibodies, T lymphocytes, and phagocytosing macrophages against the myelin of peripheral nerves, nerve roots, and plexuses.[3,4]

The incidence is between 1.6 and 1.9 per 100,000, and the mortality rate is 2–5%. Although it is slightly more common in adults above the age of 40, it does occur in children. Early recognition of GBS is important because of the rapidity and severity of progression; some 10–20% of patients require ventilator assistance during their course. Approximately 85% of patients make excellent clinical recovery with skilled medical and nursing care, but 10–15% are left with some degree of residual disability and about 5% experience a chronic relapsing course.[1] Recently, a syndrome clinically indistinguishable from acute GBS has been described.[14] Electrophysiologic studies, however, show severe axonal neuropathy. Long-term recovery has been poor in this subgroup of patients.

CLINICAL FEATURES

In 60–70% of cases, the precipitating event is an upper respiratory or gastrointestinal viral infection.[5] Cytomegalovirus is one of the more common (30%) among a host of viruses to be implicated, including Epstein-Barr virus (infectious mononucleosis), rubella, measles, mumps, hepatitis A and B, and echovirus. Bacterial infections, vaccinations, surgery, and traumatic injury may also be antecedents of the disease.

Following the presumed initiating event by a few days to a month (most typically 7–10 days), 55% of patients experience paresthesia and/or pain in the legs, which may be accompanied by tenderness of the muscles to palpation. This is followed in hours to a few days by a progressive weakness of both legs simultaneously and usually symmetrically in degree, ascending to involve the trunk, arms, cranial nerves, and muscles of respiration. Those most at risk for the development of respiratory failure are patients with severe quadriplegia and a predominantly proximal distribution of weakness.[5] Distal leg muscles are usually affected earlier than proximal muscles, but the reverse may occur. The motor deficit may commence in the arms and descend to the legs, or may appear (5%) only after the development of cranial nerve palsies. The time from the onset of neurologic symptoms to the maximum deficit may be a matter of hours; however, usually it is 1–2 weeks and rarely is as long as a month.

There is invariably an early severe diminution or total absence of the deep tendon reflexes, frequently with preservation of the superficial reflexes (abdominal and cremasteric). GBS cannot be diagnosed if the tendon reflexes are not so affected. It is very helpful in establishing the diagnosis to look carefully for the peripheral loss of sensation that occurs in about 80% of patients. Position, vibration, and light touch and less commonly pain and temperature sense are usually slightly diminished but may be affected severely.

A facial palsy of the lower motor neuron pattern is seen in 55% of patients, most commonly bilaterally. The lower cranial nerves are affected in 45%, causing dysarthria, dysphonia, and dysphagia with compromise of the upper airway. Extraocular palsies are present in 15–20%, and nystagmus and poor reactivity of the pupils to light are rarely described. Papilledema is occasionally seen.

Ataxia may be a prominent feature, and when associated with a variable degree of ophthalmoplegia it bears the eponym Miller-Fisher syndrome.[6] Myoclonus, asterixis, tremors of the extremities, and a continuous vermiform movement of the facial muscles termed myokymia have all been reported.

Autonomic dysfunction with abnormal sweating patterns, significant arrhythmias, postural hypotension, hypertension, and tachycardia is not infrequent (5%).[8] Electrolyte disturbances, most notably those of sodium with excess or insufficient antidiuretic hormone secretion, and a membranous glomerulonephritis are occasionally observed.[9] Loss of sphincter function is rare and usually transient. Abnormalities of the plantar response may occur but should be viewed with caution and a high index of suspicion for other pathology.

EVALUATION

An elevated CSF protein concentration with a low mononuclear cell count is a laboratory hallmark of the illness. The protein concentration becomes elevated usually in the second to third week, although it may rise earlier, and persists well into the phase of clinical resolution. The concentration ranges from 50 to 1000 mg% but is most commonly 100–300 mg%. The lymphocyte count is less than 10 cells/mm^3 in 85% of cases, but it may be as high as 50 and rarely, assuming the clinical setting is unequivocal, may be higher. The cells disappear with clinical improvement. The presence of CSF polymorphonuclear leukocytes casts doubt upon the diagnosis. The glucose and bacteriologic analyses of the CSF are normal.

Abnormalities of nerve conduction velocities (NCV) and electromyography are present in 90% of patients after 2–3 weeks.[10] Sensory and motor nerve conduction are slowed. The degree of slowing of nerve conduction does not necessarily correlate with the duration or severity of the weakness. The electromyographic (EMG) findings are characterized by diminished numbers of motor unit potentials during maximal contraction, and by muscle fibrillation that varies in proportion to the severity of atrophy resulting from extension of the destructive process to axonal degeneration.[10]

DIFFERENTIAL DIAGNOSIS

Corynebacterium diphtheriae exotoxin causes a cranial nerve symptom complex of palatal paralysis, dysarthria, and a loss of facial sensation and movement early in its course, followed by ciliary paralysis with loss of accommodation and blurred vision. It may go on to develop a rapidly evolving symmetrical, ascending paralysis after a delay of some weeks. The underlying pharyngeal infection and clinical evolution of diphtheria are distinctive. *Botulism,* caused by the presynaptic neuromuscular blocking exotoxin of *Clostridium botulinum,* produces a polyneuropathy similar to GBS. However, there are no sensory symptoms, it is usually heralded by oculomotor paresis and symptoms referable to the lower cranial nerve nuclei, and is usually associated with gastrointestinal upset occurring within 48 hours of ingestion of contaminated food. Loss of pupillary reflexes, a rarity in GBS, occurs regularly in botulism. *Tick paralysis,* caused by the injection into the host of a neurotoxin by the offending tick, may mimic GBS closely. Paresthesias may herald the onset of a severe and rapid ascending paralysis, areflexia, and often ataxia, but there is no objective sensory deficit and the spinal fluid is normal. Diagnosis is established by locating the tick, or by obtaining a history of tick exposure in the preceding few days. *Poliomyelitis* is usually markedly asymmetrical, not associated with sensory abnormalities, progresses during the febrile stage to its maximum in 2 days to a week, and is frequently associated with retention of urine and segmental loss of cutaneous and tendon reflexes. Coarse muscle fibrillations, onset in 2–3 weeks of muscle atrophy, and CSF pleocytosis are usual. It does not, for practical purposes, occur in individuals who have been immunized against all three infective strains. *Acute intermittent porphyria* may present with polyneuropathy, confusion, and acute abdominal pain, but the autosomal dominant transmission and the presence of porphobilinogen, delta-aminolevulinic acid, and porphyrins in the urine confirm the diagnosis.

The Miller-Fisher variant needs to be differentiated from Wernicke's encephalopathy (ataxia, nystagmus, oculomotor paresis, and confusion), and although the ataxic form of GBS is often initially diagnosed as hysteria, the widespread areflexia should alert the physician. Bell's palsy and basilar meningitis or encephalitis are possibilities when cranial nerve involvement is early. Acute spinal cord compression, as from epidural abscess, and acute transverse myelitis should be considered in the differential diagnosis. Prominent, early urinary retention, transverse sensory level over the trunk, and Babinski's responses are the important pointers to spinal cord injury, but tendon reflexes may be hypoactive. Myasthenia gravis, the Eaton-Lambert syndrome, polymyositis, and periodic paralysis from disturbances of potassium, phosphate, or thyroid metabolism may cause an acute onset of weakness, but the distinction can usually be made on clinical grounds.

MANAGEMENT

Emergency management of a suspected case of GBS should include consideration of the causes and differential diagnosis outlined; a spinal tap; admission to the hospital; and close observation of vital signs, particularly the respiratory capacity. Forced vital capacity should be measured on admission and repeatedly in patients with the rapidly evolving paralyses or those with prominent proximal weakness or cranial nerve involvement. Arterial blood gases are frequently misleading, because they may remain within normal range as lung mechanics rapidly fail. A vital capacity below 15 ml/kg requires intensive care unit management, and elective intubation must be considered. Ventilator dependence may last for weeks to months and thus necessitate tracheostomy. Nutritional fluid and electrolyte balance should be monitored and maintained. The syndrome of inappropriate antidiuretic hormone (SIADH) or diabetes insipidus may occur. Physical therapy and nursing care are important to prevent contractures, bedsores, and deep venous thrombosis. The use of prophylactic low-dose heparin is indicated for the prevention of thromboembolism, which remains a significant cause of mortality. Acute dysautonomia affecting cardiovascular reflexes is another potential cause of death. Postural hypotension, labile hypertension, and cardiac arrhythmias should be monitored and managed conservatively. Vasoactive drugs may cause an excessive and unpredictable response. Depolarizing muscle relaxants should not be used during intubation or general anesthesia because of their association in this illness with ventricular tachycardia and fibrillation.

The weight of evidence is that corticosteroids are not efficacious in this disease and may be detrimental, and the benefit of their use is outweighed by the potential side effects.[11]

A multicenter study has demonstrated major improvements in the outcome of severe acute GBS with the use of plasmapheresis.[12] When used within a week of onset in patients who are unable to walk unhelped, bed- or chair-bound, or ventilator dependent, significant impact has been found in terms of fewer days on the ventilator and shorter time for independent walking. Thus, for the severely affected, acute GBS patients plasmapheresis is recommended provided staff and ICU facilities with experience in plasmapheresis are available. The role of plasmapheresis for patients seen much later in the disease or for those less severely affected has not yet been defined. Particular care is needed when employing plasmapheresis in patients with prominent autonomic instability.[13]

Immunosuppressive therapy is a hypothetical possibility not currently recommended. Severe depression of mood in the acute and prolonged phases is frequent, particularly in ventilator-dependent patients, and ongoing supportive counseling should be viewed as part of the overall care.

KEY FEATURES

GUILLAIN-BARRÉ SYNDROME

GBS is an autoimmune disorder leading to widespread destruction of myelin sheaths of peripheral nerves, mediated by humoral and cellular immune mechanisms.

Clinical Features
1. Rapid evolution of symmetrical paralysis of extremities as well as truncal and faciobulbar muscles
2. Widespread loss of tendon reflexes
3. Frequent association with distal sensory impairment
4. Dysautonomia, usually manifested by postural hypotension and persistent tachycardia
5. Miller-Fisher variant has prominent ataxia and ocular palsies

Diagnostic Tests
A. CSF
   1. Elevated protein (50–1000 mg%)
   2. Minimal increase in mononuclear cells ($<50/mm^3$)
   3. Normal glucose
   4. May be normal early in the course
B. EMG and NCV
   1. Widespread marked slowing of motor and sensory nerve conduction velocities

C. CBC, ESR
  1. Electrolytes, renal and liver function tests are usually normal but may provide clue to underlying disease. Differential diagnosis may be confirmed by monospot, urine for porphyrins, creatinine kinase, and thyroid functions.

Treatment
  A. Symptomatic
  1. Supportive therapy is the cornerstone
  2. Assisted ventilation and respiratory care
  3. Low-dose heparin
  4. Physical therapy
  5. Monitoring and conservative management of dysautonomia
  6. Monitoring and maintenance of nutritional, fluid, and electrolyte balance
  B. Specific
  1. Current regimen of corticosteroids and cytotoxic drugs not shown to be beneficial
  2. Plasmapheresis early in course

REFERENCES

1. Haymaker W, Kernohan JW: The Landry-Guillain-Barré syndrome. A clinicopathological report of fifty fatal cases and a critique of the literature. Medicine (Baltimore) 28:59–141, 1949.
   Landmark article. Remains a classic, although diagnostic criteria differ from current usage, and some cases sound like porphyria.

2. Asbury AK: Diagnostic considerations in Guillain-Barré syndrome. Ann Neurol 9(suppl):1–5, 1981.
   Defines the clinical criteria and the variations acceptable for the diagnosis of GBS.

3. Prineas JW: Pathology of the Guillain-Barré Syndrome. Ann Neurol 9(suppl):6–19, 1981.
   Discrete foci of segmental demyelination occur throughout the peripheral nervous system, with myelin being the specific target of immune attack. Destruction is effected by macrophages in the presence of lymphocytes, and in particularly severe instances, axonal damage also results. This is a precise and well-referenced discussion. (Also: Asbury AK, Arnason BG, Adams RD: The inflammatory lesion in idiopathic polyneuritis. Its role in pathogenesis. Medicine (Baltimore) 48:173–215, 1969.)

4. Iqbal A, Oger JJF, Arnason BG: Cell-mediated immunity in idiopathic polyneuritis. Ann Neurol 9(suppl):65–69, 1981.
   Discusses the relative roles of cell-mediated and humoral immunity in GBS. Studies are quoted in which lymphocyte transfer induces experimental allergic neuritis (the animal model of GBS). The possibility is emphasized that more than one type of immune response may occur to cause GBS.

5. Kennedy RH, et al: Guillain-Barré syndrome. A 42 year epidemiologic and clinical study. Mayo Clinic Proc 53:93–99, 1978.
   Forty cases are studied. Incidence of 1.7 per 100,000. Slightly more frequent in >40 years age group. Seventy per cent of patients had antecedent infections. Sixty-eight per cent had onset in the legs, 20% in the arms, and 8% in the cranial nerves. There was bilateral involvement in 98%, all had leg weakness, 95% had weakness in arms, 58% had

bulbar symptoms, and 10% had respiratory failure. Complete recovery occurred in 78%. There was a single case of recurrence. Eight-six per cent of 36 spinal taps had protein concentration >50 mg/100 ml, and 89% had less than 4 white cells/mm³.

6. Fisher CM: An unusual variant of idiopathic polyneuritis (syndrome of ophthalmoplegia, ataxia and areflexia). N Engl J Med 255:57–65, 1956.
   First dilineation of the symptom complex as a syndrome, and its relation to GBS.

7. Gracey DR: Respiratory failure in Guillain-Barré syndrome. A 6 year experience. Mayo Clinic Proc 57:742–746, 1982.
   Study of 79 patients. Twenty-seven per cent were admitted to respiratory intensive care unit. Sixteen per cent required intubation, all leading to tracheostomy, lasting from 10 to 104 days (average 50 ± 27 days). Complications were related to care of the tracheostomy. There was a 49% mortality rate.

8. Tuck RR, McLeod JG: Autonomic dysfunction in Guillain-Barré syndrome. J Neurol Neurosurg Psychiatry 44:983–990, 1981.
   Tests of heart rate, blood pressure, response to Valsalva's maneuver, baroreflex sensitivity, and sweating revealed varying degrees of autonomic nervous system dysfunction in all seven patients. Severity is not related to the degree of motor or sensory deficit. Demyelinating lesions have been of sympathetic and parasympathetic nerves.

9. Rodriguez-Iturbe G, et al: Acute glomerulonephritis in the Guillain-Barré-Strohl syndrome. Report of nine cases. Ann Intern Med 78:391–395, 1983.
   Each of nine patients studied developed acute glomerulonephritis with GBS. The clinical manifestations of hypertension, edema, and microscopic hematuria were minimal, but the diagnosis was confirmed by renal biopsy in eight cases. In two cases, there was histologic evidence of progressive changes toward chronicity. (Also: Talamo TS, Borochovitz D: Membranous granulonephritis associated with the Guillain-Barré syndrome. Am J Clin Pathol 78:563–566, 1982.)

10. McLeod JG: Electrophysiological studies in the Guillain-Barré syndrome. Ann Neurol 9(suppl):20–27, 1981.
    Ninety per cent of 114 patients had abnormal studies. Sensory and motor nerve conduction were slowed or completely blocked, and distal motor latencies were prolonged. The F wave latency was increased and conduction velocity slowed. Electromyographic evidence of fibrillation was sparse, except in the presence of axonal degeneration and muscle atrophy, in which case this finding may be marked. (Also: Brown WF, Feasby TE: Conduction block and denervation in Guillain-Barré polyneuropathy. Brain 107:219–239, 1984.)

11. Hughes RAC, Kadlubowski M, Hufschmidt A: Treatment of acute inflammatory polyneuropathy. Ann Neurol 9(suppl):125–133, 1981.
    Comprehensive, well-referenced overview of currently available supportive and reportedly specific therapy.

12. The Guillain-Barré syndrome study group: Plasmapheresis and acute Guillain-Barré syndrome. Neurology 35:1096–1104, 1985.
    This important study demonstrated major positive impact of plasmapheresis on the course of severe acute GBS. Two hundred forty-five patients from several institutions in the United States and Canada were studied and given phasmapheresis or conventional therapy in an unblinded, randomized fashion. Statistically significant differences occurred in favor of plasmapheresis patients in terms of outcome at 6 months, time to independent walking, time on ventilator, and time to improve one grade of strength. The benefit was particularly notable for patients who required mechanical ventilation after entering the study and in whom treatment was started within a week of onset. In the setting of experienced ICU management, the risks of treatment were reasonable.

13. Rodnitzky RL, Goeken JA: Complications of plasma exchange in neurological patients. Arch Neurol 39:350–354, 1982.

Sobering reminder that this regimen is not without risk, particularly for hypotension, arrhythmias, sepsis, and hemolysis.

14. Feasby TE, Gilbert JJ, Brown CF, et al: Acute axonal form of Guillain-Barré polyneuropathy. Brain 109:1115–1126, 1986.

The patients in this report had the usual clinical picture of acute Guillain-Barré syndrome. Electrophysiologic studies showed severe axonal neuropathy as opposed to the predominantly demyelinating picture usually seen. The recovery of neurologic function was poor. This may be considered as a distinct acute axonal polyneuropathy of unknown etiology clinically resembling acute GBS.

Coma

Harold B. Schiff, M.D.

Coma is defined as a disturbance of consciousness in which the patient cannot be aroused by any stimulus no matter how vigorous; coma ends with the return of any form of responsiveness. The patient will then progress through various levels of disordered consciousness until a clear sensorium is finally attained.[1]

Alertness requires the normal functioning of the reticular activating system (RAS). The ascending RAS is a highly complex polysynaptic fiber system that passes from the upper pons through the midbrain into the thalamic regions bilaterally. A lesion below the level of the upper pons or a unilateral destructive lesion at or above the level of the thalamus will not cause obtundation. In between these two areas, however, the RAS is remarkably vulnerable. Either anatomic or biochemical disturbances may result in a pathologic state of consciousness. Anatomic lesions, such as small infarcts in the reticular core of the brain stem, may result in prolonged coma. Alternatively, a unilateral supratentorial space occupying lesion may force the medial uncal portion of the temporal lobe through the tentorial notch, distorting the RAS in the core of the brain stem and producing an alteration in consciousness. In a herniation syndrome, the RAS is often the first brain stem structure to be affected.

The sequential loss of CNS function, beginning with the cortex, upper brain stem, midbrain, pons, and finally medulla, is known as a rostral-caudal progression. Depending on the direction of the herniation syndrome, other neighborhood signs become apparent and are helpful in localizing the direction and degree of herniation. The herniated uncus would compress the ipsilateral oculomotor nerve; the parasympathetic pupillar motor fibers, being superficially placed and most susceptible to compression, produce an ipsilateral dilated pupil that is unresponsive to light. If the herniated uncus forces the midbrain against the narrow ridge of the contralateral tentorial margin, motor fibers within the cerebral peduncle of the midbrain are compressed. These fibers then cross at the level of the cervicomedullary junction, and thus a hemiparesis is noted on the same side as the supratentorial mass lesion.

An understanding of the rostral-caudal progression of a herniation syndrome makes anatomic localization quite accurate. By using the parameters of eye signs, respiratory function, and motor activity, an accurate clinical assessment can be made. This assessment is most helpful in differentiating anatomic lesions from those caused by pharmacologic or biochemical disturbances—the primary diagnostic step in evaluating the comatose patient.

CLINICAL EVALUATION

Examination of the pupils should include size, symmetry, and response to light. In the diencephalic stage, both pupils tend to be small. A magnifying glass may be necessary to see if the pupillary response to light is preserved. In uncal herniation, compression of the oculomotor nerve will present with a progressive pupillary dilatation (relative overactivity of the sympathetic system) until finally a widely dilated unreactive pupil is noted. The diencephalic stage is thus characterized either by unilateral pupillary dilatation (as with unilateral herniation syndromes) or by symmetrical small pupils that respond to light (in midline herniation or most toxic/metabolic encephalopathies). Once the deterioration involves the midbrain, the pupils are no longer reactive to light; they tend to be in the midposition and may not change even with progression of the syndrome to the pontine and medullary phase of deterioration.

In the diencephalic stage of coma, the doll's eyes maneuver may become overly facile. In a normal conscious individual, if the head is passively turned to the right the eyes will move to the right; in the diencephalic stage, the eyes will move to the left. With progression to the mesencephalic stage, the oculovestibular reflex is no longer facile and a stronger stimulus may be necessary. With the head raised 30 degrees on the body, 40 ml of ice water instilled over 30 seconds into the external ear canal (after checking for an intact tympanic membrane) will produce conjugate deviation of the eye to the side of the stimulation. With the lesion at the level of the pons or below, there is no response to the doll's eye maneuver or to ice water caloric stimulation.

Conjugate eye movement is also helpful in determining the level of the lesion. In an acute hemispheric lesion with destruction of the fibers from the frontal center for conjugate gaze, there will be a relative overactivity of the contralateral center causing conjugate deviation of the eyes toward the injured hemisphere. Therefore, the eyes will deviate toward the side of the lesion and away from an associated hemiplegia. These fibers for contralateral conjugate gaze cross in the midbrain; thus with a lesion in the brain stem below the level of the midbrain, the eyes may conjugately deviate away from the site of the lesion and toward the hemiplegia.

The respiratory pattern is also helpful in determining the level of CNS function. In the diencephalic stage of rostral-caudal deterioration, normal or slow periodic respirations, including Cheyne-Stokes respirations, are noted. At the level of midbrain dysfunction, 40/minute central neurogenic hyperventilation occurs. With pontine damage, central neurogenic hyperventilation disappears and, paradoxically, breathing appears more normal. A pause at peak inspiration (apneustic breathing) is characteristic of pontine level respiration. With progression to the medulla, breathing becomes atactic, irregular, and unpredictable. At this point, respiratory arrest is imminent.

The motor system is the last parameter and is monitored by observing spontaneous movements and the response to painful stimuli. In the diencephalic stage, there is effective movement away from painful stimuli but the range of passive movements in the limbs is limited by counterholding-gegenhalten (paratonia). In this stage, bilateral decorticate posture may rarely be seen. This consists of a posture of adduction at the shoulder with flexion at the elbow, wrists, and fingers, with extensor posturing of the lower extremities; however, decorticate posturing is rarely complete. At the level of the midbrain, decerebrate postures appear. Initially these may be only fragmentary postures: with the patient's arms placed across the abdomen and a painful stimulus applied to the sternum, the patient may consistently seek the painful stimulus with only one limb, indicating hemiplegia of the opposite side. If the patient's forearms extend away from the painful stimulus or pronate even slightly, this is suggestive of decerebration and thus dysfunction at the mesencephalic level. A full-blown decerebration occurs with extension and pronation of the upper extremities and extension of the lower extremities. With destruction at the level of the pons or below, decerebration will disappear and the limbs will become flaccid with no response to noxious stimuli.

With these parameters of the examination in mind, one can quickly localize the level of nervous system dysfunction and begin consideration of the major diagnostic categories.

DIFFERENTIAL DIAGNOSIS

The most important diagnostic consideration is to determine whether the alteration of consciousness is primarily due to an intracranial structural lesion or to a systemic toxic-metabolic disorder.[2,3]

Intracranial structural lesions may or may not present with focal or lateralizing signs. With an expanding intracranial lesion, the patient will classically follow the rostral-caudal progression of a herniation syndrome. The major categories of intracranial processes with focal brain dysfunction include trauma, intraparenchymal hemorrhages, tumors, infarcts, and certain forms of infection. Parenchymal hematomas and isodense subdural hematomas are diagnostic entities that should be kept in mind, and a repeat CT scan or arteriogram may be necessary for full evaluation.[4]

Spontaneous parenchymal hemorrhages associated with hypertension, bleeding diatheses, leukemias, hepatic disease, and so forth are usually sudden in onset and may evolve over several days. Pontine hemorrhages, usually in the face of hypertension, present a clinical picture different from that seen with the rostral-caudal deterioration. There is bilateral flaccid paralysis of the limbs, and the doll's eye maneuver and ice water calorics will be negative. However, vertical gaze may remain, owing to the intact midbrain centers. Vertical conjugate eye movements and ocular bobbing are reliable localizing signs, along with pinpoint pupils, which require a magnifying glass to confirm the response to light. Cerebellar hemorrhages, commonly seen in hypertension, are most important to identify, because again, patients do not present with a classic rostral-caudal progression. Patients present with acute ataxia (truncal or hemiataxia), nausea, vomiting, and severe headache. Nystagmus is usually present, and there may be forced deviation of the gaze opposite to the side of the hematoma. Prompt recognition in this syndrome is essential, because a mass lesion compressing the medullary respiratory centers directly may result in sudden death.

Diagnostic dilemmas may occur with posterior fossa tumors, presenting with an upward herniation syndrome of central neurogenic hyperventilation; loss of upgaze and small, fixed pupils; or a foramen magnum herniation with sudden respiratory arrest. Pituitary apoplexy with headaches, visual loss, stiff neck, obtundation, ocular palsies, and acute hypotension may occur with spontaneous hemorrhagic necrosis of a pituitary adenoma. Treatment must include steroid replacement.

Infarcts do not, as a rule, produce lethargy; however, massive hemispheric infarction may produce a herniation syndrome. Brain stem infarcts interrupting the RAS may produce lasting coma. In the locked-in syndrome, with bilateral destruction of the brain stem motor pathways, the patient is unable to move; he remains conscious and able to comprehend but may only be able to communicate by means of eye blinks. Herpes encephalitis may produce a focal mass lesion, classically involving the temporal tip with surrounding edema, and may cause an uncal herniation syndrome.

Subarachnoid hemorrhage, meningitis, encephalitis, or any cause of acute hydrocephalus may cause coma with no focal or lateralizing signs. These disease processes serve as a forceful reminder that all comatose patients must have their spinal fluid examined unless there is a contraindication to lumbar puncture. CT scan is advisable prior to lumbar puncture, unless the patient presents with an acute meningitis.

Patients with toxic-metabolic encephalopathies do not present with a classic rostral-caudal localization. Patients characteristically do not have lateralizing signs; they may present with focal signs (e.g., decerebration, etc.), but the focal signs are *scattered* throughout the neuroaxis and generally do not follow the rostral-caudal progression. Drug overdose and endogenous metabolic derangements are the most common causes. All toxic-metabolic encephalopathies except anoxic encephalopathy and those from drugs having specific effects on the pupil will spare the pupillary light response regardless of the stage of rostral-caudal deterioration. Specific drugs, e.g., glutethimide (Doriden), may cause unresponsive pupils because of their atropine-like effects. Morphine will produce pupillary constriction.

Signs of old and inapparent CNS lesions may become apparent in the face of a metabolic encephalopathy; focal seizures may occur, and widespread involuntary small-amplitude myoclonic jerks may be noted. The clinical differentiation of structural from metabolic causes of coma pivots around a clearly progressive anatomic localization of the rostral-caudal syndrome. Intracranial mass lesions by and large follow exactly this syndrome, whereas the signs of a toxic-metabolic encephalopathy are much more patchy.

MANAGEMENT

The initial management of a patient presenting in coma requires the establishment of an airway and the maintenance of vital signs followed by the empirical treatment of immediately reversible causes of coma with IV administration of 50 ml of 50% glucose, 100 mg of thiamine, and 1 ampule of a morphine antagonist such as naloxone. In the face of multiple trauma, cervical spine films should be taken prior to the clinical evaluation because the doll's head maneuver might result in cervical cord damage. The next step would be to establish the level of CNS function by means of the clinical examination, and then the differential diagnosis can be established. Standard blood tests and toxic screen of the urine and serum should be performed, and depending on the outcome a CT scan and a lumbar puncture should be considered. The treatment of raised intracranial pressure depends on the underlying pathology; for example, with a subdural, epidural, or intraparenchymal hematoma, surgical drainage and placement of an intracranial pressure monitoring device may be helpful. In the acute phase, hyperventilation (to keep the PCO_2 at 28 mmHg), dexamethasone (Decadron), and/or mannitol may be required. Long-term management requires attention to the bladder, skin, cornea, joints and tendons, and peripheral nerve pressure points; as well as the respiratory, alimentation, and hydration status of the patient. Careful monitoring of the level of CNS functioning over time will document a gradual improvement; a plateau or deterioration of CNS function is an indication for a thorough re-evaluation of the patient.[5-10]

KEY FEATURES

Definition
Coma is defined as the disturbance of consciousness in which the patient cannot be aroused by any stimulus no matter how vigorous.

Pathogenesis
Alertness requires normal functioning of the ascending reticular activating system (RAS). A lesion below the upper pons or a unilateral lesion of the thalamus or above will not cause coma.

Clinical Evaluation
The primary diagnostic step in evaluating the comatose patient is aimed at differentiating anatomic lesions from those caused by toxic-metabolic disturbances.

Differential Diagnosis
1. Structural lesions with focal signs: trauma, intraparenchymal hemorrhage, tumor, infarcts, abscess, hematoma.
2. Structural lesions without focal signs: subarachnoid hemorrhage, meningitis, encephalitis, hydrocephalus.
3. Toxic-metabolic encephalopathies.

Treatment and Management
1. Stabilization and support of vital functions.
2. Treatment of immediately reversible causes of coma, including administration of glucose, thiamine, and a narcotic antagonist (naloxone).
3. Establishing the level of CNS function and the etiology of the coma.
4. Intermediate and long-range prognosis and plans.

REFERENCES

1. Plum F, Posner JB: Diagnosis of Stupor and Coma, 3rd ed. Philadelphia, FA Davis, 1980.
   This volume is the standard text on coma. It discusses the pathophysiology, signs, and symptoms of coma and describes in detail the structural and metabolic causes of coma.

2. Caromma JJ, Simon RP: The comatose patient: A diagnostic approach and treatment. Int Anesth Clin 17(2/3):3–18, 1979.
   This is a succinct discussion of the diagnostic approach to coma with discussions on the regulation of consciousness and the pathophysiology of coma. It includes an outline of the emergency evaluation and treatment of the comatose patient.

3. Sabin TD: Coma and the acute confusional state in the emergency room. Med Clin N Am 65(1):15–32, 1981.
   This is perhaps a slightly more detailed approach in the assessment and management of the acutely comatose patient.

4. Levin HS, Benton AL, Grossman RG: Neurobehavioral Consequences of Closed Head Injury. New York and Oxford, Oxford University Press, 1982.
   This volume covers head injury. Chapters of particular interest include pathophysiologic mechanisms, outcome, social recovery, and rehabilitation in head trauma. It provides significant insight into the intermediate and long-term problems facing the physician managing severely brain-injured patients.

5. Jennett B, Plum F: Persistent vegetative state after brain damage. Lancet 1:734–737, 1979.
   This article provides an excellent clinical description and discusses the terminology of patients who survive coma but never exhibit demonstrable cortical function.

6. Segarra JM: Cerebral vascular disease and behavior. I. The syndrome of the mesencephalic artery (basilar artery bifurcation). Arch Neurol 22:408–418, 1970.
   This article describes the pathogenesis of the akinetic mute, reviews the clinical symptomatology, and discusses the clinicoanatomic relationships and the differential diagnosis of akinetic states.

7. Westmoreland BF, Klass DW, Sharborough FW, Reagon TJ: Alpha-coma. Electroencephalographic, clinical, pathological and etiological correlations. Arch Neurol 32:713–718, 1975.
   The authors describe clinical and pathologic findings in patients who are noted to have alpha coma on EEG. They discuss the relationship of the "normal waking EEG" of comatose patients to the underlying etiology and outcome.

8. Rosenberg G, Wogensen K, Starr A: Auditory brain-stem and middle- and long-latency evoked potentials in coma. Arch Neurol 41:835–838, 1984.
   This article describes the neurologic assessment, auditory brain stem–evoked responses, and outcome of 25 comatose patients studied acutely following various causes of coma. The study shows that there is no direct relationship between outcome and pattern of evoked responses. The authors note that the predictability of outcome depends not only on the pattern of evoked responses but also on the cause of the coma. They do not advocate that auditory-evoked responses be used as a reliable tool in the assessment of the outcome of coma.

9. American Medical Association: Guidelines for the determination of death: Report of medical consultants on the diagnosis of death to the President's Commission for the Study of Ethical Problems in Medicine and Biomedical and Behavioral Research. JAMA 246:2184–2186, 1981.
   This article discusses the neurologic and ethical issues in the determination of death and lists criteria for determination of brain death.

10. Loewy EH: Treatment decisions in the mentally impaired (editorial). N Engl J Med 317:1465–1469, 1987.
    Thoughtful discussion of issues that arise in the management of neurologically impaired (but not brain-dead) individuals.

Acute Confusional States

Harold B. Schiff, M.D.

Acute confusional state can be defined as an acquired incapacity to think with customary speed and clarity.[1-3] Patients are unable to maintain a coherent stream of thought. Their general behavior and speech reflect an inappropriate sequencing of ideas and an inability to rank the priority of stimuli. This inability to distinguish between relevant and irrelevant stimuli results in a disintegration of the patient's adaptation with the environment. These patients may present with a wide range of abnormal behaviors, including somnolence, hallucinations, motor hyperactivity, assaultiveness, and extreme states of panic or fear, and these states should be considered a medical emergency.

CLINICAL FEATURES

Confusional states are characterized by fluctuating disturbances of attention, thought, perception, psychomotor and autonomic activity, and sleep-wake cycle.[4]

Attentional Deficits. Disturbances include difficulties in attaining and/or maintaining attention. Patients may show marked distractibility, responding equally to all auditory, visual, and kinesthetic stimuli.

Thought Disorder. Cognitive deficits result in an incoherent stream of thought. Patients may be aware of this and complain of being "confused" or "unable to get it together" and have difficulty in organizing recent and remote memory into an orderly sequence. Spatial disorientation may be expressed in reduplicative paramnesia, especially of place, the patient insisting that the hospital room is a branch of the main hospital located near his home. Temporal disorientation occurs when events from the past are directly related to the present. Association of unrelated events may create the appearance of confabulation. Although memory disturbances and disorientation are clearly evident in spontaneous conversational speech, the patient may do remarkably well on formal memory testing.

Delusions do occur, and vague feelings of apprehension may develop into paranoid delusions. The classic schneiderian delusions of thought insertion, withdrawal, control, and broadcasting are rare.

Perceptual Disturbances. Misinterpretations, illusions, and hallucinations are not uncommon, as typified in delirium tremens. Patients frequently do not acknowledge these symptoms unless directly questioned. Markings on the wall may be misinterpreted as crawling insects; sounds may be perceived as fire alarms or gun shots. Inadvertent accident or death may result from patients' acting on these misinterpretations. Hallucinations may occur in all sensory modalities but visual and auditory hallucinations are most common.

Psychomotor and Autonomic Activity. Patients may be hyperaroused, requiring minimal sleep, and may demonstrate increased speech output and heightened emotional tone. Alternatively, patients may be withdrawn and quiet with empty, vague speech. Language disturbance with word finding difficulty, circumlocution, and perseveration is not uncommon, and abnormal writing with perseveration, misspelling of ordinary words, and lack of regard for lines is characteristic.

Disturbances in the Sleep-Wake Cycle. This is an invariable feature of confusional states. Patients may present in a hypersomnolent state, whereas others remain awake for days. A complete inversion of the sleep-wake cycle is also not uncommon.

Fluctuation of Symptomatology. This is the most characteristic feature of the confusional state, with fluctuations in cognitive and behavioral functions over a 24-hour cycle and also from day to day. Patients may appear remarkably intact at one moment, only to become a major behavior problem at the next. Patients usually function less well in the early morning, following a nap, or at sundown. Such fluctuation is rare in any other disorder of the mental status.

PATHOPHYSIOLOGY

Confusional states appear to occur with a wide variety of CNS and systemic diseases.[5] A pathophysiologic mechanism has yet to be established. Regional cerebral blood flow and cerebral metabolism studies have been inconclusive but suggest that a generalized decrease in cerebral metabolism is not the basis for acute confusional states, as initially suggested. Serum thyroxine, ACTH, and growth hormone concentrations were found to be abnormal in confusional states, but these disturbances are not considered to be clinically significant. CSF analysis has shown abnormalities of 5-hydroxyindoleacetic acid (5-HIAA) and homovanillic acid (HVA) (serotonin and dopamine breakdown products), but the significance of these neurotransmitter abnormalities is uncertain. However, a clear association has been shown between acute confusional states and infarction in the territory of the right middle cerebral artery, involving the frontal and parietal lobes; and the posterior cerebral artery territory, involving the right fusiform, calcarine, and hippocampal region. An hypothesis has been forwarded that may be applicable to acute confusional states and would account for the diversity of causes that produce this clinical syndrome. Mesulam postulates a CNS network, involving a disturbance in the integration of stimuli, at one or more of a number of specific CNS sites: the reticular activating system, the limbic system, and the polymodal association areas of the cortex. Biochemical disturbances, the most common cause of confusional states, would probably act at the level of the reticular activating system; epileptiform and endocrine abnormalities may well be operative at the level of the limbic system, and certainly the ischemic lesions do conform with the cortical association areas as hypothesized.[6] This theory could explain a number of issues concerning the etiology, clinical signs, and outcome of confusional states; however, it remains to be tested and verified.

ETIOLOGY

The etiology of acute confusional states can be divided into those of focal central nervous system origin, and those secondary to a generalized toxic metabolic disorder. An etiologic classification in Table 1 is presented purely as an example of the long list of agents associated with confusional states to emphasize the large variety of disorders that may produce such a state. Common central nervous system disorders include trauma, seizures, infection, infarction, nutritional problems, mass lesions, and dementias.[7,8]

Head trauma and seizures frequently result in a variable period of a confusional state, often with agitation.[9] An acute confusional state may be the first presenting symptom of a vasculitis or encephalitis. Elderly and demented patients are particularly prone to present with acute confusion, the degenerated brain being sensitive to even slight changes in the metabolic milieu. An intracranial space-occupying lesion (such as a tumor or subdural hematoma) and right hemisphere strokes or transient ischemic attacks may present with acute confusion. In these instances, computed tomography (CT) may demonstrate the anatomic abnormality, but a scan performed too early may miss an infarct or possibly a tumor. Nevertheless, toxic or metabolic disturbances are the most common cause of confusional states.

LABORATORY INVESTIGATIONS

The work-up of an acutely confused patient is outlined in Table 2. However, the priority of specific tests should reflect each individual clinical presentation. A lumbar puncture (LP) should always be performed unless there is a specific contraindication, such as signs of increased intracranial pressure. A prior CT scan is desirable, especially in the face of a history of head trauma or lateralizing neurologic signs; however, when meningitis is

Table 1.   ETIOLOGIC AGENTS IN ACUTE CONFUSIONAL STATES

Head Trauma

Injury by Physical Agents
1. Heat stroke
2. Radiation
3. Electrocution

Infections and Inflammation
1. *Systemic:* pneumonia, typhoid, typhus, acute rheumatic fever, malaria, influenza, brucellosis, infectious mononucleosis, infectious hepatitis, subacute bacterial endocarditis, bacteremia, septicemia, Rocky Mountain spotted fever, Legionnaire's disease
2. *Intracranial:* acute, subacute, and chronic
   a. Viral encephalitis; aseptic meningitis; rabies; human immunodeficiency virus (HIV) disease
   b. Bacterial meningitis, meningococcal, pneumococcal, *Haemophilus influenzae,* etc.
   c. Tuberculous meningitis
   d. Neurosyphilis
   e. Fungal infections; cryptococcosis, coccidioidomycosis, histoplasmosis, moniliasis, mucormycosis
   f. Protozoal infections: toxoplasma encephalitis, cerebral malaria
   g. Trichinosis

Hypersensitivity and Autoimmune Disorders
1. Serum sickness
2. Systemic lupus erythematosus
3. Polyarteritis nodosa
4. Rheumatoid arthritis
5. Postinfectious and postvaccinal encephalomyelitis

Intoxication and Withdrawal Syndromes of Drugs and Toxins
1. Drug: anticholinergic agents, sedative-hypnotics, digitalis derivatives, opiates, corticosteroids, salicylates, antibiotics, anticonvulsants, antiarrhythmic and antihypertensive drugs, antineoplastic agents, cimetidine, lithium, antiparkinsonian agents, disulfiram, indomethacin, phencyclidine
2. Alcohol: ethyl and methyl
3. Industrial toxins; carbon disulfide, organic solvents, methyl chloride and bromide, heavy metals, organophosphorus, insecticides, carbon monoxide, gasoline, glue, ether, and nitrous oxide

Other Toxins
1. Snake bite
2. Poisonous plants and mushrooms

Metabolic Disorders, Nutritional and Hormonal
1. Hypoxia
2. Hypoglycemia
3. Hepatic, renal, pancreatic, pulmonary insufficiency (encephalopathy)
4. Avitaminosis: nicotinic acid, thiamine, cyanocobalamin (vitamin B_{12}), folate, pyridoxine
5. Hypervitaminosis: intoxication by vitamin A or D
6. Hormonal disorders: hyperinsulinism, hyperthyroidism, hypothyroidism, hypopituitarism, hyperparathyroidism
7. Disorders of fluid and electrolyte metabolism
   a. Dehydration, water intoxication
   b. Alkalosis, acidosis
   c. Hypernatremia, hyponatremia, hypercalcemia, hypocalcemia, hypomagnesemia
8. Errors of metabolism
   a. Porphyria
   b. Carcinoid syndrome

Table continued on following page

Table 1.   ETIOLOGIC AGENTS IN ACUTE CONFUSIONAL STATES *Continued*

Vascular Disorders
1. Migraine
2. Cerebrovascular disorders
   a. Transient ischemic attacks
   b. Hypertensive encephalopathy
   c. Infarcts in right middle cerebral or posterior cerebral artery territory
3. Cardiovascular disorders
   a. Myocardial infarction
   b. Congestive heart failure
   c. Cardiac arrhythmias
4. Hematologic
   a. Pernicious anemia
   b. Polycythemia
   c. Thrombotic thrombocytopenic purpura

Cerebral Degenerative Disorders
1. Multiple sclerosis

Tumors
1. Intracranial: parenchymal or extraparenchymal space occupying lesions (primary or secondary)
2. Nonmetastatic effects of cancer: limbic encephalitis

Table 2.   LABORATORY STUDIES IN ACUTE CONFUSIONAL STATES

CBC, erythrocyte sedimentation rate
PT/PTT
Electrolytes, urea, creatinine, Mg^{++}, Ca^{++}
Fasting blood glucose and 2-hour postprandial blood glucose
Serum albumin and globulin
Bilirubin
LDH, SGOT, creatine kinase, alkaline phosphatase
Serum ammonia daily $\times$ 3 days
Toxic screen
Urine analysis
Vitamin B_{12}
Folate
T_3, T_4
Heavy metal screen (including lead and mercury)
Blood cortisol
Protein electrophoresis
ANA, C_3 complement
VDRL
Purified protein derivative
Chest radiograph
ECG
CT scan without and with contrast material
Lumbar puncture with CSF Gram's stain; India ink stain;
   culture; protein, glucose, and immunologic studies
EEG

suspected the LP should not be delayed by the CT scan. Neurologic consultation may aid in the selection of the appropriate diagnostic tests.

TREATMENT AND MANAGEMENT

Once the cause is identified, the underlying abnormality should be corrected. Because medication is frequently a cause of confusional states, the most effective initial approach is to discontinue, whenever possible, all medications while correcting other metabolic disturbances. Acute confusional states are usually short lived, and supportive management is the most important means of treatment. Behavior management of an acutely confused patient usually presents a more significant problem but one that requires specialized nursing care rather than specific pharmacotherapy.[10] The more belligerent patient may require padded bed rails and physical restraints. However, patients do best unrestrained in a restricted environment such as in a geriatric chair in a private room. Reassurance and positive reinforcement from the staff, large calendars, a bedside lamp, and a radio are invaluable orienting stimuli. Only when these measures fail should pharmacotherapy be used. Antipsychotics, e.g., thioridazine (Mellaril) or haloperidol (Haldol), may be more effective than sedatives or anxiolytics. Beta adrenergic blockers such as propranolol may be effective in agitated and belligerent patients. Antihistamines are sedating and sometimes useful. The initial dosage of all drugs ought to be low with gradual increments, because these medications may precipitate a paradoxical reaction of markedly increased behavioral disturbance.

KEY FEATURES

An acute confusional state can be defined as an acquired incapacity to think with customary speed and clarity and an inability to maintain a coherent stream of thought.

Clinical Features
1. Attentional deficits
2. Thought disorder
3. Peceptual disturbance
4. Psychomotor and autonomic activity
5. Disturbance of the sleep-wake cycle
6. Fluctuations in symptomatology

Pathophysiology
Yet to be established, but probably involving the reticular activating system, the limbic system, and the cortical association areas.

Etiology
Nonspecific: almost any physiologic disturbance may result in this syndrome.

Management
1. Treat the underlying cause
2. Behavioral-nursing management in a safe, restricted environment
3. Pharmacologic: only as a last resort—antipsychotics, e.g., Mellaril or Haldol, in low doses

REFERENCES

1. Engel GL, Romano J: Delirium, a syndrome of cerebral insufficiency. J Chron Dis 9:260–277, 1959.
   This classic article on acute confusional states gives a broad discussion of the syndrome and a detailed clinical description. However, subsequent work by Sokoloff (1975) and Bergland and coworkers (1977) have challenged the ideas of the pathogenesis of confusional states; Obrecht and colleagues (1979) have also added significant information on the value of EEG in acute confusional states. However, this rather lengthy article remains well worth reading.

2. Berrios GE: Delirium and confusion in the 19th century: A conceptual history. Br J Psychiatr 139:439–444, 1981.
   This article provides a broad historical background to acute confusional states.

3. Lipowski ZJ: Delirium updated. Comp Psychiatr 21(3):190–196, 1980.
   Lipowski summarizes his work on acute confusional states. A more detailed account can be found in his book Delirium, *published by Charles C Thomas (1980). Lipowski and Folstein are the foremost psychiatrists working in this field.*

4. Adams RD, Victor M: Delirium and other acute confusional states *In* Adams RD, Victor M (eds): Principles of Neurology. New York, McGraw-Hill, 1981.
   In this chapter, Adams and Victor provide a neurologic viewpoint on the pathogenesis and clinical features of the acute confusional states.

5. American Psychiatric Association: Diagnostic and Statistical Manual of Mental Disorders, 3rd ed. Washington, DC, APA, 1980, pp 104–107.
   The diagnostic criteria for acute confusional states are summarized. These diagnostic criteria have been formulated and tested and are currently used in the clinical setting, predominantly by the psychiatric community.

6. Banki CM, Vojnik M: Comparative simultaneous measurement of cerebrospinal fluid 5-hydroxyindoleacetic acid and blood serotonin levels in delirium tremens and clozapine induced delirious reaction. J Neurol Neurosurg Psychiatr 41:420–424, 1978.
   This article describes the finding of raised CSF 5-hydroxyindoleacetic acid and simultaneously reduced blood 5-hydroxytryptophan in 11 female patients with delirium tremens and 9 schizophrenic women with clozapine-induced acute delirium. The levels of 5-HIAA were found to be significantly raised as compared with a control group. It demonstrated that after clinical recovery values returned to normal. These findings are suggested by the findings of Johansson and colleagues (1972) and raise the possibility that serotonin may be an important neurotransmitter in the pathogenesis of acute confusional states.

7. Mesulam M, Waxman SG, Geschwind N, Sabin TD: Acute confusional states with right middle cerebral artery infarctions. J Neurol Neurosurg Psychiatr 39:84–89, 1976.

Mesulam and coworkers provide the first account of the anatomic basic for acute confusional states. Subsequent articles by Horenstein and colleagues (1967) and Medina and coworkers (1974) provide further evidence that acute confusional states may result from focal right hemisphere lesions—a principle that is further expanded in the following reference.

8. Mesulam M: A cortical network for directed attention and unilateral neglect. Ann Neurol 10:309–325, 1981.

This article, although primarily addressing attention and neglect, has direct relevance to acute confusional states. The section on anatomy and pathogenesis provides a detailed description of a network hypothesis that is most relevant when applied to acute confusional states.

9. Obrecht R, Akhomia FOA, Scott DF: Value of EEG in acute confusional states. J Neurol Neurosurg Psychiatr 42:75–77, 1979.

This article summarizes the electroencephalographic findings from 95 patients over a 3-year period. The study concludes that EEG is a useful tool for deciding whether confusional states are primarily due to an intracranial process secondary to a toxic-metabolic disturbance. The authors point out the nonspecificity of the EEG; it is not invariably abnormal, and there are no pathognomonic EEG findings in acute confusional states.

10. Sabin TD: Coma and the confusional state in the emergency room. Med Clin North Am 65(1):25–32, 1981.

This relatively short article provides a solid approach to the initial management of a patient with acute confusional state. It concentrates on the clinical features, the differential diagnosis, and the methods of evaluation.

Management of Acute Head Injury

Edward Fischer, M.D.

Head injury is both common and diverse in its manifestations. Clinical problems may include coma, cranial nerve palsies, meningitis, headaches, stroke syndromes, dementia, and behavioral abnormalities. With this diverse clinical presentation, physicians are often insecure in identifying those patients likely to deteriorate. This article outlines the application of the Glasgow Coma Scale (GCS) to objective categorization of head-injured patients and to rapid identification of those needing urgent care. Diagnostic evaluation appropriate to degree of GCS severity and therapeutic modalities are discussed.

GENERAL ASSESSMENT OF THE HEAD-INJURED PATIENT

A secure, adequate airway and circulation are the first priorities in all patients. An unstable neck fracture must be assumed until proved otherwise. Stabilization of the neck with a cervical collar or sandbags must be maintained until radiographs showing all seven cervical vertebrae are scrutinized. A general physical examination will identify associated injuries that are often present, such as hemothorax, pneumothorax, splenic rupture, and fractures of long bones. Bimanual, gentle palpation of the head will reveal swelling, laceration, or bone depression. Physical signs of basal skull fracture may include ecchymosis over the mastoid process or under the eyes, bluish discoloration behind the ear, perforation and bleeding from the tympanic membrane, and watery discharge from the ear or nose. Nasal discharge of fluid may be evident only in the upright posture. A positive dipstick test for glucose in this fluid can help to identify it as cerebral spinal fluid (CSF).

NEUROLOGIC EXAMINATION

The neurologic examination should be brief and pertinent. A GCS rating is assigned at the earliest possible moment. The rest of the neurologic examination is tailored to each patient, depending on the severity of injury, and includes observations on level of consciousness, cranial nerves, and motor and sensory functions.

The Glasgow Coma Scale (GCS) categorizes head-injured patients on the basis of simple clinical observation (Fig. 1). Three functions are assessed: eye opening, verbal response, and motor response. If the eyes open spontaneously, score 4; to voice only, score 3; to pain only (sternal rub, distal nail bed pressure), score 2; and if they do not open at all, score 1. If the verbal response is normal and oriented, score 5; conversational but confused, score 4; with short words only, score 3; moans and groans only, score 2; and no response, score 1. If the motor response is appropriate to simple commands, score 6; no response to command but patient pushes away a painful stimulus, score 5; withdrawal to pain only, score 4; decorticate response to pain, score 3; decerebrate response to pain, score 2; and no response to pain, score 1. The best possible score is 15, and the worst is 3, even if the patient is dead. Head injury resulting in a GCS rating of 8 or less is severe and carries a mortality rate of approximately 50%. Scores between 9 and 12 are of moderate severity, and 13–15 are mild. Only the best response on the best side is scored (e.g., if the patient is hemiplegic, score the moving side). Demonstrated inter-user reliability of the scale allows its use by nurses, physicians, and paramedics and gives each group a common language about

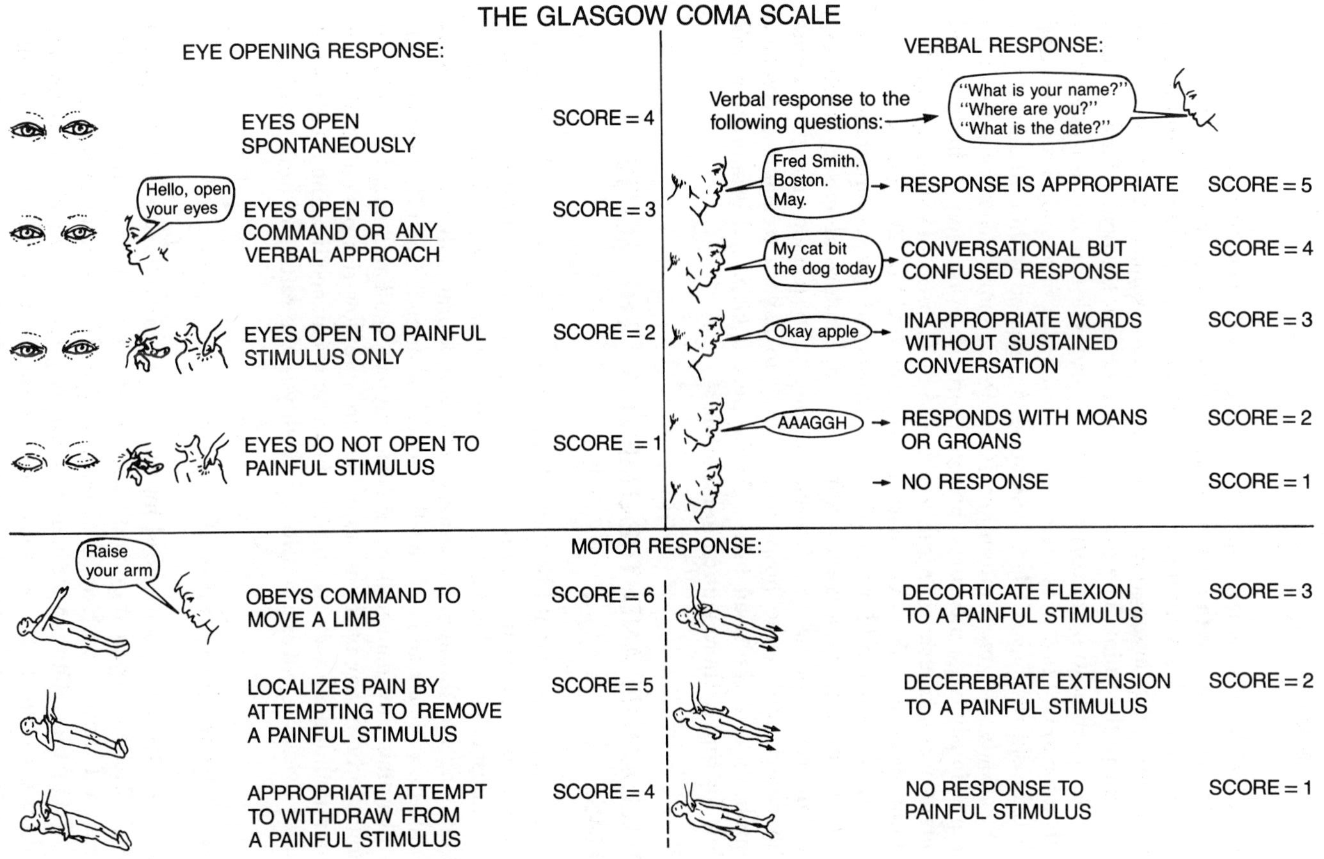

Figure 1. The Glasgow coma scale.

the patient for discussion among themselves. Deterioration of the score to a lower level may be the first warning of clinically important change.

Patients with severe injury (GCS of 8 or less) need urgent attention and often emergency intervention. Therefore, the examination should be succinct and to the point. The examiner should check the ocular fundus, pupil size and reaction to light, corneal reflexes, gag reflex, motor movements on both sides to nail bed pressure in hands and feet, deep tendon reflexes, and the Babinski response. The examination is repeated within 30 minutes.

Patients with moderate injury (GCS 9–12) should have, in addition to the previously cited measures, a more thorough evaluation of the level and content of consciousness. Attention should be focused on any complaint the patient may have. The examination is repeated within 30 minutes.

Patients with mild injury (GCS 13–15) should have comprehensive examination of mental status and cranial nerve and motor and sensory functions. The importance of the first examination cannot be stressed enough: patients who deteriorate in the hospital are likely to have a treatable secondary complication of the head injury. The repeated GCS and examination will allow for timely therapeutic intervention.

EVALUATION AND TREATMENT IN THE ACUTE PHASE

Management should be individualized and based on as thorough a history and physical examination as possible. A noncontrast head CT scan is the mainstay of evaluation. It is noninvasive and extremely sensitive in identifying life threatening lesions such as epidural, subdural, or intracerebral hematomas and focal or diffuse cerebral edema. The CT scan is crucial in planning the management of head injury. Skull radiography has been shown to be of low utility in a defined group of low-risk patients and is not recommended for such patients.[12] Magnetic resonance imaging (MRI) is not widely available but is a sensitive modality in the setting of brain trauma.[13]

Severe Head Injury (GCS of 8 or less)

Patients with severe head injury have a mortality rate of between 50 and 70%. Rapid evaluation and stabilization are the keys to improved outcome. CT scan is performed as early as possible, without losing time on plain skull films. Other tests include spine, chest, and abdominal radiographs and toxic screen. In the setting of hypotension, extracerebral causes should be sought (e.g., abdominal paracentesis for splenic rupture). Management is first directed at airway maintenance; endotracheal intubation is performed, or nasotracheal intubation is used, if possible, when strong suspicion of cervical injury exists and the likelihood of basal skull fracture is low. This is followed by hyperventilation to achieve an arterial PCO_2 of 25–30 mmHg. The head of the bed is elevated to 30 degrees, and once intravenous access is established, fluid restriction is maintained. Patients in this category are so likely to have underlying brain swelling that dexamethasone 10 mg intravenously is given as a bolus, then every six hours, with the dose tapered off over three days if there are indications of normal intracranial pressure (ICP) or over one week if ICP remains elevated. Signs of rising ICP (deterioration of the GCS or enlarging, sluggishly reacting pupil) are treated with mannitol intravenously in a dose of 1 gm/kg body weight over 20–30 minutes. Naloxone, thiamine, and 50% dextrose are given intravenously for potentially treatable predisposing conditions. As indicated by the CT scan, intracranial hematomas are evacuated as necessary. ICP monitoring with an epidural sensor, a subarachnoid bolt, or an intraventricular catheter is a prerequisite for management where facilities and expertise in the use of these devices exist. ICP measurement is essential to further treatment with mannitol or with barbiturates if the pressures remain high. These patients are at risk for delayed brain swelling or delayed intracranial bleeding. For this reason, the CT scan is repeated within 24 hours if the GCS rating remains the same or deteriorates. Modern management of severe head injury also involves invasive monitoring of hemodynamics in an intensive care unit setting. Support of central venous and systemic pressures can improve outcome. This is especially true when standard measures such as dehydration therapy and barbiturate coma can provoke significant systemic hypotension and cardiac suppression.

Moderate Head Injury (GCS 9–12)

Patients with moderate head injury frequently deteriorate from a treatable complication of head injury. Skull radiographs may be obtained in the emergency room. Although a normal film does not exclude significant underlying pathology, linear or other fractures indicate a high risk for delayed intracranial bleeding like an epidural hematoma. If the GCS rating does not improve or actually deteriorates, an immediate CT scan is obtained regardless of the skull film findings. A toxic screen should be obtained and naloxone, thiamine, and 50% dextrose administered. Clinical observations are made at least hourly with GCS assignments. The head of the bed is elevated 30 degrees, fluid is restricted, and fevers are controlled because the accompanying cerebral vasodilation will elevate the ICP. Depressed skull fractures and more than one clinical generalized seizure are indications for loading with phenytoin (Dilantin) intravenously or orally by nasogastric tube.

Mild Head Injury (GCS 13–15)

Patients with mild head injury are most likely to do well. Skull films are optional, depending on complaints and clinical suspicion. If a small object caused injury, look for depressed skull fracture on the films, because these patients can be alert at admission. CT scan is indicated when there is no clinical improvement within 24 hours. Those patients with a GCS rating of 15 and a normal neurologic examination may be sent home with frequent awakening by the family for evaluation. A printed sheet with warning signs of raised ICP should be provided to the family. If the patient is disoriented or has persistent, severe headaches with no one reliable at home, it is best to observe the patient for 24 hours in the hospital. It is not unusual for epidural hematoma to have a prolonged "lucid interval" while the hematoma slowly enlarges to the danger point. However, this should be quite evident in most cases within the 24-hour observation period. Restriction of oral fluid intake and elevation of the head 30 degrees are recommended.

DELAYED COMPLICATIONS OF HEAD INJURY

The likelihood of seizure is 50% if trauma results in disruption of the dura, and long-term anticonvulsant therapy is recommended for such patients. For those with diffuse contusions on CT scan, treatment for 1 year is usually recommended. Those patients with early seizures (within 1 week) should be treated and re-evaluated at approximately 1 year. Patients with seizures after the first week will likely need life-long treatment.

One must suspect meningitis from basilar skull fracture in head trauma patients with fever, even several weeks after the injury. It is usually preferable to perform a CT scan first and then lumbar puncture (LP) if there are no contraindications.

Intermittent rage attacks or periods of unusual behavior for which the patient has poor recall should raise the possibility of temperal lobe epilepsy, because the temporal poles are often contused in head injury. Confused behavior with no other findings should lead to careful electrolyte evaluation for complications such as inappropriate secretion of ADH or diabetes insipidus. Progressive deterioration of intellectual function with poor memory, difficulty in walking, and urinary incontinence should suggest post-traumatic normal pressure hydrocephalus. These patients require CT scan, radioisotope cisternography, and a shunt procedure if the diagnosis is established.

Rare causes of delayed rapid deterioration of patients include delayed intracerebral hemorrhage (most likely to occur after 7–21 days), chronic subdural hematoma (3–6 weeks later), and post-traumatic pseudoaneurysm (months to years later).

AREAS OF DIFFICULTY IN THE MANAGEMENT OF HEAD INJURY

The vast majority of severely head-injured patients are intoxicated at the time of their injury. A frequent but serious mistake is to assume that the obtunded head-injured patient is "just drunk." The GCS is helpful in this situation. Unless the patient has been drinking up to the time of admission and while on the accident floor, the initial GCS rating should improve, because alcohol is metabolized in the body. Therefore, a GCS value that stays the same or worsens should be evaluated with CT scan. Skull films will identify those patients with a skull fracture, which should be evaluated with CT scan immediately. Plain skull films do not eliminate the possibility of serious intracranial pathology, which will be indicated by an unchanging or deteriorating GCS.

All patients with significant head injury should be kept fluid restricted in an effort to control brain edema. Of course, severe volume depletion should be avoided with its attendant hypotension and renal failure. The ideal fluid for maintenance is normal saline; hypotonic solutions such as dextrose and water should be avoided because these may exacerbate brain swelling.

Much controversy surrounds the use of steroids in head injury. However, most experienced clinicians use short-course steroid therapy in severe head injury and in moderate or mild head injury with CT evidence of brain swelling. The dosage should be the equivalent of 10 mg of dexamethasone initially, then 6 mg every six hours, tapered over three days if the intracranial pressure is normal or if the patient is moderately or mildly injured, and tapered over one week if the intracranial pressure is elevated.

Skull radiographs can be helpful, although in severe head injury the CT scan has priority. But even here, skull films will aid in locating skull fractures that will determine proper placement of cervical traction devices if these are needed and will help the neurosurgeon plan the craniotomy. In moderately or mildly injured patients, depressed fracture (which can be present without alteration of consciousness) and linear fractures will alert the physician to potential delayed intracranial hematomas. The most important point to remember, however, is that normal skull films do not exclude the possibility of intracranial pathology.

Agitated behavior often accompanies acute head injury and has a strong correlation with subarachnoid blood and, at times, with incipient brain herniation. These patients should be gently restrained but not sedated, and the agitation should be seen as a sign that warrants continued close observation.

KEY FEATURES

A. General assessment of the head-injured patient
   1. Maintain adequate airway and circulation
   2. Stabilize the cervical spine
   3. General physical examination
B. Neurologic examination
   1. Glasgow Coma Scale assignment, sequentially
      a. 8 or less: severe; 50% mortality
      b. 9–12: moderate; high risk for deterioration
      c. 13–15: mild; best prognosis
C. Investigation and management of acute head injury
   1. Glasgow Coma Scale rating of 8 or less: severe head injury
      a. High mortality rate
      b. Rapid evaluation and stabilization, with intubation, hyperventilation, elevation of head of the bed, fluid restriction, naloxone (Narcan), thiamine, 50% dextrose, and steroids, mannitol if signs of progressive rise in ICP
      c. CT scan early, surgical decompression early if indicated and monitor ICP
      d. Repeat CT in 24 hours
      e. Hemodynamic monitoring and support
   2. Glasgow Coma Scale rating of 9–12: moderate head injury
      a. High risk of deterioration from treatable secondary complications
      b. Skull films in emergency room if possible
      c. If skull fracture present or if GCS value same or worse, early CT and toxic screen
      d. Elevate head of bed, restrict fluids, administer short course of steroids
      e. Load with phenytoin (Dilatin) if indicated
   3. Glasgow Coma Scale rating of 13–15: mild head injury
      a. Close clinical observation
      b. Skull films optional
      c. CT scan if no clinical improvement in 24 hours
      d. Outpatient follow-up only with appropriate home setting and head injury symptom sheet
D. Delayed complications
   1. Seizures
   2. Fever
   3. Behavioral disorders
   4. Sudden onset headaches may indicate delayed intracranial bleeding

BIBLIOGRAPHY

1. Stuart GG, et al: Severe head injury managed without intracranial pressure monitoring. J Neurosurg 59:601–605, 1983.
   The outcome of 100 prospectively studied severely head-injured patients without ICP monitoring compares favorably with those series of patients with ICP monitoring.

2. Jennett B, Teasdale G: Management of Head Injuries. Philadelphia, FA Davis, 1981.
   A comprehensive, practical overview of head injury management with strongly stated approaches.

3. Cooper PR (ed): Head Injury. Baltimore, Williams and Wilkins, 1982.
   A presentation of the multifaceted nature of head injury management issues; well referenced.

4. Teasdale G, Jennett B: Assessment and prognosis of coma after head injury. Lancet 2:81–84, 1974.
   A detailed presentation of the Glasgow Coma Scale.

5. Teasdale G, Knill-Jones R, Van der Sande J: Observer variability in assessing impaired consciousness and coma. J Neurol Neurosurg Psychiat 41:603–610, 1978.
   The Glasgow Coma Scale has excellent inter-user reliability, especially among different levels of the health care profession.

6. Braakman R, Schouter HJA, et al: Megadose steroids in severe head injury. Results of a prospective double blind clinical trial. J Neurosurg 58:326–330, 1983.
   High-dose dexamethasone has no effect on outcome in severe head injury.

7. Cooper PR, Ho V: Role of emergency skull x-ray films in the evaluation of the head-injured patient: A retrospective study. Neurosurgery 13:136–140, 1983.
   Only 1 patient out of 207 returned to hospital after skull fracture and delayed deterioration from epidural hematoma. Skull films are not cost effective or useful in predicting deterioration from intracranial mass lesions when performed to identify linear skull fractures.

8. Coonley-Hoganson R, Sachs N, et al: Sequelae associated with head injuries in patients who were not hospitalized: A follow-up survey. Neurosurgery 14:315–317, 1984.
   The results of this study show the persistence of sequelae (headaches, dizziness, nausea) in the majority of patients with head injury not associated with brain involvement.

9. Rosner MJ, Newsome HH, Becker DP: Mechanical brain injury: The sympathoadrenal response. J Neurosurg 61:76–86, 1984.
   Increased sympathoadrenal discharge resulting from severe head injury may cause blood pressure, cardiac rhythm, and glucose metabolism problems.

10. Fife D, Jagger J: The contribution of brain injury to the overall injury severity of brain injured patients. Neurosurg 60:697–699, 1984.
    Brain injury severity was closely related to overall injury severity in a group of hospitalized head-injured patients, more so than injury severity for all other body organs.

11. Eisenberg HM, Frankowski RF, et al: High-dose barbiturate control of elevated intracranial pressure in patients with severe head injury. J Neurosurg 69:15–23, 1988.
    High-dose barbiturates can be effective in an appropriate, experienced setting, where factors such as systemic hypotension can be controlled.

12. Masters SJ, McClean PM, Arcarese JS, et al: Skull X-ray examinations after head trauma. Recommendations by a multidisciplinary panel and validation study. N Engl J Med 316:84–91, 1987.
13. Gentry LR, Godersky JC, Thompson B: MR imaging of head trauma: Review of the distribution and radiopathologic features of traumatic lesions. AJR 150:663–672, 1988.

Spinal Cord Compression

Robert Goldman, M.D.
Fereydoun Shahrokhi, M.D.

Spinal cord compression is frequently a medical or surgical emergency. Unfortunately, the likelihood of successful intervention is greatly reduced by the time the diagnosis is obvious. Thus, the primary challenge lies in establishing the diagnosis early.

The common causes of spinal cord compression include cervical spondylosis and degenerative disk disease, spinal and epidural metastases, spinal epidural abscess or hematoma, and trauma. Less common causes include primary spinal tumors, syringomyelia, spinal arteriovenous malformation, spinal arachnoiditis, and fungal or parasitic infections. Multiple sclerosis, subacute combined degeneration as a result of vitamin B_{12} deficiency, and Guillain-Barré syndrome can occasionally be confused with spinal cord compression.

Symptoms and signs will depend upon the anatomic level and the chronicity of the lesion. Pain is an important symptom of spinal cord compression. The pain may be located over the spine or may radiate across the trunk or to an extremity, owing to root involvement.[1] In addition, there may be weakness, numbness, or paresthesia and difficulty in walking or with balance. Urinary symptoms usually may occur in the more advanced stages and require urgent evaluation.

The physical examination in a patient with a history suggesting spinal cord compression begins with a thorough general examination. Examination of the back should note the presence of paraspinal tenderness, muscle spasm, and limitation of movement. Neurologic examination centers on motor, reflex, sensory, and autonomic changes. Acute complete spinal cord transection will initially cause a flaccid paralysis, with areflexia and anesthesia below the level of the transection, and absent plantar responses. In 3–6 weeks, this will gradually be replaced by a spastic paralysis, with hyperreflexia and upgoing toes. Partial spinal cord transection will produce varying features. Characteristic partial syndromes include the following: Hemisection of the cord results in the Brown-Séquard syndrome, with ipsilateral paralysis and corticospinal signs and contralateral loss of pinprick and temperature sensation. Anterior cord damage results in paralysis with moderate loss of pinprick and light touch and relative preservation of vibration and position sense. The central cervical cord syndrome is characterized by weakness, with the hands more affected than the shoulders and with variable sensory loss.

The severity and rate of progression of the symptoms and signs, together with initial assessment as to the likely cause, will determine the rapidity with which the work-up is to be undertaken. Development of symptoms and signs over a period of hours to days, particularly in cases in which there is suspicion of a malignancy or infection, will require immediate definitive evaluation, whereas clinical development over months without recent progression can be evaluated less urgently. However, suspected spinal cord compression should receive prompt attention in any case, as even stable patients can deteriorate abruptly.

The definitive laboratory test for evaluation of suspected spinal cord compression is contrast myelography. Advantages include the fact that the blockage to the flow of CSF can be studied in the entire spinal cord and a lumbar puncture is not routinely performed until the time of myelography. If a complete block above the site of puncture is demonstrated, the only way to determine the upper limit of the block is to inject dye in the cervical region through a cisternal puncture. If an overlying soft tissue infection in the lumbar region is suspected, a lumbar puncture is contraindicated, owing to the risk of causing a meningitis. In this case, a cervical puncture is performed. If a block is demonstrated, dye can be left in the subarachnoid space, allowing subsequent radiologic examination without repeat lumbar puncture.

Other diagnostic studies that may be helpful in establishing the diagnosis of cord compression prior to myelography include plain radiographs of the spine. These may show a malignant or infectious process. A radionuclide bone scan may show these earlier in the course of the illness. CT scan of the spine is now the best readily available noninvasive radiologic modality for the diagnosis of spine, nerve root, and spinal cord disease. Magnetic resonance imaging (MRI) poorly visualizes bone but effectively identifies lesions of the bone marrow or those compromising the spinal cord and may supplant other diagnostic tests for some indications.[11] CSF analysis is an important adjunct of myelography, especially when cord compression occurs as a result of infection or malignancy.

Cervical spondylosis in common in the elderly and may be associated with a progressive myelopathy.[2] Both compression and ischemia of the spinal cord are thought to be involved in the pathogenesis. In a patient with a cervical myelopathy, the diagnosis is suggested by evidence of significant degenerative disease on cervical spine radiographs with decreased anteroposterior diameter of the spinal cord on the lateral views, and by exclusion of other causes. Diagnosis is confirmed by myelography. Conservative treatment consists of a cervical collar, physical therapy, and anti-inflammatory medication. Surgery may be helpful and is indicated when there are signs of significant or recent progression of myelopathy.

Acute intervertebral disk herniation in cervical spondylosis or as an isolated event in younger patients can cause cervical cord compression. Disk herniation is more commonly lateral than central, causing spinal root compression and radicular pain in the upper extremity. Cord compression is less common and is caused by a central or a large lateral disk. The common sites for disk prolapse are C6–C7 and C5–C6.[3] Diagnosis is corroborated by cervical spine radiographs; spinal CT scan; and, when surgery is being considered, a myelogram. In the absence of myelopathy, the treatment is usually conservative, with bed rest, anti-inflammatory/analgesic therapy; heat; immobilization with a cervical collar; and, at times, traction. Significant neurologic deficit or persistent pain may be indications for surgical excision of the disk. Acute central disk herniation with signs of myelopathy from spinal cord compression is an indication for urgent surgery.

Tumors are a common cause of spinal cord compression, although primary spinal tumors remain quite rare. Metastatic malignant disease is a more common cause of morbidity and generally presents in a more acute fashion.[4] Common primary tumors include lung, breast, prostate, and renal cell carcinomas.[4] Most (85%) of such cases will involve metastases to the bone, and as such may produce abnormalities on plain radiographs or bone scan. Hematologic malignancies will often cause spinal cord compression without involving the vertebra.

Outcome in this group of patients with malignant disease is strongly dependent upon how early treatment is instituted.[5] Therefore, any symptoms or signs of spinal cord compression in a patient with known or suspected cancer deserve immediate evaluation. Indications for immediate myelography include a history of progressive weakness or evidence of a new neurologic deficit. Patients with a normal examination but abnormal spinal radiographs should have myelographic examination urgently. Patients with both normal examination and normal radiographs are observed closely, with consideration given to elective myelography or bone scan.

Treatment consists of steroids; radiation therapy; surgery; and, in some cases, chemotherapy. Steroids are used initially in most cases. Chemotherapy is generally not an immediate treatment, though it may be quite efficacious in certain cases.[6] The efficacy of radiation therapy, surgery, or a combination has been investigated, and though there is no single definitive study, the general consensus is that in most cases radiation therapy is as effective as surgery and may be safer in most instances.[4] Combination therapy is no more effective than radiation alone. Specific indications for surgery include (1) tissue needed for diagnosis, (2) progression of deficit while patient is receiving radiation therapy, (3) radiation therapy not available, and (4) previous radiation therapy to the allowable limit.

Spinal epidural or subdural abscess may be difficult to diagnose early. Epidural abscess is suggested by the triad of back pain, local spine tenderness, and fever.[7] Common sources of infection include furuncle, respiratory tract infection, and dental or vertebral osteomyelitis. Associated conditions include diabetes mellitus, intravenous drug abuse, and history of back trauma or surgery. *Staphylococcus aureus* is the most common pathogen.[7] Pott's disease leading to spinal cord compression is now rare, but it needs to be considered.

In the evaluation of such patients, the plain spine radiographs may show evidence of vertebral osteomyelitis. CSF analysis may show evidence of a parameningeal infection, with elevated protein and a moderate number of white blood cells. Again, suspicion of an overlying soft tissue infection contraindicates a lumbar puncture. Treatment consists of antibiotics followed by immediate laminectomy and drainage.

Spinal epidural or subdural hematoma is suggested by back pain and appropriate neurologic deficit. The diagnosis should be considered in patients who have recently undergone a lumbar puncture, even in the absence of a coagulopathy.[8] Treatment consists of correction of any bleeding disorder and, in some cases, surgical evacuation of the hematoma.

Although not a cause of direct spinal cord compression, meningeal infections are a medically treatable cause of progressive spinal cord dysfunction. Such infections include various fungi, parasites, and syphilis.[9,10] If there is suspicion of such an infection in the face of a progressive spinal lesion, and CSF is confirmatory with low glucose concentration in addition to high protein and WBC, treatment should be started immediately and further evaluation is not usually warranted.

KEY FEATURES

Once the diagnosis of spinal cord compression is obvious, chances for successful therapy are reduced. Therefore, one must maintain a high level of suspicion in order to allow for treatment early in the course of the disease.

Back pain is a prominent symptom, with progression to radicular pain, weakness, and paralysis. The neurologic deficit will depend upon the anatomic level and location of the lesion.

Once the diagnosis of spinal cord compression is suspected, urgent neurologic evaluation is required. The speed with which a definitive diagnosis needs to be made will depend upon the severity and rate of progression of the neurologic symptoms and signs.

Cervical spondylosis and chronic herniated intervertebral disks are usually treated conservatively initially, but may eventually require surgery. Acute herniation of a cervical disk, with resultant neurologic deficit, may require urgent surgery. For compression associated with metastatic malignancy, steroids and radiation therapy are the mainstay of treatment. Epidural abscess is treated with antibiotics and surgical drainaged. Epidural hematoma requires correction of any coagulopathy and surgical drainage.

REFERENCES

1. Harries B: Spinal cord compression. Br Med J *1*:611–614, 673–677, 1970.

   An excellent review of the pathophysiology, clinical presentation, common causes, and treatment of spinal cord compression.

2. Nurick S: The natural history and the results of surgical treatment of the spinal cord disorder associated with cervical spondylosis. Brain 95:101–102, 1972.

   Ninety-one patients were followed. In most cases, the process is benign. Surgery is recommended primarily for those with progressive disability.

3. Yoss RE, et al: Significance of symptoms and signs in localization of involved root in cervical disc protrusion. Neurology 7:673–683, 1959.

   Ten patients with confirmed protrusions of a single cervical disk were studied. In 87 of them, the lesion was accurately localized on the basis of history and neurologic examination.

4. Gilbert RW, Kim JH, Posner JB: Epidural spinal cord compression from metastatic tumor: Diagnosis and treatment. Ann Neurol 3:40–51, 1978.

   A study of 235 cases of spinal cord compression by metastatic epidural tumor. Though the study was uncontrolled, outcome as judged by ability to ambulate was the same with radiation therapy as with decompression laminectomy followed by radiation therapy.

5. Rodichof LD, et al: Early diagnosis of spinal epidural metastases. Am J Med 70:1181–1188, 1981.

   Patients who presented with myelopathy had a high incidence of complete block and a poor outcome, whereas patients presenting with back pain, normal examination, and abnormal radiographs often had early epidural compression, which was more amenable to therapy.

6. Posner JB, Howieson J, Cuitkovic E: "Disappearing" spinal cord compression: Oncolytic effect of glucocorticoids (and other chemotherapeutic agents) on epidural metastases. Ann Neurol 2:409–413, 1977.

   Article presents four cases of epidural metastases that were relieved by treatment with steroids alone, or in combination with chemotherapy.

7. Baker AS, et al: Spinal epidural abscess. N Engl J Med 293:463–468, 1975.

   Clinical course and outcome of 39 cases of spinal epidural abscess are reviewed.

8. Kirkpatrick D, Goodman SJ: Combined subarachnoid and subdural hematoma following lumbar puncture. Surg Neurol 3:109–111, 1975.

   Article presents a case of spinal subarachnoid and subdural hematoma following a lumbar puncture in the absence of a coagulopathy. Stresses the features of spinal hematomas, which are localized back pain, rapidly progressive myelopathy, and poor prognosis without immediate surgical decompression.

9. Singh A, et al: Paraplegia in cysticercosis: Case of spinal cysticercosis with paraplegia (India). Br Med J 2:684–685, 1966.

   Report of a case. Spinal fluid was acellular with low glucose. Myelogram showed spinal cord compression.

10. Bird A: Acute spinal schistosomiasis. Neurology 14:647–656, 1964.

    Article describes six cases. Pathology was either a granuloma compression of the spinal cord or microscopic involvement of the spinal cord producing a myelitis.

11. Posner JB: Mechanical lesions of the spine and related structures. *In* Wyngaarden JB, Smith LH (eds.): Cecil Textbook of Medicine, 18th ed. Philadelphia, WB Saunders Co., 1988, pp 2247–2258.

    Excellent general discussion of anatomy, physiology, diagnosis and treatment of lesions of the spine.

Epilepsy

Fereydoun Shahrokhi, M.D.

A seizure, according to Hughlings Jackson's nineteenth century definition, consists of sudden excessive discharge of gray matter of the central nervous system. Seizures occur intermittently at irregular intervals, usually lasting each for seconds to minutes. They may occur as a single event, a single cluster, or may continue for a lifetime. The major types of seizures include the following:[1,2]

1. Simple partial (focal, motor, or sensory) seizures without impairment of consciousness.
2. Complex partial seizures (psychomotor or temporal lobe epilepsy) with impairment of awareness, perceptual, and emotional experiences and involuntary automatic behavior such as lip smacking, chewing, running, or laughing.
3. Petit mal (absence seizures), involving a sudden interruption of awareness associated with a staring spell, lasting less than 30 seconds, with minimal motor manifestations and a typical 3-Hz generalized spike-wave pattern on electroencephalogram (EEG).
4. Tonic-clonic or grand mal seizures with sudden loss of consciousness, 10–20 second generalized stiffness (tonic), and falling to the ground, followed by a few minutes of violent rhythmic (clonic) jerking of the body and extremities, and then a quiet comatose state for another few minutes. Finally, sleep or postictal confusion follow and may last minutes to hours. There may be urinary and fecal incontinence and biting of the tongue or buccal mucosa.

5. Myoclonic seizures with single lightning-fast jerks that may be generalized or segmental.
6. Status epilepticus with repeated or very prolonged grand mal, petit mal, or focal seizures without recovery between the attacks.

Possible causes of epilepsy are summarized in Table 1.

DIAGNOSIS

The diagnosis of seizure is made by history from a witness or by an EEG in the ictal or interictal state showing focal or generalized paroxysmal (epileptiform) discharges, i.e., spikes, spike-wave, sharp-wave, or bursts of abnormal rhythms. A complete history, examination and EEG, CT scan with and without contrast, lumbar puncture, screening blood tests, and chest radiograph are needed for evaluation of the systemic or CNS diseases that may be the cause of the seizures. Positron-emission tomography (PET) scan and magnetic resonance imaging (MRI) are useful adjunctive diagnostic procedures.

TREATMENT

The acute treatment of a single seizure during its occurrence involves gentle prevention of injuries and maintenance of an open airway. Recurrent seizures require chronic antiepileptic treatment (Tables 2 and 3). Seizure disorders from the toxic and metabolic encephalopathies may respond to

Table 1.   POSSIBLE CAUSES OF EPILEPSY

1. Idiopathic epilepsy	
a. Primary generalized epilepsy with a hereditary tendency	Grand mal, petit mal, myoclonic epilepsy
b. No causes are found or recorded	Generalized or focal seizures
2. Head trauma	Including birth injuries
3. Cerebral vasoanoxia	Including perinatal hypoxia
4. Intracranial tumors	
5. Intracranial infections	Meningitis, abscess, subdural empyema, viral encephalitis, granulomas, Jakob-Creutzfeldt disease, toxoplasmosis
6. Cerebrovascular disease	Intracerebral bleed, arteriovenous malformation, lupus cerebritis, cortical vein thrombosis, acute embolism, old stroke
7. Congenital, hereditary	Cerebral palsy, tuberous sclerosis, porencephaly
8. Degenerative disease	Rarely in Alzheimer's disease
9. Metabolic and toxic	Hypoglycemia, hyponatremia, hypocalcemia, uremic myoclonic twitch syndrome, dialysis, toxemia of pregnancy, porphyria, hepatic encephalopathy, neuroleptic disease, theophylline, drug withdrawal syndromes

Table 2.   EFFECTIVE DRUGS IN VARIOUS SEIZURE TYPES

1. Tonic-clonic (grand mal): Phenytoin, phenobarbital, carbamazepine, primidone, and valproic acid (as a secondary drug)
2. Simple partial: Phenytoin, phenobarbital, carbamazepine, primidone
3. Complex partial (psychomotor seizures, temporal lobe epilepsy): Carbamazepine, primidone, phenytoin (reportedly does not prevent kindling), phenobarbital (reportedly not as effective)
4. Myoclonic seizures: clonazepam, valproic acid, diazepam, phenytoin, 5-hydroxytryptophan with carbidopa
5. Petit mal: Ethosuximide, valproic acid

metabolic correction, obviating the need for specific anticonvulsant therapy, although some patients may, during the acute phase, require such treatment.

The recurrence risk following a single seizure or a single cluster of seizures in an afebrile adult is approximately 30% over 3 years.[3] The risk is reportedly lower in patients with seizure resulting from acute metabolic dysfunction and higher in patients with an anatomic CNS lesion. Patients must be informed that it is illegal for them to drive until they are seizure-free for a certain period of time (1–2 years in the United States, depending on the state).

Anticonvulsants given chronically for recurrent epilepsy are usually continued until the patient is seizure-free for 3–5 years. Anticonvulsants should be tapered slowly over 2–4 months rather than stopped abruptly, to avoid status epilepticus. Anticonvulsant therapy is usually initiated with one medication and a second drug is added only after high blood levels (not high doses) fail to produce satisfactory control. One must keep in mind that the most common cause of anticonvulsant failure is noncompliance.

Seizures in alcoholic patients may be caused by withdrawal (rum fits) or by head trauma, hypoglycemia, hyponatremia, meningitis, brain tumor, or idiopathic epilepsy, among others.[4-6] This necessitates a full work-up in an alcoholic with recent onset of seizures or with poorly documented prior evaluation. Virtually all seizures that are due to alcohol withdrawal occur within 48 hours of withdrawal or diminished consumption.[5] Approximately 40% are single seizures, and the rest are clusters of two to four seizures in a 6-hour period. There is no consensus regarding the chronic management of patients with recurrent alcohol withdrawal seizures, but we believe that such treatment is usually futile and may be dangerous. However, prophylactic treatment with phenobarbital, chlordiazepoxide (Librium), paraldehyde, lorazepam (Ativan), or phenytoin (Dilantin) in addition to the treatment of hypomagnesemia and other metabolic problems may be very effective in the first few days.[6,7]

Chronic prophylactic anticonvulsant therapy is usually given to patients with brain tumor, because such patients have a 35% chance of developing epilepsy. The risk of epilepsy after head trauma is 5–60%, depending on the nature and severity of the injury.[8] The peak incidence of post-traumatic

Table 3. COMMON ANTIEPILEPTIC DRUGS

Drug	Adult Daily Dose (mg)	Pediatric Daily Dose (mg/kg)	Therapeutic Blood Level (μg/ml)	Half-life	Days to Achieve Steady State Blood Levels
Phenobarbital	60–150	4–6	15–50	3–4 days	14–21
Phenytoin (Dilantin)	300–500	5–10	10–20	1 day	7–10
Carbamazepine (Tegretol)	600–1200*†	10–25	4–12	12–35 hours	3–4
Primidone (Mysoline)	750–1500*†	10–25	5–15	16–18 hours	4–7
Valproic acid (Depakene)	1000–3000*	15–60	50–100	8–12 hours	4
Clonazepam (Clonopin)	1.5–20.0†	0.05–0.2	20–80 ng/ml	1–2 days	5–7
Ethosuximide (Zarontin)	750–1500	15–35	40–100	1–3 days	7–10
Diazepam (Valium)	10–20 mg% IV in status	0.15–0.5 mg/kg or up to 10 mg for status	0.1–1.0	1–3 days	4–10

*Because of the short half-life, must be given in divided doses.
†Start with a low dose and work up to seizure control or toxicity.

522

epilepsy is at about 9 months, and 80–90% of epilepsies start within 2 years after trauma. Most patients with severe head injuries are given 1–2 years of prophylactic daily doses of anticonvulsants. The incidence of seizures is low in ischemic strokes but high in intracerebral hemorrhage and arteriovenous malformation (AVM) and very high in cerebral abscess. Prophylactic anticonvulsant therapy is indicated for intracerebral hemorrhage, AVM, or abscess.

Idiopathic seizure disorder consists of two groups. The first includes so-called primary generalized epilepsy with inherited predisposition for petit mal, grand mal, and/or epileptic myoclonus. Patients may develop one or more types of these seizures, and petit mal usually resolves spontaneously in adolescence. Frequently, however, these patients develop grand mal seizures. Complete cessation or control of the primary seizure disorder by the fourth decade of life is not uncommon. However, antiepileptic anticonvulsant treatment is continued until the patient is seizure-free for 3–5 years. The second type of idiopathic epilepsy has no documented inheritance and may be related to various causes such as birth injury, hypoxia, or other factors that have escaped diagnosis.

In pregnant epileptics, the risk of grand mal seizures to the baby and the mother outweighs the risk of anticonvulsant therapy. However, these drugs are suspected of causing various malformations, including cleft palate, and heart defects when administered in the first trimester. Congenital malformations initially attributed to phenytoin use during pregnancy have not been confirmed in subsequent studies and are seen with the use of other anticonvulsant medications. Of the newer agents, valproic acid has been shown to be teratogenic in animals, but carbamazepine has not been associated with a significant teratogenic risk.[23] Trimethadione is highly teratogenic and should be avoided. During pregnancy, the anticonvulsant blood levels significantly and progressively drop,[9] owing to weight gain, impaired GI absorption, higher plasma clearance rate, hormonal changes, retention of water and sodium, accelerated drug metabolism, and administration of supplemental folic acid. The blood level of any anticonvulsant given during pregnancy must be maintained carefullly and the dose adjusted accordingly.

STATUS EPILEPTICUS

Status epilepticus refers to very prolonged or very frequent seizures without recovery between the attacks. The seizures may be grand mal, petit mal, simple, or complex partial. Tonic-clonic status is a neurologic emergency with a mortality rate of over 10–12% and risk of serious morbidity including a persistent vegetative state. The causes include idiopathic seizures, head trauma, intracranial infections, cerebral vascular diseases, brain tumors, metabolic encephalopathies, cerebral hypoxia, withdrawal from alcohol, benzodiazepines and barbiturates, administration of theophylline, and, perhaps, most important, withdrawal from anticonvulsant medications.[12] Generalized seizures lasting for more than a few hours have, in well-oxygenated and metabolically stable laboratory animals, resulted in ischemic neuronal changes and scattered petechial hemorrhages.[10] The factors contributing to neuronal damage appear to include increased metabolic demand, decreased energy supplies, lactic acidosis, brain edema, mitochondrial swelling, increased free radicals from peroxidation of membranes, disturbance of protein synthesis, noxiously high calcium influx, late hypotension, hypoglycemia, and hyperthermia.[10,11] Cardiorespiratory failure; renal failure from hypotension, myoglobinuria, or acidosis; and the side effects of IV anticonvulsants are the three main causes of death.

Status epilepticus should be managed by a team of physicians, preferably in an ICU. Management should have three broad goals: (1) the maintenance of vital functions and prevention of hyperthermia, (2) the diagnosis and treatment of any precipitating factors, and (3) the control of the seizures with metabolic therapy and antiepileptic drugs.

Intubation during convulsive seizure is difficult and may cause injuries. However, if rapidly acting anticonvulsants are ineffective or if signs of respiratory depression appear, this may need to be attempted. Neuromuscular blockers may be used to help intubation or when there are multiple fractures, severe acidosis, hypoventilation, or severe myoglobinuria. The serious disadvantage of masking clinical signs of seizure by neuromuscular blocking agents may be overcome by continuous EEG monitoring.

The most commonly used drug regimens for status epilepticus are as follows:

1. IV diazepam at 2 mg/minute up to 10–20 mg total dose or until the seizures are controlled. Diazepam is a very fast-acting medication but also a very short-acting one, with a distribution half-life of only 20–40 minutes. In combination with diazepam, phenytoin, a longer-acting medicine, is used at 14–18 mg/kg given at 50 mg/minute or slower in normal saline. Intravenous phenytoin can be given most safely by infusion pump, with ECG and BP monitoring. Contraindications for IV phenytoin include significant bradycardia, sinoatrial block, second- or third-degree atrioventricular block, severe myocardial insufficiency, and perhaps age greater than 65 years. Phenytoin is fully effective in 20–30 minutes from the start of infusion. IV phenytoin should be discontinued if significant bradycardia or hypotension develops. If the seizures continue after 20–30 minutes from the time phenytoin was started, some investigators advocate the slow IV infusion of diazepam, 100 mg/500 ml D5W* at 40 ml/hour.[13,14]

---

*D5W = 5% dextrose in water.

2. Phenobarbital is an effective alternative to the combination of diazepam and phenytoin. The initial IV dose of 200–300 mg must be given at no more than 100 mg/minute but may be repeated twice at 20–30 minute intervals.[15] Phenobarbital may be given in conjunction with IV phenytoin. Respiratory suppression is the major toxicity of IV phenobarbital and may be very severe when the drug is used in conjunction with diazepam or other sedatives.

3. Paraldehyde, lidocaine, and lorazepam (Ativan) are among the secondary choices in anticonvulsants.[13] Paraldehyde may be particularly effective in alcohol withdrawal status. However, because this is an intensely corrosive agent that dissolves plastic syringes and tubing within a few minutes, its IV use is of questionable safety. Intramuscular paraldehyde (10% USP) must be given safely away from nerve trunks at an initial dose of 0.1–0.2 mg/kg. The dose may be repeated at 0.1 mg/kg every 2–4 hours. Side effects include congestive heart failure and metabolic acidosis, as well as pain and sterile abscess at injection sites. Lidocaine is given at 50–100 mg slow IV push followed by 1–2 mg/minute continuous intravenous infusion. Lorazepam, a benzodiazepine with a half-life of about 15 hours, is given in an IV or IM dose of 2.5–10.0 mg.

4. Thiopental anesthesia to produce EEG burst-suppression as an anticonvulsant and to decrease the metabolic rate may be helpful when initial measures have failed. Induced hypothermia to core temperature of 32°–35° C, acetazolamide 500 mg/day (an anticonvulsant that increases CNS CO_2 and GABA*), and IV corticosteroids (to decrease edema and free radicals) may also be helpful.[16–18]

Once the seizures are controlled, high maintenance doses of anticonvulsants such as phenytoin and/or phenobarbital are started within a few hours. Over the next few days, the doses are adjusted according to the clinical state and blood levels.

A CT scan needs to be performed at some point early in the management of status epilepticus if the cause remains uncertain. In most cases, CT can be performed after reasonable control of the vital functions and the seizures is achieved. The same is true for lumbar puncture, except when there is suspicion of meningitis.

Focal status epilepticus is at times very resistant to drug treatment. In some cases of epilepsia partialis continua, the recurrent focal motor seizures involving the face or an arm may continue for decades in spite of anticonvulsant treatment.[19] There is, however, no impairment of consciousness in these cases. Widespread unilateral continuous seizure activity and opposite

---

*GABA = gamma-aminobutyric acid.

hemiparesis, i.e., periodic lateralized epileptiform discharges (PLEDs), when associated with severe obtundation has a poor prognosis and deserves early diagnosis (by EEG) and treatment.[20-22]

KEY FEATURES

Diagnosis of seizures is made by detailed history from witnesses and EEG.

More common seizure types include simple partial (focal), complex partial (usually temporal lobe epilepsy), petit mal (usually in children), grand mal, and myoclonic epilepsy.

An etiologically oriented history, physical examination, and lab work-up are needed for seizures of recent onset. These may have to be repeated periodically during follow-up to rule out the evolution of brain tumor or other potentially treatable causes.

Treatment of status epilepticus is as follows:
A. Participation of a team of physicians, preferably in a medical ICU.
B. Stabilization and maintenance of the vital functions.
C. Prevention of hyperthermia, myoglobinuria, acidosis, and excessive movement.
D. Correction of any contributory or secondary metabolic disturbance.
E. Treatment with anticonvulsants:
    1. Anticonvulsant drugs are used intravenously.
    2. The inappropriate or overzealous treatment with anticonvulsants is one of the three main causes of death along with cardiorespiratory and renal failure.
    3. Diazepam: A short-acting agent that should be used in conjunction with another drug, usually phenytoin.
    4. IV phenytoin: induced at 50 mg/minute to a total leading dose of 14–18 mg/kg. ECG and BP monitoring are essential.
    5. Phenobarbital: used alone or in conjunction with phenytoin. Loading dose of 200–300 mg is induced at no more than 100 mg/minute. Dose may be repeated twice at 20–30 minutes.
    6. Intubation is attempted for airway protection or ventilatory insufficiency.
    7. Neuromuscular blockers may be used when there are multiple fractures, significant myoglobinuria, or possibility of cardiac failure from exertion. Because these drugs mask motor activity, they are preferably used in conjunction with continuous EEG monitoring.

REFERENCES

1. Dreifuss FE, et al: Proposal for revised clinical and electroencephalographic classification of epileptic seizures. Epilepsia 22:489–501, 1981.

More extensive details about various seizure types and their EEG abnormalities, including atonic seizures, "reflex seizures," and some others.

2. Shahrokhi F, Sabin T: Seizure disorders. *In* Noble J (ed): Textbook of General Medicine and Primary Care. Boston/Toronto, Little, Brown, 1987, pp 1431–1444.
   A review article.

3. Hauser WA, et al: Seizure recurrence after a first unprovoked seizure. N Engl J Med 307:522–528, 1982.
4. Isbell H, et al: An experimental study of the etiology of "rum fits" and delirium tremens. Q J Stud Alcohol 16:1–33, 1955.
   Ten volunteer patients consuming large daily quantities of alcohol were studied for 3 months. With withdrawal or lowered amount of alcohol, they developed tremulousness, delirium, and seizures.

5. Victor M, Brausch J: The role of abstinence in the genesis of alcoholic epilepsy. Epilepsia 8:1–20, 1967.
   An excellent article with extensive and meticulous data about alcohol withdrawal, 90% within 7–48 hours; 3% of patients developed status epilepticus. Photic stimulation during EEG produced increased excitability and photomyogenic activity as late as 130 hours.

6. Mattson RH: Effect of alcohol intake in non-alcoholic epileptics. Neurology 25:361–362, 1975 (abstract). Presented at the American Academy of Neurology Meeting, Bal Harbour, FL, 1975.
   The alcohol intake itself suppresses the EEG epileptiform activity. It is the "morning after effect" with the rapid falling of alcohol blood level that activates the seizures.

7. Kaim SC, et al: Treatment of the acute alcohol withdrawal state. A comparison of 4 drugs. Am J Psych 125:1640–1646, 1969.
   Four drugs, hydroxyzine (Vistaril), chlorpromazine, thiamine, and chlordiazepoxide (Librium), were studied in a double-blind fashion in 537 alcoholic patients in regard to their preventive effects of alcohol withdrawal, convulsions, and DTs. Chlordiazepoxide was significantly more effective than the others.

8. Jennett B, Teasdale G: Management of Head Injuries. Philadelphia, FA Davis, 1981, p 287.
9. Dam A, Dam AM: Epilepsy in pregnancy. In Tyrer JH (ed): The Treatment of Epilepsy. Philadelphia, JB Lippincott, 1980, pp 323–348.
   An excellent review of various aspects of epilepsy in pregnancy, including the treatment.

10. Meldrum BS, et al: Systemic factors in epileptic brain damage after prolonged seizures in paralyzed artificially ventilated baboons. Arch Neurol 29:82–87, 1973.
11. Meldrum BS: Metabolic factors during prolonged seizures and the relation to nerve cell death. *In* Delgado-Escueta AV, et al (eds): Status Epilepticus: Mechanisms of Brain Damage and Treatment. New York, Raven Press, 1983.
    It is hypothesized that the calcium influx to the neurons has a very significant noxious effect in neuronal death.

12. Aminoff MJ, Simon RP: Status epilepticus: Causes, clinical features and consequences in 98 patients. Am J Med 69:657–666, 1980.
    The article contains a large body of useful data, including the etiologic break-down of status epilepticus and CSF findings. CSF showed abnormal white blood cell content in several patients in the absence of a documented infection. Irregularity or alteration of anticonvulsant therapy was considered the most common cause of status. Alcohol abuse

was one of the most common causes of status. Hyperthermia was rather common and seemed to be a bad prognostic sign, in part due to increased metabolic demand.

13. Delgado-Escueta AV, et al: Management of status epilepticus. N Engl J Med 306:1337–1340, 1982.
    A good review of the treatment of status epilepticus.

14. Browne TR: Status epilepticus. *In* Browne TR, Feldman R (eds): Epilepsy: Diagnosis and Management. Boston, Little, Brown, 1983.
    A good review of the treatment of status epilepticus.

15. Goldberg MA, McIntyre HB: Barbiturates in the treatment of status epilepticus. In Delgado-Escueta AV, et al (eds): Status Epilepticus: Mechanisms of Brain Damage and Treatment. New York, Raven Press, 1983.
    An appropriate emphasis on the treatment of status epilepticus with barbiturates, including phenobarbital and pentobarbital anesthesia. This is a significant article in part because of the scarcity of articles about treatment of status with phenobarbital.

16. Orlowski JP, et al: Hypothermia and barbiturate coma for refractory status epilepticus. Crit Care Med 12:367–372, 1984.

17. Woodbury DM: Antiepileptic drugs: Carbonic anhydrase inhibitors. *In* Glaser GH, et al (eds): Antiepileptic Drugs: Mechanisms of Action. New York, Raven Press, 1983, pp 617–634.

18. Woodbury DM: Effects of chronic administration of anticonvulsant drugs, alone and in combination with desoxycorticosterone, on electroshock seizure threshold and tissue electrolytes. J Pharmacol Exp Ther 105:46–57, 1952.

19. Thomas J, et al: Epilepsia partialis continua. A review of 32 cases. Arch Neurol 34:266–275, 1977.

20. Schraeder P, et al: Seizure disorder following periodic lateralized epileptiform discharges. Epilepsia 21:647–653, 1980.

21. Chatrian GE, et al: The significance of periodic lateralized epileptiform discharges in EEG and electroencephalographic, clinical and pathological study. Electroenceph Clin Neurophysiol 17:177–193, 1964.

22. Schwartz MS, et al: The occurrence and evolution in the EEG of a lateralized periodic phenomenon. Brain 96:613–622, 1973.

23. Dalessio DJ: Seizure disorders and pregnancy. N Engl J Med 312:559–563, 1985.
    Excellent concise review of seizure disorders in pregnancy with emphasis on management issues.

SECTION 8
PULMONARY DISEASE

Adult Respiratory Distress Syndrome

Martin Joyce-Brady, M.D.

CLINICAL PRESENTATION

The adult respiratory distress syndrome (ARDS) was described in 1967 as a clinical triad of refractory hypoxemia, decreased lung compliance, and diffuse alveolar infiltrates.[1] The terms shock lung, Da Nang lung, respirator lung, stiff lung syndrome, and noncardiac pulmonary edema describe the same entity.[2] ARDS is a common and often lethal form of acute respiratory failure that occurs in an estimated 150,000 persons/year.[3] Multiple risk factors have been identified for this syndrome, with the most common being trauma, aspiration of gastric contents, multiple transfusions, pancreatitis, prolonged hypotension, diffuse infectious pneumonia, and burns.[4,5] The incidence of ARDS among at-risk patients has been observed as being from 8.9%[4] to 34%.[5] Higher risk is associated with the presence of more than one risk factor and with a direct pulmonary insult. Preventive measures in at-risk persons, particularly the use of positive end-expiratory pressure (PEEP), have not proved protective.[6]

The diagnosis of ARDS is based on the clinical triad just described in association with a possible risk factor. One must exclude hydrostatic pulmonary edema and a stable chronic pulmonary process. There is usually a latent period of 12–48 hours from the initial insult to the onset of clinical symptoms. Respiratory distress presents with tachypnea and labored breathing. This reflects reduced lung compliance caused by increased lung water. Surfactant abnormalities associated with ARDS may exacerbate this effect by raising surface tension. The measured static lung compliance is often less than 50 ml/cm H_2O, whereas a normal compliance is 100 ml/cm H_2O. The chest radiograph shows diffuse pulmonary infiltrates, as in cardiogenic pulmonary edema, but there is sparing of the costophrenic angles and an absence

529

of Kerley B lines. Arterial blood gas analysis reveals profound hypoxemia that is refractory to oxygen therapy. This manifests as a reduced partial pressure of oxygen (PaO_2), often to less than 50 mmHg, despite a fractional inspired concentration of oxygen (FIO_2) of greater than 60%. Ventilation is preserved with a normal or more often low partial pressure of carbon dioxide ($PaCO_2$), although minute ventilation is increased.[3,7,8] Hydrostatic pulmonary edema can be excluded by documenting normal filling pressures with a Swan-Ganz catheter.

PATHOPHYSIOLOGY

ARDS may represent a final common endpoint of acute lung injury from multiple causes. The injury may originate at the alveolar epithelium or the capillary endothelium and results in severe damage to the gas exchange surface. The lung injury affects all structural components and cells of the alveolar wall and is not homogeneous.[8] The acute stage is characterized by damage to epithelial and endothelial cells with interstitial edema. Increased lung vascular permeability allows leakage of water and protein from the vascular space and disrupts normal intravascular Starling's forces. Alveoli become filled with a protein-rich and often hemorrhagic exudate. The late stage shows interstitial infiltrates with inflammatory cells, thickened alveolar septa as a result of type 2 cell proliferation, and organization of intra-alveolar exudate with or without fibrosis.[3,7,8] Severe interstitial and intra-alveolar fibrosis is noted at autopsy and is felt to be a principal component of mortality.

The mechanism(s) of lung injury in ARDS remains elusive. Several investigations have suggested a role for the polymorphonuclear leukocyte in a final common pathway of acute lung injury. Complement activation by a number of factors may initiate C5a-mediated neutrophil aggregation and adherence to the pulmonary vascular endothelium. These activated neutrophils can cause acute lung injury by oxygen-metabolite dependent[8] and independent mechanisms.[9] However, ARDS does occur in neutropenic patients, suggesting that other mechanisms, either alone or in conjunction with leukocytes, can produce severe lung injury.[10,11] The diverse risk factors for ARDS suggest that multiple potential pathogenic sequences may lead to acute lung injury, whereas the clinical diagnosis is based only on an end-stage common presentation. Other inflammatory mediators such as coagulation factors, platelet aggregation and microemboli, arachidonic acid metabolites, histamine, serotonin, fibrin and fibrin degradation products, and proteolytic enzymes have all been implicated, but their role remains undefined.[3,8,12,13]

The hypoxemia seen in ARDS results predominantly from intrapulmonary right-to-left shunting that is due to alveolar flooding and collapse. It is this shunt that makes the hypoxemia refractory to increases in inspired oxygen concentration. Ventilation/perfusion (V/Q) mismatch also plays a role in the gas exchange abnormality. The multiple inert gas elimination method shows a bimodal distribution of ventilation to perfusion ratios. The low V/Q units are underventilated and overperfused. This may result from broncho-constriction or alveolar flooding and contributes to venous admixture effect. High V/Q units are overventilated and underperfused. This may result from vascular obstruction and adds to dead space ventilation. Pulmonary vascular resistance may be elevated as a result of (1) vasoconstriction induced by alveolar hypoxia and/or vasoactive mediators, (2) vascular obstruction caused by intravascular clotting, and/or (3) increased interstitial fluid pressure. In the late stages of ARDS, the presence of severe, persistent pulmonary hy-pertension or CO_2 retention indicates extensive injury and a poor progno-sis.[3,7,8]

MANAGEMENT

The goals of management are (1) to identify and remove the inciting agent(s); (2) to maintain gas exchange in the lung and *blood oxygen content*, defined as hemoglobin concentration × oxygen saturation × 1.34 ml O_2/ 100 ml blood; (3) to preserve *oxygen transport* to peripheral tissues (cardiac output × blood oxygen content) until the lung has had time for repair; and (4) to anticipate and treat complications of ARDS or its therapy.

Respiratory support is aimed at improving gas exchange and reducing the work of breathing. Intubation and mechanical ventilation within 72 hours of onset of respiratory distress are required in 90% of patients.[5] Throughout intubation, the airway should be protected by using an endotracheal tube with a low-pressure, high-compliance balloon cuff and an internal diameter of at least 8 mm. Such a tube can be maintained for 2 weeks with minimal mucosal damage, has a low resistance to airflow, and allows fiberoptic bron-choscopy if needed.[3,7,8] Mechanical ventilation requires a volume-cycled ventilator with the capacity to ventilate at high pressures. Such a ventilator is usually set to deliver a tidal volume of 12–15 ml/kg, using either the assist/ control mode or the intermittent mandatory ventilation (IMV) mode. The assist mode allows patient-initiated respiratory rates with a fixed tidal volume delivered by the ventilator. This may result in hypocarbia if the patient is tachypneic as a result of increased ventilatory drive. The IMV mode com-bines spontaneous breathing in which the rate and volume are determined by the patient with mechanical ventilation at a preset ventilator rate and volume. This may minimize hypocarbia. However, there is no defined ad-vantage of IMV over assist/control modes for ventilation.[8]

Supplemental oxygen is required to attain a PaO_2 above 60–65 mmHg to maintain blood oxygen content, but the hypoxemia is generally refractory to O_2 alone because of intrapulmonary right-to-left shunting. Positive end-expiratory pressure (PEEP) can significantly improve gas exchange and may allow adequate oxygenation at a lower FIO_2, thus reducing the risk of O_2 toxicity exacerbating lung injury.[14] PEEP increases functional residual capacity and thereby expands and maintains patency of previously collapsed alveoli throughout the respiratory cycle. These perfused units become ventilated and reduce intra-alveolar shunting, hence directly affecting the primary mechanisms of hypoxemia in this disease. The optimum level of PEEP is determined by empiric trial. PEEP is started at 5 cm H_2O and gradually increased in 2.5–5.0 cm increments until an effect on PaO_2 is noted. Improved oxygenation can be seen with PEEP levels of 5–15 cm of H_2O.[8,14,15] PEEP may not immediately improve oxygenation. Rather, this may occur more slowly over several minutes to hours.

Hemodynamic monitoring via a Swan-Ganz catheter is not routinely required in all cases of ARDS. However, it is useful (1) to guide fluid therapy, (2) to monitor cardiac filling pressures, and (3) to monitor oxygen transport to the tissues.[16,17] The measurement and interpretation of the pulmonary artery occlusion pressure (PAOP) or the pulmonary capillary wedge pressure (PCWP) in ARDS has been reviewed in detail.[18] The Swan-Ganz catheter must be in a dependent lung zone (West zone three) so that an intact fluid column exists from the pulmonary artery to the left atrium.[17,18] PEEP will affect the measurement of PAOP. O'Quin and Marini[18] have suggested that a PAOP increase of at least two thirds of a PEEP increase indicates that the catheter is in a non–zone three region and should be repositioned. A lateral chest radiograph may be helpful in determining that the catheter tip is below the left atrium. Despite the complexity involved, PEEP should not be removed during PAOP measurements because acute, and sometimes prolonged, hypoxemia may result. The PAOP should be measured at end-expiration after one has ascertained that the catheter is in a dependent region of lung.[14,16,17]

Antibiotic therapy is indicated for defined or suspected infection but not as prophylaxis.[3,7,8] Infection may be a primary cause or a complication of therapy. Recent studies emphasize potential sources for infection in ARDS. Sepsis preceding ARDS may originate from an abdominal focus, whereas sepsis complicating ARDS may result from a pulmonary source.[19] ARDS complicated by bacteremia may result from a focus of infection requiring surgical drainage, whereas nonbacteremic patients with a suspected but unidentified focus of infection usually have an occult pneumonia.[20] Sepsis is a leading cause of death, as opposed to progressive respiratory failure.

Steroid use in established ARDS remains controversial.[21] However, recent randomized prospective clinical trials of high-dose methylprednisolone (30 mg/kg q6h × 4 doses) have not been able to demonstrate either a preventive or a therapeutic effect in ARDS, particularly that as a result of sepsis.

COMPLICATIONS

Intermittent positive-pressure ventilation (IPPV) and especially PEEP are associated with three types of complications. These include (1) barotrauma, (2) V/Q mismatch, and (3) reduced cardiac output.[14,25] Barotrauma may present as pneumothorax, pneumomediastinum, or pneumoperitoneum. V/Q mismatch may result from overinflation during any part of the respiratory cycle. Reduced cardiac output, especially with PEEP, may result from (1) reduced venous return, (2) increased pulmonary vascular resistance, (3) alteration of interventricular septal geometry, and/or (4) reduced left ventricular compliance.[25] Therapy may involve volume loading, reduction of PEEP, and/or positive inotropic drugs to improve cardiac output.

Oxygen therapy is toxic to the cells of the lung.[8,26] FIO_2 above 50–60% for prolonged periods is toxic to both lung alveolar type 1 epithelium and to lung capillary endothelium.[26] It can also impair type 2 cell proliferation, which is at least one component of lung epithelial repair. Oxygen also stimulates fibroblast proliferation and collagen production, which may favor the formation of fibrosis. Excessive oxygen may also inactivate antiprotease inhibitors and enhance lung injury by toxic oxygen radicals. In addition, host lung defenses may be impaired as oxygen (1) reduces function of the pulmonary alveolar macrophage, (2) impairs mucociliary clearance and (3) enhances adherence of gram negative organisms to lung epithelium.[8] To minimize these potential problems, one attempts to use the lowest FIO_2 necessary to maintain the PaO_2 at 60–65 mmHg.

Steroid therapy, if prolonged, may impair macrophage function[8] and may deleteriously affect alveolar type 2 epithelial cell proliferation, differentiation and maturation.[27] The macrophage effects might also predispose the patient to infection, and the epithelial effects could interfere with alveolar repair processes.

Infection has been demonstrated to be a major cause of mortality in ARDS, especially with multisystem failure.[19] Given the potential impairment of pulmonary defense mechanisms, one must evaluate invasive interventions in light of potential infection risks.

OUTCOME

Despite increasingly sophisticated ventilators and hemodynamic monitoring techniques, mortality from ARDS has remained high and has not changed significantly over time. Two studies reported a case fatality rate of 65%[24] and 68%.[19] Prognosis has been evaluated in three studies. Bell and colleagues[19] reported that multiple organ failure involving the central nervous, coagulation, endocrine, gastrointestinal, and renal systems was associated with a high rate of infection and mortality. For those persons who do survive, relatively few sequelae have been observed. One evaluation revealed only mild to moderate restrictive ventilatory defects and some airway hyperreactivity in survivors.[29] Another study using exercise testing revealed an increased alveolar-arterial gradient in all survivors, suggesting some degree of permanent lung injury.[30]

KEY FEATURES

The adult respiratory distress syndrome (ARDS) has been defined clinically by the triad of (1) refractory hypoxemia, (2) decreased lung compliance, and (3) diffuse alveolar infiltrates once a stable chronic pulmonary process and hydrostatic pulmonary edema have been excluded.

Common risk factors for the development of ARDS include the following:

1. Trauma
2. Sepsis
3. Aspiration of gastric contents
4. Multiple transfusions
5. Pancreatitis
6. Prolonged hypotension
7. Diffuse pneumonia
8. Burns

ARDS ususally presents clinically as tachypnea and labored breathing, reflecting a reduced lung compliance.

Arterial blood gases generally reveal preserved ventilation with profound hypoxemia resistant to supplemental oxygen.

Chest radiographs demonstrate diffuse pulmonary infiltrates with sparing of the costophrenic angles and an absence of Kerley B lines.

Pulmonary artery catheterization shows normal or reduced left-sided cardiac filling pressures.

ARDS most likely represents the final common clinical pathway of a number of diverse pulmonary insults.

The acute stage is typified by endothelial and/or epithelial cell damage with interstitial edema.

In later stages, alveoli fill with protein-rich exudates, inflammatory cells appear, and type 2 cells proliferate.

Organization of exudates and fibrosis may ensue.

Hypoxemia results predominantly from intrapulmonary right-to-left shunting, with a lesser contribution from ventilation-perfusion mismatch.

Management is directed at (1) identifying and removing inciting factors, (2) optimizing gas exchange and blood oxygen content, and (3) preserving oxygen transport.

The vast majority of patients require intubation and mechanical ventilation.

Supplemental oxygen is required to attain PaO_2 ⩾60–65 mmHg.

Positive end-expiratory pressure (PEEP) can significantly improve gas exchange and may allow a reduction of FIO_2 to minimize the added risk of oxygen toxicity.

Prognosis may correlate with the response to PEEP.

Hemodynamic monitoring is an adjunctive measure that can be used (1) to exclude hydrostatic pulmonary edema, (2) to guide fluid management, and (3) to optimize cardiac output and oxygen transport.

Antibiotic therapy is indicated for suspected or documented infection but not as prophylaxis.

Costicosteroids do not appear to be beneficial.

Complications of mechanical ventilation, PEEP, oxygen therapy, and steroids are common.

Despite advances in critical care, the case fatality rate of ARDS remains high (65–68%), and is associated with multiple organ system failure and infection.

Survivors generally manifest evidence of only limited pulmonary defects.

REFERENCES

1. Ashbaugh DG, Bigelow DB, Petty TL: Acute respiratory distress in adults. Lancet 2:319, 1967.
2. Petty TL, Fowler AA: Another look at the adult respiratory distress syndrome. Chest 82:98–104, 1982.
3. Bernard GR, Brigham KL: The adult respiratory distress syndrome. Ann Rev Med 36:195–205, 1985.
4. Fowler AA, Hamman RF, Good JT, Benson KN, Baird M, Eberle D, Petty TL, Hyers TM: Adult respiratory distress syndrome: Risk with common predispositions. Ann Intern Med 98:593–597, 1983.
5. Pepe PG, Potkin RT, Reus DH, Hudson LD, Carico CJ: Clinical predictors of the adult respiratory distress syndrome. Am J Surg 144:124–130, 1982.
6. Rounds S, Brody JS: Putting PEEP in perspective. N Engl J Med 311:323–325, 1984.
7. Divertee MB: The adult respiratory distress syndrome. Mayo Clinic Proc 57:371–378, 1982.
8. Rinaldo JE, Rogers BM: The adult respiratory distress syndrome: Changing concepts of lung injury and repair. N Engl J Med 306:900–909, 1982.
9. Simon RH, DeHart PD, Todd RF: Neutrophil-induced injury of cat pulmonary alveolar epithelial cells. J Clin Invest 78:1375–1386, 1986.
10. Maunden RJ, Hackman RC, Riff E, Albert RK, Springmeyer SC: Occurrence of the adult respiratory distress syndrome in neutropenic patients. Am Rev Resp Dis 133:313–316, 1986.
11. Onigbene FP, Martin SE, Parker MM, Schlesinger T, Roach P, Burch C, Shelhamer JH, Parrillo JE: Adult respiratory distress syndrome in patients with severe neutropenia. N Engl J Med 315:547–551, 1986.
12. Heffner JE, Sahn SA, Repine JE: The role of platelets in the adult respiratory distress syndrome. Am Rev Resp Dis 135:482–492, 1987.
13. Tate RM, Repine JE: Neutrophils and the adult respiratory distress syndrome. Am Rev Resp Dis 128:552–559, 1983.
14. Weisman IM, Rinaldo JE, Rogers RM: PEEP in adult respiratory failure. N Engl J Med 307:1381–1384, 1982.
15. Lamy M, Fallat RJ, Koeniger E, Dietrich H, Ratliff JL, Eberhart RC, Tucker HJ, Hill JD: Pathologic features and mechanisms of hypoxemia in adult respiratory distress syndrome. Am Rev Resp Dis 114:267–284, 1976.

16. Prewitt RN, Matthay MA, Chignonc M: Hemodynamic monitoring in the adult respiratory distress syndrome. Clin Chest Med 4:251, 1983.
17. Wiedmann HP, Matthay MA, Matthay RA: Cardiovascular-pulmonary monitoring in the intensive care unit. Chest 85:537–549, 656–668, 1984.
18. O'Quin R, Marini JJ: Pulmonary artery occlusion pressure: Clinical physiology, measurement and interpretation. Am Rev Resp Dis 128:319–326, 1983.
19. Bell RC, Coalson JJ, Smith JD, Johanson WG: Multiple organ system failure and infection in the adult respiratory distress syndrome. Ann Intern Med 99:293–298, 1983.
20. Montgomery AB, Stager MA, Carrico CJ, Hudson LD: Causes of mortality of patients with the adult respiratory distress syndrome. Am Rev Resp Dis 132:485–489, 1985.
21. Nicholson DP: Corticosteroid in treatment of septic shock and adult respiratory distress syndrome. Med Clin North Am 67:717–724, 1983.
22. Bernard GR, Luce JM, Sprung CL, et al: High-dose corticosteroids in patients with the adult respiratory distress syndrome. N Engl J Med 317:1565–1570, 1987.
23. Bone RC, Fisher CJ Jr, Clemmer TP, et al: Early methylprednisolone treatment for septic syndrome and the adult respiratory distress syndrome. Chest 92:1032–1036, 1987.
24. Luce JM, Marks JD, Montgomery AB, et al: Methylprednisolone does not prevent the adult respiratory distress syndrome or improve mortality in patients with septic shock. Am Rev Resp Dis 135 (abstract), 1987.
25. Pick RA, Handler JB, Friedman AS: The cardiovascular effects of positive end-expiratory pressure. Chest 82:345–350, 1982.
26. Jackson RM: Pulmonary oxygen toxicity. Chest 88:900–905, 1985.
27. Smith LJ, Brody JS: Influence of methylprednisolone on mouse alveolar type 2 cell response to acute lung injury. Am Rev Resp Dis 123:459–464, 1981.
28. Fowler AA, Hamman RF, Zerbe GO, Benson KN, Hyers TM: Adult respiratory distress syndrome: Prognosis after onset. Am Rev Resp Dis 132:472–478, 1985.
29. Rotman HH, Laville TF, et al: Long term physiologic consequences of the adult respiratory distress syndrome. Chest 72:190–192, 1977.
30. Elliot CG, Morros AH, Cengiz M: Pulmonary function and exercise gas exchange in survivors of the adult respiratory distress syndrome. Am Rev Resp Dis 123:492–495, 1981.
31. Andreaudis N, Petty TL: Adult respiratory distress syndrome: Problems and prognosis. Am Rev Resp Dis 132:1344–1346, 1985.

Aspiration Syndromes

James J. Heffernan, M.D.

Aspiration of upper airway secretions, particulate matter, and the associated oropharyngeal bacterial flora is the precipitating event in most instances of bacterial pneumonia. Factors that predispose a patient to aspiration include altered mental status, dysphagia, trauma, and pre-existing upper airway infection. Although aspiration itself is sufficient to produce pneumonia in normal lungs, certain host factors facilitate the development of infection: compromised mucosal defenses, increased alveolar water, and anatomic lesions with or without bronchial obstruction. Pneumonia arising after aspiration may yield pure or mixed cultures of aerobic, facultative, and/or anaerobic organisms. In normal adults, anaerobic bacteria are found in oropharyngeal secretions at threefold to tenfold higher concentrations than aerobes, 10^8 vs. 10^7 organisms/ml.[1,2] In the setting of severe periodontal disease the concentration of anaerobic bacteria may approach 10^{11}/ml in gingivitis exudate, whereas in edentulous patients the ratio of anaerobic to aerobic bacteria may drop to unity.[2] The composition of the aerobic and facultative component may vary tremendously as a result of host factors, clinical setting, physical environment, and time of year.[1,5]

Although aspiration is the common etiologic thread in lower respiratory tract infections arising from aerobic or anaerobic bacteria, the term "aspiration pneumonia" implies, by common usage, a predominant role for the usual anaerobic inhabitants of the oropharynx. Several anaerobic pleuropulmonary aspiration syndromes are described: (1) aspiration pneumonia, (2) lung abscess, (3) necrotizing pneumonia, and (4) empyema. There is, in fact, much overlap among these syndromes, and the distinctions are somewhat arbitrary. Moreover, similar patterns of disease may be produced by aerobic bacteria in the setting of aspiration or by entirely different mechanisms.

The principal organisms recovered by transtracheal (or rarely percutaneous) aspiration, thoracentesis, or blood culture or in pathologic specimens from patients with clinically defined aspiration syndromes have included, in order of decreasing frequency, *Bacteroides melaninogenicus, Fusobacterium nucleatum,* Peptostreptococcus, Peptococcus, *Bacteroides fragilis,* and microaerophilic streptococci; aerobic isolates have been obtained less commonly than any of the just-listed species. A wide variety of other anaerobic species have also been identified, albeit at lower frequencies. In most instances, appropriately obtained cultures produce mixed flora of anaerobes alone, or of anaerobes and aerobes. In the landmark series by Bartlett and Finegold, anaerobic organisms were recovered at a rate of 2.3–2.8 species/case, compared with a rate of 0.4–0.9 aerobic species/case.[1] However, aerobic species, especially *Staphylococcus aureus* and gram negative enteric organisms, are much more commonly recovered in the setting of hospital-acquired aspiration pneumonia.[2,4,5,7]

Simple aspiration pneumonitis is the most common of the anaerobic pleuropulmonary infections, accounting for 30–65% of cases in reviews of aspiration-associated lower respiratory tract infections confirmed by culture of transtracheal aspirates.[1,6,7] The best prospectively obtained data demonstrate that 50% of such infections are cases of simple pneumonitis.[7] However, the actual prevalence of this entity is unknown and likely grossly underestimated for several reasons: (1) early disease is in many ways clinically indistinguishable from community-acquired pneumonia caused by common aerobic pathogens; (2) transtracheal aspirates or other suitable culture materials are seldom obtained; (3) anaerobic culture techniques are often not applied; and (4) empiric therapy with a variety of antimicrobial agents is often promptly effective.[1,5,8]

Simple aspiration pneumonitis generally presents as an acute febrile illness with symptoms referable to a pulmonary source of infection—cough, dyspnea, and chest pain. Most patients have been symptomatic for 1–5 days at the time of presentation, and the mean peak rectal temperature is 102.4° F.[1,7,8] Putrid sputum production is uncommon, occurring in only 9–18% of cases of uncomplicated pneumonitis in the larger series;[1,8] anaerobic bacteremia is rare, found in less than 2% of instances.[1] The mean peak leukocyte count is 14,000–17,000.[1,7,8] Examination and radiographic evaluation demonstrate infiltrates in segments favored by dependency—the posterior segments of the upper lobes and the superior segments of the lower lobes following aspiration while the patient is recumbent, and the basilar segments of the lower lobes after aspiration in the upright position.[1,8] An observed episode of aspiration or, more commonly, a predisposition to aspiration can be documented in the majority of cases, with altered mental status reported at rates of 55–85%, periodontal disease described in up to two thirds, and dysphagia in 15%.[1,7,8] Causes of compromised consciousness include alcoholism, drug intoxication, general anesthesia, seizures, stroke, cardiac arrest/shock, metabolic coma, and central nervous system infection. Anaerobic pneumonitis is often associated with underlying lung pathology, especially evident in the high prevalence rates of bronchogenic carcinoma (8–17%) among patients with such infections.[1,8] Comparison of the clinical features of a series of cases of anaerobic pneumonitis with those of a control group of patients with pneumococcal pneumonia has revealed only limited differences.[8]

Simple aspiration pneumonitis generally responds promptly to appropriate antimicrobial therapy with defervescence over 2–3 days and clearing of chest radiographic abnormalities in 3–5 weeks.[1,8] However, despite appropriate treatment, up to 20% of cases may progress to abscess formation or necrotizing pneumonia.[1,8] The case fatality rate from infection alone is 6–14%, although a similar number of patients die from associated conditions.

That lung abscess and necrotizing pneumonia represent complications of simple anaerobic pneumonitis is suggested by the differences in duration of symptoms before presentation (12 and 10 days, respectively) for the "complicated" infections vs. 3–5 days for simple pneumonitis.[1,7,8] This is further substantiated by the well-documented later development of abscess and necrotizing pneumonia in a subset of patients presenting with simple pneumonitis.[8] In most series, primary lung abscess is defined as a single or dominant cavity of >2 cm diameter in the appropriate clinical setting, whereas the diagnosis of necrotizing pneumonia requires the presence of a suppurative process involving more than one lobe with the demonstration of multiple small cavities.[1,5] Necrotizing pneumonia does indeed appear to be a more virulent clinical expression, or simply a later stage, of aspiration pneumonitis, attended by high fever (mean peak 102.4° F), striking leukocytosis (mean peak WBC 24,200), persistent fever despite treatment, long time for cure (median 46 days), and a case fatality rate from infection alone of 18%.[1,5] Putrid sputum production occurs in the majority of cases, and weight loss and anemia are common, markers of more chronic and/or more severe infection than simple pneumonitis. Predisposing characteristics are the same as those for the other aspiration syndromes.

Anaerobic lung abscess occurs in a population similarly at risk for aspiration. Although most, if not all, cases arise in the setting of a pre-existing aspiration pneumonitis, most patients present with clinical features suggesting a somewhat more indolent albeit debilitating illness. The fever and WBC peaks tend to be lower (101.8° F and 14,400, respectively), duration of symptoms longer (12 days, mean), and weight loss and anemia more prevalent at presentation.[1,9] Two thirds of patients demonstrate a cavity on initial chest radiograph, whereas one third develop an abscess while under care for an underlying pneumonitis.[1] Cough, dyspnea, and chest pain are common, as is production of putrid sputum, the latter occurring in 48–76% of cases.[1,9] Massive hemoptysis, brain abscess, and acute pyopneumothorax are potential catastrophic complications. In the prechemotherapeutic era, one third of patients died, one third developed debilitating or recurrent disease, and one third recovered.[12] In the past several decades, antibiotics have supplanted surgery as the primary mode of therapy and the direct mortality of lung abscess is now less than 10%, although indirect mortality remains at a similar level (approximately 10%).

Empyema may complicate any of the clinical subgroups of anaerobic pulmonary parenchymal infection, and was described in one third of cases across the board in the largest review to date.[1] Subsequent studies have suggested somewhat lower rates; nonetheless, mixed anaerobic infection is today the most common cause of empyema. The clinical features of this entity are intimately bound to those of the underlying parenchymal process, and the mortality and morbidity directly attributable to empyema are difficult to quantify. Thoracostomy tube drainage or a more extensive surgical procedure, in addition to high-dose antibiotics, has been required to effect cure in the large majority of instances. Empyema presages a long febrile period (median 19 days) and protracted time for cure (median 142 days).

A related aspiration syndrome that does not fall fully under the preceding rubric is aspiration of gastric contents.[2,3] With this entity, the severity and type of pulmonary injury, the tempo of illness, and the prognosis are most critically dependent on the pH of the aspirate, its volume, the particulate content, and, less significantly, on the bacterial flora. Aspiration of neutral liquids results in pulmonary edema and congestion, secondary bronchospasm and hypoxemia. With appropriate supportive care, recovery is prompt and complete. When the pH of the aspirate falls below 2.5, a severe chemical pneumonitis ensues, with hemorrhage, granulocytic reaction, and necrosis; the case fatality rate is 25% when the pH of the aspirate is 1.8–2.5 and approaches 100% at pH <1.8. Residual lung damage can generally be demonstrated in survivors after acid aspiration. Immediate suffocation may result from aspiration of large particulate matter. Smaller particles stimulate a granulomatous reaction within 48 hours, following an initial hemorrhagic, granulocytic response of variable intensity. Infection often complicates aspiration of gastric contents. In such cases, the flora is usually that of the upper airway and any of the infectious aspiration syndromes may result.

DIAGNOSIS

The presumptive diagnosis of anaerobic pleuropulmonary infection rests on proper interpretation of the clinical features described previously and is generally a straightforward exercise. Other clinical entities can produce similar findings: aerobic bacteria, especially hospital-acquired staphylococci and gram negative enteric organisms, can produce necrotizing lesions by the mechanisms of aspiration, bacteremic seeding, or deposition of septic emboli; carcinoma, tuberculosis, and, less commonly, fungi may produce cavitary lesions that may be confused with or complicated by anaerobic bacterial infection; and empyema may result from transdiaphragmatic spread of intra-abdominal infection. Hence, bacterial confirmation is desirable in cases of suspected anaerobic pleuropulmonary infection. Blood cultures are positive only in rare instances, and empyema fluid is available in only a minority of cases. Under usual circumstances, transtracheal aspiration is the procedure of choice for bacteriologic confirmation because sputum obtained by expectoration, nasotracheal suctioning, or bronchoscopy is, perforce, contaminated by passage through the oropharynx. Grossly putrid sputum suggests a necrotizing anaerobic infection, although the actual site may lie in the upper airway. Suction recovery from the trachea of fluid with a low pH or high glucose content or of food matter substantiates aspiration but does not directly address the question of infection. When appropriate anaerobic and aerobic culture techniques are utilized, specimens obtained by transtracheal aspiration yield the correct bacteriologic diagnosis in the vast majority of instances.[1,2,5–8] False negative cultures are exceedingly rare, and false positive cultures occur at rates <5%, especially when anaerobic organisms are implicated. Anaerobic species alone are recovered in the majority of cases of community-acquired aspiration disease (60%), and mixed aerobic-anaerobic infection occurs in another 30%; with hospital-acquired infection, aerobic species alone may account for up to one third of cases. Protected bronchoscopic brush sampling and percutaneous lung aspiration are infrequently used alternatives to transtracheal aspiration. Basic radiographic techniques may not be able to distinguish empyema from parenchymal infection; ultrasonography or computed tomography much improves this determination. Thoracentesis should always be performed when empyema is present or strongly suspected. Bronchoscopy is seldom indicated early in the disease course, and then usually to relieve suspected obstruction; if the response to standard management is inadequate or if the original diagnosis is questioned, bronchoscopy may contribute important information, especially in the settings of carcinoma or unusual infection.

MANAGEMENT

The cornerstone of management of anaerobic pleuropulmonary infection is antibiotic therapy. In the past 35 years, a wide variety of antimicrobial agents have been used with varying degrees of effectiveness. By the early 1970s, penicillin G was accepted as the drug of choice, demonstrating in vitro efficacy against the majority of oropharyngeal anaerobic species as well as clinical effectiveness even in the 15% of cases in which penicillin resistant B. fragilis was implicated. Penicillin V and a variety of extended spectrum penicillins—ampicillin, amoxicillin, carbenicillin, ticarcillin, piperacillin, mezlocillin, azlocillin—are similarly effective against oropharyngeal anaerobes, as are first-generation cephalosporins, although none of these agents demonstrate significant activity against B. fragilis in vitro. The antistaphylococcal penicillins are not comparably effective, lacking activity against gram negative anaerobic species as well as against B. fragilis. Tetracycline and chloramphenicol have activity against many of the causative species and were used to good effect in early trials. Vancomycin and erythromycin are not acceptable on the basis of antimicrobial spectrum. Of note, clindamycin has shown reliable in vitro efficacy against all the implicated anaerobic species as well as clinical effectiveness comparable, and possibly superior, to penicillin;[1,5,7–12] cefoxitin, with activity against B. fragilis, is another alternative to penicillin, as is metronidazole.[13]

On the basis of clinical experience and cost, the standard of treatment for anaerobic pleuropulmonary infection has been parenteral penicillin G at moderate to high dosage (10–20 million U/day) until clinical improvement and defervescence, followed by oral penicillin V 500–750 mg PO q6h to resolution. A prospective controlled trial of clindamycin vs. penicillin has challenged the primacy of the standard in the setting of lung abscess.[11] It is clear that clindamycin 600 mg IV q6–8h and thereafter 300–450 mg PO q6h is at least as effective as the comparable penicillin regimen and may be attended by a significantly lower failure rate. The combination of metronidazole with amoxicillin or ampicillin, both administered orally, has been used effectively, but this regimen has not been compared formally in a prospective trial against penicillin G or clindamycin.[13]

Because of the high representation of aerobic species, especially staphylococci and gram negative enteric organisms, among cases of hospital-acquired aspiration pneumonitis, initial antibiotic coverage should include agents effective against such pathogens. Only a rare patient with anaerobic pleuropulmonary infection requires intubation, although oxygen therapy, bronchodilators, and physiotherapy are often beneficial. Empyema requires thoracostomy tube drainage and sometimes a more extensive surgical intervention. Indications for bronchoscopy are as noted previously. Patients with the complication of massive hemoptysis may benefit from bronchoscopic intervention prior to or in place of surgery. The presence of acute pyopneumothorax obligates emergent thoracostomy tube placement. A lung abscess that fails to respond to conservative medical management may be successfully treated by percutaneous catheter drainage or thoracotomy with pulmonary resection.[14]

KEY FEATURES

Anaerobic lung infection results from aspiration of polymicrobial oropharyngeal flora.

Predisposition to aspiration and/or anatomic abnormalities (of lung or upper aerodigestive tract) are present in the vast majority of instances.

Arbitrarily defined disease entities include (1) simple aspiration pneumonitis, (2) necrotizing pneumonia, and (3) lung abscess; (4) empyema may complicate any of these.

Diagnosis is based on history or suspicion of aspiration; clinical features; and acquisition of appropriate bacteriologic specimens, usually by transtracheal aspiration.

Oropharyngeal anaerobic species account for an overwhelming majority of community-acquired cases; infection is generally polymicrobial.

Staphylococci, gram negative enteric bacilli, and pseudomonads are often implicated in hospital-acquired cases, frequently in mixed flora with anaerobes.

Treatment of choice for anaerobic pleuropulmonary infection is penicillin G or clindamycin; cefoxitin is an acceptable alternative consideration, as is metronidazole.

Empyema requires thoracostomy tube drainage; lung abscess rarely requires surgical resection.

Long courses of therapy are necessary for complicated infections.

Case fatality rates are 6–18% from infection, with similar mortality from associated conditions.

Aspiration of gastric contents results in a chemical pneumonitis, the severity of which is most critically dependent on the pH of the aspirated inoculum.

REFERENCES

1. Bartlett JG, Finegold SM: Anaerobic infections of the lung and pleural space. Am Rev Resp Dis *110*:56, 1974.

    Landmark review of this topic with detailed clinical, laboratory, radiographic, and bacteriologic data from 143 cases, grouped by type of infection. Predisposing conditions were identified in 90% of cases. Prospectively obtained data are cited that clearly establish the predominant role of anaerobic bacteria in these clinical syndromes. Penicillin G is recommended as the antibiotic of choice; ampicillin, clindamycin, and chloramphenicol are considered acceptable alternatives.

2. Bartlett JG, Gorbach SL: The triple threat of aspiration pneumonia. Chest 68:560, 1975.

    General discussion using a classification based on the aspiration inoculum: (1) toxic fluids—chemical pneumonitis; (2) bacterial pathogens—bacterial infection; and (3) inert substances—airway obstruction. Stresses the role of pH and volume in aspiration of gastric contents. Again emphasizes the predominant role played by anaerobic organisms in the development of aspiration-related infection, but also emphasizes the difference between community-acquired and hospital-acquired disease, with aerobic organisms, especially gram negative bacilli and staphylococci, more often isolated in the latter setting (albeit usually with anaerobes).

3. Wynne JW, Modell JH: Respiratory aspiration of gastric contents. Ann Intern Med 87:466, 1977.

    Detailed review of human and animal studies. Distinguishes acid from non-acid aspiration, citing the critical pH of 2.5 as a threshold for severe injury. There is a brief discussion of infectious complications. The authors stress that (1) there are no conclusive clinical or experimental data on which to base the use of steroids in the setting of aspiration, and (2) antibiotics are best withheld until established infection is documented.

4. Valenti WM, Trudell RG, Bentley DW: Gram-negative oropharyngeal colonization in the aged. N Engl J Med 298:1108, 1978.

    Oropharyngeal colonization with gram negative bacilli in 407 elderly subjects increased with level of care: 9% in independent apartment dwellers, 12% in residents of private nursing homes, 37% in patients in skilled-nursing facilities, and 60% in acute hospital ward patients. Common organisms included Klebsiella species (41% of isolates), Escherichia coli (24%), and Enterobacter species (14%). Respiratory disease and bedridden state contributed most to colonization.

5. Johanson WG, Harris GD: Aspiration pneumonia, anaerobic infections, and lung abscess. Med Clin North Am 64:385, 1980.

    Concise, clinically oriented review of aspiration-associated infections. The authors stress the predominant role of anaerobic organisms but also distinguish between community- and hospital-acquired disease, with aerobic species identified as sole (36%) or contributing (47%) flora much more commonly in the latter clinical setting. Penicillin is cited as the drug of choice for anaerobic infection, with a caution to consider aerobic species in the appropriate setting and treat accordingly.

6. Gonzalez CB, Calia F: Bacteriologic flora of aspiration-induced pulmonary infections. Arch Intern Med *135*:711, 1975.

    Three indicators of aspiration were defined and applied to a group of hospitalized patients with pneumonia and/or lung abscess. Cultures obtained by transtracheal aspiration or thoracentesis yielded anaerobic organisms in 17 of 17 patients with two or more indicators of aspiration and in 6 of 17 patients with none or one such indicator. Two or more bacterial isolates were recovered from 16 of 17 patients in the former group but from fewer than half of patients in the latter group.

7. Bartlett JG, Gorbach SL, Finegold SM: The bacteriology of aspiration pneumonia. JAMA 56:202, 1974.
   Prospective study of 54 cases of pulmonary infection following aspiration. Culture materials were obtained by transtracheal aspiration, thoracentesis, or blood sampling. Anaerobic species were recovered in all but four instances and were the only pathogens identified in 25 cases (46%). B. fragilis was identified in 9 cases, and gram negative enteric bacilli and pseudomonads were common among those whose infection was acquired in the hospital. Treatment directed against only the anaerobic component of mixed aerobic-anaerobic infections was effective.

8. Bartlett JG: Anaerobic bacterial pneumonitis. Am Rev Resp Dis 119:19, 1979.
   Forty-six patients with anaerobic bacterial pneumonitis confirmed by culture of trans-tracheal aspirates were compared with 46 patients with similarly confirmed pneumococcal pneumonia. Presenting characteristics, response to therapy, and mortality rates were similar. A history of shaking chills was highly specific for pneumococcal disease. Features associated with anaerobic infection included longer duration of symptoms, predisposition to aspiration, and bronchogenic carcinoma. Putrid sputum was noted in only two cases of anaerobic pneumonitis, whereas bacteremia was documented exclusively with pneumococcal disease. Nine cases of anaerobic infection progressed to abscess formation despite antibiotic treatment.

9. Barnett TH, Herring CL: Lung abscess—initial and late results of medical therapy. Arch Intern Med 127:217, 1971.
   Retrospective review of 63 cases of "nonspecific" pyogenic lung abscess. Patients were treated with penicillin G (2.4 million U/day) and either tetracycline or chloramphenicol; three patients received erythromycin or novobiocin in place of penicillin. Putrid sputum was noted in 76% and hemoptysis in 43% of cases. Initial results of therapy were deemed satisfactory in 43 cases. Unsatisfactory outcome correlated with long disease course before treatment and larger abscesses. Late recurrences were predicted by failure to resolve cavity to less than 2 cm during initial treatment.

10. Bartlett JG, Gorbach SL: Treatment of aspiration pneumonia and primary lung abscess; penicillin G vs. clindamycin. JAMA 234:935, 1975.
    Retrospective review of response of anaerobic pneumonia/lung abscess to parenteral penicillin G (49 cases) vs. clindamycin (35 cases). Both agents were found to be highly effective (75% and 84% cure rates, respectively); no statistically significant differences in outcome were noted.

11. Levison ME, Mangura CT, Lorber B, et al: Clindamycin compared with penicillin for the treatment of anaerobic lung abscess. Ann Intern Med 98:466, 1983.
    Prospective, randomized, multicenter clinical trial of clindamycin vs. penicillin G in the treatment of anaerobic lung abscess. No treatment failures occurred in 13 patients followed to completion of planned therapy on clindamycin, whereas only 8 of 15 patients followed to the end of the study on penicillin fulfilled criteria for cure. Clindamycin-treated patients demonstrated significantly shorter duration of fever and less tendency to extend their infection. The authors stress the possible role of increasing pencillin resistance among oropharyngeal anaerobes.

12. Bartlett JG, Gorbach SL: Penicillin or clindamycin for primary lung abscess? (editorial). Ann Intern Med 98:546, 1983.
    Editorial response to reference No. 11. Criticizes small patient numbers, drop out rate, and, most importantly, the arbitrariness of defined endpoints but acknowledges that

clindamycin may now represent optimum therapy for this problem, especially in severely ill patients.

13. Neild JE, Eykyn SJ, Phillips I: Lung abscess and empyema. Quart J Med 57:875, 1985.
    British series of 48 patients, 17 with abscess and 31 with empyema. Bacterial flora similar to that reported in American series but for the absence of B. fragilis. Eighteen of 101 anaerobic isolates resistant to penicillin. Details of antibiotic therapy not reported but success described with regimen of amoxicillin (or ampicillin) and metronidazole and appropriate drainage procedures. The authors advocate use of antibiotics other than penicillin but do not document treatment failures with penicillin although one patient relapsed on metronidazole alone.

14. Parker LA, Melton JW, Delany DJ, Yankaskas B: Percutaneous small bore catheter drainage in the management of lung abscesses. Chest 92:213, 1987.
    Six patients with lung abscess who failed to respond to conservative medical management were successfully treated by percutaneous catheter drainage coupled to continued antibiotic therapy, thus avoiding thoracotomy and pulmonary resection.

Asthma

Joseph Miaskiewicz, M.D.

Asthma is defined as a hypersensitivity of the airways to various stimuli, causing a reversible narrowing of the trachea and bronchi, which can change as a result of therapy or spontaneously.[1] In the United States, this disease occurs in approximately 3% of the population. It accounts for 28 million physician visits per year and results in 183,000 yearly hospital admissions. If treated appropriately, there is almost no immediate mortality.[2]

The mechanism of bronchial constriction has not been fully elucidated. It can be precipitated by allergens, mediators, pharmacologic agents, air pollution, ingested substances, physical agents, and other factors. The mast cell and nervous system are felt to play key roles in hyperreactivity. When stimulated, the mast cell releases factors such as leukotrienes, platelet activating factor, eosinophilic chemotactic factor, neutrophilic chemotactic factor, and histamine. The actions of these substances are felt to be responsible for bronchoconstriction. In addition, mediator release can occur from or be modulated by epithelial cells, eosinophils, neutrophils, or mononuclear cells.

Within the next few hours to days, there is a cellular infiltration of eosinophils, neutrophils, macrophages, monocytes, and plasma cells. Other mediators such as serotonin; prostaglandins F_2 and D_2; leukotrienes C_4, E_4, and D_4; kinins; hydroxy-eicosatetraenoic acids (HETE); and thromboxane are released, which further constrict bronchi. The T cell is also felt to play a role in bronchoconstriction.[4] It is important for the production of IgE as well as plays a possible role in mediator release and in cell-mediated immunity. There are also a number of neurologic influences over bronchomotor tone. Increases in vagal or cholinergic tone cause bronchoconstriction. This appears to occur at the level of smooth muscle. There is also evidence to suggest that mast cells are innervated by cholinergic fibers. Stimulation of beta-2 fibers leads to bronchodilatation. Alpha fibers, although few in the lung, cause bronchoconstriction. Basal motor tone is felt to be mediated by a balance between vagal and beta motor tone.

Classically asthma has been divided into two categories, although patients may fall anywhere along a broad spectrum of clinical disease. "Extrinsic asthma" usually occurs in children. There is a known history of allergy to multiple allergens with positive skin tests and elevated serum IgE. These patients tend to have intermittent asthma attacks. "Intrinsic asthma" tends to occur in older patients, who generally lack a history of multiple allergies or positive skin tests to allergens. These patients tend to have more continuous attacks.

Regardless of the mode of precipitation, asthma manifests as a mix of four primary pathologic features: (1) the bronchial smooth muscle is contracted and hypertrophied; (2) there is vasodilatation and edema; (3) the distal bronchioles are plugged with tenacious mucus secondary to increased mucous production, and (4) eosinophils and neutrophils are present.

Clinically, patients present with an unproductive cough, wheezing, and dyspnea. One must consider the differential diagnosis of large airway obstruction, tumors, acute bronchitis, chronic obstructive pulmonary disease, "cardiac asthma," and pulmonary embolus. A meticulous history concerning the time and events initiating the current attack as well as past events is most useful. Cough alone may be the major symptom. On physical examination, there is evidence of hyperinflation, inspiratory/expiratory rhonchi and wheezes, decreased air movement, and prolonged expiration. Pulsus paradoxus (>10 mmHg drop in BP on inspiration) is a very important measure of the severity of an attack.[5] Sputum examination may demonstrate Curschmann's spirals, Charcot-Leyden crystals, mucopurulence, and eosinophils. A peripheral blood smear may also reveal eosinophilia. Arterial blood gases will usually demonstrate hypoxemia (secondary to perfusion-ventilation mismatch) and hypocapnia with a slight respiratory alkalosis.[6] However, if the attack is severe, one can see a normal or slightly acidotic pH as well as normal or slightly elevated PCO_2. Blood gases are indispensable in demonstrating the severity of an attack and do not necessarily correlate with the clinical picture. Thus, it is vital to obtain blood gases on at least all admitted patients. Chest radiographs will usually show hyperinflation, and their main value is to rule out other causes of wheezing.[7] Pulmonary function testing will show a decrease in forced expiratory volume in 1 second (FEV_1) and in tidal volume (TV) (the ratio of FEV_1 to TV is also usually decreased) with an increase in residual volume. Spirometry may be too difficult to perform in the acutely ill patient. Peak expiratory flow rate (PEFR) has been shown to be an equally effective measure of airway obstruction in asthma.

The evaluation of the asthmatic in the emergency room and his disposition is frequently difficult.[8] The best predictors of severity are objective and include pulsus paradoxus (>18 mmHg), heart rate (>120 beats/minute), respiratory rate (>30 breaths/minute), PEFR (<120 L/minute), accessory muscle use, diaphoresis, and an abnormal blood gas. Wheezing does not correlate well with the severity of an attack; thus if a patient "clears," there must also be evidence of improvement by other objective data. One must also consider how the patient perceives the progress or lack thereof in response to therapy.[9]

Status asthmaticus is defined as asthma not responsive to conventional therapy. It can occur in up to 10% of all asthmatics. The mortality rate is 1–2% (if mechanically ventilated, 10–20%). Frequently these patients have a prodromal period, which is treated in an emergency room; such patients are sent home, with subsequent worsening asthma.[10] The PO_2 is usually 40–60 mmHg, and the PEFR is <80 L/minute. These patients require aggressive and well-monitored management.

The therapy of asthma should include identification of provoking factors, hydration, and supportive care such as supplemental O_2, chest therapy, and antibiotics. Medications available for acute and maintenance therapy include methylxanthines, beta adrenergic stimulants, corticosteroids, cromolyn sodium, anticholinergics, and possibly calcium channel blockers.[11] Methylxanthines are a class of drugs that inhibit phosphodiesterase, thereby decreasing mast cell mediator release as well as smooth muscle contraction. These drugs are well tolerated and have traditionally formed the cornerstone of maintenance therapy. Beta stimulants are especially useful in the acute setting; some are more beta-2 specific, whereas others stimulate both beta and alpha receptors. They must be used very cautiously in elderly patients or those with coronary artery disease but are rapidly effective and most likely to produce immediate benefit in the acute setting. Corticosteroids are also very useful but have many serious long-term side effects. In the acute setting, corticosteroids have been shown to be a very useful form of therapy with few side effects.[12] Anticholinergics are still under investigation for use in asthma. These drugs appear to dilate the larger airways more than the smaller ones. Side effects such as drying of secretions, decreased mucociliary transport, and increased heart rate are not limiting factors when useful doses of inhaled atropine and ipratropium are used.[13] Cromolyn sodium has been shown to stabilize mast cell membranes and increase cAMP in lymphocytes. This drug was cumbersome to administer in its solid form but is now available as a liquid and in metered dose inhalers. It is most useful in steroid dependent patients or in stable asthmatics who are allergen sensitive. Calcium channel blockers seem to decrease smooth muscle contraction and mast cell mediator release. With currently available drugs, this effect is not clinically significant but could become so as new calcium channel blockers are made available.[14]

KEY FEATURES

Evaluation of asthma consists of the following:

1. Careful history taking with emphasis on current and previous attacks
2. Physical examination confirming the diagnosis of asthma
3. Sputum examination
4. Peak expiratory flow rate determination
5. Arterial blood gas
6. Chest radiograph if there is any doubt about the diagnosis

MANAGEMENT OF ASTHMA IN THE EMERGENCY ROOM

Time (minutes)	Treatment
0	Epinephrine 0.3 ml of 1:1000 dilution SC (contraindicated in cases of known coronary artery disease or age 45 years old)
	Isoetharine 0.5 ml or metaproterenol 0.3 ml in 2.5 ml normal saline via nebulizer
	Aminophylline 5–6 mg/kg IV bolus over 20 minutes. (If the patient has not been previously taking an aminophylline preparation.) Followed by 0.6–0.9 mg/kg continuous IV infusion. This should be initiated without the bolus if prior aminophylline preparation has been taken and appropriately adjusted when the theophylline level returns.
20	Epinephrine 0.3 ml of 1:1000 dilution SC
40	Epinephrine 0.3 ml of 1:1000 dilution SC
120	Isoetharine 0.5 ml in 2.5 ml normal saline via nebulizer
240	Isoetharine 0.5 ml in 2.5 ml normal saline via nebulizer

If the patient has not almost returned to baseline after this therapy, admission should be strongly considered. It appears that steroids may play an important role in the acute therapy of asthma; although the data are limited, a corticosteroid could be considered at time 0 of this management scheme in the absence of contraindications to this drug.

REFERENCES

1. American Thoracic Society: Chronic bronchitis, asthma, and pulmonary emphysema. Am Rev Respir Dis 85:762, 1962.
   A statement by the Committee on Diagnostic Standards for Nontuberculous Respiratory Diseases. This includes definitions and classification of chronic bronchitis, asthma, and pulmonary emphysema.

2. McCombs RP, Lowell FC, Ohman JL: Myths, morbidity, and mortality in asthma. JAMA 242:1521, 1979.
   Reviews some aspects of the socioeconomic impact of asthma, as well as commonly held myths about asthma.

3. Boushey HA, Holtzman MJ, Sheller JR, Nadel JA: Bronchial hyperreactivity. Am Rev Respir Dis 121:389, 1980.
   Extensive, well written review of the mechanisms of bronchial hyperreactivity and their relation to various respiratory diseases.

4. Gerblich AA, Campbell AE, Schuyler MR: Changes in T-lymphocyte subpopulations after antigenic bronchial provocation in asthmatics. N Engl J Med 310:1349, 1984.
   A study of seven extrinsic asthmatics who underwent bronchoprovocation. Changes in T cell subpopulations were quantitated. A relevant antigen, methacholine, and an irrelevant antigen were used on all seven patients. Changes in T cell subpopulations were noted only when asthmatics were antigenically stimulated.

5. Shim C, Williams HM: Pulsus paradoxus in asthma. Lancet 1:530, 1978.
   A study of 308 episodes of acute asthma in 93 patients. The presence of pulsus paradoxus and its degree correlated well with the severity of airway obstruction in most cases.

6. McFadden ER, Lyons HA: Arterial blood gas tension in asthma. N Engl J Med 278:1027, 1968.
   Arterial blood gas was measured in 101 asthmatics during acute exacerbations. The findings of these measurements are reported.

7. Findley LJ, Sahn SA: The value of chest roentgenograms in acute asthma in adults. Chest 80:535, 1981.
   Chest radiographs taken routinely on 90 patients admitted with asthma were reviewed. Chest radiographs are only indicated when the acute asthmatic exacerbation appears to be complicated.

8. Kelson SG, Kelson DP, Fleegler BF, Jones RC, Rodman T: Emergency room assessment and treatment of patients with acute asthma. Am J Med 64:622, 1978.
   Adequacy of conventional approach is considered. Article reports on a study of 102 asthmatics with acute exacerbations and their assessment, therapy, and clinical outcome over a 10-day follow-up period.

9. Shim CS, Williams MH: Evaluation of the severity of asthma. Patients versus physicians. Am J Med 68:11, 1980.
   This study shows that patients are better at predicting their PEFR than are physicians and can better tell on a day to day basis the direction of their therapy.

10. Rebuck AS, Read J: Assessment and management of severe asthma. Am J Med 57:788, 1971.
    Sixty-six hospitalized asthmatics were studied. Characteristics and therapy of status asthmaticus are presented.

11. Webb-Johnson DC, Chin B, Andrews JL: Bronchodilator therapy. N Engl J Med 297:476, 758, 1977.
    Excellent review article about most aspects of drugs used in bronchodilator therapy.

12. Littenberg B, Gluck EH: A controlled trial of methylprednisolone in emergency treatment of asthma. N Eng J Med 314:150, 1986.
    A randomized, double-blind, placebo controlled study of 97 patients in the emergency room. Forty-eight patients received methylprednisolone and 49 were given placebo. There were significantly fewer admissions in the methylprednisolone group.

13. Snow RM, Miller WC, Blair HT, Rice DL: Inhaled atropine in asthma. Ann Allergy 42:286, 1979.
    Atropine was given via nebulizer to ten asthmatics. Atropine appears to dilate the larger airways. It was as effective as beta agonists and had few of the expected side effects.

14. Middleton E: Newer drugs in management. Calcium antagonists. Chest 87:79s, 1985.
    Review of the current role of calcium antagonists in asthma.

Acute Respiratory Failure in Chronic Obstructive Pulmonary Disease

Martin Joyce-Brady, M.D.

DEFINITION

Acute respiratory failure is defined by a PaO_2 (arterial partial pressure of oxygen) of less than 50 mmHg, or a $PaCO_2$ (arterial partial pressure of carbon dioxide) greater than 50 mmHg with an arterial pH of less than 7.35. This potentially life-threatening syndrome may result from disorders of the central nervous system, the spinal cord, the neuromuscular system, the thorax and pleura, the upper airway, the cardiovascular system, or the lower airway and alveoli.[1] This discussion addresses acute respiratory failure in chronic obstructive pulmonary disease (COPD).

PATHOLOGY

Chronic obstructive pulmonary disorders include chronic bronchitis, chronic asthma, and emphysema. The hallmark of these disorders is chronic airflow obstruction as a result of a combination of increased airway secretions, bronchoconstriction, and loss of lung elastic recoil, all of which increase airway resistance. This pathology results in increased work of breathing and decreased airflow rates. The respiratory muscles are placed at a mechanical disadvantage because air trapping and hyperinflation alter the length-tension index.[2,3] Gas exchange is disrupted because of severe ventilation-perfusion mismatching (V/Q mismatch), which reduces PaO_2 in excess of $PaCO_2$. Airflow obstruction is quantitated by spirometry during a forced expiration that initially reveals a reduced forced expiratory volume in the first second of exhalation (FEV_1) with preservation of the forced vital capacity (FVC), so that the FEV_1:FVC ratio is reduced. Carbon dioxide retention does not usually occur until the FEV_1 is below 1 L, and even then it is not seen in all patients.[4] Arterial blood gases are essential in differentiating acute from chronic changes in PaO_2, $PaCO_2$, and arterial pH as a guide for therapeutic intervention.

Acute decompensation in COPD is characterized by a further increase in airflow obstruction and in the work of breathing. Arterial blood gases reveal worsening hypoxemia and increased alveolar-arterial gradient for O_2 (A-a gradient) and/or hypercapnia above baseline.[2] Acute decompensation may result from a viral or a bacterial infection of the upper or lower respiratory tract, air pollution, or cigarette smoking.[5] In addition, complications such as pneumothorax, hydrothorax, electrolyte imbalance, acid-base imbalance, drug-induced respiratory depression, pulmonary embolism, congestive heart failure, rib fractures, and upper airway obstruction should be evaluated. Oftentimes, however, such specific causes for acute decompensation cannot be identified. The patient presents only with a change in the color, consistency, or volume of airway secretions or with the symptom of increased dyspnea on exertion.[2] Physical examination may only reveal expiratory wheezing, use of accessory muscles of respiration, hyperresonance of the chest, distant breath sounds, and occasionally bibasilar rales.[2] Extrapulmonary signs may include a change in mental status, asterixis, or right-sided congestive heart failure. The pattern of breathing appears to be altered both in stable COPD patients with CO_2 retention[4,6] and in most COPD patients during the acute exacerbation.[7] This pattern is rapid, shallow breathing. Although the minute ventilation (respiratory rate × tidal volume) may be unchanged, the reduced tidal volume will increase the dead space to tidal volume ratio (VD/VT). Alveolar ventilation is reduced, and hypercapnia results. The stimulus for such breathing is not totally understood but may arise directly from alveolar hypoxia and from airway or parenchymal receptors.

MANAGEMENT

Management of the acute exacerbation of COPD with respiratory failure is directed at (1) correction of hypoxemia and (2) reduction in the work of breathing. Most patients can be managed without intubation.[8] The goal of *oxygen* therapy is to relieve severe hypoxemia without inducing severe respiratory acidosis. Relief of alveolar hypoxia enhances bronchodilatation and vasodilatation, thereby improving airflow and reducing right ventricular afterload. Increased arterial oxygenation will improve cardiac function and tissue oxygen delivery (cardiac output × blood oxygen content). Increased oxygen delivery will also improve central nervous system function;[2] correct metabolic acidosis;[4] and reduce antidiuretic hormone secretion, which impairs free water excretion from the kidneys.[2] Supplemental oxygen is delivered with an air entrainment (Venturi) mask by gradually increasing the fractional concentration of oxygen (FIO_2) until the PaO_2 reaches 60–65 mmHg. Further hypercapnia may result, but this is acceptable so long as the arterial pH remains above 7.25. If severe hypercapnia occurs during oxygen therapy, one should avoid a precipitous reduction of the FIO_2 because severe alveolar hypoxia will result. The alveolar air equation for $PAO_2 = (PB - PH_2O) FIO_2 - 1.25 PaCO_2$. Alveolar hypoxia will result in further arterial hypoxemia. If the hypercapnia fails to decline with mild reduction in the FIO_2, mechanical ventilation may be required.

Just as the etiology of CO_2 retention in the stable COPD patient remains elusive, the etiology of CO_2 retention with O_2 therapy in acute decompensation is also unclear.[7] The classic teaching emphasizes a disordered control of respiration whereby hypoxemia assumes the primary stimulus to respiration as the CO_2 stimulus becomes blunted. Removal of the hypoxemic stimulus with overaggressive oxygen therapy allows unopposed hypercarbia to ensue. One might then expect a correlation between the correction of hypoxemia and increased CO_2 retention. Aubier and colleagues have examined the role of central respiratory drive during acute respiratory failure in COPD before and after oxygen therapy.[7] Central respiratory drive was assessed using the mouth occlusion pressure technique. Central respiratory drive was acutely elevated during the exacerbation, and although a reduction was noted with O_2 therapy, drive remained elevated *above* the baseline level obtained during a stable state. Relief of hypoxemia did not correlate with a depressed respiratory drive. The observed hypercarbia appeared to correlate with an altered pattern of breathing associated with the acute exacerbation. This pattern is rapid, shallow breathing that reduces alveolar ventilation and increases VD/VT. Therapy with O_2 correlated with a reduction in the respiratory rate, but the reduced tidal volume that was due to shallow breathing was unchanged. Hence, the increased VD/VT was unchanged. Increased CO_2 production, which was not measured in this study, could also have played a role. These results suggest that CO_2 retention in acute exacerbations associated with oxygen therapy is more complicated than the removal of a hypoxemic stimulus alone.[7]

Bronchodilators remain an integral part of therapy because additional reversible airflow obstruction occurs during exacerbations. Intravenous the-ophylline and aerosolized beta-2 agonists provide additive effects and are used in concert. Theophylline also enhances respiratory muscle contractility, increases the resistance of respiratory muscles to fatigue, and augments the ventilatory response to hypoxemia. Theophylline clearance will be reduced in heart failure and liver disease, and doses will have to be reduced. Mon-itoring serum levels guides therapy.[9,10] Beta agonists also enhance mucocil-iary clearance,[9] which aids removal of airway secretions. Aerosolized para-sympatholytic drugs in concert with theophylline and sympathomimetics are also useful for bronchodilation of large airways.[10,11]

Steroid therapy also has a defined role during exacerbations, despite its dubious value in the stable COPD patient.[8] Doses equivalent to meth-ylprednisolone 0.5 mg/kg q6h should be used for 72 hours. Larger doses do not appear to be beneficial.

Antibiotic therapy during exacerbations remains empiric and is often employed despite a lack of proven efficacy.[5] These do not include exacer-bations that are due to pneumonia. A controlled trial of tetracycline therapy found no benefit.[12] However, therapy based on sputum Gram's stain is usually employed.

Additional therapy is selective. *Diuretics* may be useful in the hyper-volemic patient[13] and in the treatment of right-sided and/or left-sided con-gestive heart failure. Cardiac glycosides are only useful if left-sided failure is present.[14] Chest physical therapy may be useful in the acutely ill patient with large volumes of secretions. Otherwise, it is not beneficial and may induce bronchoconstriction and hypoxemia.[15] Respiratory stimulants may be counterproductive, because respiratory drive is already maximal and therapy should be directed at reducing respiratory muscle activity.[7] Nutritional sup-port would appear warranted, as malnutrition in advanced COPD is prev-alent and affects respiratory and nonrespiratory muscles equally. However, it is not clear that malnutrition alone can precipitate acute respiratory failure nor that nutritional repletion will reverse respiratory muscle dysfunction.[16] Hence nutritional therapy in the acute stage is often minimal, but in chronic failure requiring mechanical ventilatory assistance, therapy is often initiated. Phlebotomy is reserved for the patient with severe right-sided congestive heart failure and hematocrits over 60%. One should only remove 300–500 ml of blood at a time.[13]

The indications for *mechanical ventilation* are (1) severe hypoxemia (PaO_2 less than 40 mmHg) with respiratory acidosis and altered mental status, (2) failure of conservative therapy to correct hypoxemia without further res-piratory acidosis, (3) onset of respiratory muscle fatigue, and (4) inability of the patient to expectorate copious airway secretions.[2] The clinical signs por-tending incipient respiratory muscle fatigue are (1) increasing respiratory rate, (2) respiratory alternans (altering thoracic and abdominal breathing), and (3) abdominal paradox (inward motion of the abdominal wall with inspiration).[3,17] The patient should be repeatedly evaluated and may require assisted ventilation if fatigue is noted. Mechanical ventilation in either the assist/control or the intermittent mandatory ventilation (IMV) mode can be used. One should avoid hyperventilation in the hypercapneic patient, because severe metabolic alkalosis will occur. Instead, one should maintain the baseline $PaCO_2$ during mechanical ventilation.

PROGNOSIS

Despite the aberrations noted during the acute exacerbation of COPD, the prognosis is not altered from that of the stable COPD patient. Martin and colleagues reported a 94% survival during acute exacerbations (excluding pneumonia) and a 72% two-year survival. Only 1 patient of 36 in their study required mechanical ventilation.[8,18] Hence, the prognosis is good and conservative management is the norm for acute respiratory failure in chronic obstructive pulmonary disease.

KEY FEATURES

Acute respiratory failure is defined as:

1. PaO_2 ≤50 mmHg *or*
2. $PaCO_2$ ≥50 mmHG *and* arterial pH ≤7.35

Pathophysiology of chronic obstructive pulmonary disease:

1. Increased airway secretions
2. Bronchoconstriction   Increased airway resistance
3. Loss of lung elastic recoil

Manifests as increased work of breathing and decreased airflow rates.

Air trapping affects respiratory muscle action.

Ventilation-perfusion mismatch reduces PaO_2 in excess of $PaCO_2$.

FEV_1 is reduced and FVC preserved.

Acute decompensation results in worsening of baseline abnormalities.

Common causes of decompensation include viral and bacterial infection, air pollution, and cigarette smoking; numerous other causes must also be considered.

Clinical features include the following:

1. Rapid, shallow breathing
2. Expiratory wheezing
3. Use of accessory respiratory muscles
4. Hyperresonance

5. Rales
6. Altered mental status
7. Asterixis
8. Right-sided congestive heart failure

Dead space to tidal volume ratio (VD/VT) is increased with an exacerbation.

Increased CO_2 retention may result from altered breathing patterns, increased VD/VT, and/or reduced hypoxemic drive.

Oxygen therapy is the mainstay of management:

1. Best administered by Venturi mask to increase PaO_2 to 60–65 mmHg
2. Patient can tolerate increased $PaCO_2$ so long as pH ≥ 7.25.

Benefits of increased oxygenation include bronchodilatation, vasodilatation, improved cardiac function, improved mental status, reduced metabolic acidosis, and enhanced free water excretion.

Other interventions for acute respiratory failure complicating COPD including the following:

1. *Bronchodilators*
2. *Corticosteroids*
3. *Antibiotics* for established infection
4. *Diuretics* in hypervolemic patients
5. *Nutritional support* for prolonged exacerbation requiring mechanical ventilation
6. *Phlebotomy* for hematocrit >60%
7. *Cardiac glycosides* if left-sided congestive failure present

Mechanical ventilation is indicated for:

1. PaO_2 ≤ 40 with respiratory acidosis and altered mental status
2. Failure of conservative therapy to correct hypoxemia without unacceptable worsening of respiratory acidosis
3. Incipient respiratory muscle fatigue:
   a. Increasing respiratory rate
   b. Respiratory alternans
   c. Abdominal paradox
4. Inability of patient to expectorate copious airway secretions

Acute prognosis is good with appropriate management.

REFERENCES

1. Balk R, Bone RC: Classification of acute respiratory failure. Med Clin North Am 67(3):551–556, 1983.
2. Francis PB: Acute respiratory failure in obstructive lung disease. Med Clin North Am 67(3):657–668, 1983.
3. Macklem PT: Respiratory muscles: The vital pump. Chest 78:753–758, 1980.
4. Javaheri S, Blum J, Kasemi H: Pattern of breathing and carbon dioxide retention in chronic obstructive pulmonary disease. Am J Med 71:228–234, 1981.
5. Tager I, Speizer F: Role of infection in chronic bronchitis. N Engl J Med 292:563–571, 1975.

6. Skatrud JB, Dempsey JA, Bhansuli P, Irvin C: Determinants of chronic carbon dioxide retention and its correction in humans. J Clin Invest 65:813–821, 1980.
7. Aubier M, Murciano D, Fournier M, Milic-Emili J, Pariente R, Derenne JP: Central respiratory drive in acute respiratory failure of patients with chronic obstructive pulmonary disease. Am Rev Respir Dis 122:191–199, 1980.
8. Albert RK, Martin TR, Lewis SW: Controlled trial of methylprednisolone in patients with chronic bronchitis and acute respiratory insufficiency. Ann Intern Med 92:753, 1984.
9. Bukowski M, Nakatsu K, Munt P: Theophylline reassessed. Ann Intern Med 101:63–73, 1984.
10. Paterson JW, Woolcock AJ, Shenfield GM: Bronchodilator drugs. Am Rev Respir Dis 120:1149–1188, 1979.
11. Lefcoe NM, Toogood JH, Biennerhassett G, et al: The addition of an aerosol anticholinergic agent to oral beta agonist plus theophylline in asthma and bronchitis. Chest 82:300, 1982.
12. Nicotra MB, Rivers M, Awe RJ: Antibiotic therapy of acute exacerbations of chronic bronchitis: A controlled study using tetracycline. Ann Intern Med 97:18, 1982.
13. Gertz I, Hedenstierna G, Wester PO: Improvement in pulmonary function with diuretic therapy in the hypervolemic and polycythemic patient with chronic obstructive pulmonary disease. Chest 75:146–151, 1979.
14. Mathur PN, Powles ACP, Pugsley SO, McEwan MP, Campbell EJM: Effect of digoxin on right ventricular function in severe chronic airflow obstruction. Ann Intern Med 95:283–288, 1981.
15. Kirilloff L, Owens G, Rogers R, Mazzoco M: Does chest physical therapy work? Chest 88:437–444, 1985.
16. Rochester DF, Esau SA: Malnutrition and the respiratory system. Chest 85:411–415, 1984.
17. Cohen C, Zagelbaum G, Gross D, Roussos C, Macklem PT: Clinical manifestations of inspiratory muscle fatigue. Am J Med 73:308–316, 1982.
18. Martin TR, Lewis SW, Albert RK: The prognosis of patients with chronic obstructive pulmonary disease after hospitalization for acute respiratory failure. Chest 82:310–314, 1982.

Hemoptysis

Gary R. Garber, M.D.

The observation by Hippocrates, "the spitting of pus follows the spitting of blood, consumption follows the spitting of this and death follows consumption," gives ancient documentation of the significance of hemoptysis in intrathoracic disease.[1] Today, hemoptysis is still recognized as a serious symptom; however, modern methods in management have diminished its mortality. Hemoptysis, as seen in a pulmonary referral practice, may make up as many as 10% of patients.

The major danger in hemoptysis is not exsanguination, but rather asphyxiation as a result of aspiration of large amounts of blood. Therefore, it is imperative to sort out those patients who need emergent attention. Massive hemoptysis, variously defined as between 200–600 ml blood/24 hours, carries a mortality rate of 20–70%, depending on cause and therapy.[2,3,12]

Other authors suggest that hemoptysis should be regarded as massive if it causes respiratory distress, anemia or hypotension, regardless of the volume expectorated.[4]

The major causes of massive hemoptysis, in descending order of frequency, are active pulmonary tuberculosis, bronchiectasis, necrotizing pneumonias, lung abscesses, and lung cancer (for more extensive list, see reference 5). The pathophysiology behind inflammatory and cancerous lesions accounting for most major hemoptysis was demonstrated in the early 1950s.[6,7] Low-pressure pulmonary arterial branches are thrombosed in inflamed areas, whereas bronchial arterial vessels and collaterals enlarge. These thin-walled, high-pressure vessels traverse inflamed and necrotic areas and bleed massively once ruptured.

A careful history, physical examination, and several simple laboratory studies are key in evaluating patients with hemoptysis and can often lead to etiologic diagnoses. Certain cause and effect combinations are observed frequently in practice: hypertension and epistaxis; coarse rales at the bases of the lungs and bronchiectasis; mitral stenosis and exertional hemoptysis; phlebitis and pulmonary infarction; and clubbing and lung cancer. Therefore, the history should include (1) amount and appearance of blood, including color, fluidity, and clots; (2) duration of bleeding; (3) cough, dry or productive, before or after blood was noticed; (4) chest pain, substernal or pleuritic; (5) relation of bleeding to rest, exertion, or position; (6) history of lung or heart disease; and (7) smoking habits.

Serious bleeding from a peptic ulcer or varices is rarely confused with hemoptysis. Epistaxis and minor bleeding from the gingiva or nasopharynx may be confusing. Therefore, the physical examination should not be limited to the chest. Useful signs are clubbing, weight loss, abdominal masses, and vascular spiders. Mirror laryngoscopy and oropharyngeal examination are necessary to rule out upper airway causes. Laboratory tests are limited to hematocrit, leukocyte count, coagulation studies, blood gas determination, urinalysis, electrocardiogram, chest radiograph, sputum analysis (acid-fast bacilli, Gram's stain, and cytologic examination), and a perfusion lung scan if the radiograph is normal.

Initial management includes establishment of two large-bore intravenous catheters for fluid resuscitation and nasal oxygen. In massive hemoptysis or with a weak cough, the patient should be positioned with the bleeding lung in the dependent position. If the site is unknown, Trendelenburg's position is adequate to increase drainage.

Definitive treatment is often difficult. The bleeding vessels in massive hemorrhages are not amenable to local therapy (cautery), and bleeding sites are rarely directly visualized. Control of massive hemorrhage is best accomplished emergently with a rigid bronchoscope that has adequate suction capacity to remove large quantities of blood. With submassive hemoptysis, the timing of bronchoscopy is less urgent. Although active bleeding localization was increased 10–40% with early fiberoptic bronchoscopy (within 48 hours), therapeutic and clinical outcomes were not changed.[8] Fiberoptic bronchoscopy identifies a cause of hemoptysis in a quarter of cases when the chest roentgenogram is normal or nonlocalizing.[13]

There are only a limited set of therapeutic options in the massively bleeding patient. The bleeding must be stopped, or aspiration will quickly lead to death. Surgical removal of the affected segment, lobe, or lung was formerly definitive therapy. There is a very high operative mortality rate in actively bleeding patients or in patients with either unknown or low pulmonary reserve.[9] Therefore, several successful methods to stabilize the patient have been developed. Selective bronchial intubation of the unaffected lung allows for airway protection and minimizes aspiration. The double-lumen Carlens tube is difficult to place and is no longer generally used. Endobronchial tamponade with a Fogarty's catheter placed under fiberoptic bronchoscopy is very successful in controlling massive hemoptysis.[10] Hurwitz reported that iced saline lavage of the affected segment controlled bleeding in all cases of massive hemoptysis, allowing time for adequate medical treatment or pre-surgical evaluation.[3,9] Remy, using angiographically guided bronchial artery, pulmonary artery, and systemic nonbronchial artery embolization, controlled massive hemoptysis in close to 70% of acutely bleeding patients.[11] Follow-up over 1–8 years showed a 50% relapse in hemoptysis. The high relapse rate was felt to be secondary to recanalization of the reabsorbable embolized material and inadequate treatment of the underlying conditions. Of note, several tuberculous cavities and most aspergillomas were associated with rebleeding within 18 months, suggesting a high-risk subgroup.

Treatment of the underlying cause of hemoptysis is imperative in controlling rebleeding. Every day that a person is on antituberculous or broad-spectrum antibiotics (for cystic fibrosis, bronchiectasis, pneumonias, or abscesses), the risk of rebleeding decreases and, if surgery is necessary, operative mortality decreases. Antitussives may be used for persistent violent cough. Oversedation should be avoided, because this may lead to aspiration and atelectasis. Surgery is indicated for refractory or recurrent hemoptysis. Early resection of cavitary lesions (especially aspergillomas) has been suggested, because there is a higher incidence of early, massive rebleeding.

Careful attention to history, physical examination, and basic management principles, organized in an efficient manner, can lead to successful control of hemoptysis.

KEY FEATURES

I. Massive hemoptysis: 200–600 ml/24 hour or respiratory distress, anemia, or hypotension

II. Evaluation
  A. History
    1. Amount, color, fluidity, clots
    2. Duration
    3. Presence of dry or productive cough
    4. Chest pain, substernal or pleuritic
    5. Relation to rest, exertion
    6. Weight loss
    7. Lung or heart disease, smoking
  B. Physical
    1. Lungs: localized wheezes
    2. Clubbing, masses, vascular spiders
    3. Mirror laryngoscopy and oropharynx inspection
  C. Laboratory values
    1. Hct, WBC, prothrombin time
    2. Blood gas determination, urinalysis, ECG
    3. Chest radiograph
    4. Sputum (acid-fast bacilli, Gram's stain, cytologic examination)
III. Management
  A. General
    1. Large-bore IV with saline or Ringer's lactate
    2. Oxygen
    3. Bleeding lung in dependent position
  B. Localize bleeding with rigid bronchoscope if patient is massively bleeding
  C. Selective bronchial intubation for airway protection
  D. Control bleeding
    1. Iced saline lavage
    2. Endobronchial tamponade
    3. Arterial embolization
  E. Treat underlying cause
  F. Antitussives: avoid oversedation
  G. Surgery
    1. Uncontrolled or recurrent hemoptysis
    2. Aspergilloma

REFERENCES

1. Pursel SE, Lindskog GE: Hemoptysis: A clinical evaluation of 105 patients examined consecutively on a thoracic surgical service. Am Rev Resp Dis 84:329, 1961.
    Good review of the causes of hemoptysis focusing on initial evaluation, history, physical examination and etiology.

2. Crocco JA, et al: Massive hemoptysis. Arch Intern Med 121:495, 1968.
    Study defined elevated mortality in patients with over 600 ml/16 hour hemoptysis; 23% mortality if treated surgically, 75% if treated medically (did not use modern medical innovations).

3. Conlan AA, Hurwitz SS, et al: Massive hemoptysis: Review of 123 cases. J Thorac Cardiovasc Surg 85:120, 1983.
    Excellent current review of management. Demonstrates value of endobronchial iced saline lavage and embolization to stabilize patients prior to definitive surgery if needed.

Noted eight sudden deaths from engulfing hemorrhage while awaiting endoscopy. This demands the quick, efficient use of hospital resources in these patients.

4. Bobrowitz ID, Ramakrishna S, Shim Y-S: Comparison of medical vs surgical treatment of major hemoptysis. Arch Intern Med 143:1343, 1983.
   Review of massive hemoptysis in 82 medically and 31 surgically treated patients. Excluding nonoperative candidates, mortality was similar and 87% of major hemoptysis stopped within 4 days with conservative therapy. Surgery was indicated in medically uncontrolled hemoptysis.

5. William L, et al: The management of hemoptysis: A statement by the committee on therapy. Am Rev Resp Dis 93:471, 1966.
   Extensive differential diagnosis and good review of the initial evaluation of patients with hemoptysis.

6. Marchand P, Gilroy JC, Wilson VH: An anatomical study of the bronchial vascular system and its variation in disease. Thorax 5:207, 1950.
   First description of the abnormal vasculature supplying inflammatory lesions in lungs. Demonstrated that bronchial arteries supply abscesses and that large, thin-walled anastomoses exist between bronchial and pulmonary arteries in abscesses and bronchiectasis.

7. Cudkowicz L: The blood supply of the lung in pulmonary tuberculosis. Thorax 7:270, 1952.
   Shows same findings in TB as those reported in reference 6, along with aneurysm formation in bronchial arteries.

8. Gong H, Salvatierra C: Clinical efficacy of early and delayed fiberoptic bronchoscopy in patients with hemoptysis. Am Rev Resp Dis 124:221, 1981.
   Demonstrated that in nonmassive hemoptysis, early bronchoscopy (within 48 hours of presentation) did not change therapeutic or clinical outcomes. Definitive diagnosis by early or late bronchoscopy occurred primarily with neoplasm.

9. Conlon AA, Hurwitz SS: Management of massive hemoptysis with the rigid bronchoscope and cold saline lavage. Thorax 35:901, 1980.
   Describes excellent results with cold saline lavage.

10. Lee BC, et al: Flexible fiberoptic bronchoscopy and endobronchial tamponade in the management of massive hemoptysis. Chest 70:589, 1976.

11. Remy J, et al: Treatment of hemoptysis by embolization of bronchial arteries. Radiology 122:33, 1977.
    Remy has the most published experience with bronchial artery embolization and has very good results. Forty-one of forty-nine patients with hemoptysis were acutely controlled. Complications were very low. The only absolute contraindication is an anterior spinal artery arising from the intercostal artery system, which could lead to accidental spinal infarction by embolization.

12. Corey R, Khin MH: Major and massive hemoptysis: Reassessment of conservative management. Am J Med Sci 294:301, 1987.
    Retrospective review of 33 patients with major (≥200 ml/24 hr) and 26 with massive hemoptysis (≥1000 ml/24 hr). The overall mortality rate was 31% (18/59). Mortality was greatest for those with a malignancy (59% died) or those who bled ≥1000 ml/24 hr (58% died). The series included only a small number of patients with tuberculosis. Conservative management is recommended for most patients.

13. Poe RH, Israel RH, Marin MG, et al: Utility of fiberoptic bronchoscopy in patients with hemoptysis and a nonlocalizing chest roentgenogram. Chest 93:70, 1988.

Review of 196 patients with hemoptysis and a normal or nonlocalizing chest roentgenogram who underwent fiberoptic bronchoscopy. A specific cause for the hemoptysis was identified in 23% of cases. Bleeding in excess of 30 ml/day was associated with an increase in overall diagnostic yield, while age ≥50, male sex, and smoking of ≥40 pack years best predicted a diagnosis of malignancy.

Diseases of the Pleura

Martin Joyce-Brady, M.D.

ANATOMY

The pleura is a thin layer of connective tissue that lines the surface of the thoracic cage, the diaphragm, and the mediastinum as the parietal pleura and reflects to line the entire surface of the lung parenchyma as the visceral pleura. The parietal and the visceral pleura join at the hilum and extend to the diaphragm as the pulmonary ligament.[1] Flattened mesothelial cells line both pleural surfaces. Their microvilli provide a large absorptive surface and produce lubrication to reduce the work of breathing. Lymphatic channels are abundant beneath the mesothelium. Along the parietal pleura of the lower mediastinum and the infracostal region, direct pleurolymphatic communications, known as stomas, exist. Particulate matter and cells are cleared via these stomas.[1,2]

The parietal pleura has a systemic blood supply and a sensory innervation. It is easily stripped from the chest wall. In contrast, the visceral pleura has primarily a pulmonary blood supply and no sensory innervation. It is more highly vascularized and is tightly attached to the lung parenchyma. The fluid dynamics in the pleural space promote a new flow of fluid from the parietal pleura into the pleural space with resorption along the visceral pleura.[1]

PATHOLOGY

Pleural disease is most often a secondary phenomenon resulting from an extrapleural process. It presents as the abnormal accumulation of fluid or gas or as a solid mass in the pleural space.

Fluid

A fluid accumulation in the pleural space is called a pleural effusion. Effusions are traditionally classified as transudate or exudate, based on their protein or lactate dehydrogenase (LDH) content.[3,4] An exudate contains a pleural fluid protein/serum protein ratio ≥ 0.5, a pleural LDH/serum LDH of ≥ 0.6, or a pleural fluid LDH $\geq$ two thirds of the upper limit of normal for serum LDH. A transudate results from altered hydrostatic forces that enhance flow across the pleura into the pleural space or impair resorption from the pleural space. Hence, the protein content of the fluid is low. A transudative effusion often results from congestive heart failure, nephrosis, cirrhosis, and/or hypoalbuminemia. Therapy is directed at the primary disease and not the pleural surface. In contrast, an exudate may result from direct damage to the pleural surface and adjoining tissue induced by disease or from lymphatic obstruction. The etiology of an exudate is more extensive and, in general, includes disease of the lung parenchyma, systemic disease with pleural involvement, intra-abdominal and pelvic diseases, and primary pleural disease. Analysis of the pleural fluid or direct examination of pleural tissue may establish the cause of an exudate. Fluid examination can include, in addition to protein and LDH measurements, total cell counts; differential leukocyte count, glucose and amylase concentrations; Gram's stain, acid-fast stain; fungal stains; culture for aerobic, anaerobic, mycobacterial and fungal organisms; and cytologic study.

Cells

A blood-tinged effusion results from as little as 5000–10,000 RBC/mm³ and is nondiagnostic. In contrast, a grossly bloody effusion is usually associated with greater than 100,000 RBC/mm³. This commonly results from trauma, malignancy, or pulmonary embolism.[5]

Exudative effusions usually have greater than 1000 WBC/mm³. Mesothelial cells shed from the pleural surface are also present. An absence of these cells indicates extensive pleural surface involvement by a disease process, as seen with pleural tuberculosis,[6] although this may also occur in empyema and in some malignancies.[5,7]

A predominance of polymorphonuclear leukocytes (greater than 50%) results from acute inflammation and has numerous causes. Acute infection must be differentiated from noninfectious inflammatory disease. A transudative effusion that is due to congestive heart failure with a predominance of polymorphonuclear leukocytes should raise the suspicion of pulmonary embolism.[7] Eosinophils and basophils are nondiagnostic, although plasma cell accumulations may be due to multiple myeloma or plasmacytomas.[5,7]

In the absence of active inflammation, any chronic pleural effusion will show mainly lymphocytes.[8] The differential diagnosis is frequently reduced to granulomatous (especially tuberculous) versus malignant disease of the pleura. Tuberculous effusions are usually acid-fast smear and culture negative, whereas malignant effusions from all causes will have a positive cytologic finding in 50% of cases.[4] When pleural fluid analysis of an exudate is unrevealing, examination of the pleural surface by percutaneous closed needle biopsy may provide a diagnosis.[9] One must also recall that malignancy may produce an effusion without direct pleural involvement by causing lymphatic or bronchial obstruction, in which case examination of the pleural surface will not provide a diagnosis.[8]

Biochemical

A pleural fluid glucose concentration of less than 60 mg/dl suggests empyema; complicated parapneumonic effusion; or effusion as a result of rheumatoid arthritis, tuberculosis, or malignancy.[7] Rheumatoid arthritis produces an extremely low glucose level, usually less than 25 mg/dl, by impairing glucose transport across the pleural surface.[10] An increased amylase activity is found in pancreatitis (pancreatic isoenzyme), esophageal rupture (salivary gland isoenzyme), or malignancy. Pleural fluid pH usually reflects arterial pH, but it may be reduced in an effusion secondary to adjacent pneumonia (parapneumonic effusion) and in an effusion that is due to rheumatoid arthritis, tuberculosis, or malignancy.[7]

Further evaluation of pleural fluid in selected instances includes the following: A positive LE cell preparation is pathognomonic of systemic lupus erythematosus. The presence of rheumatoid factor is nonspecific and is found in rheumatoid arthritis, pneumonia, tuberculosis, and malignancy. Elevated hyaluronic acid is seen in some malignant mesotheliomas. Lipid analysis of turbid or milky appearing fluid for triglyceride and cholesterol will differentiate a chylous versus a pseudochylous effusion (see later discussion).[7]

Culture

If infection is a possible cause of an exudative pleural effusion, the fluid should be cultured for aerobic and anaerobic bacteria. Mycobacterial and fungal cultures should also be performed if these organisms are suspected. Pleural space infection is most commonly due to anaerobic bacteria, but *Staphylococcus aureus, Streptococcus pneumoniae, Streptococcus pyogenes,* and gram negative organisms are also causative.[11] Less common agents are *Mycobacterium tuberculosis,* nontuberculous mycobacteria, Actinomyces species, Nocardia species, and fungi.[12]

Percutaneous Pleural Biopsy

Percutaneous pleural biopsy allows direct analysis of the parietal pleura.[4] This procedure is often used to differentiate pleural tuberculosis from malignancy. Both disorders produce a lymphocytic exudative effusion that may have a low glucose concentration. If the pleural fluid cytologic examination is negative, malignancy cannot be excluded. The biopsy is performed using a closed needle technique and should include three to five specimens. These should be examined by acid-fast smear and culture for tuberculosis and also by routine histologic study for possible malignancy. Because involvement of the pleura is often patchy, examination of the parietal pleura on three separate occasions may be necessary to establish a diagnosis. Tuberculosis can be diagnosed in 90% of cases, whereas malignancy can be diagnosed in 68%.[4]

Despite these diagnostic evaluations, the etiology of 15–20% of exudates remains unclear. If tuberculosis or malignancy is still suspected, the direct visualization of the pleural surface with pleuroscopy or thoracotomy may provide an answer.[9] The Mayo Clinic reported that an exudate undiagnosed at thoracotomy remained so, and did not recur in 60% of their cases. A diagnosis became apparent from 12 days to 6 years post-thoracotomy in 35% of the cases and was usually malignancy.[13]

Thoracic Empyema and Parapneumonic Effusion

An empyema, by definition, is the accumulation of pus in a cavity of the body. This results from an acute inflammatory response that is almost invariably infectious in origin but need not be so. No exact number of polymorphonuclear leukocytes has been accepted to define an empyema. From a bacteriologic point of view, an empyema is an exudate with a positive bacterial culture. An exudate resulting from a contiguous pneumonia is called a parapneumonic effusion. A parapneumonic effusion is sterile on culture but may subsequently grow organisms and thereby evolve into an empyema.

An empyema may be caused by (1) a contiguous inflammatory process of the lung (pneumonia, lung abscess), the diaphragm (subdiaphragmatic abscess), the esophagus (esophageal rupture into the pleural space), or the mediastinum (acute mediastinitis); (2) contamination of the pleural space during a diagnostic or surgical procedure involving the pleura; (3) trauma; or (4) a spontaneous occurrence. Spontaneous infection may be associated with a subclinical pneumonia.[14] The progression of an empyema has been divided into three stages. The exudative stage involves the formation of a sterile effusion that is due to a process listed previously and can be called a parapneumonic effusion. The fibrinopurulent stage involves infection of the effusion by an offending organism with the accumulation of leukocytes and fibrin in the pleural space. This results in the formation of loculations that contain the infection. The pleural fluid pH and glucose concentration are reduced by leukocyte phagocytosis and bacterial metabolism, and the LDH content rises. The organizing stage involves the pleural space from the visceral and parietal pleural surface with the formation of a pleural peel.[14,15]

The management of pleural space infection involves (1) identification of the offending organism, (2) treatment with antibiotics, (3) locating the source of the pleural space infection, and (4) deciding on the need and type of pleural space drainage. Identification of the organisms involves specific cultures (see previous discussion). Antibiotic therapy is initially based on Gram's stain results and clinical suspicion of the most likely agent(s) of infection. Culture and sensitivity data are used to adjust therapy as they become available. The decision for drainage may be based on the size, the appearance, or the biochemical characteristics of the pleural fluid. Optimal management of pleural space infection should prevent further complications. These include the formation of empyema necessitatis (spontaneous drainage of an empyema into the chest wall), a bronchopleural fistula (from rupture of an empyema into the lung), a thick pleural peel that may prevent adequate sterilization and may impair lung function, uncontrolled pleural sepsis, pericarditis, mediastinal abscess, and osteomyelitis of the ribs or sternum.[14,15]

Concerning the management of parapneumonic effusions, Light has recommended the following guidelines, based on his experience:[14,15] He emphasizes optimal management with the use of closed tube drainage for a parapneumonic effusion that he defines as complicated (definition follows), in order to prevent further potential morbidity and mortality.

Small parapneumonic effusions, which measure less than 10 mm from the inside of the chest wall to the bottom of the lung, do not usually require thoracentesis. They should resolve with treatment of the primary pneumonia. This may not necessarily apply to an effusion of another cause, as listed previously.

For larger parapneumonic effusions, if the diagnostic thoracentesis yields pus or has a positive Gram's stain, immediate closed tube thoracostomy drainage is used.

If the fluid is not frank pus or if the Gram's stain is negative, pleural fluid pH, glucose, and LDH are used to guide therapy. An effusion with a pH of 7.00 and a glucose concentration of less than 40 mg/dl is called a complicated parapneumonic effusion because it is unlikely to resolve spontaneously. Light also uses closed tube thoracostomy to drain this effusion at the onset of treatment.

An effusion with a pH of 7.20, a glucose level of greater than 40 mg/dl, and an LDH of less than 1000 IU/ml will usually resolve with therapy for the primary pneumonia. Hence further drainage is not used unless another indication arises, such as a large effusion resulting in respiratory symptoms.

For an effusion with a pH between 7.00 and 7.20 and an LDH of greater than 1000 IU/ml, clinical judgment is required. If the effusion is small and the pH is closer to 7.20, serial thoracentesis every 12–24 hours may be successful drainage. However, for larger effusions with a pH closer to 7.00, closed tube thoracostomy may be more successful. Once a chest tube is inserted, it should be maintained until the drainage is less than 50 ml/24 hours. If the tube fails to fluctuate with respiration, it is nonfunctional and should be removed or repositioned if still needed. This approach should be successful in the management of most parapneumonic effusions and purportedly can reduce the incidence of further complications. Occasionally, owing to multiple loculations or to late drainage, the lung may fail to reexpand fully or infected locules may persist. Such a patient may ultimately require further surgical intervention such as open drainage or decortication for cure.[14,15] However, if the patient's fever and toxicity have largely resolved, these collections can clear spontaneously with continued antimicrobial therapy.

An exception to this outline of chest tube drainage involves an effusion produced by a malignancy in which the tumor is obstructing a mainstem or lobar airway. Under this condition, the lung will be unable to fill the pleural space once a chest tube is inserted and the patient will be unnecessarily burdened with the tube. Such a condition is best treated with antibiotic therapy and concomitant radiation therapy to the obstructed airway. If the obstruction is relieved, chest tube drainage can be initiated. If the obstruction persists, antibiotic therapy alone should be continued.[14]

Chylothorax

Chylothorax is the accumulation of chyle in the pleural space. This is due to injury or obstruction of the thoracic duct, usually from trauma or malignancy (especially lymphoma and metastatic tumor). The fluid has a milky appearance and a high triglyceride content, which is greater than 400 mg/dl. A chylothorax should be distinguished from a pseudochylous effusion, which is high in cholesterol. A pseudochylous effusion is found in any chronic exudative effusion and is mostly due to tuberculosis or rheumatoid arthritis.[16]

Gas

A pneumothorax is the abnormal accumulation of gas in the pleural space. This results from penetration of the parietal or visceral pleura either spontaneously or traumatically. Spontaneous pneumothorax results from rupture of the visceral pleura. It most frequently occurs in healthy persons, usually males under 40 years of age, as a result of a ruptured bleb, commonly in the apex of the lung. There is a 50% recurrence rate within two years, and 75% will recur on the same side as the initial pneumothorax. After two recurrences on the same side, surgical pleurodesis may be indicated. Spontaneous pneumothorax also occurs in persons with underlying suppurative or interstitial lung disease. It is not an infrequent occurrence in emphysema, cystic fibrosis, or eosinophilic granuloma (histiocytosis X). Thirdly, spontaneous pneumothorax may rarely occur in women during menses (catamenial pneumothorax). The woman is usually over 30 years of age, and the pneumothorax occurs within 48 hours after the onset of menses. It is more common in the right hemithorax. In this instance, therapy is directed at suppression of ovulation. If ovulation is resumed, pleurodesis may be required to prevent recurrence.

Traumatic pneumothorax may occur as a complication of diagnostic and therapeutic maneuvers that violate the pleural space, such as thoracentesis, percutaneous pleural biopsy, transthoracic needle biopsy, and central venous cannulation. It also occurs in the setting of penetrating and nonpenetrating injuries to the chest wall, diaphragm, or mediastinal structures.

Therapy for pneumothorax is guided by the mechanism of injury, the associated symptoms, the presence of underlying disease, and the size of the pneumothorax. Large pneumothoraces associated with penetrating chest or abdominal trauma and during positive pressure mechanical ventilation are treated with closed tube thoracostomy. In patients with underlying lung disease and limited lung function, even a small pneumothorax may produce respiratory symptoms or cardiovascular compromise and will require drainage. Many pneumothoraces induced during diagnostic procedures result from disruption of the parietal pleura and may be drained with a small-bore catheter or simply observed for spontaneous resolution. An asymptomatic spontaneous pneumothorax in a healthy person can be allowed to resorb spontaneously if it is less than 15–30% of the volume of the hemithorax. Beyond 15–30%, however, the time needed for resorption of gas may exceed 10 days and drainage is usually employed to prevent a potential complication of incomplete lung expansion. A tension pneumothorax is a life-threatening complication that results from the accumulation of air under positive pressure in the pleural space. This may complicate any cause of pneumothorax. The positive pleural pressure impedes venous return and cardiac output. Immediate pleural space decompression is indicated.[17]

Solid

Fibrothorax is the abnormal accumulation and organization of fibrin into a nonelastic fibrous tissue. It is usually a complication of a previous empyema or hemothorax. If severe, it may impair mechanics in the ipsilateral as well as the contralateral lung. Respiratory embarrassment is treated with decortication.[18]

Calcification of the pleura may result from an old empyema, hemothorax, pneumothorax therapy for tuberculosis, or asbestos exposure.[18]

Tumors

Metastatic involvement of the pleural space is common, especially from breast, lung, ovarian, and lymphatic cancer.[19] Primary tumors are rare and are usually mesotheliomas. Most of these are malignant, but some are benign. The distinction is often difficult. The benign form presents as a localized mass and usually arises from the visceral pleura. It may be associated with hypertrophic osteoarthropathy and clubbing and is treated by surgical excision. In contrast, malignant mesothelioma is associated with asbestos exposure and presents with diffuse involvement of the pleura. It has a poor prognosis, with few therapeutic options at present.[20]

KEY FEATURES

Anatomy and Physiology of the Normal Pleura

The pleurae are thin connective tissue layers with mesothelial surface cells lining the intrathoracic space.

The visceral pleura is tightly adherent to the lung surface, has primarily a pulmonary blood supply, and has no sensory innervation.

The parietal pleura lines the thoracic cage, mediastinum, and superior surface of the diaphragm; is only loosely adherent; and has a systemic blood supply and innervation.

Fluid dynamics promote a net flow of fluid from the parietal pleura into the pleural space with resorption by the visceral pleura.

Pathologic Conditions

Pleural Effusions

Transudative pleural effusions are low in protein content and arise from altered hydrostatic forces, generally in the clinical settings of congestive heart failure, nephrosis, cirrhosis, and/or hypoalbuminemia of other causes.

Exudative effusions are defined by the following:

1. Pleural fluid protein/serum protein ≥.5, or
2. Pleural fluid LDH/serum LDH ≥.6, or
3. Pleural fluid LDH ≥two to three times upper limit of normal serum LDH.

Exudates may arise from pleural disease or from a wide variety of systemic processes.

Grossly bloody pleural effusions generally result from trauma, malignancy, or pulmonary embolism.

A paucity of mesothelial cells in an exudative effusion suggests extensive pleural surface pathology, as with tuberculosis.

A predominance of polymorphonuclear leukocytes in an exudative effusion suggests acute infection or other inflammatory processes.

Eosinophils and basophils are nondiagnostic; plasma cells in pleural fluid are associated with plasma cell dyscrasias.

Low pleural fluid glucose concentration usually occurs in the clinical settings of infection, rheumatoid arthritis, tuberculosis, or malignancy.

Fluid complement levels and an LE preparation may substantiate the diagnosis of connective tissue disease; rheumatoid factor is nondiagnostic.

Increased pleural fluid amylase levels suggest pancreatitis, esophageal rupture or malignancy.

Turpid and/or milky appearing fluid may represent a chylous effusion (high in triglycerides, resulting from lymphatic obstruction) or pseudochylous effusion (high in cholesterol, from any chronic exudate).

Empyema thoracis generally results from contiguous infection, usually of the lung; diagnosis rest on pleural fluid cell count, Gram's stain, and culture.

Treatment of thoracic empyema includes the administration of appropriate antibiotics and drainage of the pleural space, usually with a closed chest tube. Multiple chest tube placements and/or surgical breakdown of loculations are often necessary.

Parapneumonic effusions result from contiguous pneumonia.

Complicated parapneumonic effusions, defined by pH $\leq$7.00–7.20, glucose $\leq$40 mg/dl, and/or LDH $\geq$1000 IU/ml, require treatment as for empyema.

The diagnosis of pleural malignancy or tuberculosis may require pleural biopsy.

Pneumothorax

Pneumothorax most commonly arises spontaneously from rupture of a visceral pleural bleb in an otherwise healthy young person.

Recurrences of spontaneous pneumothorax are common (50%), generally on the same side (75%).

Pneumothorax may also occur in association with trauma, or complicate diagnostic procedures.

Therapy is guided by mechanism of injury, size, associated symptoms, and presence of underlying disease.

All pneumothoraces $\geq$15–30% of the hemithorax volume or of any extent during positive pressure ventilation require closed chest tube thoracostomy.

Tension pneumothorax is a life-threatening emergency and requires immediate decompression.

Mass Lesions

Fibrothorax generally occurs as a complication of previous empyema or hemothorax and may necessitate decortication.

Calcification of the pleura may complicate numerous pleural diseases.

Metastatic involvement of the pleura occurs most commonly with carcinomas of the breast, lung, or ovary, and with lymphomas.

Benign mesotheliomas usually present as isolated mass lesions of the visceral pleura.

Malignant mesotheliomas usually present with diffuse involvement of the pleura in individuals with a history of previous exposure to asbestos.

REFERENCES

1. Black LF: The pleural space and pleural fluid. Mayo Clinic Proc 47:493, 1972.
2. Wang NS: The preformed stomas connecting the pleural cavity and the lymphatics in the parietal pleura. Am Rev Resp Dis 111:12–20, 1975.
3. Light RW, MacGregor MI, Luchsinger PC, Ball WC: Pleural effusions: The diagnostic separation of transudates and exudates. Ann Intern Med 77:507–513, 1972.
4. Health and Policy Committee, American College of Physicians: Diagnostic thoracentesis and pleural biopsy in pleural effusions. Ann Intern Med 103:799–802, 1985.
5. Light RW, Erozan YS, Ball WC: Cells in pleural fluid. Arch Intern Med 132:854–860, 1973.
6. Spriggs AI, Boddington MM: Absence of mesothelial cells from tuberculous pleural effusions. Thorax 15:169–171, 1960.
7. Light RW: Pleural effusions. Med Clin North Am 61:1339–1351, 1977.
8. Sahn SA: Malignant pleural effusions. Clin Chest Med 6:113–125, 1985.
9. Gunnels JJ: Perplexing pleural effusion. Chest 74:390–393, 1978.
10. Dodson WH, Hollingsworth JW: Pleural effusion in rheumatoid arthritis. N Engl J Med 275:1333–1342, 1966.
11. Bartlett JG, Gorbach SL, Thadepalli H, Finegold SM: Bacteriology of empyema. Lancet 1:338–340, 1974.
12. George RB, Penn RL, Kinasewitz GT: Mycobacterial, fungal, actinomycotic and nocardial infections of the pleura. Clin Chest Med 6:63–76, 1985.
13. Ryan CJ, Rodgers RF, Unni KK, Hepper NG: Outcome of patients with pleural effusion of indeterminate cause at thoracotomy. Mayo Clinic Proc 56:145–149, 1981.
14. Light RW: Parapneumonic effusions and empyema. Clin Chest Med 6:55–62, 1985.
15. Light RW: Management of parapneumonic effusions. Arch Intern Med 141:1339–1341, 1981.
16. Bessone L, Ferguson T, Buford T: Chylothorax. Ann Thorac Surg 12:527–550, 1971.
17. Jenkinson SG: Pneumothorax. Clin Chest Med 6:153–161, 1985.
18. Hinshaw HC, Murray JF (eds): Diseases of the Chest, 4th ed. Philadelphia, WB Saunders Co, 1980, pp 911–912.
19. Leff A, Hopwell P, Castello J: Pleural effusion from malignancy. Ann Intern Med 88:532–537, 1978.
20. Antman KH: Malignant mesothelioma. N Engl J Med 303:200–202, 1980.

Smoke Inhalation and Carbon Monoxide Poisoning

David Schwartz, M.D.

Since Boston's Coconut Grove fire in 1942, in which nearly 500 patrons of a nightclub perished, smoke inhalation injury and carbon monoxide poisoning have become well-recognized causes of morbidity and mortality among burn victims. In fact, 50% of fire-related deaths in the United States are a direct result of smoke exposure. At least three factors (thermal, chemical, and carbon monoxide) are involved in the pathogenesis of smoke-induced injury. An understanding of these factors will allow one to develop a rational therapeutic approach to the patient suffering from smoke inhalation.[1,2,3,7]

Thermal burns are almost always limited to the upper respiratory tract (above the larynx). The lower respiratory tract is protected by a very efficient heat exchanging mechanism between the nasopharyngeal and hypopharyngeal regions and by the relative low heat capacity in hot dry air. Even superheated dry air will be cooled before reaching the larynx. On the other hand, as one increases the moisture content of air, the heat capacity increases proportionately and may override the heat exchange mechanisms of the upper respiratory tract. Steam, with a heat capacity of 4000 times that of hot dry air, may cause thermal injury to the lower respiratory tract. Thermal burns to the upper airway serve as a marker for a significant exposure, and if they are either extensive or associated with marked edema, one must consider early intubation (preferably nasotracheal) to avoid upper airway occlusion.

Chemical fumes have become a major concern and account for the lower respiratory tract complications seen within the first 24 hours. Burning of synthetic products (such as nylon, asphalt, polyurethane, polyvinylchloride, and others) will release toxic fumes (ammonia, sulfur dioxide, chlorine, hydrogen chloride, phosgene, aldehydes, nitrogen dioxide, and cyanide), which when inhaled may exert direct toxic effects (e.g., cyanide poisoning, of mitochondrial electron transport compounding the effect of carbon monoxide by impairing oxygen utilization[7]) or may react with water to produce strong acids or alkalis. These agents cause an intense inflammatory reaction wtih mucosal edema that may extend into the bronchiolar or alveolar epithelium.

In addition, ciliary motion and surfactant activity are markedly depressed. Within hours of exposure, the patient may slough his or her bronchial mucosa and develop a necrotizing bronchiolitis and intra-alveolar hemorrhage. Early on, these patients may be clinically asymptomatic with mild bronchospasm but within 24 hours of exposure can develop adult respiratory distress syndrome (ARDS) or infectious respiratory complications.[4] Early treatment with steroids and prophylactic antibiotics has not been shown to alter the course of these complications.[5,8] One must observe and treat the patient supportively, adding antibiotics when microbiologic evidence supports this course of action.

Carbon monoxide is felt to be the most common cause of death in burn victims.[6] This odorless, nonirritating gas is given off with the incomplete combustion of carbon-containing materials (wood, coal, gasoline, and other organic substances). Thus in addition to burn victims and fire fighters, coal miners, smelters, police, toll booth workers, and mechanics are at risk for carbon monoxide poisoning. Its high affinity for hemoglobin (200 times that of oxygen) displaces oxygen from hemoglobin-binding sites and shifts the oxygen dissociation curve to the left. Although the PaO_2 remains normal, the oxygen content is markedly diminished. The best measure of carbon monoxide exposure is the carboxyhemoglobin level. The oxyhemoglobin saturation is reliable only if it is a measured saturation in a machine that can detect carboxyhemoglobin. The clinical sign of cherry red nailbeds is not at all reliable. Carboxyhemoglobin levels will provide a rough guide to the severity of exposure (mild, <20%; moderate, 20–40%; severe, >40%) and will be predictive of CNS changes (headaches, confusion, coma). The half-life of carboxyhemoglobin is normally 4 hours, but elimination may be hastened three- to fourfold by applying 100% O_2 rebreathing apparatus. Hyperbaric oxygen, if available, will decrease the half-life to 30 minutes.

Evaluation of the smoke-exposed patient should revolve around the three etiologic factors (thermal, chemical, and carbon monoxide) responsible for respiratory-related morbidity and mortality. On examination, one must assess patency of the upper airway and if significant upper airway burns are visualized, early intubation is recommended. In the event of a significant smoke exposure, the patient should be hospitalized for at least 24 hours and observed for the delayed complications related to chemical fume exposure. Lastly, one must first treat the patient with 100% rebreathing apparatus and then assay for carbon monoxide poisoning via a carboxyhemoglobin level. Risk factors predictive of a clinically significant exposure requiring observation include steam exposure, exposure to plastic fumes, singed facial hair, oropharyngeal burns, and asymptomatic carboxyhemoglobin level >20%.

KEY FEATURES

MANAGEMENT OF SMOKE INHALATION AND CARBON MONOXIDE POISONING

Etiology	Clinical Concern	Therapeutic Options
Thermal	Upper airway obstruction	Observe patient Early intubation
Chemical	Lower airway:inflammation, atelectasis, bronchospasm, bronchiolitis, pneumonia, or ARDS	Observe patient and treat with supportive measures (steroids and prophylactic antibiotics have not been effective)
Carbon monoxide	Tissue ischemia (CNS and cardiac)	100% O_2 rebreathing mask Hyperbaric oxygen

COHb Level	Symptoms
<20%	Headaches, tinnitis, disinhibition, nausea
20–40%	Weakness, depressed mental status, vomiting
>40%	Coma, cardiac arrhythmias, death

High-Risk Patients

Steam exposure
Exposure to plastic fumes
Singed facial hair
Oropharyngeal burns
Symptomatic carboxyhemoglobin levels >20%
Underlying cardiopulmonary disease

REFERENCES

1. Mellins RB, Park S: Respiratory complications of smoke inhalation in victims of fires. J Pediatr 87:1, 1975.
    A very complete review examining the thermal, chemical, and carbon monoxide related toxicities of smoke inhalation. Therapeutic options are considered, and preventive measures are reviewed.

2. Trunkey DD: Inhalation injury. Surg Clin North Am 58:1132, 1978.
3. Crapo RO: Smoke-inhalation injuries. JAMA 246:1694, 1981.
4. McArdle CS, Finlay WEI: Pulmonary complications following smoke inhalation. Br J Anaesth 47:618, 1975.
    Presents two cases of smoke inhalation (without significant cutaneous burns) complicated by ARDS. The pathophysiology and therapeutic options are discussed.

5. Levine B, Petroff P, Slade I, Pruitt B: Prospective trials of dexamethasone and aerosolized gentamicin in the treatment of inhalation injury in the burned patient. J Trauma 18:188, 1978.
    Two prospective, randomized, placebo-controlled intervention trials were performed—one with dexamethasone (20 mg IV × 3 days), and the other with aerosolized

gentamicin (80 mg tid × 10 days). Thirty burn victims were allotted to each trial. Smoke inhalation injury was defined via xenon scan or bronchoscopy. Neither trial noted significant changes in mortality, pulmonary complications, or infectious complications.

6. Winter P, Miller J: Carbon monoxide poisoning. JAMA 236:1502, 1976.
   Reviews the pathophysiology, symptomatology, and therapeutic options in carbon monoxide poisoning.

7. Cahalane M, Demling RH: Early respiratory abnormalities from smoke inhalation. JAMA 251:771, 1984.
   Excellent concise summary article with cogent discussion of clinical features and pathophysiology. Brief review of therapy.

8. Robinson NB, Hudson LD, Riem M, et al: Steroid therapy following isolated smoke inhalation injury. J Trauma 22:876, 1982.
   Retrospective review of clinical course of smoke inhalation survivors of two Las Vegas hotel fires. Few serious complications among those admitted to area hospitals for observation; no difference in outcome noted between those treated or not treated with corticosteroids.

Tuberculosis

Martin Joyce-Brady, M.D.

Tuberculosis is a chronic granulomatous disease caused by an obligate aerobic, slow-growing, acid-fast bacillus known as *Mycobacterium tuberculosis*.[1,2] This "white plague" has been the scourge of humankind for centuries. A decline in morbidity and mortality from tuberculosis paralleled an improving socioeconomic status in developing countries and preceded both bacille Calmette-Guérin (BCG) vaccination and modern chemotherapy.[3] The disease remains a problem in undeveloped nations and within the United States afflicts the indigent, the homeless, the imprisoned, the malnourished, and the immunocompromised host.[1] There are still more than 20,000 new cases reported per year and approximately 1800 deaths per year. Extrapulmonary disease accounts for 8–10% of these cases.[4,5] Prior to the AIDS epidemic, the epidemiology in the United States had shifted from a prevalence in children, pregnant women, and young adults to involve more middle-aged to elderly adults.[1] Epidemics of primary disease among elderly nursing home populations have been described.[5] From 1963 to 1984, the incidence rate of tuberculosis declined annually, but this decline abruptly ended in 1985 and the incidence rate increased by 2.6% in 1986. This increase has been attributed, in part, to recent immigrants of Hispanic and Asian/Pacific Islander origin and to the AIDS epidemic.[6]

PATHOGENESIS

Tuberculosis is a disease of humans.[1,2] It is contracted by inhaling tubercle bacilli in droplet nuclei produced during coughing by a diseased person. The bacilli reach lung alveoli, usually in lower lung zones, where ventilation is greater.[3] In the nonimmune host, the ensuing inflammatory response consists of neutrophils and macrophages. With time a granuloma will form in which central caseation may occur. During this initial phase, tubercle bacilli enter peripheral lung lymphatics, which then drain into hilar and mediastinal lymph nodes and may produce adenopathy. They also enter the bloodstream, and this transient bacteremia inoculates extrapulmonary sites. The pulmonary process results in a primary complex that includes a pulmonary tubercle and an enlarged regional lymph node. There may be minimal to no symptoms at this time. In the immunocompetent host, this primary complex heals sometimes with calcification as a result of a cellular immune response that occurs within 2–6 weeks of the initial exposure. A PPD skin test (see later discussion) will reveal a delayed hypersensitivity reaction and serves to identify the host as infected by *Mycobacterium tuberculosis*. There is no evidence of tissue necrosis or acid-fast organisms in host secretions at this time. Tuberculous disease, as opposed to infection, is diagnosed by acid-fast smear and culture of organisms from an involved site. In the immunocompromised host and in some immunocompetent individuals, *progressive primary disease* may develop in the form of lung parenchymal necrosis (cavitation), bronchogenic spread throughout the lung, tuberculous pneumonia, generalized adenopathy, or miliary disease. The PPD skin test may be unreactive in these persons. In contrast, disease may develop in the immune host at a later point in time as a result of *reactivation* of foci inoculated during the primary infection. Exogenous reinfection is probably rare. Reactivation tends to occur in areas of high oxygen tension, which favors growth of the organism. These sites include the lung apices, the epiphyses of long bones, the vertebral bodies, the kidneys, the meninges, the pericardium, the peritoneum, the bone marrow, the liver, and the spleen. The initial process is insidious but eventually produces fever, night sweats, and weight loss. Within the lungs, reactivation commonly occurs in the posterior segment of the right upper lobe or the superior segment of a lower lobe. Tuberculosis of the pleura may occur in primary and reactivation tuberculosis.[7] The mechanism of pleural involvement appears to be a combined seeding of the cavity with tubercle bacilli and a host hypersensitivity reaction to the organism or its products. Disease may present as a pleuritis, an exudative pleural effusion, or an empyema. The pleural effusion is believed to result primarily from the host hypersensitivity reaction. As such, organisms are rarely present in the pleural fluid and biopsy of the parietal pleura for acid-fast smear and culture is usually required for diagnosis. It is important to diagnose and treat a tuberculous pleural effusion because even though it tends to resolve spontaneously, untreated persons have a high risk of developing reactivation disease, which is estimated to be 30% within five years. A tuberculous empyema results from rupture of a subpleural parenchymal cavity directly into the pleural space. This results in a bronchopleural fistula and a frank empyema.[7]

DIAGNOSIS OF TUBERCULOUS INFECTION AND DISEASE

The diagnosis of tuberculosis has been hampered by a declining awareness of the disease among health care professionals,[1] by an increasing prevalence of extrapulmonary disease,[1] and by atypical presentations of pulmonary disease.[8]

Tuberculous infection is identified by the PPD skin test.[1,9,10] PPD is a purified protein derivative of *Mycobacterium tuberculosis*. Forty-eight hours after placement of a 5 TU* PPD (intermediate strength), the test is interpreted as negative if there is less than 5 mm induration, questionable if 5–10 mm, and positive if greater than 10 mm. However, in the setting of a recent exposure to an infectious person, a 5–10 mm PPD in a previously healthy skin test negative person should be interpreted as meaningful.[1,9,10] A 1 TU PPD (first strength) is reserved for suspected sensitized persons. A 250 TU (second-strength) is used only for maximal evidence of a true negative test in excluding the diagnosis of tuberculosis.[1] Physicians must be aware of the following pitfalls in interpreting the PPD skin test. First, cross-reactivity with nontuberculous mycobacteria results in a false positive reaction. This is a prevalent problem in the southeastern United States and a common cause of an intermediate reaction. Second, false negative reactions also occur. In patients with active disease, 10–35% have a negative PPD on their first evaluation. A false negative PPD skin test may result from: (1) an extradermal injection of antigen, (2) an erroneous reading of induration, (3) an improper source of antigen material, or (4) a host-related phenomenon that results in impaired cell-mediated immunity. These include miliary disease, lymphoproliferative disease, advanced age, malnutrition, recent viral infections, antiviral vaccinations, corticosteroid use, immunosuppressive therapy, or the acquired immune deficiency syndrome (AIDS).[11] Third, the booster phenomenon results in a falsely positive interpretation of PPD skin test conversion. The booster phenomenon is faced during screening and occurs in previously infected persons in whom reactivity to PPD has waned. During the initial screening PPD skin test, an insignificant response may be noted

---

*TU = tuberculin unit.

that serves to stimulate some reactivity. The person is falsely categorized as a nonreactor, and during a follow-up test as soon as one to a few weeks later, an anamnestic response may occur with greater than 10 mm induration. The person is then incorrectly labeled a recent converter and may be exposed to a potentially toxic prophylactic chemotherapeutic regimen. This response occurs in all ages but is more prevalent with increasing age, as is the risk of adverse side effects to drugs. It can be avoided in adults who are periodically retested by repeating the skin test within 1 week when an initially negative or insignificant result is obtained.[1,9] A positive result indicates true positivity, not skin test conversion, and is suggestive of the booster phenomenon.

Within the guidelines just listed, skin test reactivity indicates infection by *Mycobacterium tuberculosis*. Such individuals must then be evaluated for tuberculous disease. Disease is diagnosed by acid-fast smear and culture of organisms from an involved site. The acid-fast smear and the culture provide complementary information. The smear is rapid and easy to perform but must be viewed as presumptive evidence of disease because false positive results may occur with nontuberculous mycobacteria and nonmycobacterial acid-fast organisms. The culture data are delayed, as the organism requires 4–6 weeks for growth. However, the culture provides the definitive diagnosis and allows drug sensitivity testing.[1,11]

TUBERCULOSIS CONTROL

Effective, safe, self-administered outpatient chemotherapy is the rule for antituberculous therapy today.[1,11,12] Hospitalization is reserved for diagnostic purposes and incapacitating illness. Chemotherapy is indicated for infected as well as diseased persons. Tuberculosis control is concentrated on (1) identifying persons at risk for infection and preventing infection, (2) identifying persons who are infected and preventing disease, and (3) identifying diseased persons and rendering them noninfectious.[1]

Prevention of Infection

The use of BCG vaccine remains controversial. It plays little role in tuberculosis control in the United States, where most disease arises in persons who are already infected.[1,11] On average, a newly diagnosed person with tuberculous disease has infected fewer than five persons prior to diagnosis. Once chemotherapy is begun, little if any further transmission occurs.[12] The major emphasis on infection prevention in the United States, then, is the identification and treatment of diseased persons.

Treatment of Infection

Treatment of infected persons is an integral part of tuberculosis control, since new cases of disease arise from such persons, especially if the chest radiograph reveals previous stable parenchymal involvement.[1,11,12] Therapy involves isoniazid, which presumably sterilizes the inactive tuberculous foci. Twelve months of isoniazid preventive therapy has been shown to reduce the incidence of subsequent disease.[1] In the case of a person with a positive PPD and an abnormal chest radiograph, the physician must be certain that the radiographic changes are stable and that the patient has no symptoms or signs of disease before initiating preventive therapy with isoniazid alone. If there is any doubt as to the presence of disease, the patient should be fully evaluated by obtaining appropriate acid-fast smears and cultures of specimens. One should begin therapy for disease until culture results and further clinical evaluation over time allow a firm distinction of infection versus disease. Isoniazid preventive therapy does have a risk of hepatitis and cannot be used indiscriminately. The hepatitis appears to be age related. It is rare below 20 years of age. From 20 to 30 years, it is 0.3%/patient/year. From ages 36–49 and 50–64, it is 1.2% and 2.3%, respectively. Therapy is recommended for the following groups, in order of priority, by the American Thoracic Society:[11]

1. Household members and other close contacts or potentially infectious cases. Children and newborns must be evaluated carefully.
2. Newly infected persons who have converted their skin test from negative to positive within 2 years of a known negative test. These persons are called recent converters.
3. Persons with past tuberculosis that has not been treated with adequate chemotherapy.
4. Persons with a positive PPD and an abnormal chest x-ray. *The chest x-ray must show nonprogressive (previous) disease with negative bacteriology and a stable parenchymal lesion,* not merely isolated calcification or pleural thickening. Reactivation rates range from 0.5–5% per year in this group.
5. A significant skin test associated with certain diseases. These include silicosis, diabetes mellitus, prolonged therapy with corticosteroids, immunosuppressive therapy, some hematologic and reticuloendothelial diseases such as leukemia and Hodgkin's disease, AIDS (including persons with antibodies to the HIV virus), end-stage renal disease, and situations associated with rapid weight loss or chronic malnutrition (such as intestinal bypass surgery for obesity, the postgastrectomy state, chronic peptic ulcer disease, chronic malabsorption syndromes, and carcinoma of the oropharynx and upper GI tract complicated by poor oral nutrition).
6. A positive PPD in persons less than 35 years old without any of the above risk factors.

The duration of preventive therapy for infection is 6–12 months.[11] A European trial of prevention showed no benefit for longer therapy. Six months of therapy was equal to 12 months in persons with stable fibrotic lesions less than 2 cm in diameter, but only 66% effective for larger lesions.[12] For patients who are noncompliant or at risk for hepatitis, therapy for less than 1 year may be beneficial. The issue of an isoniazid-resistant source case complicates preventive therapy. Options include (1) give isoniazid in hope of an *in vivo* efficacy, (2) observe the patient without any therapy, or (3) prescribe a different therapy.[1,11] There are no data for non-isoniazid regimens at present. For immunosuppressed hosts and children, therapy may be initiated with rifampin and ethambutol for 6–12 months. Otherwise, rifampin alone for 9 months is recommended.[1,11] In all cases, therapy is monitored by monthly clinical evaluation for symptoms or signs of drug toxicity. Routine liver function tests are monitored in persons at high risk for drug toxicity.

Treatment of Disease

Therapy is based on disease severity, suspicion of drug resistance, associated social or medical problems, and suspected drug toxicity.[1,11,12] There may be three distinct populations of organisms to kill: a slow-growing intracellular group in an acid milieu (mainly within macrophages); a group inside a caseous focus in a neutral milieu; and a large, actively growing extracellular group in a slightly alkaline milieu.[14] These three populations have a broad range of metabolic activity from least to most active, respectively. Because the tubercle bacillus is only susceptible to a drug during replication, there is a broad range of drug susceptibility. Chemotherapy must avoid the selection of drug-resistant organisms within the large extracellular group and must inactivate the slow-growing groups within caseous foci and within macrophages. Spontaneous resistance to a drug tends to occur in one tenth of organisms.[6] The probability of simultaneous resistance in one organism to two drugs[13] is 1×10. Because the total organism load/individual rarely exceeds 10, at least two drugs are used to treat disease.[10,14] The actively growing extracellular organisms are killed quickly by drugs; however, the slow-growing organisms require more prolonged therapy (i.e., months) for effective removal. There are at least ten drugs available to treat tuberculous disease. Isoniazid, rifampin, streptomycin, viomycin, capreomycin, ethionamide, pyrazinamide, and para-aminosalicylic acid are bactericidal agents. Ethambutol and cycloserine are bacteriostatic agents.[14] Isoniazid and rifampin are effective against all three groups of organisms. Pyrazinamide is most effective in an acid milieu (i.e., against the intracellular organisms). Streptomycin is most effective in an alkaline milieu (i.e., the extracellular organisms).[14] Regimens used to treat pulmonary disease are also used for extrapulmonary disease.[1,11,12] Isoniazid plus rifampin for 9 months with or without ethambutol or streptomycin for the first 2–8 weeks is effective therapy *if the sputum culture is negative for the final 6 months of therapy.* The relapse rate is less than 3%. Vitamin B_6 therapy to prevent isoniazid-associated peripheral neuropathy is reserved for the nutritionally deficient person.[1] Therapeutic monitoring emphasizes patient education and supervision with less performance of routine laboratory tests except in groups at high risk for drug toxicity. An intermittent, biweekly supervised regimen of isoniazid and rifampin for noncompliant persons is also effective treatment *if* the organisms are sensitive to the drugs *and* the person has completed a daily course of therapy for the first 4–8 weeks. If isoniazid or rifampin cannot be used because of drug-resistant organisms or drug toxicity problems, at least two new drugs are used for 18–24 months. The 9-month regimen cited previously is also known as short-course therapy, and newer regimens directed at even shorter duration of therapy, 6 months or less, are under evaluation. The most recent recommendations also include a 6-month regimen of isoniazid, rifampin, and pyrazinamide for the first 2 months, followed by isoniazid and rifampin for 4 months in selected patients if the organisms are sensitive to these drugs and the patient is compliant.[11]

Disease involving the meninges or pericardium is usually treated with three drugs with the addition of steroids if the inflammatory response is resulting in clinical problems with management.[1] The issue of drug-resistant organisms is a real problem and is variable in the United States. Practitioners are advised to seek information from local sources on prevalence data for drug resistance. One should suspect drug resistance in (1) patients from ethnic groups with a high prevalence of drug-resistant organisms; (2) persons previously treated for tuberculosis, (3) individuals with persistently culture positive sputums after 3 months of therapy; and (4) patients with known exposure to a drug-resistant group. Therapy for these groups should include at least three drugs until drug sensitivity data allow a change. Isoniazid is generally discontinued if drug resistance is found.[1]

Drug Toxicity and Interactions

The clinician must be aware of drug toxicity and interactions.[1,11,12] *Isoniazid* may cause hepatitis or a peripheral neuropathy. The neuropathy appears to involve an interference with pyridoxine metabolism. This vitamin is given with therapy when diabetes, uremia, alcoholism, and malnutrition are present. Phenytoin levels will increase while the patient is on isoniazid and may produce toxicity. Phenytoin levels should be monitored during the induction of therapy. *Rifampin* commonly causes GI upset and less commonly induces a skin rash, hepatitis, or thrombocytopenia. Rifampin is excreted in all body fluids, and the patient should be alerted to the orange color that will be present in the urine. Lastly, rifampin induces mixed function oxidases. This will complicate therapy with sodium warfarin (Coumadin), oral contraceptive drugs, steroids, methadone, oral hypoglycemic agents, digitoxin, and cyclosporine. *Pyrazinamide* may cause hepatitis and hyperuricemia. *Ethambutol* levels are increased in renal failure. This drug also may cause a retrobulbar neuritis that is dose related. It occurs in fewer than 1% of patients if 15 mg/kg of drug is used. Incidence rises when 25 mg/kg is used. *Streptomycin, kanamycin, and capreomycin* may cause nephrotoxicity or ototoxicity. *Para-aminosalicylic* acid causes GI upset and hypersensitivity phenomena. *Cycloserine* may cause behavioral abnormalities, seizures, and a peripheral neuropathy. Anticipation of these interactions and careful drug selection will minimize complications during therapy for tuberculosis.[1,11,12,15]

Special Treatment Circumstances

During pregnancy, therapy for active disease should be initiated without delay because the risk of complications from disease treatment are outweighed by the risk of the disease.[1,11,12,16] Isoniazid and ethambutol are safe to use. Pyridoxine is recommended with isoniazid therapy during pregnancy.[11] Rifampin may be safe, but experience is limited. Aminoglycoside therapy causes fetal ototoxicity and should be avoided. Ethionamide is teratogenic and hence contraindicated. Data for other drugs are limited. Isoniazid, rifampin, and streptomycin are all secreted into breast milk but do not produce toxicity in the nursing newborn.[11] Therapy for infection can be started after delivery unless the mother is a recent PPD skin test converter or a household contact of a diseased person, in which case therapy should be initiated after the first trimester with isoniazid.[11] If uncertainty exists, the patient should be referred to a public health authority.

In persons with renal disease, one must monitor aminoglycoside levels carefully and perhaps avoid ethambutol because levels cannot be checked easily.[1] Concomitant hepatic disease is problematic. In general, one should use a regimen with the least number of hepatotoxic drugs and monitor therapy carefully. Complications do not appear to be increased in these patients.[11,17,18] Lastly, chemotherapy has virtually eliminated surgical therapy in this disease except to treat complications such as a tuberculous empyema with a bronchopleural fistula. The historical and therapeutic role of surgery has been reviewed elsewhere.[19]

Although the most common mycobacterial species that causes disease in AIDS is *M. avium* complex, *M. tuberculosis* is also increasing. PPD skin testing is recommended in all persons with HIV infection or with AIDS. In hopes of preventing disease, persons who have a positive PPD or who have a history of a positive PPD should be evaluated for preventive therapy regardless of age, once active disease has been ruled out.[20] The presence of extrapulmonary tuberculosis in patients with HIV infection indicates a diagnosis of AIDS. The lungs remain the most common site of tuberculous disease in patients with AIDS, and unlike many other of their respiratory tract infections, it is treatable. Treatment guidelines have been outlined by the American Thoracic Society.[20] In patients with AIDS, tuberculous disease does appear to respond to therapy, but survival is frequently limited by concomitant disease.[22,23]

KEY FEATURES

Tuberculosis (TB) is a chronic granulomatous disease caused by *Mycobacterium tuberculosis*.

Twenty thousand new cases and 1800 deaths occur annually from TB in the United States.

Infection is contracted by inhalation of tubercle bacilli in droplet nuclei and generally results in a self-limited inflammatory process involving lung and regional lymph nodes (primary complex).

Disease may result from a progressive primary process or, more commonly, from reactivation of foci inoculated during primary infection (sometimes decades later).

Clinical manifestations of tuberculous disease include tuberculous pneumonia with or without parenchymal cavitation, generally involving the superior segment of a lower lobe or posterior segment of an upper lobe; pleural effusion or empyema; and intrathoracic or generalized lymphadenopathy.

Extrapulmonary disease occurs in 8–10% of cases, usually at sites of high oxygen tension: epiphyses of long bones, vertebral bodies, kidneys, meninges, pericardium, peritoneum, bone marrow, liver, and spleen.

Infection is diagnosed by use of the PPD skin test; the primary complex is infrequently noted radiographically.

False positive and false negative results and the booster phenomenon may complicate interpretation of PPD skin test activity.

Disease is diagnosed when acid-fast smear and culture from an involved site yield *M. tuberculosis*.

Tuberculosis control efforts are focused on (1) identifying persons at risk and preventing infection, (2) identifying infected persons and preventing disease, and (3) identifying diseased persons and rendering them noninfectious.

Treatment of infection with isoniazid (INH) prevents progression to tuberculous disease and is recommended for:

1. Household members/close contacts, especially infants and children, of potentially infectious persons
2. Newly infected individuals (recent converters)
3. Those with past TB and a history of inadequate treatment
4. Persons with a positive PPD and an abnormal chest radiograph (nonprogressive disease with negative bacteriologic findings only)
5. Persons with a positive skin test and certain underlying diseases or immunosuppressive therapy (see text)

6. A positive skin test in persons less than 35 years of age

Such prophylactic therapy is effective when administered for 6–12 months; treatment of infection from an INH-resistant source is problematic.

First-line treatment of established tuberculous disease includes the administration of INH and rifampin for 9 months with or without ethambutol or streptomycin for the first 2–8 weeks.

In the settings of drug resistance to or patient toxicity from INH or rifampin, at least two new drugs should be substituted for a treatment duration of 18–24 months.

Drug resistance should be considered in:

1. Patients from ethnic groups with a high prevalence of drug resistance
2. Persons previously treated for TB
3. Individuals with persistently positive sputum cultures after 3 months of therapy
4. Persons with known exposure to drug-resistant disease

Chemotherapeutic agents effective against *M. tuberculosis,* other than those previously mentioned, include pyrazinamide, para-aminosalicylic acid, viomycin, capreomycin, ethionamide, and cycloserine. All currently available agents can produce serious toxic effects.

REFERENCES

1. Glassroth J, Robins A, Snider DE Jr: Tuberculosis in the 1980's. N Engl J Med 302:1441–1450, 1980.
2. Dannenburg AM: Pathogenesis of pulmonary tuberculosis. In Green GMG, Daniel TM, Ball WCB (eds): Koch Centennial Supplement. Am Rev Resp Dis 125(Part 2):25–29, 1982.
3. Middlebrook G: Tuberculosis and medical science. In Green GMG, Daniel TM, Ball WCB (eds): Koch Centennial Supplement. Am Rev Resp Dis 125(Part 2):5–7, 1982.
4. Centers for Disease Control: Tuberculosis in the United States, 1984. Morbid Mortal Wkly Rep 34(21):299–307, 1985.
5. Stead W: Tuberculosis among elderly persons: An outbreak in a nursing home. Ann Intern Med 94:606–610, 1981.
6. Centers for Disease Control: Tuberculosis, final date—United States, 1986. MMWR 36(50.51):817–820, 1988.
7. Hinshaw HC, Murray JF: Diseases of the Chest, 4th ed. Philadelphia, WB Saunders Co, 1980, pp 298–355.
8. Khan M, Kovnat D, Bacchus B, Whitcomb M, Brody J, Snider G: Clinical and roentgenographic spectrum of pulmonary tuberculosis in the adult. Am J Med 62:31–38, 1977.
9. Snider DE: The tuberculin skin test. In Green GMG, Daniel TM, Ball WCB (eds): Koch Centennial Supplement. Am Rev Resp Dis 125(Part 2):108–118, 1982.
10. Snider DE: The tuberculin skin test. Am Rev Resp Dis 124:356–363, 1981.
11. Official Statement of the American Thoracic Society: Treatment of tuberculosis and tuberculosis infection in adults and children. Am Rev Resp Dis 134:355–363, 1986.
12. Snider DE, Cohn D, Davidson P, Hershfield E, Smith M, Sutton F: Standard therapy for tuberculosis 1985. Chest 87(suppl):105–135, 1984.
13. Gunnels J, Bates J, Swinsoil H: Infectivity of sputum positive tuberculosis patients on chemotherapy. Am Rev Resp Dis 109:323–330, 1974.
14. Comstock G: New data on preventive treatment with isoniazid. Ann Intern Med 98:663–665, 1983.
15. Van Scoy RE, Wilhowske CJ: Antituberculous agents. Mayo Clin Proc 62:1129–1136, 1987.

16. Dutt AK, Stead WW: Present chemotherapy for tuberculosis. J Infect Dis *146*:698–704, 1982.
17. Snider DE: Pregnancy and tuberculosis. Chest *86*(suppl):105–135, 1984.
18. Cross FS, Long MW, Banner AJ, Snider DE: Rifampin-isoniazid therapy of alcoholic and nonalcoholic tuberculosis patients in a U.S. Public Health Service Cooperative therapy trial. Am Rev Resp Dis *122*:319, 1980.
19. Gaensler EA: The surgery for pulmonary tuberculosis. *In* Green GMG, Daniel TM, Ball WCB (eds): Koch Centennial Supplement. Am Rev Resp Dis *125*(Part 2):73–84, 1982.
20. Snider DE, Hopewell PC, Mills J, Reichman LB: Mycobacterioses and the acquired immunodeficiency syndrome. Am Rev Resp Dis *136*:492–496, 1987.
21. Centers for Disease Control: Revision of the CDC Surveillance Case definition for acquired immunodeficiency syndrome. MMWR *36*(1 Suppl):3S–14S, 1987.
22. Louie E, Rice LB, Holzman RS: Tuberculosis in non-Haitian patients with acquired immunodeficiency syndrome. Chest *90*:542–545, 1986.
23. Chaisson RE, Schecter GF, Theuer CP, Rutherford GW, Echenberg DF, Hopewell PC: Tuberculosis in patients with the acquired immunodeficiency syndrome. Am Rev Resp Dis *136*:570–574, 1987.

SECTION 9
RHEUMATOLOGY AND IMMUNOLOGY

Approach to the Patient with Acute Rheumatic Disease

David Felson, M.D.

Acute arthritis is symptomatic joint inflammation lasting less than 6 weeks. It can be subdivided into acute monarthritis (arthritis affecting one joint), oligoarticular arthritis (arthritis affecting two to four joints, usually asymmetrically), or polyarticular arthritis (affecting four or more joints in a symmetrical distribution). Some patients who state they have arthritis and complain of joint pain actually have tendinitis, periarthritis, or bursitis (see article on soft tissue rheumatism).

The key to the successful diagnosis of acute arthritis lies in a systematic approach:[1,2] first, determine whether the arthritis is monarthritis, oligoarticular arthritis, or polyarticular arthritis, and next factor in the demographic status of the patient and the duration of symptoms. Synovial fluid examination and selected laboratory tests can be used to corroborate the clinical diagnosis.

Acute monarthritis commonly affects the knee, but it can occur in any joint and has a number of possible causes. Nongonococcal bacterial arthritis[6] usually presents as an acute monarthritis developing over several days, often in a previously abnormal or damaged joint. Because bacterial arthritis can swiftly and irreversibly destroy a joint, rapid diagnosis and commencement of therapy are critical; therefore, all patients with acute monarthritis should be examined for fever, skin lesions, and possible sources of infection. Synovial fluid examination, which is mandatory if this diagnosis is suspected, shows greater than 50,000 WBC/mm^3, a low glucose concentration, and a positive culture or Gram's stain. The most common causes are *Staphylococcus aureus* and Streptococcus, but gram negative organisms may seed an abnormal joint during a bacteremia from another source. Gonococcal arthritis[7] has a spectrum of manifestations ranging from acute monarthritis often with a positive joint fluid culture to a diffuse periarthritis with skin lesions and an occasional positive blood culture.

Osteoarthritis, a common cause of monarthritis, occurs in knees and hips or in joints already impaired, most often afflicts the elderly, and usually has been intermittently symptomatic for several years. Synovial fluid typically shows a WBC count of less than $1000/mm^3$. Acute trauma with cartilage damage can cause a monarticular arthritis that usually resolves with rest. Synovial fluid may be bloody, and fractures may coexist. In adult men and postmenopausal women, gout is a possible cause of acute monarthritis, affecting the great toe, ankles, feet, and knees (see *Crystal-Induced Arthritis*). Pseudogout (also described in *Crystal-Induced Arthritis*) can cause an acute monarthritis, especially in elderly patients, and most often affects the knee. In gout and pseudogout, the presence of birefringent crystals in the synovial fluid is diagnostic. Acute hemorrhagic arthritis can occur in patients with bleeding diatheses. Rarely, systemic lupus erythematosus (SLE), rheumatoid arthritis, or other major connective tissue diseases begin as an acute monarthritis or with so-called palindromic rheumatism, in which monarthritis or oligoarticular episodic attacks arise acutely and resolve completely.

Acute oligoarticular arthritis may be caused by many diseases that also cause symmetrical polyarthritis, including rheumatoid arthritis, gout, and pseudogout. Seronegative spondyloarthropathies, which include ankylosing spondylitis, Reiter's syndrome, psoriatic arthritis, and the arthritis associated with inflammatory bowel disease, are usually oligoarticular and predominantly affect men. Although it usually initially involves the spine causing morning stiffness in the back, ankylosing spondylitis is an inflammatory arthritis that can affect the extremities. Reiter's syndrome usually begins in lower extremity joints, especially the knees or ankles. Coexistent symptoms include urethritis, which may cause dysuria or a urethral discharge; a scaly erythematous rash on the palms and soles (keratoderma blennorrhagicum); a rash on the penis (circinate balanitis); iritis or conjunctivitis; and shallow, nontender oral ulcers. Psoriatic arthritis has a variety of peripheral joint and spinal manifestations and is associated with psoriatic nail involvement in 80% of patients. Inflammatory bowel disease can be accompanied by arthritis affecting large lower extremity joints. Infectious diarrhea caused by Salmonella, Shigella, Yersinia, and Campylobacter can lead to an acute reactive arthritis resembling Reiter's syndrome. Unique features of all spondyloarthropathies are the frequent inflammation of tendon site insertions in the lower extremities, especially the Achilles tendon; and the presence of sausage digits, signifying inflammation of the digital tendon sheaths. HLA-B27 is increased in those spondyloarthropathies in which there is spinal involvement.

Despite a long list of causes,[3] acute symmetrical polyarthritis often has an immune complex pathogenesis. Clinically, most patients have bilateral symmetrical aching and stiffness in the small joints of the hands and feet. Viral arthritis[5] and serum sickness are the most common causes of acute polyarthritis in children and young adults. Usually secondary to rubella or hepatitis B infection,[4] viral arthritis is almost always symmetrical, lasts less than 6 weeks, and is occasionally associated with a viral rash or preceding upper respiratory symptoms. In hepatitis B,[4] the arthritis is frequently accompanied by an urticarial rash and tender hepatomegaly with rising hepatic transaminases. Hepatitis B surface antigen is invariably positive. Serum sickness is also frequently heralded by a rash with symptoms occurring up to 2 weeks after exposure to an immunogen, often penicillin. Erythema nodosum, a painful nodular rash in the lower legs, can be associated with a lower extremity symmetrical polyarthritis. Some patients with acute sarcoidosis[10] have erythema nodosum, symmetrical arthritis, and hilar adenopathy on chest radiograph, a triad called Löfgren's syndrome. Although in recent years it has become rare, acute rheumatic fever[12] can cause an acute polyarthritis and should be considered if the patient lives in a crowded environment and if fever or carditis is present. Serial antistreptolysin-O (ASLO) titers should be elevated, reflecting recent streptococcal infection. Lyme disease[8] is caused by a spirochete that is transmitted by the bite of the tick *Ixodes dammini*, which inhabits coastal New England and Great Lakes regions. Clinically, it is manifested by a gradually enlarging annular rash, erythema chronicum migrans, fever, malaise, and headache, with occasional evidence of meningeal irritation. In the first weeks, a migratory polyarthritis may occur; later, attacks may localize to one large joint, especially the knee.[9] Early Lyme disease responds to tetracycline or penicillin therapy.

Another cause of polyarthritis, hypertrophic pulmonary osteoarthropathy,[11] occurs in patients with congenital heart disease or lung disease, especially pulmonary malignancy. It causes a lower extremity arthritis, distal long-bone tenderness, and often clubbing.

In elderly patients with symmetrical polyarthritis, gout, pseudogout, and polyarticular osteoarthritis should be considered. In these diseases, the arthritis is often not truly symmetrical despite the patient's complaint of arthritis "all over."

Rheumatoid arthritis, SLE, and other major connective tissue diseases, which usually cause symmetrical polyarthritis, may affect any age group. Although patients with connective tissue disease often visit physicians early in their course, it is frequently easier to reach a definitive diagnosis later when a clear-cut disease pattern evolves. Seventy-five per cent of patients with rheumatoid arthritis have positive rheumatoid factors, and most have elevated sedimentation rates.

If arthritis has persisted for more than 6 weeks, the diagnostic possibilities change. A chronic monarthritis may be secondary to tumor or tuberculosis but is not likely to be caused by an acute bacterial infection or gout, both of which are illnesses of shorter duration. A chronic symmetrical polyarthritis may be due to rheumatoid arthritis or SLE; viral arthritis and serum sickness generally remit and do not become chronic.

KEY FEATURES

APPROACH TO ACUTE ARTHRITIS
(Joint Inflammation of Less Than 6 Weeks' Duration)
Causes of Acute Monarthritis

All Ages	*Middle-Aged and Elderly*
Bacterial arthritis	Gout
Post-traumatic arthritis	Pseudogout
Acute hemorrhagic arthritis associated with bleeding diathesis	Osteoarthritis exacerbation
Early rheumatoid arthritis	

Causes of Acute Oligoarthritis
(2–4 joints, usually in asymmetrical distribution)

All Ages	*Middle-Aged and Elderly*
Reactive arthritis secondary to Yersinia, Shigella, Salmonella, Campylobacter	Gout
Almost all causes of polyarthritis can begin with oligoarthritis	Pseudogout
Seronegative spondyloarthropathies	

Causes of Acute Polyarthritis
(4 or more joints in symmetrical distribution)

All Ages	*Middle-Aged and Elderly*
Serum sickness	Gout
Viral arthritis	Pseudogout
Early rheumatoid arthritis	Polyarticular osteoarthritis
Hypertrophic pulmonary osteoarthropathy	
Acute sarcoidosis (Löfgren's syndrome)	
Erythema nodosum	
Lyme disease	
Acute rheumatic fever	

REFERENCES

1. Moskowitz RW: Clinical Rheumatology, A Problem-Oriented Approach. Philadelphia, Lea & Febiger, 1975, p 331.
   Excellent introductory text with chapters organized not by diseases, but rather by patient presentation, including chapters on acute monarthritis and acute polyarthritis.

2. Kelley WN, Harris ED Jr, Ruddy S, Sledge CB (eds): Textbook of Rheumatology, 2nd ed. Philadelphia, WB Saunders Co, 1985.
   Several chapters in this standard text deal with evaluating arthritis patients.

3. Hoffman GS: Polyarthritis: The differential diagnosis of rheumatoid arthritis. Semin Arthritis Rheum 8:115, 1978.
    Fine discussion of the causes of polyarthritis.

4. Duffy J, Lidsky MD, Sharp JT, et al: Polyarthritis, polyarteritis, and hepatitis B. Medicine 55:19, 1976.
    Arthritis and rash occur in the preicteric phase, caused by immune complex deposition at a time of antigen excess. Vasculitis occurs later.

5. Hyer FH, Gottlieb NL: Rheumatic disorders associated with viral infection. Semin Arthritis Rheum 8:17, 1978.
    Literature review on viral arthritides, most common of which is rubella. Live attenuated rubella vaccine can also cause arthritis, as can many other viruses, including varicella; mumps; certain adeno- and echoviruses; and the Epstein-Barr virus, associated with infectious mononucleosis.

6. Goldenberg DL, Reed JL: Bacterial arthritis. N Engl J Med 312:764, 1985.
    Review incorporating large clinical series. Staphylococcus was the most common organism with Streptococcus and gram negative bacilli also frequent. Most patients presented with monarticular arthritis and purulent joint fluid. Fever, present in 78%, was often low-grade, and Gram's stain was positive in most patients, especially those with staphylococcal infections (75%). Synovial fluid culture was almost always positive.

7. O'Brien JP, Goldenberg DL, Rice PA: Disseminated gonococcal infection: A prospective analysis of 49 patients and a review of pathophysiology and immune mechanisms. Medicine 62:395, 1983.
    Best recent review. Two groups of patients, one with monarticular septic arthritis, and the second with periarthritis, skin lesions, and occasional positive blood cultures.

8. Goldings EA, Jericho J: Lyme disease. Clin Rheum Dis 12:343, 1986.
    Fine review of clinical features by stage of disease; laboratory findings, including antibody titers to the causative spirochete; and treatment options.

9. Steere AC, Schoen RT, Taylor E: The clinical evolution of Lyme arthritis. Ann Intern Med 107:725, 1987.
    Fifty-five untreated patients with erythema chronicum migrans were followed 6 years on average. Twenty-eight (51%) developed episodic arthritis, usually in large joints (knees, shoulders, ankles), which waned in frequency over time. Ten (18%) had arthralgias alone, especially early in disease. Six (11%) developed chronic arthritis. Of note, 20–40% of patients do not remember antecedent skin rash.

10. James DG, Neville E, Carstairs LS: Bone and joint sarcoidosis. Semin Arthritis Rheum 6:53, 1976.
    Reviews acute and chronic sarcoidosis. Acute disease usually occurs in young women, is often associated with erythema nodosum and hilar adenopathy, and has a good prognosis. Erythema nodosum has a multitude of causes, which are discussed.

11. Segal AM, Mackenzie AH; Hypertrophic osteoarthropathy: A 10-year retrospective analysis. Semin Arthritis Rheum 12:220–232, 1982.
    Describes 16 patients with hypertrophic osteoarthropathy and pulmonary neoplasm. Most had musculoskeletal symptoms before cancer diagnosis. Thickening and furrowing of the scalp, tender distal long bones with periosteal elevation on radiograph, clubbing, and noninflammatory synovial fluid were common features. Twelve of sixteen patients had symmetrical knee and ankle arthritis, but hand involvement was also common. Other disease associations are reviewed.

12. Persellin RH: Acute rheumatic fever: Changing manifestations (editorial). Ann Intern Med 89:1002, 1978.

In adults, carditis, rash, subcutaneous nodules, and chorea are rare and acute rheumatic fever is usually manifested as arthritis alone, most often affecting lower extremity joints and migratory or additive. Bursitis and tendinitis can be prominent.

Soft Tissue Rheumatism

David Felson, M.D.

Soft tissue rheumatism, which includes tendinitis, bursitis, and compression neuropathy, constitutes one of the most common diagnostic problems in outpatient medical practice. Although soft tissue rheumatism affects nonarticular areas, patients often complain of pain in joints. Arthritis can easily be ruled out, however, by a careful physical examination. Most importantly, pain on passive range of motion is present in patients with synovitis but absent in those with bursitis or tendinitis. Pain on active and resisted motion is often present in both nonarticular and articular disease.

The shoulder is a common site of tendinitis and bursitis, which combined cause 90% of shoulder pain.[1,2] With man's evolutionary development of upright posture, the shoulder joint no longer suffers from the trauma of weight bearing, and, with increased shoulder motion, injury affects mainly periarticular structures (Figs. 1 and 2). The rotator cuff tendons, especially the supraspinatus and infraspinatus, along with the biceps tendon are affected most often. The rotator cuff arises from the scapula, inserts in the proximal humerus, and is active in shoulder abduction. It is vulnerable to impingement by the coracoacromial ligament, which lies directly above the humeral head. Strain and compression may lead to degeneration and occasional calcification of the rotator cuff tendons near their insertion on the humeral head.[8] The subacromial bursa lies just above the rotator cuff and separates these tendons from the acromion. Calcium deposited in a tendon may be extruded into the bursa and cause bursal inflammation. Alternatively, tendinitis of one or several of the rotator cuff muscles may occur without an associated bursitis. The biceps tendon, active in arm flexion, may become inflamed separately or can be part of a generalized shoulder periarthritis.

Patients with shoulder tendinitis or bursitis complain of shoulder pain. This pain is worsened by movement of the extremity, frequently radiates down the lateral aspect of the arm, and can cause sleeplessness if the patient awakens when turning onto the affected side. In bursitis, diffuse tenderness may be present on examination, and, unlike tendinitis or bursitis in other

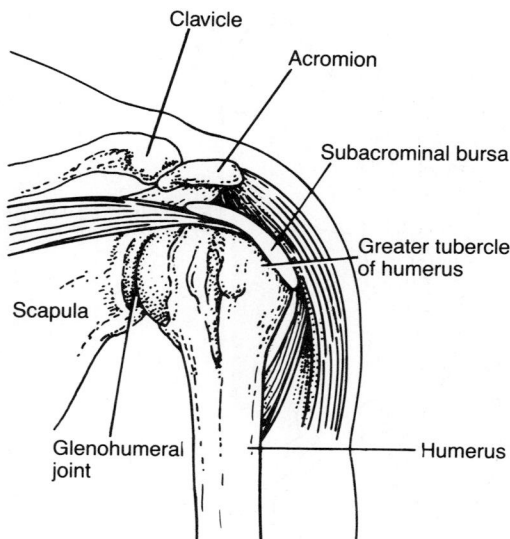

Figure 1. Anterior view of shoulder anatomy. Subacromial bursa lies deep to the deltoid muscle and between the supraspinatus muscle, which inserts on the greater tubercle, and the acromion.

sites, passive movement may be painful. If tendinitis predominates, resisted abduction (supraspinatus) or flexion (biceps) may cause pain.

It is important to identify other causes of shoulder pain. Arthritis of the cervical spine can produce referred pain in the shoulder, with symptoms often localized to the trapezius muscle and worsened by activities requiring neck movement, such as driving a car or looking up. True shoulder joint arthritis causes shoulder pain also, but patients with it often have evidence of systemic arthritis. The presence of fever may indicate a shoulder joint infection. Acute trauma is not usually a precipitant of tendinitis or bursitis, and their occurrence should raise suspicion of a fracture or dislocation. Also diaphragmatic disease, chest pathology, and ischemic heart disease can cause referred shoulder pain.

Therapy for shoulder tendinitis/bursitis consists of salicylates or a non-steroidal anti-inflammatory agent in high dose.[3] Local heat or ice often relieves pain and associated muscle spasm. Regular passive range of motion exercises prevent the development of a frozen shoulder[4] and shoulder-hand syndrome,[10] both of which are especially likely to occur in elderly or diabetic patients. If initial therapy is unsuccessful, a steroid injection at the site of pain may help.[12]

Soft tissue rheumatism also occurs frequently in the elbow region. The olecranon bursa lies between the skin and the olecranon process of the ulna. Repeated minor trauma is the most frequent cause of olecranon bursitis, but other etiologic factors include gout, pseudogout, and infection.[9] Patients with olecranon bursitis complain of pain and swelling in the elbow, but on

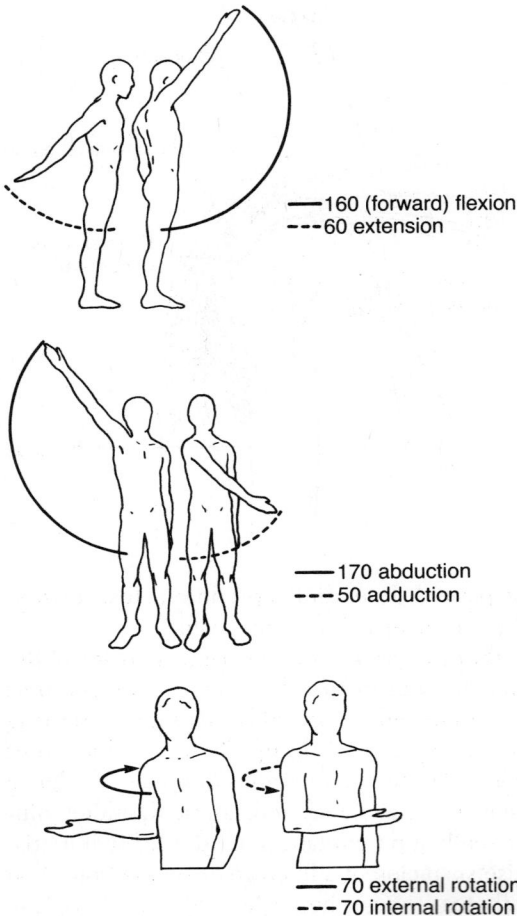

—160 (forward) flexion
---60 extension

Figure 2. Normal range of motion of the shoulder.

—170 abduction
---50 adduction

—70 external rotation
--- 70 internal rotation

examination, elbow motion is normal and usually painless. Even so, there is often dramatic swelling with superficial fluctuance over the olecranon bursa. Aspiration of bursal fluid may reveal crystals or evidence of infection. Traumatic olecranon bursitis can be treated with a protective pad to prevent further trauma.

Lateral epicondylitis, also called tennis elbow, is an inflammation of the conjoined tendons of the hand extensors at their origin, the lateral epicondyle of the humerus. Symptoms include pain in the elbow despite full and painless elbow range of motion. There is tenderness on palpation of the lateral epicondyle, especially if wrist extension is resisted simultaneously. Putting the inflamed area to rest, one of the fundamental precepts of rheumatic disease care, is the mainstay of therapy. The wrist should be splinted, and nonsteroidal anti-inflammatory agents or salicylates are useful as adjunctive therapy. The conjoined tendons of the wrist flexors originate from the medial epicondyle of the humerus, and this can also be the site of tendinitis, the result being medial epicondylitis, or golfer's elbow. Treatment is similar to that for lateral epicondylitis.

Nonarticular rheumatic problems often affect the hand. De Quervain's tenosynovitis consists of inflammation of the tendon sheath covering the two tendons that extend and abduct the thumb. The patient complains of pain over the radial aspect of the wrist, and tenderness is present over the tendon sheath that lies just proximal to the radial styloid. In Finkelstein's maneuver, the examiner stretches the affected tendons and elicits pain by having the patient put his thumb inside a closed fist while forcing the wrist into ulnar deviation. Treatment consists of a hand splint with a thumb post to ensure immobility. The use of nonsteroidal anti-inflammatory agents or salicylates may also be helpful.

A common cause of hand and forearm pain is compression of the median nerve inside the wrist flexor retinaculum, causing carpal tunnel syndrome.[7] Although carpal tunnel syndrome is often idiopathic, hypothyroidism, diabetes, and inflammatory arthritis are possible causes. Patients experience paresthesias and numbness in the region innervated by the median nerve, including the palmar surface of the thumb and digits two, three, and the radial half of the fourth digit. Examination reveals loss of sensation in this distribution. The median nerve also innervates the abductor pollicis brevis, which forms the muscular prominence in the palm proximal to the thumb, and carpal tunnel syndrome can lead to atrophy of this area. Sensory symptoms may be elicited by tapping on the median nerve in the middle of the flexor side of the wrist (Tinel's sign) or by forceably hyperflexing the wrist for up to a minute (Phalen's maneuver). However, these tests may be normal in a large percentage of those with carpal tunnel syndrome. The diagnosis may be confirmed by electromyogram and nerve conduction studies. Initial treatment consists of wrist splinting and nonsteroidal anti-inflammatory agents when inflammation is present. If this is unsuccessful, steroid injection into the carpal tunnel may afford relief. If medical therapy fails, surgery to release pressure in the carpal tunnel may be indicated.

Nonarticular rheumatism also occurs commonly in the lower extremities. Some examples of bursitis include trochanteric bursitis, popliteal cyst swelling (Baker's cyst),[11] and retrocalcaneal bursitis. Tendinitis can occur in the hamstring muscles and the Achilles tendon. Compression neuropathies include meralgia paresthetica, a compression of the lateral femoral cutaneous nerve causing paresthesias in the lateral thigh; peroneal nerve compression, which can cause foot drop; and tarsal tunnel syndrome,[6] which is associated with paresthesias and pain on the bottom of the foot.

Fibromyalgia[5] is a common syndrome in women characterized by chronic generalized aching with evidence on physical examination of multiple tender nonarticular points. Tender sites often cluster in muscular areas of the neck, shoulders, and back. This syndrome may be related to intrusion of alpha waves into stage 4 non-REM sleep producing a sleep disorder that is frequently symptomatic. Low doses of tricyclic antidepressants ameliorate the pain, presumably because of their salutary effect on the sleep disorder.

KEY FEATURES

Shoulder Tendinitis/Bursitis
Tendinitis and bursitis are the most common causes of shoulder pain.

Symptoms
1. Shoulder pain, worsened by activities requiring shoulder movement, including dressing, reaching up to shelves, and combing hair.
2. Pain can radiate down lateral aspect of arm.

Examination
1. Shoulder tenderness can be localized or diffuse.
2. Passive range of motion may be restricted and is often painful, especially abduction and external rotation.
3. Resisted active motion elicits pain if tendinitis/bursitis is present.

Radiographs
1. Shoulder often normal, but flecks of calcium may be present at site of rotator cuff insertions near humeral head.

Treatment
1. Aspirin or nonsteroidal anti-inflammatory agent in high dose.
2. Passive range of motion exercises to preserve range of motion.
3. Heat or ice to relieve pain and muscle spasm.
4. Steroid injection if initial therapy fails.

REFERENCES

1. Cailliet R: Shoulder Pain, 2nd ed. Philadelphia, FA Davis, 1981, p 113.
   This book gives a complete overview of the differential diagnosis of shoulder pain and is especially valuable for its description of rotator cuff disease and drawings of three-dimensional anatomy.

2. Bland JH, et al: The painful shoulder. Semin Arthritis Rheum 7:21, 1977.

Thorough treatise on musculoskeletal shoulder pain with fine diagrams and discussion of physical examination and therapy.

3. Cogen L, et al: Medical management of the painful shoulder. Bull Rheum Dis 32:54, 1982.
    Brief monograph detailing therapeutic alternatives.

4. Rizk TE, Pinals RS: Frozen shoulder. Semin Arthritis Rheum 11:440, 1982.
    A frozen shoulder is one that is severely limited in motion and diffusely painful, even at night. It is often preceded by subacromial bursitis and immobilization and occurs most often in the elderly. Treatment can include anti-inflammatory medicines, steroid injections, and suprascapular nerve block. Range of motion exercises are required to re-establish normal shoulder function.

5. Goldenberg DL: Fibromyalgia syndrome; an emerging but controversial condition. JAMA 257:2782, 1987.
    Symptoms in patients with this common syndrome include diffuse aching and stiffness, fatigue, and sleep disturbance. Seventy to ninety per cent are women, usually between 20 and 50 years old. On examination, multiple tender points are present, but laboratory tests are usually normal. A history of depression is common, although many patients have no psychiatric problems. Low doses of nightly amitriptyline or cyclobenzaprine are effective treatments.

6. Delisa JA, Saeed MA: The tarsal tunnel syndrome. Muscle and Nerve 6:664, 1983.
    This is an uncommon syndrome caused by entrapment of the tibial nerve posterior and inferior to the medial malleolus before it innervates the sole of the foot. Symptoms include paresthesias and pain over the sole, especially after prolonged walking or standing. Definitive diagnosis is made by electromyographic and nerve conduction studies.

7. Gelberman RH, et al: The carpal tunnel syndrome; a study of carpal canal pressures. J Bone Joint Surg 63:380, 1981.
    Carpal canal pressures were elevated in 15 patients with carpal tunnel syndrome, as compared with 12 controls. Pressure increased further with wrist flexion and fell with carpal tunnel surgery.

8. Canoso JJ: Bursae, tendons, and ligaments. Clin Rheum Dis 7:189, 1981.
    Definitive review of embryology, histology, and pathology of soft tissue disease. Location of tendon ruptures depends on the amount and rapidity with which strain is applied.

9. Raddatz DA, Hoffman GS, Franck WA: Septic bursitis: Presentation, treatment and prognosis. J Rheumatol 14:1160, 1987.
    Forty-nine cases of septic bursitis are reported, most in olecranon (63%) or prepatellar (27%) bursae. Common risk factors were skin breakage or repeated trauma, and Staphylococcus aureus was usually (78%) cultured. Bursal fluid cultures were positive in 48 of 49 cases. Fluid leukocyte count was variable, but there was always a predominance of neutrophils. Cellulitis near the bursa and edema of the extremity were common concomitant findings. Parenteral therapy was more often successful than oral therapy (50% relapse rate with the latter), but resolution in all patients took at least several weeks.

10. Kozin F, et al: The reflex sympathetic dystrophy syndrome—I. Clinical and histologic studies: Evidence of bilaterality, response to corticosteroids and articular involvement. Am J Med 60:321, 1976.
    The classic description of this syndrome, also called the shoulder-hand syndrome. It consists of pain and swelling in an extremity associated with trophic skin changes, vasomotor instability, pain in the ipsilateral shoulder, and a precipitating event such as a stroke or myocardial infarction. Eleven patients described had joint synovitis, and although symptoms were unilateral, the contralateral side usually evidenced inflammatory changes also.

11. Wigley RD: Popliteal cysts: Variations on a theme of Baker. Semin Arthritis Rheum 12:1, 1982.

Baker's cysts are fluid accumulations in the gastrocnemius-semimembranous bursa in the medial popliteal space behind the knee. These may cause symptoms by enlargement, dissection, or rupture into the calf, the last problem called pseudothrombophlebitis. Cysts usually communicate with the knee joint. Helpful diagnostic tests include ultrasound and knee arthrography.

12. Petri M, Dobrow R, Neiman R, Whiting-O'Keefe Q, Seaman WE: Randomized, double-blind, placebo-controlled study of the treatment of the painful shoulder. Arthritis Rheum 30:1040, 1987.

One hundred patients with shoulder bursitis/tendinitis with symptoms lasting about 4 months were randomized to placebo or regimens including naproxen or steroid injections. Steroid injections were significantly more effective than placebo or naproxen in ameliorating shoulder pain and were better than placebo on all parameters of improvement. When compared with placebo, naproxen caused improved motion, better function, and an improved clinical index. Patients with limited motion, functional impairment, and severe pain at trial onset did worse regardless of treatment.

Acute Low Back Pain

David Felson, M.D.

At some point in their lives, 70–80% of the population will experience low back pain. Such pain is usually caused by derangement of the muscles, ligaments, joints, or bones of the lower back. Although the disk and its encasing annulus fibrosis are not pain sensitive, contiguous structures such as the posterior longitudinal ligament, dural sheath, facet joints, and paraspinal muscles contain pain fibers.[1,2] Pain often emanates from more than one site. For example, facet joint arthritis with associated synovial swelling may impinge on the adjacent nerve root causing dural irritation, and this may initiate painful localized muscle spasm. In acute musculoskeletal low back pain, it is frequently impossible to pinpoint the specific source of pain. In addition to locally derived symptoms, disorders in the chest, abdomen, and genitourinary tract may cause referred pain in the low back. Infections and tumors of the vertebral bodies and disk spaces may cause back pain as well.

Pain often begins suddenly after lifting, bending over, or doing hard work. Even if nerve root impingement is absent, this pain may be referred into the buttocks or thigh.[3] Characteristically, in disease of the upper lumbar spine, pain is referred to the groin and anterior thigh, whereas lower lumbar involvement is felt in the posterior thigh. Nerve root impingement by an acute disk is often heralded by pain radiating below the knee or by sudden neurologic deficits such as foot drop. Low back pain of musculoskeletal origin is usually relieved by recumbency and exacerbated by sitting or bending over.

Back pain that does not conform to these characteristic symptom patterns or that is associated with symptoms outside the back should raise suspicion of other disease. For example, the simultaneous onset of urinary incontinence or retention with back pain may signify central posterior disk herniation in cauda equina roots, a syndrome that may require quick surgical intervention. Ankylosing spondylitis, an inflammatory arthritis of the spine, causes back pain that usually begins insidiously, is worse in the morning, and is relieved by movement.[6] It most often afflicts young men and is associated with intermittent iritis and peripheral arthritis or tendinitis.[7] Also, in patients with osteomyelitis, septic diskitis, or epidural abscess, fever often accompanies back pain.[4,5] Such infections occur most often in drug addicts or immunocompromised hosts. Finally, patients with malignancies may present initially with low back pain and weight loss; multiple myeloma and metastatic lung and breast or colon cancer are the most common causes.

In acute back pain, physical examination focuses on uncovering evidence of neurologic impairment or disk disease. Many patients with acute pain have muscle spasm, paraspinal tenderness, and pain on passive lumbar flexion, but these findings are not especially helpful diagnostically. A neurologic examination yields clues regarding disk-related nerve impingement. Common disk lesions are at L4–L5 and L5–S1. An L5–S1 disk impinging against the S1 nerve root may cause depression of the ankle reflex and weakness of the gastrocnemius muscle. With an L5 nerve root lesion, the patient often has weakness of ankle and great toe dorsiflexion and hypoesthesia over the dorsum of the foot. An L4 lesion can cause loss of the patellar tendon reflex.

Straight leg raising stretches the ipsilateral sciatic nerve and lumbosacral roots. If the dura mater surrounding these roots is inflamed and irritated by disk impingement, this maneuver will cause pain in the ipsilateral back, buttocks, and lower posterior thigh.[8] If straight leg raising causes pain on the contralateral side, a positive "crossed straight leg raising test," the likelihood of disk disease on the side of the pain is high. The presence of midline back tenderness often indicates an infection or tumor of the spine or a vertebral compression fracture. A careful cardiorespiratory, abdominal, and genitourinary examination, including a rectal examination, should be performed.

For most patients with back pain for the first time, lumbosacral spine radiographs are not indicated.[9] Such x-rays are normal in cases of muscular spasm or ligamentous disease and are usually unrevealing in acute disk disease. Specific radiographic findings such as osteophytes, narrow disk spaces, or spondylolisthesis (anteroposterior slippage of vertebral bodies out of alignment) often do not predict the source of the pain and rarely alter therapy. Finally, lumbosacral radiographs are costly and carry with them the risk of gonadal radiation exposure. Despite these contraindications, back films are needed in the small minority of patients with severe back trauma or falls because of the possibility of transverse process or vertebral body compression fractures. Also, physicians treating patients with back pain and fever need radiographs to evaluate possible vertebral osteomyelitis. In elderly patients with weight loss, radiographs may reveal metastatic disease. In patients with possible ankylosing spondylitis, a single pelvis film to view the sacroiliac joints is indicated. The erythrocyte sedimentation rate (ESR) may be elevated in patients with infection, malignancy, or ankylosing spondylitis. A urinalysis and examination of the stool for occult blood should be performed when indicated.

Therapy of the patient with acute musculoskeletal low back pain should emphasize three points. First and most importantly, the patient needs bed rest. This should be as complete and restricted as possible for at least 2 days,[10] perhaps longer if radicular symptoms or signs are present. After that, the patient may sit up in a supported chair for brief periods and then gradually resume normal activity. Second, as back pain begins to resolve, the patient should start performing William's exercises, especially pelvic tilt and abdominal wall strengthening exercises twice daily (Fig. 1). Exercises strengthen extra-axial postural support and alter the biomechanics of weight bearing in the spine. The third and probably least important aspect of treatment is medication. Analgestic drugs, nonsteroidal anti-inflammatory agents, and muscle relaxants are all effective. Corsets that encompass the whole abdomen from rib cage to pelvis are more effective in chronic recurrent back pain than in acute pain. Heating pads or ice therapy may be useful, especially for patients with prominent paraspinal muscle spasm.

The prognosis for most patients with acute back pain, even those with radiculopathy secondary to disk disease, is excellent. Symptoms usually resolve fully within 1 month, and patients are often completely well in 1–2

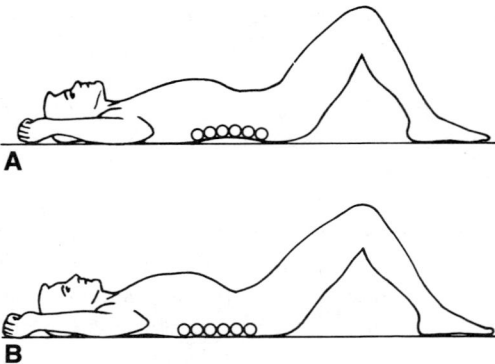

Figure 1. Combined pelvic tilt–abdominal strengthening exercise (William's exercise). A, Normal position. B, With buttocks and abdominal muscles tightened.

weeks.[3] For the approximately 10% of patients who have continuous or recurrent back pain, surgery may be considered.

KEY FEATURES

Symptoms

1. Acute onset after bending, lifting, or physical exertion
2. Pain in lower back and/or buttocks and/or posterior thigh
3. Pain exacerbated by sitting, bending; ameliorated by bed rest

Physical Examination

1. Muscle spasm and paraspinal tenderness characteristic
2. Neurologic abnormalities (foot drop, reflex changes) suggestive of disk disease

Laboratory

1. Lumbosacral spine radiographs not necessary in most patients
2. Blood tests usually normal

Differential Diagnosis

1. Vertebral osteomyelitis or septic diskitis: fever often present; ESR increased; midline spinal tenderness may be present; radiograph often diagnostic
2. Metastatic disease: weight loss may be present; patient usually elderly; radiograph often suggests the diagnosis
3. Ankylosing spondylitis: pain or stiffness worse in the morning, onset insidious, and usually relieved by exercise and motion
4. Referred pain from chest, abdomen, genitourinary tract: patients often have symptoms and signs referable to the organ system involved

Treatment

1. Bed rest for at least 3–5 days
2. William's exercises when pain begins to resolve
3. Heating pad or ice pack for muscle spasm
4. Medication: analgesics, muscle relaxants, nonsteroidal agents all effective

REFERENCES

1. Cailliet R: Low Back Pain Syndrome, 3rd ed. Philadelphia, FA Davis, 1981, p 230.

A thorough, lucid treatise on the causes, findings, and therapies of mechanical low back pain. Emphasizes anatomy and biomechanics of the use of exercises in therapy. Diagrams are outstanding. Cailliet's theory that all mechanical pain is secondary to excessive lordosis is controversial.

2. Macnab I: Backache. Baltimore, Williams and Wilkins, 1977, p 235.
   Fine book by a respected practitioner, including a systemic approach to back pain. Many helpful illustrations.

3. Frymoyer JW: Back pain and sciatica. N Engl J Med 318:219, 1988.
   Good review with clinical approach based on duration of symptoms: 0–6 weeks, acute; 6 weeks–3 months, subacute; ≥ 3 months, chronic. Sciatica that occasionally accompanies low back pain is pain in the distribution of a lumbar nerve root often accompanied by neurologic deficits.

4. Baker AS, et al: Spinal epidural abscess. N Engl J Med 293:463, 1975.
   Twenty of thirty-nine patients had symptoms for less than 2 weeks, and this group often progressed rapidly from back pain to weakness to paraparesis. Staphylococcus was the most common organism. All patients had localized back pain and tenderness.

5. Waldvogel FA, Vasey H: Osteomyelitis: The past decade. N Engl J Med 303:360, 1980.
   Contains excellent review of vertebral osteomyelitis. Patients are usually over age 55; Staphylococcus aureus and Enterobacteriaceae are the most frequent organisms, the latter from urinary tract sources. Posterior extension may lead to cord compression in as many as 18%. Radiographs are first positive at 2–8 weeks, showing piecemeal destruction of vertebral end-plate.

6. Calin A, et al: Clinical history as a screening test for ankylosing spondylitis. JAMA 237:2613, 1977.
   Five questions were found to be 95% sensitive and 76% specific in discriminating patients with ankylosing spondylitis from those with mechanical back pain. These include morning stiffness, insidious onset, improvement with exercise, discomfort for 3 months or more, and age of onset under 40 years.

7. Khan MA, Kushner I: Diagnosis of ankylosing spondylitis. *In* Cohen AS (ed): Progress in Clinical Rheumatology, Vol I. New York, Grune and Stratton, 1984, pp 145–178.
   Fine readable clinical review by prominent investigators in the field. Focuses on differential diagnosis of radiographic abnormalities and atypical presentations, especially common in women and children (often have initial peripheral or cervical symptoms).

8. Hall H: Examination of the patient with low back pain. Bull Rheum Dis 33(4):1, 1983.
   Thorough review of physical examination maneuvers to pinpoint source of pain in those with recurrent or chronic back pain.

9. Deyo RA, Diehl AK: Lumbar spine films in primary care: Current use and effects of selective ordering criteria. J Gen Intern Med 1:20, 1986.
   Spinal radiographs rarely provided useful diagnostic information in those with acute pain. Their yield was highest when they were obtained only in those over age 50 and when there was a history of serious trauma, fever, known cancer, alcohol abuse, steroid therapy, pain at rest, unexplained weight loss, a neuromotor deficit, or a history suggesting ankylosing spondylitis. Oblique projections were rarely helpful (although in chronic or recurrent pain, they may be).

10. Deyo RA, Diehl AK, Rosenthal M: How many days of bedrest for acute low back pain? A randomized clinical trial. N Engl J Med 315:1064, 1986 (see also accompanying editorial on p 1090).
    Two hundred three patients, most with uncomplicated acute low back pain, were

randomized to two or seven days of bed rest. At three weeks and three months of follow-up, outcomes did not differ with respect to pain or functional improvement. Those assigned to the seven-day regimen missed significantly more work, even though most of them failed to comply with the prolonged bed rest regimen. Even those who stayed in bed for five to eight days did no better than those staying in bed for two. In those with uncomplicated acute back pain, a short period of prescribed bed rest may be sufficient to relieve pain and minimize loss of work.

Acute Presentations of Common Rheumatic Disorders

Chad Deal, M.D.

Connective tissue diseases are generally chronic and indolent in nature, but if acute, they may present as medical emergencies. Certain chronic rheumatic diseases may also have clinical features that require immediate intervention. Atlantoaxial subluxation in rheumatoid arthritis (RA) may cause spinal cord compression and myelopathy. Patients with systemic lupus erythematosus (SLE) may present with acute neurologic involvement. Septic arthritis is also a medical emergency and is discussed in a subsequent article.

Cervical myelopathy as a result of RA may present as a medical emergency or be an asymptomatic radiologic abnormality. Atlantoaxial subluxation (AAS), defined as a distance of greater than 3 mm between the arch of the atlas and the odontoid process of the axis with the neck flexed, may cause cord compression and acute neurologic signs. Sudden death from AAS is well described. Most patients with AAS do not have neurologic deficits, and the degree of AAS correlates poorly with the degree of neurologic involvement. Neurologic findings secondary to AAS and cord compression include increased deep tendon reflexes, paresthesias, decreased vibratory sense, motor weakness, and urinary retention. Medical management with a soft cervical collar is frequently used for symptomatic relief but has not been shown to be effective in preventing subluxation or neurologic progression. Surgical management for progressive neurologic impairment involves posterior fusion for stabilization. Reported rates of neurologic improvement after fusion range from 42 to 92%, with a 20–33% rate of nonunion and an 8–20% operative mortality.[1-4]

Patients with *ankylosing spondylitis* may also develop a myelopathy as a result of spinal fractures (often after trivial trauma) that cause spinal cord compression. Fractures are sometimes difficult to visualize on plain radiographs and tomograms are often required. Fractures are usually in the cervical region. Conservative management includes cervical traction and cervical collar. Surgical fusion is reserved for those cases with progressive neurologic involvement despite medical management.[5]

Dorsal tenosynovitis is a frequent manifestation of rheumatoid arthritis and can result in tendon rupture, most commonly of the extensor tendons of the fourth and fifth fingers. Any acute tendon rupture should be treated with urgency, within 1–2 weeks, since single ruptures are often followed by ruptures of other tendons and multiple ruptures are more difficult to treat surgically. Dorsal tenosynovectomy, resection of the distal ulna, and tendon transfer are the treatments of choice.[6]

A Baker's cyst is a communication between the gastrocnemius-semimembranous bursa and the knee joint. These cysts are common in RA and may enlarge, dissect into the calf, or rupture, causing calf pain and swelling that may be difficult to distinguish from thrombophlebitis. Although a ruptured Baker's cyst is not a medical emergency, it may predispose the patient to secondary thrombophlebitis and coexistence of phlebitis and Baker's cyst has been reported. The most important initial goal of treatment is to differentiate phlebitis from cyst rupture. Often the clinician will elect to perform a venogram prior to an arthrogram to rule out phlebitis. Treatment is then directed at reducing inflammation in the joint by arthrocentesis and synovial fluid removal, injection of steroids into the joint (after checking for infection), oral anti-inflammatory agents, and bed rest.[7,8]

SLE may present with acute manifestations that require prompt intervention. Pulmonary hemorrhage and pericardial effusions large enough to cause tamponade may occur and require immediate treatment. Cytopenias, thrombocytopenia, and neutropenia may cause bleeding or infection and may require prompt treatment. Central nervous system (CNS) manifestations of SLE include seizures, strokes, hemiplegias, and acute organic brain syndromes, all occurring in the setting of active SLE. CNS infections must be ruled out by lumbar puncture. Spinal fluid pleocytosis is often present even without infection, and may require antibiotic coverage until cultures are negative. High doses of corticosteroid therapy, although not shown to be clearly effective, are used in acute cerebritis.[9,10] Vasculitis in SLE may cause acute renal failure or rapidly progressive glomerulonephritis and an active urine sediment. Vasculitis of the celiac vessels may cause perforation of the bowel and present as a surgical emergency. Mesenteric vasculitis without perforation may be difficult to distinguish from serositis, which is common in SLE. High doses of steroids are used for vasculitic complications of SLE.[11] Central nervous system vasculitis in SLE may present with focal findings. Angiograms should be considered in these patients, since cytotoxic drugs may be required.

Renal disease in systemic sclerosis may present acutely with malignant hypertension and rapidly progressive renal failure. This syndrome is associated with high renin levels. Captopril, an angiotensin-converting enzyme inhibitor, has been used to control the blood pressure with some success, as have other antihypertensive agents.[12] Other connective tissue diseases, such as SLE and Wegener's granulomatosis, may present with rapidly progressive renal failure, which requires immediate diagnosis and treatment.

Temporal arteritis may present as an acute medical and ophthalmologic emergency. Blindness as a consequence of ophthalmic arteritis is usually preceded by local signs and symptoms of arteritis such as headache, temporal artery tenderness, and jaw claudication. Once blindness ensues, it is usually irreversible and without treatment may progress to involve the contralateral side. Any patient with clinical signs or symptoms of temporal arteritis should have a temporal artery biopsy and will require immediate treatment with high-dose corticosteroids.[13] A number of patients with temporal arteritis may present with polymyalgia rheumatica (PMR). Thus, PMR patients without localized symptoms should carefully followed.

Polymyositis may present with such extensive involvement of muscles that respiratory function is compromised and ventilatory support is required. Severe cardiac muscle involvement may cause arrhythmias or congestive heart failure. Treatment includes high doses of steroids or immunosuppressive agents.[14]

KEY FEATURES

A. Cervical myelopathy
  1. Rheumatoid arthritis
    a. Atlantoaxial subluxation (AAS) commonly present on radiographs, occasionally symptomatic (sudden death, long tract signs).
    b. Treatment with soft cervical collar for symptomatic relief, cervical fusion for progressive neuropathy.
  2. Ankylosing spondylitis
    a. Myelopathy after fracture, usually cervical spine, often after minor trauma.
B. Dorsal tenosynovitis
  1. Causes tendon rupture, most commonly of fourth and fifth extensor tendons. Early tenosynovectomy essential to prevent further ruptures and for good surgical outcome.
C. Baker's cyst
  1. Enlarged gastrocnemius-semimembranous bursa. May dissect or rupture into the calf and present as thrombosis or predispose patient to thrombosis. Venogram and arthrogram are useful in this setting. Treatment is directed at reducing inflammation.
D. Systemic lupus erythematosus (SLE)
  1. Neurologic sequalae include seizures, strokes, hemiplegias, and

acute organic brain syndrome. Must rule out infection with spinal tap. Treatment with high-dose steroids.
2. Vasculitis may cause acute renal failure or rapidly progressive glomerulonephritis. Celiac involvement may present as an acute abdomen. Vasculitis of acral parts may cause infarction and gangrene. Treatment with high-dose steroids.
  E. Systemic sclerosis
1. Malignant hypertension and renal failure occur and are treated with aggressive antihypertensive therapy (captopril is useful).
  F. Temporal arteritis
1. Blindness may arise from vasculitis of ophthalmic artery. If signs of local arteritis are present (headache, jaw claudication), treatment should be instituted immediately, and temporal artery biopsy scheduled.
  G. Polymyositis
1. Muscle weakness may be so severe as to compromise respiratory function, or may cause cardiac failure or arrhythmias.

REFERENCES

1. Mikulowski P, Willheim FA, Rotmil P, Olsen I: Sudden death in rheumatoid arthritis with atlanto-axial dislocation. Acta Med Scan 198:445–451, 1975.
    Autopsy of 11 patients with severe atlantoaxial dislocation. Sudden death occurred in 7 patients. Neurologic signs correlated poorly with risk of fatal atlantoaxial dislocation. Cord compression was found at autopsy in all 11 cases.

2. Lipson SJ: Rheumatoid arthritis of the cervical spine. Clin Orth Rel Res 182:143–149, 1984.
    Anterior atlantoaxial subluxation (AAS) was the most common subluxation and was found in 11–46% of autopsy studies of RA patients. The primary indication for surgical intervention is neurologic abnormality; preoperative skeletal traction is used. Posterior fusion is most commonly performed with neurologic improvement in 42–92%, nonunion in 20–33%, and operative mortality in 8–20%.

3. Stevens JC, Cartlidge NEF, Saunders M, Appleby A, Hall M, Shaw DA: Atlanto-axial subluxation and cervical myelopathy in rheumatoid arthritis. Quart J Med 40:391–408, 1971.
    Excellent review of atlantoaxial joint anatomy and the pathology of atlantoaxial subluxation (AAS). Incidence of AAS in RA is 19–35%. AAS was more common in severe, seropositive RA, occurred as early as 3 years after onset of disease, and correlated poorly with neck symptoms and signs. Twenty-four of 36 patients with AAS had pyramidal tract signs.

4. Breedveld FC, Algra PR, Vielroye CJ, et al: Magnetic resonance imaging in the evaluation of patients with rheumatoid arthritis and subluxations of the cervical spine. Arthritis Rheum 30:624–630, 1987.
    A review of 21 patients divided into groups based on presence of myelopathic signs. MRI was as good as myelography for assessing cord distortions. No correlation was found between vertebral dislocation on plain x-rays and the presence of cord distortion on MRI.

5. Hunter T, Dubo HIC: Spinal fractures complicating ankylosing spondylitis—a long term follow-up study. Arthritis Rheum 26:751–759, 1983.
    Twenty patients with ankylosing spondylitis and spinal fractures were studied; 14 were diagnosed immediately. Nine of 14 fractures occurred after minor falls; 3 patients

died within five days. Nine patients were followed long term. All were treated with cervical traction and collar. Three patients had complete cord lesions, six had incomplete lesions. All nine fractures obtained bone union. No patient had progressive neurologic deficit. Three patients with complete cord lesions had no recovery, three with incomplete cord lesions made major recoveries, and three died of unrelated causes. Spinal epidural hematoma is a complication of fracture and of surgical fusion. Surgical fusion is reserved for patients with progressive neurologic defects.

6. Millender LH, Nalebuff EA: Preventative surgery tenosynovectomy and synovectomy. Orth Clin North Am 6:765–792, 1975.

    Reviews indications for tenosynovectomy prior to tendon rupture as well as surgical technique. Extensor tendon ruptures are most common, usually involving the fourth and fifth finger tendons as they pass over a subluxed ulna. Extensor lag may be minimal if a single tendon is ruptured. Double and triple tendon ruptures are more difficult to treat with tendon transfers.

7. Katz RSM, Zizic TM, Arnold P, Stevens MB: The pseudothrombophlebitis syndrome. Medicine 56:151–164, 1977.

    Of 62 patients with Baker's cysts, 34 had signs and symptoms that were phlebitis-like. Thirty-one patients had inflammatory arthritis, and three patients had a noninflammatory disorder. Thirty-one had a knee effusion, only 16 had a palpable popliteal mass, 14 had a positive Homans sign, and no patient had a palpable cord. Eighteen of 34 cysts had dissected by arthrogram; 7 were intact, 5 had ruptured, and 4 had dissected and ruptured.

8. Gordon GV, Edell S, Brogadir SP, et al: Baker's cyst and true thrombophlebitis: Report of two cases and a review of the literature. Arch Intern Med 139:40–42, 1979.

    Two cases of simultaneous ruptured Baker's cyst and thrombophlebitis. In addition, five other cases had venograms that showed compression of the popliteal vein. The authors do not advocate venogram in all cases but emphasize the need for a venogram if there is doubt concerning diagnosis.

9. Adelman DC, Saltiel E, Klinenberg JR: The neuropsychiatric manifestations of systemic lupus erythematosus: An overview. Semin Arthritis Rheum 15:185–199, 1986.

    A literature review of CNS-SLE, including clinical, pathologic, diagnostic, and treatment modalities.

10. Feinglass EJ, Arnett FC, Dorsch CA, et al: Neuropsychiatric manifestations of systemic lupus erythematosus: Diagnosis, clinical spectrum and relationship to other features of the disease. Medicine 55:323–339, 1976.

    Thirty-seven per cent of patients (52 of 140) had CNS disease, 17 had seizures, 16 had long tract signs, 10 had cranial nerve abnormalities, 5 had cerebellar signs, 1 had a meningitis picture, and 2 had papilledema. Eighty-five per cent of neurologic events occurred in a setting of active disease. Spinal fluid was abnormal in 14 (32%), with increased protein in 6, increased protein and WBC in 4, and increased WBC alone in 1. Vasculitis and thrombocytopenia correlated with CNS disease activity.

11. Zizic TM, Shulman LE, Stevens MB: Colonic perforation in systemic lupus erythematosus. Medicine 54:411–426, 1975.

    Five colonic perforations are reviewed from the authors' series of 107 patients with SLE. Mesenteric arteritis was the cause and always occurred in the setting of active SLE. Abdominal syndrome was characterized by insidious onset of intermittent, colicky lower abdominal pain. Rebound tenderness was variable and late. Four of 5 patients died.

12. Traub YB, Shapiro AP, Rodnan GB, et al: Hypertension and renal failure (scleroderma renal crisis) in progressive systemic sclerosis—review of a 25 year experience with 68 cases. Medicine 62:335–352, 1983.

Renal crisis was characterized by abrupt onset of hypertension, grade 3–4 retinopathy, increased plasma renin concentrations, and rapid deterioration in renal function. Mortality rate prior to 1971 was 100% at one year. Aggressive management of blood pressure, especially using captopril, renal dialysis and nephrectomy, in selected anuric patients has improved prognosis dramatically.

13. Goodman BW: Temporal arteritis. Am J Med 67:839–852, 1979.
    Blindness in various series ranged from 7 to 60%. Most patients have definite indications of their arteritis for months prior to blindness. Visual symptoms such as blurred vision, amaurosis fugax, and diplopia may precede blindness. Blindness is usually irreversible and without treatment may involve the contralateral eye in a short time.

14. Bohan A, Peter JB, Bowman RL, Pearson CM: A computer assisted analysis of 153 patients with polymyositis and dermatomyositis. Medicine 56:255–286, 1977.
    Good general review of the subject. Approximately 1% of patients died of cardiovascular involvement (high-grade block, heart failure, arrhythmias). One per cent died of severe muscle weakness (respiratory failure). Treatment with steroids or steroids plus methotrexate for resistant cases is advocated.

Anaphylaxis

Chad Deal, M.D.

Anaphylaxis is a true allergic emergency. The term anaphylaxis is usually reserved for a systemic syndrome that occurs soon after exposure to an agent and is mediated by an immunologic mechanism (IgE). Anaphylactoid reactions may have a similar constellation of signs and symptoms (and treatment modalities), but an immunologic basis has not been conclusively demonstrated (non–IgE-mediated events such as radiocontrast or aspirin reactions).[1]

The organ manifestations of anaphylaxis are as follows: skin—erythema, pruritus, urticaria, and angioedema; gastrointestinal—pain, vomiting, and diarrhea; cardiovascular—hypotension; and respiratory—bronchospasm and laryngeal edema. No specific pattern of anaphylaxis occurs in humans, and any combination of organ system manifestations may occur. Rarely a patient may present with only cardiovascular collapse or bronchospasm.[2–4]

A large number of agents have been reported to cause anaphylaxis, and they are broadly divided into three categories: proteins—antitoxins, food, venoms, and chymopapain; polysaccharides—dextran; and haptens—penicillin. Antibiotics, especially penicillin, and venoms are the leading causes of death from anaphylaxis.[5,6]

The pathophysiologic mechanism of anaphylaxis is an antigen-IgE interaction that triggers mast cells and basophils to release vasoactive substances such as histamine and leukotrienes. A number of substances and physical stimuli have the capability of causing release of mediators from mast cells on a non-IgE basis, including activated complement components, IgG, immune complexes, radiocontrast materials, dextran, and exercise.[7,8] Aspirin and other nonsteroidal anti-inflammatory agents are postulated to cause ana-phylactoid reactions by inhibition of cyclo-oxygenase and resultant shunting of arachidonic acid metabolism to the lipoxygenase pathway.[9] So-called id-iopathic anaphylaxis refers to anaphylaxis of unknown cause with no iden-tifiable agent provoking attacks.[10]

The clinical evaluation of a person with anaphylaxis should proceed quickly. The cause of the anaphylactic reaction and its route of administration should be determined. The tempo of progression of the attack may aid in predicting severity. Cardiovascular and respiratory systems should be as-sessed and blood pressure and ventilation maintained. If the offending agent entered an extremity, a tourniquet may be applied to occlude venous and lymphatic return. Pressure should be released for 30 seconds every 3 minutes to ensure adequate circulation. Aqueous epinephrine, 1:1000 dilution, 0.1–0.2 ml should be injected into the site to impede absorption of the agent, along with 0.2–0.4 ml subcutaneously. If shock is present, 1 ml of epinephrine, 1:10,000 dilution, can be given slowly intravenously. Because the half-life of epinephrine is short, doses may need to be repeated every 15 minutes. Diphenhydramine, 50 mg orally, intramuscularly (IM), or in-travenously (IV), can be given but should not be the sole agent used in anaphylaxis. Because laryngeal edema is a potentially fatal complication, endotracheal intubation may be necessary. If there is any doubt about the cause of laryngeal obstruction, direct visualization of the airway is indicated to rule out foreign body, tumor, and so forth. Oxygen is an adjunct if res-piratory complications are present, and fluid administration with normal saline is employed if hypotension occurs. If bronchospasm does not respond to epinephrine, IV aminophylline should be administered in standard doses. Steroids are not indicated for acute treatment of anaphylaxis because their onset of action is 4–6 hours, but they may be effective for delayed mani-festations.

If a causative agent can be identified, subsequent exposure should be avoided. In the case of anaphylaxis to venoms or inhaled allergens, immu-notherapy (after appropriate skin testing) with weekly injection of specific allergens is effective in preventing recurrence of anaphylaxis.[11] If radiocon-trast dyes have caused an anaphylactoid episode in the past and a dye study is required, prednisone 50 mg PO q6h for three doses plus diphenhydramine (Benadryl) 50 mg IM 30 minutes prior to the procedure, reduces but does not eliminate the risk of recurrence.[12] A sizable fraction (10%) of hospitalized patients claim allergy to penicillin. If a patient with a history of anaphylaxis to penicillin is skin test negative to both major and minor determinants, the chance of an acute allergic reaction to pencillin is 2%.[13] If penicillin must be given to a patient at risk for anaphylaxis, rapid desensitization can be accomplished by oral, intradermal, or IV routes in 4–6 hours.[14] In cases when no agent can be identified to cause the anaphylactic episode, skin testing may be appropriate.

KEY FEATURES

Definition and Pathophysiology

1. A systemic syndrome with multiple organ system manifestations, including: skin—urticaria, angioedema; pulmonary—bronchospasm; cardiovascular—hypotension; and gastrointestinal—vomiting, pain, diarrhea

2. IgE mediated

3. Anaphylactoid reactions non–IgE-mediated (dyes, aspirin, complement, dextran, exercise)

Therapy

1. Ascertain cause and location of entry

2. Use tourniquet plus local epinephrine if on extremity

3. Aqueous epinephrine 1:1000, 0.2–0.5 ml SC; repeat every 15 min as necessary. 1:10,000, 1 ml IV may be given if shock ensues

4. Protect airway and tissue perfusion

5. Diphenhydramine 50 mg PO, IM, or IV

6. IV fluids with normal saline

6. Steroids for late manifestations

Prophylaxis

1. Avoidance

2. Immunotherapy for venoms or inhaled allergens

3. Prednisone 50 mg PO q6h for three doses, plus Benadryl 50 mg IM 30 minutes prior to dye procedure

4. Rapid desentization for penicillin if indicated

REFERENCES

1. Patterson R, Valentine M: Anaphylaxis and related allergic emergencies including reactions due to insect stings. *In* Primer of Allergic and Immunologic Disease. JAMA 248:2637–2645, 1982.
   Review of the most common agents causing anaphylaxis, clinical manifestations of anaphylaxis, and treatment modalities.

2. Delage C, Irey NS: Anaphylactic deaths: A clinicopathologic study of 43 cases. J Forensic Sci 17:525–540, 1972.
   Classic study of 43 cases of fatal anaphylaxis. Penicillin, radiographic dyes, and local anesthetics caused all but two of the reactions. Eighty-four per cent of the patients received the offending agent parenterally. Eighty-six per cent had anaphylaxis within 20 minutes after exposure. Most patients had multi-organ manifestations, but a few had only a single manifestation. Respiratory failure and circulatory failure were the most common causes of death.

3. Smith PL, Kagey-Sobotka A, Bleeck ER, et al: Physiologic manifestations of human anaphylaxis. J Clin Invest 66:1072–1080, 1980.
   Report of 14 patients who had systemic reactions after venom challenge, three with hypotension. None of these three patients had bronchospasm or cutaneous lesions. Histamine levels were elevated in 60% of sting patients without correlation to cutaneous manifestations; one of three patients with hypotension had values similar to those of other, nonhypotensive patients. Patients with hypotension had low Factor VIII and fibrinogen, consistent with intravascular coagulation. Two of three patients with hypotension responded poorly to epinephrine.

4. James LP, Austen KF: Fatal systemic anaphylaxis in man. N Engl J Med 270:597–603, 1964.
   Report of six patients with fatal anaphylaxis at autopsy. Respiratory system failure was cause for death in all but one. One patient had a normal respiratory tree and died from cardiovascular collapse.

5. Austen KF: The anaphylactic syndrome. In Samter M (ed): Immunologic Disease. Boston, Little, Brown, 1978, pp 885–899.
   Textbook review article of anaphylaxis, including pathophysiology, etiologic agents, and treatment.

6. Sheffer AL: Anaphylaxis. J Allergy Clin Immunol 75:227–233, 1985.
   A review article of anaphylaxis.

7. Sheffer AL, Austen KF: Exercise-induced anaphylaxis. J Allergy Clin Immunol 66:106–111, 1980.
   Characterizes a syndrome in 16 patients of exertion-related pruritus, urticaria, asthma, and hypotension. The syndrome did not occur with each exercise experience and might have been made worse by eating prior to exercise. A family history of atopy was present in 11 of 16, but the patients were skin test negative to usual allergens.

8. Liberman P, Siele RL, Taylor WW: Anaphylactoid reactions to iodinated contrast material. J Allergy Clin Immunol 62:174–180, 1978.
   Reviews the pathogenesis of anaphylactoid reactions to dyes. Dyes cause histamine release in vivo and in vitro, although to a lesser extent than do pollens. Depletion of cellular histamine has also been demonstrated.

9. Patterson R, Anderson J: Allergic reaction to drugs and biologic agents. In Primer of Allergic and Immunologic Disease. JAMA 248:2637–2645, 1982.
   Excellent review of drug allergies, including aspirin, insulin, dyes, local anesthetics, and penicillin. Includes desensitization schedules for penicillin and insulin. Also covers the immunologic basis for drug allergy.

10. Sonin, L, Grammer LC, Greenberger PA, Patterson R: Idiopathic anaphylaxis: A clinical summary. Ann Intern Med 99:634–635, 1983.
    Studies on a group of 50 patients with an anaphylactic syndrome for which no cause could be identified. All patients had urticaria or angioedema; 66% had bronchospasm, hypotension, or GI symptoms. Thirty-four per cent had upper airway obstruction alone.

Twenty-five of 28 patients tested had positive skin tests, none to foods. Seventeen patients required alternate-day steroids to control their symptoms.

11. Lochtenstein LM, Valentine MD, Sobotha AK: Insect allergy: The state of the art. J Allergy Clin Immunol 64:5–12, 1979.

    This review covers the scientific background for venom in diagnosis and therapy. Diagnosis of insect allergy is based on history and skin test. The dose of venom used for skin testing is critical, since there is a narrow range between diagnostic and nonspecific irritant reactions. Indications for treatment are a history of severe systemic reaction and a positive skin test. Venom immunotherapy results in better than 95% rate of success. Duration of treatment is years.

12. Greenberger PA, Patterson R, Simon R, et al: Pretreatment of high risk patients requiring radiographic contrast media studies. J Allergy Clin Immunol 67:185–187, 1981.

    The risk of anaphylactoid reactions to dyes in patients with prior reaction is 17–35%. Prednisone 50 mg for three doses q6h with the final dose 1 hour prior to procedure, in addition to 50 mg of Benadryl with the last dose, reduces the risk of serious reaction to less than 1%.

13. Green GR, Rosenblum AH, Sweet LC: Evaluation of penicillin hypersensitivity: Value of clinical history and skin testing with penicillin-polylysine (PPL) and pencillin G (PenG). J Allergy Clin Immunol 60:339–345, 1977.

    A multicenter cooperative study of almost 3000 patients to study skin testing for penicillin hypersensitivity. Nineteen per cent of patients with a history of penicillin allergy had positive skin tests to PPL or PenG, vs. 7% with no history of penicillin allergy. If a history of anaphylaxis was present, 14% had positive skin tests. Three per cent of skin test negative patients challenged with penicillin had reactions, vs. 67% of skin test positive patients.

14. DeSwarte RD: Drug allergy. *In* Patterson R (ed): Allergic Diseases: Diagnosis and Management. Philadelphia, JB Lippincott, 1985, pp 609–614.

    Details rapid desensitization techniques for pencillin allergic patients in 5–6 hours. These can be performed parenterally or orally. Up to 20% of patients experience reactions, but these are usually mild. Full desensitization and treatment can usually be accomplished.

Angioedema

Chad Deal, M.D.

Hereditary angioedema (HAE) is an inherited, autosomal dominant disorder characterized by episodic swelling of the extremities, face, abdominal viscera, or airway. The most common presenting sign of illness is swelling of an extremity (75% of cases). The duration of edema is usually 1–3 days (range 4 hours to 7 days). One half of patients have their onset before age 7 years, two thirds before age 13, but onset after age 50 has been reported. A significant minority of patients will have oropharyngeal involvement at some time. Airway involvement may result in complete obstruction and is associated with significant mortality.[1]

Trauma is identified as a precipitating event in more than 50% of patients. Dental or oropharyngeal manipulation is the most common cause of airway edema necessitating tracheostomy. Occasionally an attack will begin peripherally and extend centrally to involve the airway. Airway obstruction often begins slowly, with voice changes and dysphagia preceding complete obstruction.

The biochemical abnormality responsible for development of angioedema is either absence or a low level of C1 esterase inhibitor (C1-INH), in 85% of cases; or normal levels of a functionally deficient C1-INH, in 15% of cases. C1-INH deficiency may be acquired, usually in association with a lymphoproliferative disorder such as lymphoma or leukemia. C1-INH is an inhibitor of the first component of the complement cascade. In addition, it also inhibits effector pathways of clotting, kinin formation, and fibrinolysis.[2] Laboratory confirmation of the diagnosis of HAE requires specific assays of proteins involved in the complement system. Direct measurement of C1-INH can be performed immunochemically and will be 0–50% of normal in the 85% of patients with the common form of HAE. In the remaining 15% of patients (with the variant form), who have normal levels of a functionally deficient C1-INH, a functional assay must be performed. C4 and C2, the substrates of C1 esterase, are always low during an attack and are often low between attacks. C3 and CH50 are usually normal during attacks. C1 levels are normal in HAE but low in acquired angioedema. A positive family history is helpful in making the diagnosis but was absent in 7 of 30 cases in one series.[1,11,12]

Treatment of HAE is directed toward prevention of attacks. Treatment of an acute attack is often unsatisfactory. Patients often do not respond to epinephrine, antihistamines, or steroids, although these agents should be tried in patients with oropharyngeal involvement. Antifibrinolytic and hormonal agents are of no use during an acute attack. Administration of fresh-frozen plasma (FFP) is controversial because it provides not only C1-INH but also more substrate for C1 esterase.[3] Partially purified C1-INH is effective in terminating acute attacks of HAE but is not generally available.[4] Because mortality from HAE results from airway obstruction, tracheostomy can be life saving. Factors associated with an increased risk of airway obstruction include rapid progression, an attack that begins in the oropharynx, a history of a dental or oropharyngeal procedure as a precipitating event, and the presence of dysphonia or dysphasia.

In patients whose attacks of angioedema are frequent and severe, prophylactic therapy is indicated. Two types of drugs have been used. Antifibrinolytic agents, such as epsilon-aminocaproic acid (Amicar), can prevent attacks by reducing the activity of vasoactive substances of the kinin and fibrinolytic pathways but can cause rhabdomyolysis and thrombosis.[5] Androgen derivatives such as methyltestosterone, oxymetholone, danazol, and stanozolol can also prevent attacks.[6] These agents cause an increase in the concentration of C1-INH in the serum. It is not necessary to raise the C1-INH levels to normal to prevent attacks. The lowest dose that halts attacks should be the goal. These drugs also have significant side effects, including virilization in women, neuromuscular dysfunction, hematuria, liver toxicity, and decreased spermatogenesis in men.[7-10] Stanozolol has the advantage of being 10–20 times less expensive than danazol. The dosage range for stanozolol is 0.5–6.0 mg/day, whereas for danazol the dose is 200–800 mg/day. The smallest dose effective in preventing attacks is determined by adjusting the dose downward at 8–12 week intervals. If elective surgery is planned, the stanozolol is increased to 4 mg q6h five days prior to surgery. If emergency surgery is required, the dose is increased and 2 U of FFP are administered preoperatively. Although stanozolol does not abort an acute attack, the dose is also raised to 4 mg q6h until the attack subsides and is then decreased in a slow, step-wise fashion.[10]

KEY FEATURES

A. Autosomal dominant inheritance
B. Seventy-five per cent of patients present with swelling of an extremity
C. Onset after age 50 years is rare; two thirds of patients present prior to age 13 years
D. Biochemical defect is an absolute or functional deficiency of the normal inhibitor of the first component of complement (C1 esterase inhibitor [C1-INH])
E. Prophylaxis:
    1. Antifibrinolytic agents (epsilon-aminocaproic acid), which reduce the activity of vasoactive substances
    2. Androgen derivatives raise the serum concentration of C1-INH
F. Treatment of an established attack is difficult and of variable efficacy:
    1. Epinephrine, antihistamines, steroids may ameliorate oropharyngeal involvement
    2. Use of fresh-frozen plasma (FFP) is controversial
    3. Antifibrinolytic and hormonal agents are of no use during the acute attack
    4. Tracheal intubation and/or tracheostomy may be life saving

REFERENCES

1. Frank MM, Gelfand JA, Atkinson JP: Hereditary angioedema: The clinical syndrome and its management. Ann Intern Med 84:580–593, 1976.
   Classic reference based on the NIH experience with 30 patients with HAE. Reviews the clinical syndrome, pathophysiology, laboratory diagnosis, differential diagnosis, and therapy.

2. Schapira M, Silver LD, Scott CF, et al: Prekallikrein activation and high-molecular-weight kininogen consumption in hereditary angioedema. N Engl J Med 308:1050–1053, 1983.
   Demonstrates the importance of C1-INH in the contact phase of coagulation by studying kallikrein; prekallikrein (PK); high molecular weight kininogen (HMWK); and Factors IX, XI, and XII in three patients with HAE. PK and HMWK decrease during attacks and tend to be normal between episodes. Factor XII is postulated to be the central factor for inducing attacks of HAE.

3. Pickering RJ, Good RA, Kelly JR, Gewurz H: Replacement therapy in hereditary angioedema: Successful treatment of two patients with fresh frozen plasma. Lancet 1:326–330, 1969.
   Results of fresh-frozen plasma infusion in two patients with HAE, both of whom had a dramatic and rapid response. Potential objections to the use of plasma infusions include exacerbation of the attack by providing C2 and C4 as well as the risk of hepatitis.

4. Gadek JE, Hosea SW, Gelfand JA, et al: Replacement therapy in hereditary angioedema: Successful treatment of acute episodes of angioedema with partially purified C1 inhibitor. N Engl J Med 302:542–546, 1980.
   Use of partially purified C1-INH in a non–double-blind, non-placebo study. Infusion of C1-INH in three asymptomatic patients with HAE resulted in increased C1-INH activity as well as increased C4 activity. Five patients received infusions during attacks; all had a 6-hour lag time between infusion and improvement.

5. Blohmé G: Treatment of hereditary angioneurotic edema with tranexamic acid: A random double-blind cross-over study. Acta Med Scand 192:293–298, 1972.
   Five patients with HAE were treated with epsilon-aminocaproic acid derivative in a random double-blind cross-over trial. Three of the five improved with treatment. One patient developed extensive muscle necrosis on therapy. Thrombosis is a potential complication.

6. Abramowicz M (ed): Danazol and other androgens for hereditary angioedema. Med Letter 23:83–84, 1981.
   Concise review of drug therapy for HAE.

7. Gelfand JA, Sherine RJ, Alling DW, Frank MM: Treatment of hereditary angioedema with danazol: Reversal of clinical and biochemical abnormalities. N Engl J Med 295:1444–1448, 1976.
   Nine patients with HAE were treated in a double-blind, placebo-controlled study. Of 47 placebo courses, 44 ended with attacks; during 46 danazol courses only 1 attack occurred. Side effects were minimal. C1-INH and C4 levels increased dramatically, beginning on day 1, reaching a peak at 1–2 weeks.

8. Hosea SW, Santaella ML, Brown EJ, et al: Long-term therapy of hereditary angioedema with danazol. Ann Intern Med 93:809–812, 1980.
   Report on 69 patients with HAE treated for 1–6 years with danazol. All patients

responded with a decrease in frequency and severity of attacks. Side effects were frequent and included the following:

Weight gain: 38%	*Elevated muscle enzymes: 14%*
Menometrorrhagia: 34%	*Hematuria: 13%*
Myalgias: 28%	*Hot flashes: 12%*
Headaches: 22%	*Voice deepening: 10%*
Alopecia: 17%	*Hirsutism: 8%*
Anxiety: 16%	*Heme: 8%*
Amenorrhea: 16%	*Dizziness: 6%*
Altered libido: 14%	*Nausea: 4%*

Side effects could be minimized by titrating the dose downward to lowest possible levels that achieved control of attacks.

9. Sheffer AL, Fearon OT, Austen RF: Clinical and biochemcial effects of stanozolol therapy for hereditary angioedema. J Allergy Clin Immunol 68:181–187, 1981.
   Twenty-seven patients with HAE were treated with stanozolol, an attenuated androgen, for 2 years. Stanozolol effectively controlled attacks in doses as low as 0.5 mg/day with minimal side effects. Twenty patients had side effects that were similar to those caused by danazol but that did not require interruption of therapy.

10. Mathews KP: Urticaria and angioedema. J Allergy Clin Immunol 72:1–14, 1983.
    Good review of urticaria, with section on HAE. Summarizes the treatment of HAE.

11. Stoppa-Lyonnet D, Tosi M, Laurent J, et al: Altered C1 inhibitor genes in hereditary angioedema. N Engl J Med 317:1–6, 1987.
    A study of a multigeneration family with HAE that demonstrates and identifies a defective structural gene arising from DNA rearrangements, which might allow for early diagnosis using a DNA probe.

12. Gelfand JA, Boss GR, Conley CL, et al: Acquired C1 esterase inhibitor deficiency and angioedema: A review. Medicine 58:321–328, 1979.
    An excellent review of acquired C1-INH deficiency. Ten of 15 cases were lymphoproliferative disorders; three were associated with autoimmune disorders (SLE, hemolytic anemia).

Crystal-Induced Arthritis

David Felson, M.D.

GOUT

Gout is a common cause of acute monarticular or oligoarticular arthritis in middle-aged and elderly men as well as in postmenopausal women. An acute attack occurs when synovial fluid is supersaturated with uric acid, which precipitates as crystals, inciting an inflammatory response.[1,7] Patients generally have accumulated excess stores of urate, often reflected in high serum uric acid levels. Uric acid undergoes a complex excretion process in the kidney that consists of glomerular filtration, tubular secretion, and tubular reabsorption. Patients who are underexcretors have inherited abnormalities of renal tubular transport, whereas overproducers have increased nucleic acid turnover. Drugs that cause gout, including thiazide and loop diuretics and ethambutol, do so by altering renal tubular secretion or reabsorption, thereby increasing urate body pools. Alcohol may cause hyperuricemia by increasing purine production.

Uric acid solubility decreases in lower temperatures; therefore, the cooler joints in the body (feet and ankles) are the joints most often affected by gout. With weight bearing, the great toe is subjected to tremendous trauma, which can dislodge crystals from cartilage. With subsequent recumbency, water leaves the joint space and synovial fluid becomes supersaturated with urate, precipitating a gouty attack.

Gouty arthritis usually has a rapid onset with initial attacks affecting the great toe (podagra) in more than 50% of patients. Other causes of great toe arthritis include pseudogout, trauma, metatarsalgia (especially in women who wear high-heeled shoes), Reiter's syndrome, and psoriatic arthritis (for these last two, the interphalangeal joint is frequently involved). Many patients have first attacks in large lower extremity joints, and 3%–14% have an initial polyarticular attack.[4] Diuretic use or excessive intake of alcohol[6] are frequent predisposing factors.

The acute attack may be accompanied by malaise, low-grade fever, and leukocytosis, especially in patients with polyarticular disease. In addition to the first metatarsophalangeal (MTP), joints involved, in descending order, include insteps of feet (intercuboidal joints), ankles, heels, knees, and upper extremity joints. A group of adjacent joints is often inflamed simultaneously (especially forefoot, heel, and ankle), and a gouty soft tissue inflammation mimicking infection may appear. Eventually tophi may accumulate at body sites of low temperature, including olecranon processes, pretibial surfaces, Achilles tendons, and the pinnae of the ear.

The diagnosis of gout is confirmed only when uric acid crystals, which are needle shaped and negatively birefringent, are seen in synovial fluid by polarizing microscopy. Serum uric acid concentration is often, but not always, elevated in a gouty attack.

Several different medications can be used to treat acute gout.[2] The traditional therapy is colchicine 0.5-mg tablets every hour up to a total dose of 6.0 mg, a regimen that often causes diarrhea and abdominal pain. Colchicine in a dose of 1–2 mg administered over 20 minutes can be given intravenously, a method occasionally used in hospitalized patients. Although it has little gastrointestinal toxicity, intravenous colchicine can cause a severe chemical phlebitis and should be used only in patients with good hepatic and renal function, because its accumulation is toxic to bone marrow.[10]

Indomethacin is an effective drug in treating acute gout; 50 mg is given three or four times daily with food. It should not be used in patients with peptic ulcer disease or in those with chronic congestive heart failure who are on diuretics. Other nonsteroidal anti-inflammatory drugs, including naproxen, piroxicam, tolmetin, and ibuprofen, are effective as well.

Relative joint immobilization, including avoidance of weight bearing, should be prescribed, or drug therapy may be unsuccessful as a result of repeated joint trauma. Pain and inflammation should lessen within 24–48 hours, at which point the medication can be withdrawn slowly.

Patients with gout are, in general, not at increased risk of renal insufficiency; therefore, long-term therapy is unnecessary after one attack.[3,5] The first attack is followed in 62% of patients by a period of less than 1 year before the next one, although a small minority of patients never have a recurrence. If attacks recur frequently, maintenance colchicine can be prescribed. Taken regularly, colchicine, 0.5 mg one to three times daily, can prevent gouty attacks.

A urate-lowering drug should also be given to those patients with repeated attacks. If, as is usually the case, the patient's 24-hour urine uric acid excretion is less than 1 gm (600 mg if on a purine-free diet), the patient is a hypoexcretor and can be treated with an agent that increases urine urate excretion. There are two such drugs, probenecid and sulfinpyrazone, both of which are safe and inexpensive.

For overproducers, allopurinol lowers serum uric acid by inhibiting xanthine oxidase, which acts in nucleic acid metabolism to decrease uric acid production, causing the urate precursor xanthine to accumulate. Allopurinol occasionally can cause hepatitis, Stevens-Johnson syndrome, and irreversible bone marrow suppression, especially in elderly patients.

PSEUDOGOUT

Although pseudogout was so named because it was felt to mimic acute gout, extensive clinical experience has revealed that pseudogout has a broad range of clinical manifestations.[8,9] Pseudogout is caused by the synovial fluid deposition of calcium pyrophosphate dihydrate (CPPD) crystals, which incite an inflammatory response. These crystals are formed and reside in articular cartilage and are shed into the synovial fluid when trauma occurs. Factors that cause crystal formation and thus predispose the patient to pseudogout attacks include osteoarthritis, gout, hyperparathyroidism, hemochromatosis, hypothyroidism, ochronosis, hypophosphatasia, hypomagnesemia, and Wilson's disease.

Clinical pseudogout is predominantly a disease of the elderly, with symptoms varying from acute and monarticular to chronic, smoldering, and polyarticular disease. The knee joint is most often affected, but pseudogout can involve shoulders, ankles, and wrists. The diagnosis is made by identifying CPPD crystals in synovial fluid. These crystals, unlike urate, are positively birefringent and rhomboid shaped. Radiographs frequently show associated cartilage calcification, known as chondrocalcinosis, which is most often seen in knees and wrists. Although the presence of chondrocalcinosis in helpful diagnostically, its association with clinical pseudogout is not absolute.

Nonsteroidal agents are the preferred therapy for acute pseudogout. Other alternatives include intra-articular steroids, joint aspiration with removal of all joint fluid, and intravenous colchicine. Arthrocentesis alone is occasionally therapeutic.

Another calcium crystal that may be a cause of inflammatory arthritis is calcium hydroxyapatite.[11] A common cause of tendinitis, hydroxyapatite is not visible by light microscopy but seems to be present in a large percentage of elderly patients with osteoarthritis-related synovial effusions. Whether it is a cause of inflammation remains to be determined.

KEY FEATURES

Gout
A. Prevalence
   1. Common in middle-aged and elderly men and postmenopausal women.
B. Symptoms and Signs
   1. Sudden onset of pain and swelling in lower extremity joint(s).
   2. Onset is often post-traumatic or postoperative.
   3. Patients taking diuretics or with history of alcohol overindulgence are predisposed to gout.
   4. Great toe most often involved; other joints include forefoot, heel, ankle, knee.
   5. Interval between attacks (intercritical period) is symptom-free.
C. Laboratory
   1. Definitely diagnosed only by demonstration of urate crystals (needle-like, with negative birefringence) in synovial fluid.
   2. Serum uric acid concentration usually elevated.
D. Therapy
   1. Medication
      a. PO colchicine 0.5 mg hourly until better (up to 6.0 mg); often causes diarrhea, abdominal cramping.
      b. IV colchicine 1–2 mg given over 20 minutes—can cause bone marrow toxicity if impaired renal or hepatic function present.

    c. PO indomethacin 50 mg tid or qid taken with food. Effective but contraindicated in ulcer disease patients or in patients with congestive heart failure on diuretics.

    d. Other nonsteroidal anti-inflammatory agents are effective.

Pseudogout

A. Common in the elderly. Several rare metabolic diseases may cause it.

B. Clinical symptoms variable. May be acute or chronic.

C. Usually affects knee. May occur in other joints.

D. Diagnosed definitely by finding calcium pyrophosphate dihydrate (CPPD) crystals in synovial fluid (parallelopiped-shaped with weakly positive birefringence).

E. Associated with chondrocalcinosis.

F. Effectively treated with nonsteroidal agents; occasionally arthrocentesis itself is therapeutic, especially if all fluid is removed.

REFERENCES

1. Kelley WN, Fox IH: Gout and related disorders of purine metabolism. *In* Kelley WN, Harris ED Jr, Ruddy S, Sledge CB (eds): Textbook of Rheumatology, 2nd ed. Philadelphia, WB Saunders Co, 1985, pp 1359–1397.
   Comprehensive review of pathogenesis, clinical presentation, and therapy with extensive discussion of renal complications of hyperuricemia.

2. Simkin PA: Management of gout. Ann Intern Med 90:812, 1979.
   Fine review of therapy for acute and chronic gout.

3. Liang MH, Fries JF: Asymptomatic hyperuricemia: The case for conservative management. Ann Intern Med 88:666, 1978.
   Classic paper arguing, using all available evidence, that the risks of hyperuricemia are small or unknown and that therapy should in most cases be eschewed.

4. Hadler NM, Franck WA, Bress NM, Robinson DR: Acute polyarticular gout. Am J Med 56:715, 1974.
   Retrospective review of patients with polyarticular gout. Fever is common, joint involvement is usually in lower extremities and asymmetrical, and patients are usually elderly.

5. Campion EW, Glynn RJ, Delabry LO: Asymptomatic hyperuricemia: Risks and consequences in the Normative Aging Study. Am J Med 82:421, 1987.
   In this study, 2046 healthy men had serum urates measured and were followed for 14.5 years. Of those with a serum urate level ≥ 9 mg/dl, the annual incidence of gout was 4.9% compared with 0.5% per year for those with values of 7.0–8.9 mg/dl. Those with high initial urate levels had no increased risk of renal deterioration.

6. Hall JT, Ball GV: Saturnine gout: A review of 42 patients. Semin Arth Rheum 11:307, 1982.
   Review of 42 patients with gout and plumbism secondary to moonshine exposure; 34 eventually developed impaired renal function. Gout involved knees in 83% of patients and wrists in 48%. Polyarticular attacks occurred in 36%.

7. Boss GR, Seegmiller JE: Hyperuricemia and gout. N Engl J Med 300:1459, 1979.

Review of pathogenesis and therapy of gout. Discussion of renal involvement and vascular disease relationship with uric acid may overly stress the risks of hyperuricemia.

8. McCarty DJ: Arthritis associated with crystals containing calcium. Med Clin North Am 70:437, 1986.
   Review of calcium pyrophosphate dihydrate (CPPD) and basic calcium phosphate (calcium hydroxyapatite) and how these crystals may cause arthritis. Spectrum of clinical disease is also discussed.

9. Doherty M: Pyrophosphate arthropathy—recent clinical advances. Ann Rheum Dis 42(suppl):38, 1983.
   Summary of fairly recent studies. Osteoarthritis and aging are the most frequent association. Elderly women may be more prone to chronic polyarticular disease, with younger men getting acute episodic monarthritis.

10. Wallace SL, Singer JZ: Review: Systemic toxicity associated with intravenous administration of colchicine—guidelines for use. J Rheumatol 15:495, 1988.
    Of nine published cases of pancytopenia or leukopenia associated with bone marrow suppression caused by colchicine, most were in elderly patients given both intravenous and oral colchicine during an attack. Authors present guidelines for use: 2–3 mg single dose with no more than 4–5 mg total dose during an attack: reduced dose if renal or hepatic disease is present or in the elderly.

11. Schumacher HR, Smolyo AP, Tse RL, Maurer K: Arthritis associated with apatite crystals. Ann Intern Med 87:411, 1977.
    Using electron microscopy, authors identified needle-shaped hydroxyapatite crystals in 11 patients, 4 with otherwise unexplained acute arthritis, 3 with degenerative joint disease exacerbation, 1 with acute arthritis while on dialysis and 3 with apatite crystals superimposed on other rheumatic diseases. Intrasynovial hydroxyapatite injections induced acute arthritis in dogs.

Septic Arthritis

Chad Deal, M.D.

Acute bacterial arthritis requires early recognition and aggressive treatment in order to prevent joint destruction and permanent disability. The clinical features of gonococcal arthritis are sufficiently unique to require separate consideration.[11] Tuberculous arthritis and fungal arthritis are rare and more insidious and are not discussed in this article.

NONGONOCOCCAL SEPTIC ARTHRITIS

Many patients who develop nongonococcal joint sepsis have predisposing factors such as altered host resistance or previous joint damage. Host factors contributing to an increased risk of infection include immunocompromise as a result of immunosuppressive therapy or any other cause. Patients with joint damage induced by previous trauma or rheumatoid arthritis constitute a high-risk group, as do intravenous (IV) drug abusers and patients with prosthetic joints.[1,2]

The majority of patients are infected by hematogenous spread, but direct inoculation and local extension from an adjacent infection are also possible causes. The patient with septic arthritis typically presents with the rapid onset of a warm, swollen, tender joint that is painful with active and passive motion. Most cases are monarticular and involve weight-bearing joints, but any joint may be affected and polyarticular involvement is well described.

If infection is suspected, an arthrocentesis must be performed immediately and the synovial fluid (SF) should be gram stained and sent for culture (both aerobic and anaerobic) and glucose as well as analyzed for white blood cells (with differential count), crystals, mucin clot, and viscosity. Gram's stain will be positive on a spun sediment in only 50–75% of cases, but cultures will almost always be positive unless the patient has previously taken antibiotics. The typical SF will have more than 50,000 white blood cells (WBCs) with 90% or more polymorphonuclear leukocytes (PMNs), but lower WBC counts are possible and PMNs may be less than 90%. SF glucose is usually more than 40 mg% lower than simultaneous serum glucose in a fasting patient. Although any organism may cause nongonococcal septic arthritis, *Staphylococcus aureus*, streptococcal species, and gram negative bacilli are most often recovered in adults. Neonates have a higher incidence of *Haemophilus influenzae* arthritis.[3,4]

Because most cases of septic arthritis are hematogenously spread, a primary souce of infection should be sought. Blood cultures, in addition to culture of any possible infected site, should be obtained prior to initiation of antibiotic therapy. Fever, peripheral blood leukocytosis, and elevated erythrocyte sedimentation rate are usually present but are not specific. The therapy for nongonococcal septic arthritis consists of antibiotic treatment, often initially intravenous, and removal of purulent effusion by drainage. Antibiotics are chosen on the basis of information obtained from Gram's stain and culture of SF and from evidence for infection elsewhere. If infection is suspected but no organism has been identified, empirical, broad-spectrum coverage should be initiated with moderate to high doses of an antistaphylococcal penicillin and an aminoglycoside until cultures return.[1,5] In children 6 months to 2 years of age when *H. influenzae* is likely, a beta-lactamase–resistant penicillin plus either ampicillin or chloramphenicol should be used. A significant amount of literature has accumulated recommending the use of broad-spectrum cephalosporins as empiric treatment of septic arthritis in any age group. Second-, third-, and fourth-generation cephalosporins have been shown to provide effective coverage. The latest antibiotic proved to be an excellent monotherapy agent is imipenem-cilastatin sodium.[10] Most clinicians treat with intravenous antibiotics for 2–4 weeks. Adequate drainage should be accomplished by either repeated closed needle aspiration or open surgical drainage. Circumstances that would necessitate open surgical drainage (or arthroscopic drainage) include: joints that are difficult to drain adequately by needle aspiration, such as shoulder or hip, or evidence that closed drainage may not be adequate, such as failure to sterilize the joint; continued high WBC count; rapid reaccumulation of fluid or loculation; and inability to remove the synovial fluid.

The most important factor in predicting outcome is rapidity of diagnosis and treatment. Patients whose diagnosis and treatment are delayed are more likely to have irreversible joint damage and permanent disability.

GONOCOCCAL ARTHRITIS

Disseminated gonococcal arthritis (DGI) is, in some medical centers, the most common form of septic arthritis. The epidemiologic and clinical features as well as treatment and prognosis differ in a number of important aspects from nongonococcal septic arthritis.

The majority of patients with DGI are women (70–80%), usually under 30 years of age, often developing disease during pregnancy or menses. Typical musculoskeletal manifestations include migratory polyarthralgias, tenosynovitis, suppurative arthritis, and skin lesions.[6]

Patients with DGI can be separated into two groups, based on the presence or absence of suppurative arthritis. Those patients with suppurative arthritis will almost never have a positive blood culture, whereas patients without suppurative arthritis will have tenosynovitis and skin lesions more frequently. These differences do not simply represent sequential stages of the same disease process, but rather they may be determined by host factors or characteristics of the infecting organism.[6]

Polyarthralgias are the most common presenting symptom in both groups. Presenting signs in patients without suppurative arthritis include fever and chills, tenosynovitis, and skin lesions. These same signs occur but in lower frequency in the suppurative arthritis group. A minority of patients in either group, perhaps 30%, will have signs or symptoms of urethritis or pelvic inflammatory disease.[7,8]

Cultures of SF, urethra and cervix, rectum, pharynx, blood, and skin should be obtained in all patients suspected of having DGI. SF cultures are positive in less than 50% of patients with suppurative arthritis, and Gram's stain of SF reveals gram negative diplococci even less frequently. Cultures of urethra and cervix will be positive in 75% of cases; blood cultures are positive in less than 25%; and skin, rectum, and pharynx cultures are positive in only 5–20% of cases. Because *Neisseria gonorrhoeae* is a fastidious organism, cultures must be plated immediately in 5–10% CO_2 atmosphere.

Cultures from areas normally inhabited by other bacteria should be plated on Thayer-Martin medium to inhibit growth of indigenous organisms. Cultures from normally sterile areas, such as SF and blood, should be plated on chocolate agar.

Treatment is often started based on clinical suspicion, since *N. gonorrhoeae* is usually not seen on Gram's stain and often not cultured. Current treatment recommendations for gonorrhea reflect the emergence of tetracycline-resistant strains and the increasing prevalence of penicillin-resistant strains. Ceftriaxone is highly effective against penicillin-resistant strains. The recommended dose is 1 gm IV daily for 7 days.[9] Alternative treatment is with aqueous penicillin G 10 million U IV daily for 3 days followed by amoxicillin 500 mg orally four times per day for 4 days. (Note: coexisting Chlamydia is not treated with ceftriaxone.) The response to treatment is often dramatic, with clinical improvement noted after the first day of treatment. Alternative outpatient treatment regimens for DGI have been published: oral ampicillin 3.5 gm initially, followed by 500 mg four times per day for 7 days. However, hospitalization is advised for unreliable patients, those with uncertain diagnoses, and those with suppurative arthritis.[8,9]

KEY FEATURES

I. Nongonococcal septic arthritis
   A. Predisposing factors
      1. Altered host resistance; chronic disease, immunosuppressed patients
      2. Previous joint damage; rheumatoid arthritis, prior surgery
   B. Route of infection
      1. Usually hematogenous
      2. Occasionally direct penetration or spread from adjacent infection
   C. Clinical signs
      1. Usually monarticular pain, swelling, warmth, redness
      2. Other areas with infection
   D. Organism
      1. *Staphylococcus aureus,* streptococcal species, gram negative bacilli most common
      2. Any organism possible
   E. Diagnosis
      1. Culture and Gram's stain of synovial fluid (SF)
      2. SF usually with WBC >50,000, 90% PMNs; SF glucose 40 mg/dl less than blood glucose
   F. Treatment
      1. IV antibiotics 2–4 weeks
      2. Penicillinase resistant pencillin 8–12 gm/day for staphylo-

cocci; aqueous penicillin G 8–12 million U/day for streptococci; aminoglycoside for gram negative organisms; penicillin plus aminoglycoside if organism unknown

   3. Adequate drainage; repeat needle aspiration, surgical drainage for hip, shoulder, or failure to drain adequately by needle
aspiration

II. Gonococcal arthritis

  A. Predisposing factors

    a. Women, pregnant or at time of menses

  B. Route of infection

    1. Usually GU, but also pharynx, rectum

    2. GU symptoms in only 30%

  C. Clinical signs: two groups

    1. Suppurative arthritis, negative blood cultures

    2. Nonsuppurative arthritis or arthralgias, positive blood cul-
tures, tenosynovitis, skin lesions

  D. Organism

    1. *Neisseria gonorrhoeae*

  E. Diagnosis

    1. Culture of blood, SF, pharynx, rectum, skin

    2. Use Thayer-Martin medium (except SF and blood—use choc-
olate agar)

    3. Often treat without specific organism based on clinical sus-
picion

  F. Treatment

    1. IV ceftriaxone 1 gm daily × 7 days

    2. Alternative treatment: IV aqueous penicillin G 10 million U
daily × 3 days, followed by amoxicillin 500 mg orally ×
4 days

    3. Alternative outpatient treatment: oral ampicillin 3.5 gm, fol-
lowed by 500 mg qid × 7 days (not recommended if patient
unreliable, if suppurative arthritis, or if uncertain diagnosis)

REFERENCES

1. Goldenberg DL, Cohen AS: Acute infectious arthritis: A review of patients with nongonococcal joint infections (with emphasis on therapy and prognosis). Am J Med 60:369,
377, 1976.

   *A review of 59 adults with acute nongonococcal septic arthritis. Reviews types of
organisms, predisposing factors, serial synovial fluid analysis, prognostic factors, and
treatment.*

2. Rosenthal J, Bole GG, Robinson WD: Acute non-gonococcal infectious arthritis: Evalaution
of risk factors, therapy and outcome. Arthritis Rheum 23:889–897, 1980.

   *A review of 63 patients (all ages) with nongonococcal joint infections. Staphylococcus
aureus was most common (59%), followed by gram negative (37%) and anaerobic (13%)
organisms. Eleven patients with prosthetic joints required removal of prostheses. About
10% required open surgical drainage after failed closed needle aspirations. Treatment
outcome and factors influencing outcome are also detailed.*

3. Nelson JD, Koontz WC: Septic arthritis in infants and children: A review of 117 cases.
Pediatrics 38:966–971, 1966.

Review of 117 children with septic arthritis. Most common organisms, in descending order, were S. aureus, H. influenzae, N. gonorrhoeae, and gram negatives. Under 6 months of age, Staphylococcus and gram negative organisms were most common; in children 6–24 months, H. influenzae was predominant.

4. Goldenberg DL, Brandt KD, Cathcart ES, Cohen AS: Acute arthritis caused by gram negative bacilli: A clinical characterization. Medicine 53:197–208, 1974.

   Thirteen cases caused by gram negative organisms are reviewed: E. coli (5), Proteus mirabilis (4), Salmonella (2), Pseudomonas (1), and E. coli plus serositis (1). Outcome was felt to be poorer than with gram positive arthritis.

5. Goldenberg DL, Brandt KD, Cohen AS, Cathcart ES: Treatment of septic arthritis. Arthritis Rheum 18:83–90, 1975.

   Fifty-nine patients with bacterial arthritis are reviewed. Predisposing factors included extra-articular infections, underlying illness, prior antibiotic therapy, immunosuppressive drugs, and prior arthritis in the affected joint.

6. O'Brien JP, Goldenberg DL, Rice PA: Disseminated gonococcal infection: A prospective analysis of 49 patients and a review of pathophysiology and immune mechanism. Medicine 62:395–406, 1983.

   Study of 49 cases of disseminated gonococcal infection. The following features were seen:

Groups	Polyarthritis	GU Signs	Tenosynovitis	Skin Lesions	+ Blood Cultures
Suppurative arthritis	68%	32%	21%	42%	0%
Nonsuppurative arthritis	60%	23%	87%	90%	43%

7. Brogadir SP, Schimmer BM, Myers AR: Spectrum of gonococcal arthritis-dermatitis syndrome. Semin Arthritis Rheum 8:177–183, 1979.

   Review of 104 patients with gonococcal arthritis-dermatitis syndrome. Includes useful data on presenting signs and symptoms, joint distribution, distribution of tenosynovitis, frequency, and sites of positive cultures.

8. Handsfield HH, Weisner PJ, Holmes KK: Treatment of the gonococcal arthritis-dermatitis syndrome. Ann Intern Med 84:661–667. 1976.

   Prospective study of 98 patients with gonococcal arthritis-dermatitis syndrome, treated with IV penicillin G, low or high dose; IV cephalosporins; oral ampicillin; or tetracycline. The response to treatment was equally rapid and complete in each group.

9. The Medical Letter on Drugs and Therapeutics: Treatment of Sexually Transmitted Diseases 30:5–10, 1988.

   Treatment recommendations for N. gonorrhoeae.

10. Sakurai M: Effect of imipenem-cilastatin sodium in thirty cases of bone and joint infection. J Antibiot 39:1947–1959, 1986.

    Review of use of imipenem-cilastatin in septic arthritis.

11. Goldenberg DL, Reed JI: Bacterial arthritis. N Engl J Med 312:764–771, 1985.

    Review of pathophysiology, diagnostic evaluation, and treatment of gonococcal and nongonococcal septic arthritis.

SECTION 10
SELECTED TOXICOLOGIC EMERGENCIES

Tricyclic Antidepressants

David Schwartz, M.D.

Tricyclic antidepressants (TCA) have become a major source of suicide attempts in adults. These compounds, which are analogues of phenothiazines, exert varying degrees of anticholinergic and adrenergic effects, peripheral alpha blockade, and quinidine-like membrane stabilization. One must understand the metabolism and pathophysiology to recognize and intervene effectively in this common clinical problem.[1,2]

In therapeutic doses, tricyclics are rapidly absorbed, distributed, and bound to body tissue. In the overdose situation, decreased peristalsis and gastric dilatation result in a delayed absorption. Once absorbed, most of these drugs are either rapidly bound to plasma proteins or stored in tissue (10–40 times the concentration in plasma). Less than 15% of the plasma concentration remains unbound (i.e., chemically active). Plasma protein binding is very much affected by pH, with decreases in pH of 0.8 units resulting in 8-fold increases in unbound chemically active drug (the inverse is also true). The drug is primarily metabolized by the hepatic microsomal system, but up to 15% of the drug may be excreted by both the gastric mucosa and the biliary tract. Urinary excretion is minimal. Owing to the delayed absorption, excessive tissue binding, variable plasma protein binding, and hepatic microsomal activity, the half-life of tricyclics in the overdosed patient may vary from 25 to 80 hours.

The clinical presentation is most clearly characterized by peripheral anticholinergic effects, CNS toxicity, and cardiovascular toxicity.[1,2,4] Within 4 hours of ingestion, a patient begins to manifest peripheral anticholinergic effects with fever, mydriasis, flushing of skin, urinary retention, and diminished peristalsis. CNS complications are mediated via central anticholinergic actions and most commonly include confusion, agitation, and hallucinations, but severely intoxicated patients may develop generalized seizure activity

625

or even become comatose. The neurologic examination may reveal hyper-reflexia with clonus and extrapyramidal signs, including nystagmus, ataxia, and dysarthria. The cardiovascular effects, mediated by a combination of anticholinergic, adrenergic, peripheral alpha blocking, and quinidine-like membrane stabilizing actions, provide a sensitive measure of tricyclic toxicity and account for most of the 5–10% mortality rate associated with this over-dose. Within 4 hours of ingestion, patients may be tachycardiac and mildly hypertensive, but as the peripheral alpha blocking actions and membrane stabilizing effects bcome active, a full 50% of patients may become hypo-tensive. Increased adrenergic tone may predispose patients to ventricular ectopy, but conduction blocks (AV blocks, QRS lengthening, and QT pro-longation), caused by the membrane stabilizing action of tricyclics, may depress cardiac output, cause complete AV block, or predispose patients to ventricular tachycardia.[1,3,5]

Decisions to hospitalize, observe, and therapeutically intervene should be based on clinical manifestations rather than on absolute serum tricyclic levels. Both the excessive degree of tissue binding and the marked effect of serum pH in altering the amount of chemically active drug diminish the predictive value of the serum tricyclic level. One should suspect the diagnosis in the overdosed patient who presents with an altered mental status, pe-ripheral anticholinergic signs (mydriasis, skin flushing, and urinary reten-tion), or an unexplained tachycardia. Patients with one of these signs should be hospitalized and observed for at least 24 hours. In a complex case in which tricyclic levels are not available to confirm the diagnosis, physostig-mine may be used to inhibit acetylcholinesterase. This will temporarily reverse the central and peripheral anticholinergic effects of tricyclics and will confirm an anticholinergic poisoning. Owing to the increased seizure activity associated with physostigmine, one should reserve this diagnostic test for the unusual situation (tricyclic levels are not available, immediate confirmation of diagnosis would alter other therapeutic options, or more information is needed from patient) and physostigmine should never be used therapeutically.

As with all overdoses, one must treat supportively and limit absorption of drug from the gut. Charcoal administration, orally or through a nasogastric tube, is the mainstay of therapy in this regard. Gastric lavage may be helpful early after ingestion. This should be followed by repetitive doses of charcoal and cathartics, which not only may serve to clear unabsorbed drug but also may increase excretion by taking advantage of enterohepatic recycling and gastric secretion.

CNS complications should not be treated with physostigmine. Seizure activity usually responds to IV diazepam, but patients may occasionally re-quire phenytoin and/or phenobarbital for adequate control. Myoclonic jerks can be bothersome but are best treated conservatively or, if necessary, with small doses of diazepam. Coma is best managed supportively with ICU nursing and early intubation.

The early cardiovascular effects (tachycardia and mild hypertension) do not require therapy. All of the other cardiovascular complications (hypotension, AV block, QRS/QT prolongation, and ventricular ectopy) should first be treated with crystalloid infusion and sodium bicarbonate or hyperventilation to increase the serum pH to at least 7.5.[1] This will rapidly decrease the amount of unbound active drug available and should reverse these complications. If this is unsuccessful, symptomatic conduction blocks must be treated with temporary pacing, hypotension should be treated with vasopressors (dopamine or norepinephrine bitartrate [Levophed]), and ventricular irritability should respond to antiarrhythmics (lidocaine or phenytoin) or cardioversion/defibrillation. Quinidine, procainamide, and disopyramide should be avoided, since they may worsen the conduction block or further depress myocardial contractility.[3,5]

Patients who have had their stomachs emptied and have normal cardiograms 6–8 hours after ingestion need not be hospitalized for medical indications. On the other hand, those with symptoms or signs must be hospitalized for at least 24 hours. Once asymptomatic for 24 hours, these patients may be discharged.

KEY FEATURES

TRICYCLIC OVERDOSE: SIGNS, PATHOPHYSIOLOGY AND THERAPEUTIC OPTIONS

Signs	Peripheral Anticholinergic	Central Anticholinergic	Adrenergic	Membrane Stabilizing	Therapeutic Options
Altered mental status		+			Supportive
Seizures		+			Diazepam/ phenytoin/phenobarbital
Tachycardia	+		+		None necessary
Hypertension			+		None necessary
Hypotension				+	Crystalloid infusion/ alkalinization/vasopressors
Conduction blocks				+	Alkalinization/ electrical pacing
Ventricular ectopy			+	+	Alkalinization/lidocaine/ phenytoin/cardioversion

REFERENCES

1. Frommer DA, Kulig KW, Marx JA, Rumack B: Tricyclic antidepressant overdose—a review. JAMA 257:521, 1987.
    Excellent review of epidemiology, pharmacology, clinical features, and management of TCA overdose.

2. Shine D: Tricyclic antidepressant. Clin Toxiciol Rev 2 (1): 1979.
    Brief but complete review of tricyclic overdoses.

3. Langon A, Van Dyke C, Tahan SR, Cohen L: Cardiovascular manifestations of tricyclic antidepressant overdoses. Am Heart J 100:458, 1980.
    Thirty-five cases of tricyclic overdoses were reported, with particular emphasis on the cardiovascular manifestations. Levels greater than 1000 mg/ml correlated with significant QRS prolongation. Sinus tachycardia was seen in 70% of patients and proved to be a reliable early sign of toxicity. Hypotension was seen in 50% of patients and was most often associated with depressed myocardial contractility but sometimes was caused by

*intravascular depletion. No malignant arrhythmias were seen, and ventricular ectopy
responded to alkalinization or lidocaine. Normal ECGs were seen in only 20% of all
patients.*

4. Langon RA: Overdose with tricyclic antidepressants. Western J Med 137:422, 1982.
    *Reviews the indications for admission and therapeutic options for the CNS and car-
    diovascular complications.*

5. Marshall JB, Forker AD: Cardiovascular effects of tricyclic antidepressant drugs: Thera-
    peutic usage, overdose, and management of complications. Am Heart J 103:401, 1982.
    *Good discussion of pathophysiology of overdose. Stresses QRS prolongation as marker
    of severe potential toxicity.*

Acetaminophen Poisoning

William Hale, M.D.

The antipyretic, analgesic drug acetaminophen is a major component
in over 200 prescription and nonprescription products. In recommended
doses, it has few side effects and is remarkably free of drug interactions.
However, the incidence of acetaminophen poisoning appears to be increasing
in the United States and although death is quite unusual, significant toxicity
occurs frequently.

In therapeutic doses, acetaminophen is rapidly absorbed and peak
plasma levels are reached in 30–60 minutes. It is primarily metabolized by
hepatic conjugation with glucuronide or sulfate and excreted via the kidneys.
Minor amounts are excreted unchanged or as mercaptopuric acid metabolites
following cytochrome P-450– mediated conjugation with hepatic glutathione.
Plasma half-life is between 1 and 3 hours.[1,2] After an acute overdose, the
glucuronide and sulfate pathways become saturated, resulting in an increased
fraction of acetaminophen metabolism by the P-450 system. The reactive
metabolites thus formed are converted to mercaptopuric acid until glutathione stores are depleted and then bind to hepatocyte macromolecules,
resulting in cell necrosis. Serious hepatotoxicity has been reported following
the ingestion of 7 gm in adults (150 mg/kg in children), and adult fatalities
have occurred with overdoses of 13 gm.[2]

The clinical course of acute acetaminophen overdose follows a consistent
pattern. Early manifestations occur 2–6 hours after ingestion and include
nausea, vomiting, diaphoresis, and lethargy. These are nonspecific findings
and are not predictive of hepatic toxicity. Recovery is rapid, and the patient
appears well in 24 hours.[2] If, however, a hepatotoxic dose was ingested,
biochemical evidence of liver damage will be apparent within 24–48 hours.

The SGOT and SGPT levels may reach several thousand units, with somewhat smaller increases in serum alkaline phosphatase. Early and severe coagulation disturbances may occur with only modest hyperbilirubinemia. Physical manifestations at this time include right-sided abdominal pain and mild hepatomegaly without splenomegaly. Histologic examination reveals centrilobular necrosis without fatty infiltration and a mild inflammatory reaction. Death as a result of fulminant hepatic necrosis is rare and occurs 4–18 days after drug ingestion.[1,2,5] Myocardial necrosis, hemorrhagic pancreatitis, and acute renal tubular necrosis have also been reported following severe overdosage.[3,7]

Management of acetaminophen overdose involves general supportive care, removal of unabsorbed drug with gastric lavage, and specific therapy with acetylcysteine (Mucomyst); the use of ipecac is not recommended because it delays the patient's ability to take and tolerate acetylcysteine. Charcoal hemoperfusion, hemodialysis, and fluid loading do not prevent or ameliorate toxicity.[6]

An oral loading dose of actylcysteine (140 mg/kg) should be given soon after admission when acetaminophen ingestion is suspected. If a blood acetaminophen level (drawn at least 4 hours after ingestion to ensure peak levels) indicates potential toxicity, 17 additional doses (70 mg/kg) should be administered at 4-hour intervals. Activated charcoal and magnesium cathartics should not be given unless another life-threatening intoxicant has been coingested, as absorption of the antidote will be impaired. If charcoal has been given, administration of acetylcysteine should be delayed 1–2 hours and the stomach lavaged until clear. A review of 662 consecutive cases of acetaminophen overdosage treated with oral acetylcysteine showed significant reductions in the severity of hepatic toxicity between those patients treated within 16 hours after ingestion and those treated between 16 and 24 hours.[5] Initiating therapy more than 24 hours after ingestion does not appear to be helpful.[4,5] Acetylcysteine is generally without serious side effects. Recovery from the acute episode is followed by the return of hepatic architecture to normal in 3–4 months, and no long-term sequelae have been reported.

KEY FEATURES

Clinical Course

Phase I (2–6 hours): Nausea, vomiting, diaphoresis. If CNS depression occurs, suspect coingestion of another agent.

Phase II (24–48 hours): Clinical symptoms subside, patient may have early RUQ discomfort. Liver function tests become abnormal.

Phase III (48–72 hours): Increases in transaminases and bilirubin levels. Coagulation abnormalities. Possible hepatic encephalopathy.

Management

1. Gastric lavage.

2. Draw liver enzymes, coagulation studies, and blood acetaminophen level at least 4 hours after ingestion.

3. Administer oral loading dose of acetylcysteine (140 mg/kg) diluted in juice or soda. (If ingestion occurred more than 24 hours prior to admission, manage supportively.)

4. If acetaminophen blood level is in potentially toxic range, continue therapy with acetylcysteine (70 mg/kg) every 4 hours for 17 doses. Otherwise, discontinue therapy.

REFERENCES

1. Ameer B, Greenblatt D: Acetaminophen. Ann Intern Med 87:202,1977.
    A concise review of the pharmacology, clinical usefulness, and toxicity of acetaminophen.

2. Black M: Acetaminophen hepatotoxicity. Gastroenterology 78:382, 1980.
    An extensive, well-referenced review of the mechanisms of acetaminophen metabolism and hepatotoxicity. The rationale for the use of acetylcysteine is established, and an overview of relevant clinical studies is given.

3. Cobden I, Record CO, Ward MK, Kerr DN: Paracetamol-induced acute renal failure in the absence of fulminant liver damage. Br Med J (Clin Res) 284:21, 1982.
    Ten patients were identified who developed acute renal failure (creatinine level greater than 4.5 mg/dl) 2–3 weeks after paracetamol (acetaminophen) overdosage without evidence of severe liver dysfunction or coingestion of nephrotoxic drugs. Renal biopsy was consistent with acute tubular necrosis, and all patients recovered. This complication occurred in approximately 1% of all paracetamol ingestions from 1974 to 1981. The pathogenesis is unclear.

4. Prescott LF, et al: Treatment of paracetamol (acetaminophen) poisoning with N-acetylcysteine. Lancet 2:432, 1977.
    Fifteen patients with acetaminophen poisoning were treated with intravenous N-acetylcysteine (300 mg/kg over 20 hours). Eleven of 12 patients treated within 10 hours of ingestion had minimal disturbances of liver function tests. Severe liver damage (SGOT greater than 1000) occurred in the other patient and in 3 patients treated between 10 and 24 hours after ingestion. One patient (early treatment group) died from a CVA.

5. Rumack BH, et al: Acetaminophen overdose. Arch Intern Med 141:380, 1981.
    Six hundred sixty-two consecutive cases of acetaminophen overdose treated with oral acetylcysteine are reported. Severe hepatic toxicity (SGOT greater than 1000) occurred in 7% of patients treated within 10 hours of ingestion, 29% of those treated 10–16 hours post-ingestion, 62% of those treated 16–24 hours post-ingestion, and 43% of those seen after 24 hours. There appears to be no benefit in starting therapy more than 24 hours after ingestion and only minimal benefit in the 15–24 hour interval.

6. Rumack BH: Acetaminophen overdose. Am J Med 75:104, 1983.
    Excellent general overview.

7. Caldarola V, Hassett JM, Hall AH, et al: Hemorrhagic pancreatitis associated with acetaminophen overdose. Am J Gastroenterol 81:579, 1986.
   Case report.

Methanol, Ethylene Glycol, and Isopropyl Alcohol

William Hale, M.D.

Methanol, ethylene glycol, and isopropyl alcohol are found singly or in combination in a large number of substances, including solvents, detergents, cements and glues, antifreeze, and disinfectants. Poisoning as a result of these substances, although uncommon, requires prompt diagnosis and specific therapy in order to prevent serious organ damage and death.

Isopropyl alcohol ingestion occurs primarily in young children and in suicidal or alcoholic adults. A survey by the Massachusetts Poison Control Center found that isopropyl alcohol was involved in 8% of all poisonings. A clear, bitter-tasting liquid, it is rapidly absorbed from the GI tract or via inhalation (most often as a result of sponge bathing) and causes acute intoxication within 30 minutes. As little as 20 ml will cause intoxication, and the lethal adult dose is between 150 and 250 ml. Acetone is the sole metabolic product of isopropyl alcohol, giving rise to marked ketonemia without, however, a significant metabolic acidosis or large increase in the anion gap. This metabolic pattern differs from that caused by intoxication with the other commonly ingested alcohols. Methanol and ethylene glycol cause severe metabolic acidosis without major ketone production, and ethanol is associated with a moderate metabolic acidosis involving primarily lactate during drinking bouts and acetoacetic and betahydroxybutyric acids during withdrawal. All four alcohols increase serum osmolality above calculated values.

Management of isopropyl alcohol intoxication varies with the severity of the ingestion. Termination of exposure by emptying the stomach with ipecac-induced emesis or gastric lavage should be performed in all patients. Because isopropyl alcohol undergoes a recirculation through gastric juice and saliva, continuous lavage has been advocated. Mild intoxications can be handled with supportive care, airway control, and intravenous fluids to correct volume imbalances. More serious ingestions require intensive care unit monitoring, mechanical ventilation, and possibly hemodialysis. Because the major toxicity of isopropyl alcohol is its sedative/anesthetic effect, there is no rationale for the administration of ethanol in the treatment of isopropyl alcohol intoxication. A retrospective review of 22 cases of severe isopropyl alcohol intoxication found that deep coma (grade III or IV) and severe hypotension were the most serious presenting signs, with a 45% mortality rate in patients with both findings.[1] An important management decision involved the use of hemodialysis for severe intoxication, and although a controlled trial comparing dialysis to conservative therapy is not available, many authorities recommend hemodialysis for patients with hypotension unresponsive to volume replacement. A serum isopropyl alcohol level greater than 400 mg/dl is a relative indication. However, it is important to realize that optimal supportive care will generally be effective if dialysis is not available.

Methanol and ethylene glycol are relatively nontoxic in small amounts, and the minimum lethal dose for each is approximately 100 ml.[2-4] They are typically ingested as a substitute for ethanol, although suicidal intent with ethylene glycol is common. Both produce drunkenness without the characteristic odor of alcohol, and toxicity is delayed 12–24 hours while the buildup of toxic metabolites occurs. Methanol is metabolized by the enzyme alcohol dehydrogenase to formaldehyde and formic acid, which, in turn, cause metabolic derangements resulting in overproduction of various organic acids. A severe metabolic acidosis results, with a markedly increased anion gap. The clinical syndrome is characterized by a depressed sensorium, seizures, early visual blurring with prominent retinal edema and hyperemia of the disk followed by blindness as a result of atrophy of the optic nerve, pancreatitis, leukocytosis, and respiratory failure. Ethylene glycol is metabolized by the same enzyme to a number of toxic metabolites, with oxalic acid as one of the end-products. As with methanol intoxication, a severe, refractory anion gap acidosis results, with very low serum bicarbonate levels. A characteristic feature of ethylene glycol poisoning is the deposition of calcium oxalate crystals throughout the body, especially the leptomeninges, blood vessels, heart, and kidneys. Calcium oxalate crystals in the urinary sediment are an important finding and in the appropriate setting are virtually diagnostic. The clinical syndrome of ethylene glycol ingestion is manifested in three stages. The initial period of intoxication is followed by CNS depression, seizures, ocular palsies, papilledema, and a toxic meningoencephalitis with pleocytosis. Metabolic acidosis, crystalluria, hypocalcemia, myopathy, and peripheral leukocytosis are also prominent. During the next 12–18 hours, cardiopulmonary failure may predominate with hypertension, pulmonary edema, and congestive heart failure. Twenty-four to 72 hours after ingestion, acute oliguric renal failure typically occurs.

The management of methanol and ethylene glycol poisoning is similar.[2-4] Because of the delay between ingestion and the onset of toxicity, gastric lavage and the instillation of charcoal are not particularly helpful. Prompt diagnosis and therapy are vital, and these substances should be suspected in all patients with severe metabolic acidosis of unclear etiology. Correction of the acidosis with sodium bicarbonate is paramount, and some authors recommend early attempts at mannitol-induced diuresis in ethylene glycol intoxications. Blocking the conversion of the parent compounds to their toxic metabolites with ethanol is a mainstay of treatment. A loading dose of 0.6 gm/kg is followed by a maintenance dose of 100–150 mg/kg/hour. Oral administration of 20–50% ethanol solution involved considerably less volume than the equivalent amount of 5–10% intravenous preparations and is recommended. Maximal enzyme inhibition requires a blood ethanol level between 100 and 200 mg/dl. Hemodialysis is the basis of definitive therapy and is extremely effective in removing both the parent compounds and their metabolites as well as in preventing solute overload from the massive doses of sodium bicarbonate frequently required. During hemodialysis, the maintenance dose of ethanol should be increased approximately threefold to keep blood levels in the appropriate range. Although poisoning with methanol or ethylene glycol usually results in significant organ damage, favorable results have been reported following vigorous therapy. Preliminary data have shown 4-methylpyrazole, an alcohol dehydrogenase inhibitor, to be effective in the treatment of ethylene glycol and/or methanol poisoning, when substituted for ethanol; there is to date only limited experience with this agent.[5]

KEY FEATURES

The major toxic effects of methanol and ethylene glycol result from metabolic derangements manifested in the production of a severe refractory anion gap acidosis. The minimum lethal dose is approximately 100 ml of either agent.

The toxicity of isopropyl alcohol arises from its activity as a sedative/anesthetic agent. Death commonly ensues after ingestion of 150–250 ml.

Ketonemia/ketonuria without a significant metabolic acidosis is the hallmark of an isopropanol ingestion.

Calcium oxalate crystals in the urinary sediment in the setting of a refractory metabolic acidosis is strongly suggestive of ethylene glycol ingestion.

Clinically significant ingestions of methanol, ethanol, ethylene glycol, and isopropanol produce an "osmolar gap."

Management of isopropyl alcohol ingestion requires aggressive support *without* ethanol administration. Hemodialysis should be performed for severe intoxication, especially in the setting of deep coma and/or hypotension with a measured level greater than 400 mg/dl.

Management of ethylene glycol or methanol ingestion requires aggressive treatment of acidosis, early administration of ethanol to achieve and maintain a blood ethanol level of 100–200 mg/dl (thereby blocking conversion of methanol and ethylene glycol), and hemodialysis.

A favorable clinical outcome generally requires prompt recognition and early aggressive treatment.

REFERENCES

1. LaCouture M, et al: Acute isopropyl alcohol intoxication. Am J Med 75:680, 1983.
    The pharmacology and toxicology of isopropyl alcohol are presented, as is a retro-spective review of 22 cases of severe poisoning. The mortality rate was 45% when deep coma and hypotension were present on admission, and the authors recommend hemodialysis when hypotension cannot be corrected with volume replacement.

2. McCoy H, et al: Severe methanol poisoning. Am J Med 67:804, 1979.
    Two patients with extremely high blood methanol levels recovered completely with aggressive ethanol therapy and hemodialysis. Oral ethanol is recommended.

3. Parry M: Ethylene glycol poisoning. Am J Med 57:143, 1974.
    Rapid correction of acidosis, ethanol blockade, early mannitol diuresis, and hemo-dialysis are stressed. Correction of hypocalcemia and treatment with thiamine and pyri-doxine to enhance conversion of ethylene glycol to less toxic metabolites were also rec-ommended.

4. Peterson C, et al: Ethylene glycol poisoning. N Engl J Med 304:21, 1981.
    A pharmocokinetic model for ethanol blockade. Loading dose: 0.6 gm/kg; maintenance dose: 109 mg/kg/hour; maintenance dose during hemodialysis: 237 mg/kg/hour. Frequent monitoring of blood ethanol levels during hemodialysis is recommended.

5. Baud FJ, Galliot M, Astier A, et al: Treatment of ethylene glycol poisoning with intravenous 4-methylpyrazole. N Engl J Med 319:97, 1988.
    Case report and review of human and animal experience with 4-methylpyrazole, an alcohol dehydrogenase inhibitor, in the treatment of ethylene glycol (or methanol) poi-soning.

Adverse Reactions to Iodinated Contrast Media

Steven W. Paskal, M.D.

Each year, approximately 8 million radiologic studies utilizing iodinated contrast media (ICM) are performed in the United States. The tri-iodinated benzoic acid derivatives diatrizoate (Renografin) and iothalamate (Conray) currently in use were introduced in the 1950s. These compounds are weak acids administered as their sodium or methylglutamine salt and have an osmolarity 5–8 times that of normal serum.

In general, toxicity from ICM can be divided into direct chemotoxicity and idiosyncratic reactions that resemble immune-mediated phenomena (anaphylactoid). Chemotoxicity, believed to be secondary to both the hyperosmolarity and the direct chemical and enzymatic effects of the dye, can occur in many organ systems. Nonionic compounds with reduced osmolarity have been introduced. These agents (iohexol, iopamidol, and ioxaglate) are associated with fewer adverse reactions but are 15–25 times more expensive than ionic agents and their role is not yet fully defined.[1,2,19]

ANAPHYLACTOID REACTIONS TO ICM

The results of several prospective surveys of ICM reactions have defined the incidence and clinical characteristics of these reactions. Most patients report transient symptoms including mild nausea, flushing, dizziness, and paresthesias immediately after contrast injection. These symptoms resolve within 5 minutes and are not severe or persistent enough to require therapy.[3] These minor, vasomotor reactions occur so commonly that preparing patients for them may eliminate anxiety that can aggravate these responses.

More severe reactions, including persistence and increased severity of the symptoms just noted; dermal reactions; and manifestations of an anaphylactoid response, including urticaria-angioedema, bronchospasm, and hypotension, occur in 5–7% of patients studied. Only one third of these patients required therapy, and 80% of these reactions were cutaneous. Life-threatening reactions were recorded in less than 1/1100 studies, and fatalities occurred in 1/40,000–1/75,000 procedures. Symptoms occurred in combination with nausea and vomiting, and cutaneous reactions often preceded more severe reactions. Symptoms generally appear within 10 minutes of contrast injection; late reactions rarely occur. Vasovagal reactions are common, and bradycardia is reported in up to two thirds of hypotensive episodes.[3–5]

Adverse reactions are seen in 10–15% of patients with a prior history of hay fever, asthma, iodine, seafood, or shellfish allergy. Patients with a history of previous adverse reactions to ICM have a three- to sixfold increased risk of reaction on re-exposure. Ten to twenty per cent of these patients will have a recurrence on re-exposure; however, reactions more severe than the first are unusual. Pretesting for sensitivity with small intravenous doses can not reliably identify those who will have a significant reaction, can result in severe reactions, and is not generally recommended.[3–5]

A premedication protocol of prednisone 50 mg orally every 6 hours for three doses ending 1 hour prior to the procedure, and diphenhydramine 50 mg intramuscularly 1 hour before the procedure has been tested in 284 patients with a history of a prior reaction. Mild adverse reactions were seen in 7.1% of procedures, with only one severe reaction occurring. This series included 84 patients with prior severe reactions; only five minor skin reactions occurred within this subset of patients.[6] These studies did not include untreated controls. The results do represent a significant reduction from the expected rate of adverse reactions, although the risk was not completely eliminated.

A large, prospective, randomized, placebo-controlled trial of pretreatment with oral methylprednisolone in patients scheduled to undergo radiologic procedures utilizing ionic contrast agents demonstrated a significant reduction in the incidence of immediate reactions with the two-dose regimen of methylprednisolone 32 mg PO 12 hours and 2 hours before challenge with contrast, but not with a single dose 2 hours beforehand; the incidence of reactions requiring treatment in the group pretreated with two doses of methylprednisolone was similar to that reported elsewhere with nonionic agents in patients not pretreated.[19]

The pathogenesis of anaphylactoid reactions to ICM has not been clearly defined. Postulated mechanisms have included (1) antigen-antibody reactions, (2) contrast-induced histamine release, and (3) psychogenic factors.[7] Current theories have focused on the activation of the complement and coagulation systems by ICM. Products of these systems can cause release of mediators from mast cells and basophils and release of bradykinin, resulting in the clinical syndromes seen.[8] Studies of these systems have shown lower baseline levels of C1-esterase inhibitor and higher levels of conversion of prekallikrein to kallikrein in nonreactors compared with reactors.[9] These studies, although preliminary, not only provide insight into the pathogenesis of these reactions but also suggest possible *in vitro* methods to identify patients at high risk.

Therapy for minor cutaneous reactions is symptomatic, with antihistamines. More severe reactions are treated as outlined for anaphylaxis, with airway control, epinephrine, bronchodilators, and fluid replacement. Vasovagal reactions should be identified and treated with atropine as needed. Because adverse reactions cannot be predicted or completely prevented with pretreatment, equipment and personnel trained to treat life-threatening anaphylactic-like reactions must be immediately available whenever ICM is utilized.

Patients with a history of prior reactions or an allergic diathesis have an increased risk of future reactions that can be reduced but not eliminated by pretreatment. The clinical benefit of the study planned and alternatives to ICM should be considered; however, clearly needed procedures should not be withheld.

RADIOCONTRAST-INDUCED ACUTE RENAL FAILURE (RCIARF)

With the introduction of the tri-iodinated contrast agents in the mid-1950s, renal complications from ICM were believed to have become rare.

In the 1970s case reports of RCIARF became more frequent, and by 1980 over 200 well-documented cases were described.[10]

A retrospective review of patients undergoing intravenous pyelography (IVP) who had pre-and post-examination creatinine determinations during a 10-month period at Strong Memorial Hospital, Rochester, New York, identified 18 individuals among 2360 IVP patients who had a creatinine (Cr) rise of greater than 1 mg/dl, for an estimated minimum incidence of 0.8%. Among nondiabetic patients with mild azotemia (serum Cr 1.5–4.5 mg/dl) there was a 3% incidence and among those with more severe underlying renal failure (serum Cr greater than 4.5 mg/dl) 31% developed RCIARF. Diabetic patients with mild baseline renal failure had a 50% incidence of RCIARF.[11] Another series showed that 75% of diabetics with a baseline serum creatinine concentration above 2.0 mg/dl (with a mean serum Cr of 8.5 mg/dl) experienced RCIARF.[12]

A retrospective study of angiographic procedures in hospitalized patients with multiple underlying medical problems demonstrated a 12% incidence of RCIARF.[13] These patients, although not clinically dehydrated, received only 5% dextrose in water intravenously during the procedure. A subsequent prospective study of 100 similar patients who received normal saline hydration prior to angiography yielded no cases of RCIARF.[14]

A more recently reported prospective study of 378 patients undergoing angiography demonstrated a 2% incidence of RCIARF in patients with normal baseline renal function, compared with 30% in those with a mean baseline serum creatinine level of 2.5 mg/dl. In this study[15] underlying diabetes mellitus (NIDDM), age, and cardiovascular disease did not increase the risk independent of renal function. Multiple myeloma also does not appear to be an independent risk factor, although the renal failure induced in these patients may be more severe and may occur by a different mechanism.[10]

The clinical course of RCIARF is characterized by oliguria in 75% of patients. Decreased urine output occurs within 24 hours of the procedure, is refractory to volume expansion or diuretics, and rarely lasts longer than 72 hours. Reduced glomerular filtration rate (GFR) as reflected by an increased serum creatinine level peaks on day 3. The overall outcome of RCIARF is good, with over 80% of patients returning to their baseline renal function within 2 weeks. Progression to chronic renal failure is unusual except in patients with severe pre-existing azotemia. Mortality is less than 5% and in most instances is related to underlying diseases.[10,16]

The diagnosis and management of RCIARF are similar to those of ARF from any cause. Careful attention must be paid to fluid and electrolyte management, and other reversible causes of renal failure should be sought (dehydration, toxic antibiotics). Occasional patients will require temporary dialysis or cation exchange resins for complications. A persistently positive nephrogram on a 24-hour post-procedure abdominal film was found to be a sensitive test for predicting RCIARF when compared with oliguria or urinalysis. However, a high false positive rate and expense make this an impractical screening test compared with serial serum creatinine determinations.[15] A low fractional excretion of sodium and low urinary sodium level have been found in patients with RCIARF.[16,17]

The pathogenesis of RCIARF has not been fully defined. Suggested causes include (1) renal hemodynamic changes and ischemic injury—ICM cause reactive renal artery vasoconstriction in contrast to the vasodilation seen in peripheral vascular beds; (2) direct renal tubular toxicity; (3) microcirculatory changes—increased blood viscosity secondary to ICM-induced RBC morphologic changes; and (4) intratubular obstruction—ICM-induced precipitation of the Tamm-Horsfall mucoprotein, the major component of renal tubular casts. Renal biopsies after ICM injection show intense vacuolization in the cytoplasm of proximal renal tubular cells; however, these changes did not correlate with the degree of renal failure after angiography and the pathology of RCIARF is unknown.[10,16]

The incidence of RCIARF in unselected populations appears to be low enough to argue against routine screening after radiography.[15] Patients with pre-existing renal insufficiency are clearly at significant risk and should be identified and followed for this complication. In all patients, the risk of RCIARF must be evaluated and alternative imaging procedures considered in high-risk individuals.

It is prudent for the physician to maintain adequate hydration in all patients studied and to limit the amount of contrast administered. Mannitol infusions with hydration may protect high-risk patients.[18] Nonionic contrast agents may also be found to have less renal toxicity than other currently available agents.[1,19]

KEY FEATURES

Immediate idiosyncratic reactions to ICM occur in 5–7% of patients studied. Less than 2% of reactions are severe enough to require therapy, and less than 0.1% are life threatening.

Although severe reactions are unusual, they cannot be predicted or completely prevented. Therefore, *proper equipment and personnel trained to manage anaphylaxis and cardiac arrest must be readily available whenever contrast media are used.*

Minor reactions can be treated symptomatically with reassurance, antihistamines, and bronchodilators. Anaphylaxis must be recognized quickly and treated aggressively, as outlined previously (see article *Anaphylaxis*). Vasovagal reactions (hypotension with bradycardia) are common and should be treated with atropine.

Patients with a history of a prior adverse reaction or an allergic diathesis have a two- to sixfold increased risk of reacting on re-exposure. Although second reactions are usually mild, this increased risk can be decreased by pretreatment with the following protocol:

1. Reassess the need for the ICM study and possible alternatives.

2. Reassure the patient that the risk of a severe reaction is small and that appropriate precautions are being followed.

3. Methylprednisolone 32 mg orally 12 and 2 hours before the study.

4. Diphenhydramine 50 mg intramuscularly 1 hour before the study.

Acute renal failure occurs in less than 3% of patients with normal renal function or mild pre-existing renal insufficiency and in approximately 30% of patients with more severe renal failure following ICM studies. Diabetics with severe renal failure are at extremely high risk for this complication.

RCIARF is usually oliguric and reversible. Fluids and electrolytes must be managed carefully. Occasionally, ion exchange resins or dialysis is needed to treat complications.

All patients should be well hydrated prior to intravascular contrast studies. Other potentially renal toxic drugs should be stopped if possible.

The risk of contrast studies should be weighed against benefits and alternative imaging procedures considered in high-risk patients.

High-risk patients should be monitored for RCIARF by serial serum creatinine determinations.

REFERENCES

1. Bettmann MA: Angiographic contrast agents: conventional and new media compared. Am J Radiol 139:787, 1982.
   Reviews the systemic, cardiac, renal, and vascular effects of conventional ionic contrast agents and compares these with the effects of new nonionic agents.

2. Junck L, Marshall WH: Neurotoxicity of radiologic contrast agents. Ann Neurol 13:469, 1983.
   Adverse effects include seizures, transient cortical blindness, brain edema, and spinal cord injury and are more common in patients with brain tumors or other processes disrupting the blood-brain barrier. Adverse effects of myelographic agents, including seizures, meningeal reactions, and transient encephalopathy, are also reviewed.

3. Witten DM, Hirsch FD, Hartman GW: Acute reactions to urographic contrast medium: Incidence, clinical characteristics and relationship to history of hypersensitivity states. Am J Radiol 119:832, 1973.
   Results of a prospective study of adverse reactions occurring in 32,964 consecutive outpatients having IVPs at the Mayo Clinic during a 27-month period.

4. Shehadi WH: Adverse reactions to intravascularly administered contrast media: A comprehensive study based on a prospective survey. Am J Radiol 124:145–152, 1975.
   Multicenter survey of 112,003 procedures with adverse reactions occurring in 5.65% of intra-arterial injections, 2.3% of intravenous pyelograms, and 10.11% of intravenous

cholangiograms. One third of patients with reactions required therapy, and 11 deaths occurred.

5. Witten DM, Reactions to urographic contrast media. JAMA 231:974, 1975.
   Author summarizes the results of his 1973 study and outlines an approach to the treatment of reactions.

6. Greenberger PA, Patterson R, Simon R, Lieberman P, Wallace W: Pretreatment of high-risk patients requiring radiographic contrast media studies. J Allergy Clin Immunol 67:185, 1981.
   Three hundred eighteen high-risk patients were pretreated with prednisone and diphenhydramine. Minor reactions occurred in 23 procedures (7.1%) and severe reaction occurred in only one patient.

7. Lieberman P, Siegle RL, Taylor WW: Anaphylactoid reactions to iodinated contrast material. J Allergy Clin Immunol 62:174, 1978.
   A review of the literature on anaphylactoid reactions discussing possible pathogenesis and an approach to the high-risk patient.

8. Lasser EC, Lang JH, Hamblin AE, Lyon SG, Howard BS: Activation systems in contrast idiosyncrasy. Invest Radiol 15 (suppl):S2–S5, 1980.
   Hypothesized schema for the pathogenesis of anaphylactoid reactions involving the complement, coagulation, and other activation systems (kinins, fibrinolysins). From a special supplement concerning a variety of topics relating to ICM.

9. Lasser EC, Lang JH, Lyon SG, Hamblin AE, Howard MM: Prekallikrein-kallikrein conversion rate as a predictor of contrast material catastrophies. Radiology 140:11, 1981.
   Describes an in vitro test used retrospectively to identify reactors with a sensitivity of 88%, a specificity of 82%, and a predictive value of 79%.

10. Mudge GH:Nephrotoxicity of urographic radiocontrast drugs. Kidney Int 18:540, 1980.
    Analysis of data from over 200 case reports of RCIARF, including unusual cases of hypersensitivity-like reactions, medullary necrosis, and proteinuria. Includes a discussion of pathogenic mechanisms and their relationship to underlying diseases.

11. Van Zee BE, Hoy WE, Talley TE, Jaenike JR: Renal injury associated with intravenous pyelography in nondiabetic and diabetic patients. Ann Intern Med 89:51, 1978.
    A chart review covering a period during which 2360 pyelograms were performed found 23 cases of ARF. Four patients with initial serum creatinine level less than 1.5 mg/dl were found; all had an underlying urologic abnormality (benign prostatic hypertrophy [BPH], lupus nephritis). Nondiabetics with serum creatinine level over 4.5 mg/dl had a 31% incidence. Related morbidity included extended hospital stays and shortened time to dialysis in a few patients with antecedent progressive azotemia.

12. Harkonen S, Kjellstrand C: Exacerbation of diabetic renal failure following intravenous pyelography. Am J Med 63:939, 1977.
    RCIARF occurred in 1 of 23 diabetics with initial serum creatinine concentration less than 2 mg/dl. Among diabetics with severe underlying renal disease, 75% developed renal failure.

13. Swartz RD, Rubin JE, Leeming BW, Silva P: Renal failure following major angiography. Am J Med 65:31, 1978.
    A retrospective review of 109 consecutive angiograms revealing a 12% incidence of RCIARF. Patients with both pre-existing renal insufficiency and impaired liver function were particularly at risk.

14. Eisenberg R, Bank W, Hegcock M: Renal failure after major angiography. Am J Med 68:43, 1980.

A prospective study of 100 consecutive angiograms in patients similar to those described in reference 13 who were hydrated with normal saline prior to and during the procedure. No cases of renal failure were found.

15. D'Elia JA, Gleason RE, Alday M, Malarick C, Godley K, Warram J, Kalany A, Weinrauch LA: Nephrotoxicity from angiographic contrast material: A prospective study. Am J Med 72:719, 1982.

Three hundred seventy-eight patients undergoing angiography were followed for changes in renal function. Nonazotemic patients had a 2% incidence, and azotemic individuals (mean sCr 2.3 mg/dl) had a 33% incidence of RCIARF. A prior history of diabetes or cardiovascular disease was not an independent risk factor.

16. Byrd L, Sherman RL: Radiocontrast-induced acute renal failure: A clinical and pathophysiologic review. Medicine 58:270–279, 1979.

The clinical courses of 23 patients with RCIARF are discussed.

17. Fang LST, Sirota RA, Ebert TH, Lichtenstein NS: Low fractional excretion of sodium with contrast media induced acute renal failure. Arch Intern Med 140:531–533, 1980.

An FE_{Na}% of less than 1% was found in all 12 patients with RCIARF studied. Similar values are seen in patients with pre-renal azotemia and acute renal tubular obstruction, in contrast to the high values found in acute renal tubular necrosis.

18. Anto HR, Chou SY, Porush JG, Shapiro WB: Infusion intravenous pyelography and renal function. Effect of hypertonic mannitol in patients with chronic renal insufficiency. Arch Intern Med 141:1652–1656, 1981.

Thirty-seven patients with severe underlying renal failure (baseline sCr greater than 3.5 mg/dl) received an infusion of 250 ml of 20% mannitol after an IVP with adequate hydration performed. Only 5 of 24 nondiabetic and 3 of 8 diabetic patients developed RCIARF, compared with an expected 70% of incidence.

19. Lasser EC, Berry CC, Talner LB, et al: Pretreatment with corticosteroids to alleviate reactions to intravenous contrast material. N Engl J Med 317:845, 1988.

Multi-institutional, randomized, placebo-controlled trial of pretreatment with corticosteroids in 6763 patients scheduled to undergo radiographic study with ionic contrast material. Pretreatment with methylprednisolone 32 mg PO 12 hours and 2 hours before challenge with contrast was associated with a significant reduction in immediate reactions to a level comparable with that reported with nonionic contrast agents (1.2% vs 0.9% requiring therapy). Accompanying editorial by MA Bettmann suggests a schema for choosing ionic agents, ionic agents with steroid pretreatment, or nonionic agents on the basis of clinical features and risk profile.

Salicylate Intoxication

Steven W. Paskal, M.D.

Although safety packaging and reductions in the total dose of flavored children's aspirin per container have caused decreases in accidental ingestions and poisoning deaths in children, salicylate intoxication remains an important clinical problem. The toxic effects of the various salicylate compounds are qualitatively identical; however, methyl salicylate (oil of wintergreen) has a relatively high concentration of salicylate and causes a disproportionate number of lethal salicylate ingestions.[1]

Absorption of orally administered salicylates occurs rapidly, primarily from the small intestine. The rate of absorption is limited primarily by tablet dissolution but is also influenced by pH and gastric emptying time. Appreciable serum concentrations are achieved within 30 minutes, with peak serum levels occurring within 2–4 hours.[2] Large doses of ingested salicylates have been reported to cause a several-hour delay in gastric emptying and prolonged pylorospasm.[3]

Absorbed salicylate compounds are rapidly hydrolyzed to salicylic acid, which is reversibly bound to albumin and other serum proteins. Biotransformation of salicylate occurs in the liver, resulting in three major metabolites—salicyluric acid and phenolic and acetyl glucuronides—and in several minor metabolites. These compounds are rapidly excreted by the kidney; however, in toxic doses these metabolic processes become saturated and the half-life of salicylate becomes markedly prolonged. In these cases, excretion of free salicylic acid becomes rate determining. At an acid pH, a greater portion of salicylate, a weak acid, is present in the nonionized form, and able to penetrate cell membranes, and renal tubular reabsorption is increased. An alkaline environment promotes ionization of salicylate and increases urine excretion fivefold.[2]

The clinical presentation of salicylate intoxication is often subtle and includes nonspecific findings, including tinnitus; nausea; vomiting; hyperpnea; hyperpyrexia; and mental status changes ranging from hyperexcitability to mild lethargy, disorientation, seizures, and coma. Salicylates stimulate the CNS respiratory center directly and cause an increased depth of respiration and, to a lesser degree, tachypnea resulting in decreased PCO_2 and respiratory alkalosis. Salicylates also have widespread primary metabolic effects, including uncoupling of oxidative phosphorylation; inhibition of Krebs cycle enzymes and amino acid metabolism; stimulation of gluconeogenesis, tissue glycolysis, and lipid metabolism; and interference with hemostatic mechanisms. These changes result in inefficient metabolism, with increased oxygen use and heat production, aminoaciduria, and formation of ketone bodies and organic acids resulting in a metabolic acidosis.[4]

The balance among this primary metabolic acidosis, the respiratory alkalosis, and their homeostatic compensatory mechanisms determines the acid-base status of the patient. It has been conventionally observed that in young children a mixed metabolic acidosis and respiratory alkalosis is seen with acidemia predominating but that most adults demonstrate a primary respiratory alkalosis. However, in a series of 67 adults seen with salicylate intoxication, only 22% of the 45 patients who had ingested just salicylates had a simple respiratory alkalosis, 56% had a mixed respiratory alkalosis and metabolic acidosis, and 20% demonstrated a simple metabolic acidosis. One third of the 67 patients had ingested a variety of other drugs, generally CNS depressants, in addition to salicylates. Only 40% of these patients showed a respiratory alkalosis (27% simple, 13% associated with a metabolic acidosis), whereas 36% had a simple metabolic acidosis and 18% had both metabolic and respiratory acidosis, in some cases associated with a normal anion gap.[5] The associated drugs may be the primary determinant of the net acid-base status, blunting salicylate-induced hyperventilation to unmask the metabolic acidosis and potentially depressing respirations enough to result in an additional respiratory acidosis.

In addition to acid-base disturbances salicylate intoxication results in significant losses of water (increased cutaneous and respiratory insensible losses, vomiting, and renal loss accompanying organic aciduria), bicarbonate, sodium, and potassium. Patients generally have an initial hyperglycemia that may be followed by hypoglycemia as carbohydrate stores are depleted.[4] Animal studies have shown that salicylates lower brain glucose levels despite normoglycemia and suggest that this phenomenon may be involved in the CNS changes that accompany severe and lethal intoxications. Glucose infusions and attempts to maintain an alkalemic state that decreases nonionized salicylate and diminishes brain salicylate levels may be protective.[6,7]

A variety of other changes may be seen with salicylate intoxications. Bleeding can occur secondary to mucosal injury and impaired platelet aggregation even at therapeutic salicylate levels. In occasional cases of severe poisoning, reversible elevations of liver enzyme levels and vitamin K responsive elevations of the prothrombin time have been reported.[3,4]

Noncardiogenic pulmonary edema has been recognized as a complication of salicylate intoxications and was found on admission in 22% of patients over 16 years of age presenting with a salicylate level greater than 30 mg/dl over a 5-year study period.[8] Patients with pulmonary edema were older, had a smoking history, had multiple underlying medical problems, and chronically ingested salicylates. The salicylate level in these patients was greater than 40 mg/dl, and neurologic abnormalities were common. Aggressive supportive care, including mechanical ventilation with positive end-expiratory pressure (PEEP), and salicylate lowering therapy were successful in clearing the pulmonary edema within 1–7 days in these patients.[8] Accompanying proteinuria and experimental studies suggest that salicylate-induced increased membrane permeability may be responsible.[9]

Salicylate toxicity must be considered in all patients with nonfocal neurologic findings, acid-base abnormalities, unexplained hyperpnea, or noncardiogenic pulmonary edema. The diagnosis was not made for up to 72 hours in 30% of 73 consecutive adults who presented over a 5-year period with levels over 25 mg/dl. These patients did not have a clear history of drug overdose, were older, and more frequently ingested salicylates chronically than those diagnosed on admission. Mortality (25%) and morbidity (including pulmonary edema in 10 patients) were higher in this group.[10]

The ferric chloride test is an extremely sensitive screening procedure for the presence of salicylic acid in urine. Addition of several drops of 10% ferric chloride to several drops of urine results in a purple color if salicylate is present; however, false positive results do occur. Commercially available reagent strips (Phenostix) react in the same manner.[1]

In cases of chronic salicylate ingestion, estimates of the amount ingested and serum salicylate levels are not generally useful in predicting the severity of the intoxication. Acute ingestions of less than 150 mg/kg of salicylate are unlikely to produce significant symptoms. Mild to moderate reactions occur with ingestions in the 150–300 mg/kg range and can often be managed in the outpatient or emergency room setting. More prolonged and severe effects are seen at doses exceeding 300 mg/kg and ingestions over 500 mg/kg are potentially lethal.[3] Blood levels obtained 6 or more hours after an acute ingestion can be plotted on the Done nomogram to estimate the severity of the intoxication.[11]

In addition to supportive care, therapy of salicylate intoxications has three objectives: (1) prevention of further absorption, (2) correction of fluid and electrolye deficits and acid-base disturbances, and (3) reduction in tissue salicylate levels. Charcoal administration (following gastric lavage in the setting of recent salicylate ingestion) is the most effective intervention to limit absorption. A study of volunteers ingesting aspirin suggests that activated charcoal and magnesium sulfate alone are more effective than ipecac in limiting the absorption of aspirin.[12] Repeated oral charcoal doses may further limit absorption of aspirin and other poisons.[14]

Dehydration occurs early in salicylate intoxications and must be corrected quickly to ensure adequate renal perfusion and urine output. Isotonic saline or lactated Ringer's solution can be used to correct volume depletion, and fluids should be continued to maintain an adequate urine output.. In view of the altered metabolic state, fluids should contain glucose unless hyperglycemia is present. Potassium depletion is common even in the presence of normal serum potassium levels, and potassium supplements should be added to the infusion once adequate urine flow is established if renal function is normal.[3]

Fluid therapy must be individualized, and serum pH, glucose, electrolytes, and the electrocardiogram should be monitored in severely intoxicated patients. Salicylates are excreted more rapidly in an alkaline urine, and alkalemia decreases tissue uptake of salicylate. Tissue levels of salicylate are elevated in the presence of acidemia, and a primary therapeutic goal should be avoidance of systemic acidosis.[6] Sodium bicarbonate 3–5 mg/kg should be administered intravenously to correct severe acidosis.

Forced diuresis and urine alkalinzation can increase salicylate elimination but are difficult to accomplish, in part because of underlying hypokalemia. Bicarbonate administration using the urine pH as an end-point can result in severe systemic alkalosis, sodium overload, increased potassium depletion, and hypocalcemic tetany.[1] Cautious administration of bicarbonate-containing fluids (1–2 meq/kg $NaHCO_3$ every 1–2 hours) while replacing potassium and monitoring urinary and serum pH may be attempted.[4] Urine alkalinzation should not be accomplished at the cost of systemic acidosis, and the use of acetazolamide to alkalinize urine can lead to more severe complications and is not generally recommended. Inadequate ventilation will increase acidemia, and assisted ventilation should be used in cases associated with respiratory depression.[6]

Hemodialysis, charcoal hemoperfusion, and peritoneal dialysis are more efficient than forced diuresis in removing salicylates and are more likely to be effective in the severely intoxicated patient. These methods should be considered in cases of refractory acidosis, coma, levels above 80–100 mg/dl, renal or cardiac insufficiency, and in patients unresponsive to conservative therapy. Hemodialysis is more efficient than peritoneal dialysis and should be used if it can be implemented without delay.[13]

KEY FEATURES

Pathophysiology

Direct Effects
    A. CNS respiratory stimulation
    B. Uncoupling of oxidative phosphorylation
    C. Inhibition of TCA cycle, amino acid metabolism
    D. Stimulation of lipid metabolism, gluconeogenesis, tissue glycolysis

Clinical Manifestations
    A. Hyperpnea, hypocapnia
    B. Varied acid-base changes
       1. Water, Na, HCO_3, K loss
       2. Hyperglycemia, possible late hypoglycemia, and decreased CNS glucose level
       3. Hyperpyrexia and diaphoresis

Diagnosis
    A. Suspect salicylate intoxication in any patient with unexplained:

      1. Acid-base abnormalities
      2. Mental status changes
      3. Hyperpnea
      4. Noncardiogenic pulmonary edema
  B. Confirm the presence of salicylic acid in urine by Phenostix or ferric chloride; add 3–5 drops of 10% ferric chloride to patient's urine:
      1. Positive for salicylates: violet/blue color
      2. Positive for ketone bodies: color disappears with boiling
      3. Phenothiazines and coal tar dyes: false positive but pinker color
      4. Plotting the serum level at a known time 6 or more hours after an acute ingestion predicts severity
      5. In chronic ingestions, serum levels or estimated ingested dose is not predictive. Follow clinical and laboratory abnormalities

Therapy

  A. Remove ingested salicylate:
      1. Gastric lavage
      2. Charcoal/MgSO$_4$ (or sorbitol)
  B. Supportive care, correct fluid and electrolytes
      1. Control the airway, support respiration if needed
      2. Correct volume depletion:
         a. Isotonic solutions with glucose followed by hypotonic fluid to maintain urine output
         b. In cases of shock or pulmonary edema, consider colloidal solutions
      3. Monitor serum electrolyes, glucose, pH, urine output and pH and ECG
      4. Give vitamin K if increased prothrombin time
  C. Promote reduction of tissue salicylate levels: Goal is an alkalemic state and alkalinized urine, which promote excretion and decrease tissue salicylate levels
      1. Correct acidemia quickly
      2. Maintain adequate respirations (do not treat the respiratory alkalosis usually seen)
      3. Forced alkaline diuresis increases excretion but is difficult to accomplish, especially in patients with more severe intoxication. It may be attempted with bicarbonate infusion with potassium repletion. Follow systemic as well as urinary pH to avoid excessive alkalemia. Watch for fluid overload, increased hypokalemia, and hypocalcemic tetany. Avoid systemic acidosis
      4. Consider dialysis if:
         a. Unresponsive acidosis; coma; level ≥80 mg/dl
         b. Associated renal or cardiac insufficiency
         c. Clinical deterioration during conservative therapy
         d. Hemodialysis is more effective than peritoneal dialysis and should be used if it can be started without delay

REFERENCES

1. Done AK, Temple AR: Treatment of salicylate poisoning. Mod Treat 8:528, 1971.
   Review of all aspects of salicylate intoxication, including specific guidelines for fluid therapy.

2. Flowere RJ, Moncada S, Vane JR: Analgesic-antipyretics and anti-inflammatory agents; drugs in the treatment of gout. *In* Goodman LS, Gilman A (eds): The pharmocologic basis of therapeutics. New York, MacMillan Publishers, 1980.
   Comprehensive review of salicylate pharmacology.

3. Seger D: Salicylates and acetaminophen. *In* Rosen P, et al (eds): Emergency Medicine: Concepts and Clinical Practice. St. Louis, CV Mosby, 1983.
   Reviews salicylate poisoning from the viewpoint of the emergency room physician.

4. Temple AR: Acute and chronic effects of aspirin toxicity and their treatment. Arch Intern Med 141:364, 1981.
   Discusses the pathophysiology of salicylate toxicity and suggests a management strategy.

5. Gabow PA, Anderson RJ, Potts DE, Schrier RW: Acid-base disturbances in the salicylate-intoxicated adult. Arch Intern Med 138:1481,1978.
   The acid-base status of 67 adults with salicylate intoxication is presented. One third of patients had ingested other drugs that contributed to the abnormalities, primarily by depressing respirations.

6. Hill JB: Salicylate intoxication. N Engl J Med 288:1110–1113, 1973.
   Systemic and urinary alkalosis decreases CNS salicylate levels and increases excretion. Therapy should be directed at promoting this state.

7. Thurston JH, Pollock PG, Warren SK, and Jones EM: Reduced brain glucose with normal plasma glucose in salicylate poisoning. J Clin Invest 49:2139–2145, 1970.
   Intraperitoneal injection of salicylate into mice decreased brain glucose by one third. Administration of glucose solutions elevated CNS glucose and increased survival.

8. Heffner JE, Sahn SA: Salicylate-induced pulmonary edema—clinical features and prognosis. Ann Intern Med 95:405, 1983.
   Eight patients in a series of 36 salicylate intoxications presented with noncardiogenic pulmonary edema; 4 required intubation and mechanical ventilation for a mean of 5.8 days; all survived.

9. Hormaechea E, Carlson RW, Rogove H, et al: Hypovolemia, pulmonary edema and protein changes in severe salicylate poisoning. Am J Med 66:1046, 1979.
   Exudative airway fluid and proteinuria suggested increased vascular permeability as the mechanism. Patients treated with crystalloidal fluids deteriorated; those treated with colloidal fluids improved.

10. Anderson RJ, Potts DE, Gabow PA, et al: Unrecognized adult salicylate intoxication. Ann Intern Med 85:745–748, 1976.
    Older patients without a clear history of drug ingestion were admitted with diagnosis of cardiopulmonary disease, encephalopathy, and acid-base disorder for up to 72 hours before the correct diagnosis was made.

11. Done AK: Significance of measurements of salicylate in blood in cases of acute ingestion. Pediatrics 26:800, 1960.

Derivation of the nomogram to predict the severity of an acute intoxication based on serum levels and time after ingestion.

12. Curtis RA, Barone J, Giacona N: Efficacy of ipecac and activated charcoal/cathartic: Prevention of salicylate absorption in a simulated overdose. Arch Intern Med *144*:48, 1984.
    Twelve healthy volunteers ingested aspirin, and the percentage of the total dose excreted in a 48-hour urine collection was recorded. Charcoal/MgSO₄ alone was most effective, with 56% recovered versus 72% for ipecac and 96% in untreated controls.

13. Schreiner GE, Teehan BP: Dialysis of poisons and drugs—annual review. Trans Amer Soc Artif Int Organs *18*:563, 1972.
    Hemodialysis removed salicylate 3–5 times faster than diuresis, 4 times faster than peritoneal dialysis, and 5–7 times faster than normal renal excretion. Indications for the use of dialysis are suggested.

14. Park GD, Spector R, Goldberg MJ, Johnson GF: Expanded role of charcoal therapy in the poisoned and overdosed patient. Arch Intern Med *146*:969, 1986.
    Review of mechanism of action and application of activated charcoal in the poisoned patient.

Beta Blocker Overdose

Edward Agura, M.D.
Robert A. Witzburg, M.D.

Beta adrenergic blocking drugs have come into widespread use throughout the world, and there has been a proportionate increase in the number of overdose cases reported in the literature.[1-7] Although most cases are mild and require only observation, a rapid progression to coma and shock may occur—often within the hour following ingestion.[8] The clinical sequence in cases of severe overdose usually begins with bradycardia and hypotension. Atropine may be effective at this point. However, rapid drug absorption, especially of propranolol, leads to rapidly rising serum levels. The ensuing pump failure and hypotension may be refractory to conventional doses of sympathomimetic drugs, and cardiac pacing may be ineffective.[7] Asystole is usually the terminal event in cases of large overdose.

Propranolol is still the most commonly prescribed beta blocker in the United States and therefore the most likely to be abused. The management of propranolol overdose can be generalized to include all cases involving beta blockers. Propranolol, however, has chemical characteristics, namely high fat solubility, that make it behave differently from other beta blockers and therefore requires special consideration.

Propranolol is a highly lipid soluble nonselective beta blocker that is rapidly absorbed and concentrated in fatty tissues.[14] It has a biologic half-life that far exceeds its serum half-life because of high affinity for the beta adrenergic receptor. This receptor avidity is also responsible for its rapid onset of action. The drug is cleared via hepatic metabolism, but enterohepatic recirculation and the presence of active metabolites prolong the biologic effect.

Although many types of cells possess beta receptors, the principal effect of beta blockade is in the cardiovascular system. The biologic effects of propranolol are mediated by decreases in cellular levels of cyclic AMP, which result in depressed myocardial contractility, decreased automaticity in pacemaker cells, and decreased conduction velocity through the atrioventricular node.[15] In addition, because of the lipid solubility of propranolol, higher doses exert a quinidine-like membrane stabilizing effect; pacemaker calls are thus further suppressed and intraventricular conduction disturbances may occur.[2] Central nervous system manifestations include coma, seizures, myoclonus, and possibly retrograde amnesia.[1,2] Overdoses with other, less lipid soluble beta blockers have not been associated with these central nervous system effects.[5,6,13]

Treatment of propranolol overdose is directed at maximizing drug excretion and minimizing the cardiovascular manifestations. Activated charcoal may be given repeatedly during the first 24 hours to minimize enterohepatic recirculation. A transvenous pacing wire should be inserted in all but the mildest cases because high-degree atrioventricular block and asystole may occur without warning at any time during the first 12 hours following ingestion.[10]

Isoproterenol, a competitive inhibitor acting at the beta receptor, is the first treatment of beta blocker–induced electromechanical dissociation. Several reports have stressed the ineffectiveness of conventional-dose isoproterenol in reversing the beta blockade; indeed, animal studies by Lucchesi[16] performed over 20 years ago demonstrated that a 30–50 fold increase in isoproterenol dose may be needed to produce a given inotropic effect in the face of beta blockade with propranolol.[1,9,12]

In one case,[1] isoproterenol was used at concentrations *10-fold* greater than usual to produce an inotropic response. At this dose, marked peripheral vasodilation occurs, requiring concomitant therapy with volume repletion and conventional doses of the mixed alpha-beta agonist norepinephrine.

Because isoproterenol is rapidly metabolized, it must be given as a continuous infusion, often for extended periods of time. Large doses may be needed: 96 mg over 12 hours in one case, 115 mg over 65 hours in another.[1,12]

Therapy with glucagon appears to be an effective adjunct to isoproterenol in the treatment of beta blocker intoxication. It has been reported that glucagon[9–11] in association with sympathomimetic drugs may be life saving, especially when used early. Glucagon, a polypeptide produced in the alpha cells of the endocrine pancreas, has long been known to act as a cardiac inotrope,[13,14,16] although its mechanism was unknown until fairly recently. Because its effects on the heart appear to mimic those of epinephrine, early theories held that it acted by releasing stored catecholamines[17] or by direct effect on the beta receptor.[18] Subsequent studies revealed that the inotropic properties of glucagon are mediated by activation of adenylate cyclase through a membrane receptor site different from the beta receptor.[16,19]

Intravenous glucagon has potent inotropic and chronotropic properties in humans at doses ranging from 3 to 10 mg and there are several reports of its successful use in beta blocker overdose.[10,11,20] Because of its short half-life (20 minutes), it is usually administered by continuous infusion at 2–5 mg/hour following the initial intravenous bolus. However, Kosinski and colleagues reported a patient who responded to a single 10-mg injection.[9] Thus, glucagon appears to be a useful adjunct in cases of circulatory collapse resulting from beta blocker overdose and its use in such cases should be considered early. Other than occasional nausea and vomiting, its side effects in the recommended dose range appear minimal. Hypoglycemia from depletion of hepatic glycogen stores has not been reported, even during extended infusions.

Phosphodiesterase inhibitors like theophylline may be used with glucagon to prolong or enhance its effect. These drugs act synergistically to elevate intracellular cyclic AMP and produce a sustained elevation of contractile force.[16] In one case, the combined use of aminophylline and glucagon allowed discontinuance of all adrenergic drugs without circulatory compromise.[1] This would be an advantage in patients in whom arrhythmias are present.

In summary, the treatment of massive beta blocker overdose accompanied by circulatory collapse should involve traditional measures first, but should these fail, rapid institution of very high dose isoproterenol and intravenous glucagon may be life saving. Hemodynamic compromise may occur within an hour of the ingestion, and intensive support may be required for periods of 1–2 days. The widespread use of beta blockers, in an ever-expanding variety of clinical circumstances, can only lead to an increasing incidence of life-threatening overdose.[21]

KEY FEATURES

Overingestion with beta blockers may be *rapidly* fatal and requires immediate medical attention.

The initial management should consist of conventional measures:

airway protection and intubation if necessary, establishment of intravenous access, and induced emesis or gastric lavage and charcoal.

Glucagon (10 mg IV) should be given *early* if hemodynamic impairment exists. A continuous infusion (2–5 mg/hour) may be needed in massive cases.

Isoproterenol is used as an adjunct to glucagon. Extremely high doses (>200 μg/minute) may be needed and can be administered by mixing at *five-fold* higher concentrations than normal.

Cardiac pacing may be urgently needed if conduction defects develop but may be ineffective as a result of electromechanical dissociation.

Lipophilic drugs, most commonly propranolol, have the characteristics of rapid absorption, prolonged excretion, and central nervous system accumulation. Myoclonus, seizures, and retrograde amnesia are signs of the last-named effect but do not necessarily indicate irreversible CNS pathology.

REFERENCES

1. Agura ED, Wexler LF, Witzburg RA: Massive propranolol overdose; successful treatment with high-dose isoproterenol and glucagon. Amer J Med 80:755-757, 1987.
    Case report describing a patient with a large acute propranolol overdose. The patient initially failed treatment with conventional doses of sympathomimetic agents but responded to high-dose therapy and supplemental treatment with glucagon. The authors use this case to illustrate the abrupt onset of hemodynamic compromise that may occur with highly lipid soluble beta blockers. This case also illustrates the use of glucagon, and there is discussion of the indications for and difficulties associated with transvenous pacemakers in these patients.

2. Buiumsohn A, Eisenberg ES, Jacob H, Rosen N, Bock J, Frishman WH: Seizures and intraventricular conduction defect in propranolol poisoning—a report of two cases. Ann Intern Med 9:860–862, 1979.
    Case report illustrating the intraventricular conduction defects that may occur as a result of the quinidine-like effects of beta blockers taken in overdose. In addition, the progressive central nervous system effects of lipid soluble beta blockers are illustrated.

3. Halloran TJ, Phillips CE: Propranolol intoxication: A severe case responding to norepinephrine therapy. Arch Intern Med 141:810–811, 1981.
    Report of a case involving hemodynamic and central nervous system effects with propranolol blood levels increased 20-fold above the therapeutic range. The patient failed to respond to conventional doses of isoproterenol and atropine but did respond to a norepinephrine infusion.

4. Kosinski EJ, Stein N, Malindzak GS, Boone E: Glucagon and propranolol toxicity (case report). Br Med J 285:1325, 1971.

5. Moller HJ: Massive intoxication wtih metoprolol (letter). Br Med J 1:222, 1976.

6. Shanahan FLJ, Counihan TB: Atenolol self-poisoning (letter) Br Med J 2:773, 1978.

7. Mattingly PC: Oxyprenolol overdose with survival (letter). Br Med J 1:776–777, 1978.

8. Elkharrat D: Beta adrenergic receptor blockade: A report of 40 cases . . . with 0% mortality. Semin Hop Paris 58:1073–1076, 1982.

9. Kosinski EJ, Malindzak GS: Glucagon and isoproterenol in reversing propranolol toxicity. Arch Intern Med 132:840–843, 1973.
    The hemodynamic properties of glucagon and isoproterenol are compared in anesthetized dogs before and after beta blockade with propranolol. The responses to glucagon

and relatively modest doses of isoproterenol were similar when the drugs were administered prior to beta blockade, but following propranolol administration glucagon enhanced my-ocardial contractility and heart rate to a greater extent than isoproterenol. The authors conclude that glucagon is clinically superior to isoproterenol in reversing the toxic effects of propranolol. No mention is made in this report of blood levels for any of the drugs administered.

10. Ward DE, Jones B: Glucagon and beta blocker toxicity. Br Med J 2:151, 1976.
11. Illingworth RN: Glucagon for beta-blocker poisoning. Practitioner 223:683–685, 1979.
12. Lagerfeet J, Matell G: Attempted suicide with 5.1 g of propranolol, Acta Med Scand 199:517–518, 1976.

A case report of historical interest in that this was a relatively early demonstration of the potentially lethal effects of large doses of lipid soluble beta blockers. This case also illustrates the occurrence of electromechanical dissociation even in patients with functioning transvenous pacemakers. This patient required combination therapy with a transvenous pacemaker and high-dose isoproterenol infusion, ultimately receiving more than 100 mg of isoproterenol over a 65-hour period.

13. Karhunen P, Hartel G: Suicidal attempt with practolol. Br Med J 2:178–179, 1973.

An early case report of an intentional overdose with a short-acting beta blocker. This case illustrates the high therapeutic index for these drugs, wtih the patient surviving blood levels 40–60 times the therapeutic range.

14. Frishman WH: Clinical pharmacology of the new beta-adrenergic blocking drugs. I. Pharmacodynamic and pharmacokinetic properties. Am Heart J 97:663–671, 1979.

A thorough review of the pharmacology of first-generation beta blockers.

15. Whitsitt LS, Lucchesi BR: Effects of beta receptor blockade and glucagon on the atrioventricular transmission system in the dog. Circ Res 23:585, 1968.

A study of the effects of propranolol and two analogues on the functional refractory period and atrioventricular conduction velocity in anesthetized dogs. The studies illustrate the beta receptors–mediated effect of propranolol, as well as an additional membrane stabilizing effect at very high doses. Small doses of glucagon were shown to reverse the cardiodepressant effects of propranolol at levels refractory to large doses of isoproterenol. The authors allude to evidence that glucagon and cardioactive catecholomines exert their stimulatory actions through differential effects on the activation of adenyl cyclase with the consequent formation of cyclic AMP.

16. Lucchesi BR: Cardiac actions of glucagon. Circ Res 22:777, 1968.

A description of glucagon effect on heart rate and contractile force in the anesthetized dog. In addition, studies of glucagon in isolated dog papillary muscle are reviewed. Glucagon increased heart rate and contractile force as well as isometric tension. Neither inotropic nor chronotropic responses to glucagon were altered by prior administration of propranolol. Pretreatment with tyramine reduced the glucagon-induced positive inotropic response, as did administration of theophylline. The studies suggest that glucagon and the catecholamines share a common mechanism of action mediated through an increase in the intracellular concentration of cyclic AMP.

17. Whitehouse FW, James TN: Chronotropic action of glucagon on the sinus node. Proc Soc Exp Biol Med 122:823, 1966.
18. Regan TJ, Lehan PH, Henneman DH, Behar A, Hellems HK: Myocardial metabolic and contractile response to glucagon and epinephrine. J Lab Clin Med 63:638, 1964.

An early study of the metabolic and contractile response to glucagon and catecholamines, suggesting erroneously that glucagon acted through direct stimulation of cardiac sympathetic nerve input or by direct effect on catecholamine receptors.

19. Levey GS, Epstein SE: Activation of adenylcyclase by glucagon in cat and human heart. Circ Res 24:151, 1979.
20. Parmley WW, Glick G, Sonnenblick EH: Cardiovascular effects of glucagon in man. N. Engl J Med 279:12, 1968.
    A summary of early human cardiac catheterization data demonstrating the effect of glucagon. In eleven patients, 3–5 mg glucagon administered intravenously resulted in increased cardiac index, mean arterial pressure, heart rate, and maximum rate of increase in left ventricular pressure. Left ventricular end-diastolic pressure and systemic vascular resistance did not change. Onset of action for intravenous glucagon was 1–3 minutes; the hemodynamic effects peaked at 5–7 minutes after administration and lasted for 10–15 minutes after a single bolus injection.

21. Ehgartner GR, Zelinka MA: Hemodynamic instability following intentional nadolol overdose. Arch Intern Med 148:801–802, 1988.
    Case report involving a long-acting beta blocker with a half-life of 20–24 hours.

Theophylline

Don L. Stromquist, M.D.

Theophylline toxicity may occur accidentally in the treatment of obstructive lung disease or as a result of intentional overdose. Iatrogenic overdose may be avoided by use of available dosing guidelines and serum drug level monitoring.[1]

Orally administered theophylline is rapidly and completely absorbed. Commonly used sustained-release preparations may continue to release theophylline for 6–24 hours after ingestion. Theophylline is metabolized almost entirely by the liver, 10% of a dose being excreted unchanged in the urine. Serum half-life of theophylline averages 6–9 hours in healthy nonsmoking adults. Half-life is significantly shorter in smokers and in children. Congestive heart failure or liver disease may markedly prolong serum half-life, with average values of 24 hours reported in patients with each disease and half-lives as high as 60–80 hours reported in some cases. Elimination of theophylline may be slower at toxic serum levels than at therapeutic levels.[1]

Therapeutic theophylline serum levels are generally considered to lie between 10–20 µg/ml, but the frequency of side effects begins to rise at 15 µg/ml. The most common adverse effects of theophylline are nausea, vomiting, and anorexia.

Life-threatening toxic effects of theophylline are seizures, cardiac arrhythmias, and hypotension. It must be emphasized that nausea and vomiting do not reliably precede serious toxicity. Frequency of serious side effects generally increases with rising serum levels, but individual responses to the drug vary widely. Susceptibility to theophylline toxicity appears to increase with age.

Theophylline-induced seizures may be persistent and refractory to therapy. Seizures are usually generalized but may be focal. Status epilepticus may occur. Seizures are generally associated with high theophylline levels but have been reported with levels as low as 25 μg/ml. Death follows theophylline-induced seizures in a high percentage of cases. Other central nervous system toxicity includes restlessness, irritability, agitation, and obtundation.[2-5]

Cardiac rhythm disturbances include sinus tachycardia, atrial premature contractions, atrial fibrillation, atrial flutter, multifocal atrial tachycardia, supraventricular tachycardia, ventricular premature contractions, ventricular fibrillation, and asystole. Arrhythmias and hypotension tend to occur at high serum levels.[3-5]

Acute oral theophylline overdose should be treated initially with activated charcoal administered orally or per nasogastric tube. Gastric lavage is helpful only for very recent ingestion, and ipecac delays or precludes definitive therapy with charcoal and is not recommended. Repeated doses of charcoal reduce the half-life of theophylline.[9] Patients with very high levels will often not tolerate oral charcoal and should undergo hemoperfusion.[4] If ingestion of a sustained-release preparation is suspected, gastric emptying should be considered up to 6–8 hours following overdose and repeated doses of charcoal for 8–24 hours or more may be useful.[4,6]

Seizures should be treated with intravenous diazepam, phenytoin, or phenobarbital. Cardiac arrhythmias should be treated with specific drugs. Hypotension may require pressor agents.

Clearance of theophylline from serum is increased several fold by charcoal column hemoperfusion. Controversy surrounds indications for hemoperfusion in theophylline overdose. Seizures, arrhythmias, or hypotension, if refractory to conventional treatment, is a definite indication for hemoperfusion. Some sources recommend hemoperfusion in any instance in which levels exceed 50–60 μg/ml and at levels as low as 30 μg/ml in the presence of liver disease, congestive heart failure, or old age.[4] The fact that life-threatening adverse effects may occur without premonitory symptoms supports this view. Other sources suggest that hemoperfusion be reserved for treatment of intractable complications alone.[5] Serial serum drug levels should be obtained in any case, because continued absorption of sustained-release theophyllines may lead to persistently high levels. Drug levels may paradoxically increase after hemoperfusion is stopped.[7] Activated charcoal given orally has been reported to hasten the clearance of an intravenous dose of theophylline, and may thus be beneficial in treatment of parenteral theophylline overdose.[4] Hemodialysis adds little to the treatment of theophylline toxicity, producing a theophylline clearance about one third to one half that of a normal adult.[8]

KEY FEATURES

Chief toxic effects of theophylline are nausea, vomiting, anorexia, seizures, cardiac arrhythmias, and hypotension.

Serious side effects may be the first sign of toxicity and are not always preceded by nausea and vomiting.

Theophylline is metabolized by the liver. Average half-life is 6–9 hours; it may be shorter in smokers and prolonged in congestive heart failure, liver disease, and old age. Sustained-release preparations may release theophylline for prolonged periods.

Treatment of theophylline toxicity should include supportive care and specific drugs for seizures and cardiac arrhythmias. Serial drug levels should be followed.

Charcoal column hemoperfusion can increase theophylline clearance dramatically and should be used in cases of intractable seizures, arrhythmias, and hypotension. It should also be considered in cases of high serum drug levels, liver disease, or congestive heart failure.

REFERENCES

1. VanDellen RG: Theophylline: Practical application of new knowledge. Mayo Clinic Proc 54:733, 1979.
   Comprehensive review of all aspects of theophylline therapy.

2. Zwillich CW, et al: Theophylline-induced seizures in adults. Ann Intern Med 82:784, 1975.
   Eight cases of seizures during theophylline therapy. Four patients died; one seizure occurred with theophylline serum level of 25 μg/ml. Comparison with patients with minor or no side effects.

3. Helliwell M and Berry D. Theophylline poisoning in adults. Br Med J 2:1114, 1979.
   Nine cases of theophylline toxicity with several cardiac arrhythmias and three seizures. All three patients with seizures died.

4. Park GD, et al: Use of hemoperfusion for treatment of theophylline intoxication. Am J Med 74:961, 1983.
   Thirty-six patients with theophylline levels greater than 30 μg/ml, of which six where treated with hemoperfusion. Indications for hemoperfusion are suggested.

5. Greenberg A, et al: Severe theophylline toxicity: Role of conservative measures, antiarrhythmic agents, and charcoal hemoperfusion. Am J Med 76:854, 1984.
   Ten patients with severe theophylline toxicity, all of whom recovered. Limited role suggested for hemoperfusion.

6. Sintek C, Hendeles L, Weinberger M: Inhibition of theophylline absorption by activated charcoal. J Pediatr 94:314, 1979.

Oral activated charcoal significantly decreased absorption of an oral dose of theophylline.

7. Connell JMC, et al: Self-poisoning with sustained-release aminophylline: Secondary rise in serum theophylline concentration after charcoal haemoperfusion. Br Med J 284:943, 1982.
8. Levy G, et al: Hemodialysis clearance of theophylline. JAMA 237:1466, 1977.
   Report of several measurements made in one patient.

9. Sessler CN, Glauser FL, Cooper KR: Treatment of theophylline toxicity with oral activated charcoal. Chest 87:325, 1985.
   Clinical series of 14 patients with theophylline overdose treated with repeated oral activated charcoal (30 gm every 2 hours for 2–4 doses). Substantial reduction in theophylline half-life for those who tolerated the therapy. Those with the highest levels vomited the charcoal and underwent hemoperfusion.

Cocaine Poisoning

Carol M. Meils, M.D.

Cocaine poisoning has increased recently; fatalities are common. Data from the U.S. National Institute on Drug Abuse point to a 91% increase in cocaine-related deaths between 1980 and 1983. The goal of this article is to review briefly the pharmacokinetics of cocaine and management of the patient presenting with cocaine poisoning.

Cocaine is an alkaloid that occurs naturally in a concentration of approximately 1% in leaves of *Erythroxylon coca,* a tree indigenous to Peru and Bolivia. The chewing of coca leaves for the effect of reducing hunger and increasing work tolerance and resistance to cold as well as for the stimulating effect on the CNS has been common practice among the populations of the Andes mountain regions of South America for many centuries. The use of coca leaves is still widespread in South America.

The past decade has seen an increase in the use of cocaine in both the United States and other countries.[22] Cocaine was introduced in Coca-Cola in 1886. In 1906, the formulation of this beverage was changed to utilize decocainized leaves. As late as 1909, a supply of cocaine-containing Coca-Cola was seized by the Federal Government. Cocaine is legally classified in the United States as a Schedule II drug ("high abuse potential with small recognized medical use"). It is estimated that cocaine sales in this country exceed $30 billion dollars a year and that cocaine-related deaths and emergency department visits have increased 200% over the past ten years, with admissions to government treatment programs increasing 500% over the same period. Some authorities are talking now of a cocaine epidemic because the use of the drug seems to be rising steadily and the pattern of use changing.[2,22] For example, nasal inhalation of cocaine or chewing of coca leaves seldom leads to addiction, whereas smoking or injecting the drug commonly does so.[2] Alkaloidal cocaine (crack or freebase) is now widely sold in the United States in a form that is suitable for smoking. Epidemic use has been reported, and overdose is frequent because of the purity of the drug, 90% vs. 20% in the powdered form of the HCl salt.

Cocaine actions depend largely on the site and route of administration. After intranasal application, peak serum levels are reached in 15–60 minutes and the drug can be detected for 4–6 hours in the plasma and on the nasal mucosa for 3 hours.[3] Serum half-life after nasal application is approximately 1 hour. Approximately 60% of the total dose is absorbed after snorting cocaine. Most of the deaths reported to date have been out of hospital sudden death in the so-called body packers, who attempt to smuggle drugs into the country in their GI tracts, or as the result of massive IV injections.[4–8] Only about 30% of an oral dose is absorbed because it is hydrolyzed in the stomach before absorption can occur. Peak serum levels are reached in 60–90 minutes. A lethal oral dose is approximately 1 gm. When the cocaine is administered IV or smoked (freebasing), absorption is 100% and peak serum levels are reached in 3–5 minutes. A lethal IV dose is approximately 20 mg.

The metabolism of cocaine is not fully understood. It is metabolized in the liver and by serum esterases to benzoylecgonine, ecgonine, norbenzoylecgonine, and norecgonine.[9] A portion of the drug passes unchanged into the urine along with the metabolic products. Cocaine has been shown to block reuptake of norepinephrine and epinephrine into nerve endings, thus increasing their availability to adrenergic receptors. It also blocks reuptake of central dopamine. This is thought to account for its sympathomimetic effect on the heart as well as for many of the neurologic disturbances, including seizures.

The clinical manifestations of cocaine overdose in humans are multisystemic and are reflections of the dramatically increased sympathetic drive and vasospasm. Cocaine intoxication and sudden death have been reported in both recreational users of the drug[6,11,21] and body packers.[7] Reported experiments suggest that seizures are a major determinant of lethality in the conscious dog model.[10] In all dogs infused with cocaine, prolonged generalized seizures developed that led to lactic acidosis and hyperthermia prior to death.

Cocaine stimulates the CNS at a number of levels. The first manifestations in humans are euphoria, restlessness, and excitement. There is some evidence that perceptual awareness and cognitive speed are increased. There may also be an increased capacity for muscular work secondary to decreased fatigue. There is evidence that repetitive administration of CNS stimulants and other compounds may be associated with progressively increasing effects on pathologic behavior and seizures rather than with development of tolerance,[12] thus putting the chronic user at increased risk for seizures. The vasomotor and vomiting centers also share in early stimulation, and sweating and vomiting occur commonly. In acute overdose, especially with the rapid onset of action experienced after administration by the IV route or by smoking, the patient may be confused and agitated and suffer paranoid delusions. Hyperreflexia is common, and tonic-clonic seizures may supervene. Hyperthermia is thought to be secondary to a central effect on the heat-regulating center in the diencephalon, compounded by intense vasoconstriction, increased muscular activity, and reduced heat radiation. Fatal pulmonary edema has been described following intravenous use.[13] The action of cocaine on the medulla results in an initial increase in rate and depth of respiration that progressively deteriorates to a rapid shallow pattern, Cheyne-Stokes breathing, and then full respiratory arrest. Fatal respiratory collapse can occur suddenly and without warning.[21]

Sudden death as a result of cardiotoxicity is thought to be due to several mechanisms. Coronary vasospasm can lead to severe ischemia and contraction band necrosis.[20] Ventricular fibrillation can occur secondary to ischemia or may be related to increased adrenergic drive. One study reported clinical and pathologic findings in seven individuals in whom nonintravenous use of cocaine was temporally related to acute myocardial infarction, ventricular tachycardia, and sudden death.[1] The authors also reviewed 19 previously reported cases of cocaine-related cardiovascular disorders. They concluded that the cardiac consequences of cocaine abuse are not unique to parenteral use; underlying heart disease is not a prerequisite to cocaine-related cardiac disorders; and the cardiac consequences are not limited to massive doses of the drug. Possible mechanisms responsible for cocaine-related cardiac toxicity include ischemia secondary to increased myocardial oxygen demand from the increased rate pressure product; however, there is little clinical support for the concept that a discrete myocardial infarction can result solely from an enhanced sympathomimetic state. The other possibility is disturbance in myocardial oxygen supply secondary to the marked vasoconstrictor effect of cocaine. Although the actual pathogenetic mechanism has not been well characterized, it is clear that cocaine can precipitate a cardiac event in persons with no predisposing constitutional factors. Even small doses of cocaine (25 mg) absorbed systemically cause an increase in pulse (20–40% above normal) and blood pressure (15–20% above normal).[14] An initial slowing of the pulse following higher-dose cocaine intoxication results from vagal effects. Hypertensive crisis can occur. Renal infarction has been described, associated with a pre-existing thrombus and mild hypertension (150/100).[15] Intestinal ischemia with necrosis necessitating bowel resection has been reported following cocaine ingestion.[16]

The mainstay of treatment is supportive care with the goal of controlling life-threatening arrhythmias, seizures, hypertension, hyperthermia, and acid-base imbalances. The possibility of a polydrug overdose must always be considered and a cocktail of thiamine, 50% dextrose in water (D50), and naloxone should be given initially. In dogs, pretreatment with diazepam prevents hyperthermia, acidemia, and moderate changes in cardiovascular parameters.[10] Parenteral diazepam is the drug of choice to control seizures acutely in humans. The treatment of the cardiovascular complications of cocaine intoxication remains controversial. Propranolol 1 mg IV over one minute up to a total of 6 mg at one-hour intervals has been used; however, there is some evidence that this is potentially dangerous, in that it selectively blocks beta receptors and leaves alpha receptors unopposed with resultant worsening hypertension.[17,18] In animal studies, pretreatment with propranolol prior to a lethal cocaine challenge modified the cardiovascular changes; however, all animals convulsed and died.[10] Lidocaine is recommended for life-threatening ventricular arrhythmias but must be used with caution because it lowers seizure threshold. Severe hypertension is best treated with sodium nitroprusside. Severe hypotension should be treated with crystalloid infusion and pressors. Either norepinephrine or dopamine is an appropriate choice.[19] In animals, pretreatment with chlorpromazine antagonized all responses induced by a potentially lethal cocaine dose;[10] however, in clinical situations the use of phenothiazines (especially chlorpromazine) and the butyrophenone haloperidol has been avoided, owing to their propensity to lower the seizure threshold. Animal study data have demonstrated protective effects of a still experimental calcium channel blocker.

The use of cocaine is increasing to epidemic proportions, and overdose is becoming a frequent occurrence because of the increased purity of the drug and its suitabilty for smoking and IV use. Management of cocaine intoxication requires prompt recognition and aggressive early support; determination of the intervention of choice for certain toxic effects of cocaine awaits further research.

KEY FEATURES

The pattern of cocaine use is changing as a result of increased availability, decreased unit price, and the prominence of freebasing with its greater addictive potential.

Cocaine actions depend on site and route of administration:

Route	Peak Level (minutes)	% Absorption
Intranasal	15–60	60
Oral	60–90	30
IV/smoking	3–5	100

Cocaine is metabolized in the liver and by serum esterases.

Its mechanism of action is to block reuptake of norepinephrine and epinephrine into nerve endings, thus increasing their availability to adrenergic receptors. It also blocks reuptake of central dopamine.

Clinical manifestations are multisystemic and reflect increased sympathetic drive and vasospasm. Reported complications include myocardial infarction, mesenteric ischemia, seizures, pulmonary edema, hyperthermia, renal infarction, and ventricular arrhythmias.

Treatment is supportive, with the goal of controlling life-threatening arrhythmias and seizures:

1. Thiamine, D50, and naloxone for altered mental status.

2. Diazepam to control seizures acutely.

3. Lidocaine for life-threatening ventricular arrhythmias.

4. The role of propranolol is controversial. It may block cardiovascular changes, but it is potentially dangerous because it selectively blocks beta receptors leaving alpha receptors unopposed.

5. Severe hypertension should be treated with sodium nitroprusside.

6. Severe hypotension should be treated with crystalloid infusion and pressors (dopamine, norepinephrine).

7. Chlorpromazine has a general protective effect but carries the theoretic risk of enhanced likelihood of seizures.

8. Calcium channel blockers have demonstrated protective effects in animal studies.

REFERENCES

1. Isner JM, Estes M, Thompson PD, Nordin MRC, Subaramanian R, Miller G, Katsas G, Sweeney K, Sturner W: Acute cardiac events temporally related to cocaine abuse. N Engl J Med 315:1438–1443, 1986.

    A report of the clinical and pathologic findings in seven people in whom nonintravenous use of cocaine was temporally related to acute cardiac events. The authors also reviewed data on 19 previously reported cases of cocaine-related cardiac events.

2. Kieber HD, Gawin FH: The spectrum of cocaine abuse and its treatment. J Clin Psychiat 45:18–21, 1984.

    A review of the changing patterns of cocaine abuse and rehabilitation.

3. Jeveid JL, Fishman MW, Schuster CR, Dekirmmenjian H, Davis JM: Cocaine plasma

concentrations. Relation to physiological and subjective effects in humans. Science 202:227–228, 1978.

Volunteers with a previous history of cocaine use were administered cocaine IV or intranasally. There was a positive relationship among peak plasma concentrations, physiologic and subjective responses, and dose administered. After intranasal use, drug levels remained elevated for a considerably longer period.

4. Bettinger J: Cocaine intoxication: Massive oral overdose. Ann Emerg Med 9(8):429–430, 1980.

    Case report of a young man presenting with new-onset seizures and development of status epilepticus secondary to rupture in his GI tract of condoms filled with cocaine.

5. Fishbain DA, Welti CV: Cocaine intoxication, delirium and death in a body packer. Ann Emerg Med 10(10):531– 532, 1981.

    Case report of acute cocaine delirium in a body packer who presented with delirium.

6. Mittleman RE, Welti CV: Death caused by recreational cocaine use. an update. JAMA 252(14): 1889–1893, 1984.

    The epidemiologic, pathologic, and toxicologic findings of 60 cocaine-related deaths from mid-1978 to 1982 were reviewed. In addition, 180 deaths in which cocaine was an incidental toxicologic finding are discussed.

7. McCarron MM, Wood JD: The cocaine body packer syndrome. Diagnosis and treatment. JAMA 250(11):1417–20, 1983.

    Report of 47 patients treated successfully with medical treatment (cathartics) and 1 patient who required surgery to remove packages obstructing the small bowel.

8. Suarez CA, Arango A, Lester JL III: Cocaine condom ingestion. Surgical treatment. JAMA 238(13):1391–1392, 1977.

    Report of one survivor and two deaths from cocaine toxicity after cocaine was packaged in condoms and deliberately ingested to avoid detection by customs officials. Surgical removal of all packages is recommended in this report.

9. Stewart DJ, Inaba T, Lucassen M, Kalow W: Cocaine metabolism, cocaine and norcocaine hydrolysis by liver and serum esterases. Clin Pharmacol Therapeut 25:464–468, 1979.

    A thorough review of cocaine metabolism.

10. Catravas JD, Waters IW: Acute cocaine intoxication in the conscious dog: Studies on the mechanism of lethality. J Pharmacol Exp Ther 217(2):350–356, 1981.

    All animals exhibited hypertension, tachycardia, increased cardiac output, hyperthermia, and acidemia when administered a lethal dose of cocaine. Chlorpromazine pretreatment antagonized all responses, and all animals survived 48 hours. Propranolol blocked the cardiovascular response, but all animals convulsed and died. Pancuronium prevented acidemia and hyperthermia—all animals survived. Diazepam prevented hyperthermia and acidemia. Authors concluded that hyperthermia is the most important contributor to death in cocaine overdose.

11. Welti CV, Wright RK: Death caused by recreational cocaine use. JAMA 241:2519–2522, 1979.

    Sixty-eight deaths associated with the recreational use of cocaine were investigated by the Medical Examiner's Office of Dade County, Florida. Twenty-four people died directly from the toxic effects of cocaine.

12. Post RM, Kopanda RT: Cocaine kindling and psychosis. Am J Psychiat 133(6):627–634, 1976.

    Evidence is reviewed that indicates that repetitive administration of CNS stimulants and other compounds may be associated with progressively increasing effects on pathologic behavior and seizures rather than with tolerance.

13. Alfred RJ, Ewer S: Fatal pulmonary edema following intravenous "freebase" cocaine use. Ann Emerg Med 10(8):441–442, 1981.
    A 35-year-old man developed extreme shortness of breath after injecting freebase cocaine. Clinical and radiographic evaluation confirmed acute pulmonary edema. The patient died 3 hours after admission.

14. Moore DC: Complications of regional anesthesia. *In* Bonican JJ (ed): Regional Anesthesia. Philadelphia, WB Saunders, 1969, pp 217–253.
    Discussion of complications seen with use of cocaine as a regional anesthetic.

15. Shaff JA: Renal infarction associated with IV cocaine use. Ann Emerg Med 13(12):1145–1147, 1984.
    A documented case of renal infarction from IV cocaine use. The authors postulate that increased adrenergic stimulation with a pre-existing arterial thrombus led to infarction.

16. Nalbandian H, Sheth N, Dietrich R, Georgiou J: Intestinal ischemia caused by cocaine ingestion: Report of two cases. Surgery 97(3):374–376, 1985.
    Two cocaine addicts who ingested large quantities of the drug developed severe abdominal symptoms and signs caused by bowel ischemia. In one patient, gangrene of the bowel necessitated repeated resections, and he eventually died. The second person suffered less severe ischemia, and the bowel returned to normal.

17. Ramoska E, Sacchetti AD: Propranolol-induced hypertension in treatment of cocaine intoxication. Ann Emerg Med 14(1):1112–1115, 1985.
    Case report of apparent cocaine toxicity and drug-mediated hypertension and tachycardia. IV propranolol was used as initial treatment, resulting in a decreased heart rate but a paroxysmal increase in blood pressure.

18. Rappolt RT Sr, Gay GR, Inaba DS, Rappolt RT Jr: Use of inderal (propranolol—Ayerst) in Ia (early stimulative) and Ib (advanced stimulative) classification of cocaine and other sympathomimetic reactions. Clin Toxicol 13(2):325–332, 1978.
    Use of propranolol in I-a and I-b classifications of cocaine and other sympathomimetic reactions.

19. Gay GR: Clinical management of acute and chronic cocaine poisoning. Ann Emerg Med 11(10):562–572, 1982.
    Review of the physiologic and pharmacologic mechanisms responsible for cocaine intoxication. The treatment strategies used at the Haight-Ashbury Free Medical Clinics are outlined.

20. Howard RE, Hueter DC, Davis GJ: Acute myocardial infarction following cocaine abuse in a young woman with normal coronary arteries. JAMA 254:95–96, 1985.
    Report of a 28-year-old cocaine addict who presented with dyspnea and chest pain after inhalation of 1.5 gm cocaine over 5 hours. The patient initially manifested ST segment elevation on ECG; a positive MB fraction of CPK (9% of 1355) returned 12 hours after admission.

21. Welti CV, Fishbain DA: Cocaine induced psychosis and sudden death in recreational cocaine users. J Forensic Sci 30(3):873–880, 1985.
    The presentation of seven recreational cocaine users who presented with acute intense paranoia is discussed. Fatal respiratory collapse occurred without warning. Five of the seven died while in police custody.

22. Jekel JF, Podelwski H, Patterson SD, Allen DF, Clark N, Cartwright P: Epidemic free-base cocaine abuse. Lancet 1:459–462, 1986.

Report of a sharp increase in the use of freebase cocaine in the Bahamas. The pattern of drug abuse and its relation to the type of cocaine used are discussed. Authors conclude that the medical epidemic of cocaine-related physical and psychological problems was related to both the increased availability of cheap cocaine and a switch from powder to freebase.

SECTION 11

MISCELLANEOUS DISORDERS

Hypothermia

Robert A. Witzburg, M.D.

Hypothermia, a frequently unrecognized disorder of temperature regulation, may threaten life, mask or mimic other diagnoses, and complicate management of other illnesses. Although the true incidence of hypothermia, defined as a core temperature less than 35° C (95° F), is unknown, it is an increasingly common clinical problem in the United States, presumably owing to changing social conditions as well as increased awareness in the medical community.[1,2]

The diagnosis of hypothermia may be elusive; the syndrome may occur in a host of clinical settings, and the standard clinical thermometer, not calibrated below 34° C, is clearly inadequate. Accidental hypothermia is most commonly seen in neonates, the elderly, and in the intoxicated or injured patient.[4] It is important to note that extreme environmental conditions are not required to produce hypothermia. Any situation in which body heat production fails to match heat loss by mechanisms of convection, conduction, and radiation will cause core temperature to fall. The combination of wet clothing and wind exposure, for example, may cause a twenty- to thirtyfold increase in the rate of heat loss to the environment, overwhelming compensatory mechanisms even in the normal host.[11] Depressed body temperature may be a feature of various endocrinologic disorders, including myxedema, hypoglycemia, hypothalamic-pituitary dysfunction, and hypoadrenalism. Disorders of the central nervous system, most commonly tumor, Wernicke's encephalopathy, trauma, and cerebrovascular disease, have been associated with hypothermia. Exposure to ethanol, barbiturates, phenothiazines, and general anesthetics may cause or potentiate hypothermia. Extensive destruction of the dermis, malnutrition, and sepsis are associated with disturbances of temperature regulation.

Falling body temperature alters essentially every bodily function, and the ultimate clinical presentation reflects a graded response to the degree of hypothermia. The basal metabolic rate falls to 50% of normal at 28° C, with an associated decrease in CO_2 production and a change in the respiratory quotient. Hypotension, although common, is rarely significant at temperatures above 28° C.[1] A progression of electrocardiographic abnormalities may be seen, including sinus bradycardia and T wave inversions, interval prolongation, J (Osborne) waves, and atrial flutter or fibrillation, followed by asystole or ventricular fibrillation at temperatures below 28° C.[5,11] Mild hypothermia with decreasing mentation, impaired cough reflex, and bronchorrhea may cause aspiration and significant pulmonary dysfunction, even though respiratory depression does not occur until body temperature is below 30° C. Acid-base abnormalities may be complex and may evolve rapidly, and interpretation of blood gas and pH measurements may require adjustment for body temperature.[1,6,15] Depressed renal tubular oxidative activity and reduced hypothalamic secretion of antidiuretic hormone with consequent reduction in sodium and water reabsorption cause a "cold diuresis" that, in combination with plasma loss, may render the patient profoundly hypovolemic and hemoconcentrated. Splenic sequestration may cause leukopenia and thrombocytopenia, and disseminated intravascular coagulation has been described. Inhibition of both insulin release and peripheral glucose uptake may cause hyperglycemia. Impaired mentation, common in mild hypothermia, may progress to virtual cessation of brain function, with electrocerebral silence occurring at 20° C.[9]

Mild hypothermia (temperature above 32° C) may be managed conservatively, with passive rewarming and a leisurely approach to differential diagnosis. Moderate to severe hypothermia, however, is associated with a 30–80% mortality rate and requires more aggressive intervention.[7,9,12] Treatment takes the form of general supportive care combined with specific rewarming techniques. Although there is considerable controversy, most recent literature advocates rapid active internal rewarming, utilizing warmed intravenous solutions, warm gastrointestinal and urinary bladder lavage, warmed respiratory gases, extracorporeal blood rewarming, peritoneal dialysis or hemodialysis, or even mediastinal irrigation.[7,8,10,11,13] One recent report suggests that magnetic loop induction hyperthermia using radio frequency, electromagnetic radiation may provide enhanced deep tissue rewarming.[14] Associated conditions, such as myxedema or adrenal insufficiency may require emergent therapy, and infectious complications may develop within the first 24–48 hours. Frostbite, pancreatitis, tissue infarctions, and adult respiratory distress syndrome are not uncommon events, and disseminated intravascular coagulation may occur up to several days after rewarming. Despite the severe consequences of deep hypothermia, among aggressively managed patients the outcome is more closely related to the presence of underlying or predisposing disease rather than to the degree of hypothermia.[3] A well-coordinated, interdisciplinary management approach may well be rewarded by full recovery.[8–11]

KEY FEATURES

Hypothermia is a frequently unrecognized complicating feature of many illnesses.

Clinical phases are as follows:

1. Mild: 33°–35° C (91°–94° F)

2. Moderate: 29°–32.5° C (84°–90° F)

3. Severe: <29° C (<84° F)

General supportive therapy should include the following:

1. ICU monitoring for moderate/severe or complicated hypothermia

2. Volume resuscitation

3. Metabolic correction

4. Treatment of tissue injury

5. Treatment of suspected sepsis

6. Treatment of suspected endocrinopathy

Active core rewarming techniques may include these interventions:

1. Warmed respiratory gas (42°–46° C)

2. Warmed IV solutions (≤40° C)

3. Warm GI and urinary bladder irrigation

4. Peritoneal dialysis (42°–46° C at entry point)

5. Hemodialysis

6. Mediastinal irrigation

7. Pleural space irrigation

REFERENCES

1. Reuler JB: Hypothermia: Pathophysiology, clinical settings, and management. Ann Intern Med 89:519, 1978.

   A systematic review of the topic with emphasis on clinical evaluation, differential diagnosis, and the choice of appropriate treatment modalities. Effects of body temperature on arterial blood gases are as follows:

	↑ 1° C*†	↓ 1° C*†
pH	↓ 0.015	↑ 0.015
P_{CO_2} (mmHg)	↑ 4.4	↓ 4.4
P_{O_2} (mmHg)	↑ 7.2	↓ 7.2

*Change with reference to 37° C.
†Per cent change of the value measured at standard 37° C.

2. Vandam LD, Burnap TK: Hypothermia. N Engl J Med 261:546, 595, 1959.
   Historical perspective.

3. Weyman AE, Greenbaum DM, Grace WJ: Accidental hypothermia in an alcoholic population. Am J Med 56:13, 1974.
   A review of 39 cases of accidental hypothermia. Mortality was dependent of the degree of hypothermia but correlated strongly with the presence of any other primary disorder.

4. Horvath SM, Rochelle RD: Hypothermia in the aged. Environ Health Persp 20:127, 1977.
   A discussion of the special problems in temperature regulation and accidental hypothermia among the elderly.

5. Trevino A, et al: The characteristic electrocardiogram of accidental hypothermia. Arch Intern Med 127:470, 1971.
   A case presentation followed by a review of the electrocardiographic findings that may be encountered at various levels of hypothermia.

6. Dula DJ: Interpreting blood gases of hypothermic patients (letter). Ann Emerg Med 9:232, 1980.
7. Marcus P: The treatment of acute accidental hypothermia: Proceedings of a symposium held at the RAF Institute of Aviation Medicine. Aviat Space Environ Med 50:823, 1979.
   Stresses the importance of a careful search for co-factors that may potentiate the physiologic effects of cold exposure, and the use of active internal warming.

8. Ledingham I, Mone JG: Treatment of accidental hypothermia: A prospective clinical study. Br Med J 280:1102, 1980.
   A 15-year study involving 44 patients with core temperatures ranging from 20° to 34° C. Mortality (12 of 44 patients) was attributable to intercurrent illness. Active internal rewarming is advocated for profound hypothermia or cases complicated by ventricular fibrillation.

9. Meriwether WD, Goodman RM: Severe accidental hypothermia with survival after rapid rewarming. Am J Med 53:505, 1972.
   Case report and review of the literature. These authors stress the importance of rapid rewarming in the management of hypothermia complications.

10. Sekar TS, et al: Survival after prolonged submersion in cold water without neurologic sequelae. Arch Intern Med 140:775, 1980.
    Report on two cases, speculating that the metabolic effects of cold exposure may protect critical tissues from injury.

11. Southwick FS, Dalglish PH: Recovery after prolonged asystolic cardiac arrest in profound hypothermia. JAMA 243:1250, 1980.
    Prolonged asystole, a common event when core temperature is below 28° C, may not represent irreversible cardiac injury if adequate cardiopulmonary support and active rewarming can be achieved. The authors suggest that asystole is a primary manifestation of hypothermia, whereas ventricular fibrillation may be secondary complication of resuscitation, precipitated by hypocapnic alkalosis, physical manipulation of the heart, and abrupt temperature changes.

12. Milner JE: Hypothermia. Ann Intern Med 89:565, 1978.
    Editorial review and comment.

13. Zell SC, Kurtz KJ: Severe exposure hypothermia: A resuscitation protocol. Ann Emerg Med 14:4, 1985.
    Specific clinical guidelines for management of severely ill hypothermia patients.

14. White JD, et al: Rewarming in accidental hypothermia: Radio wave versus inhalation therapy. Ann Emerg Med 16:50, 1987.
   Anesthetized dogs were cooled by refrigeration to a core temperature of 25° C and then rewarmed with warmed inhalation or radio frequency induction hyperthermia. The latter technique produced more rapid rewarming, and all dogs survived without sequelae.

15. Swain JA: Hypothermia and blood pH: A review. Arch Intern Med 148:1643–1646, 1988.
   A discussion of the physiologic basis for and clinical management of deleterious effects related to hypothermia-induced changes in blood pH.

Toxic Epidermal Necrolysis

Michael Rosenbaum, M.D.

Toxic epidermal necrolysis (TEN) is an acute and life-threatening mucocutaneous syndrome.[1,6] Its clinical course is initated by a prodromal phase characterized by fever, skin tenderness, and a burning sensation of the eyes and oral mucosa followed within 24 hours by a blotchy erythematous-violaceous macular rash that quickly becomes generalized and confluent. As the entire thickness of epidermis becomes necrotic, it loses its attachment to the dermis and fluid fills the potential space at the dermal-epidermal junction. Clinically apparent flaccid bullae may develop in some areas. In other areas, the "floating"epidermis tears off in large sheets, somewhat like wet tissue paper, leaving patches of exposed dermis. The epithelia of the lips, mouth, and conjunctiva are nearly always affected, and the vagina, esophagus, and trachea may be involved as well. Fever, leukocytosis (often with eosinophilia), and elevation of transaminases are to be expected. Complications of electrolyte imbalance, infection (usually pneumonia), GI bleeding, dehydration, malnutrition, and scarring of the external eye occur all too often. Mortality rates as high as 25–30% have been reported.[1,6] It takes 2 weeks for the epidermis to regenerate, so patients are quite ill for at least that period of time.

The vast majority of cases of TEN are caused by drugs. The list of agents that have been implicated is long, but the most frequent offenders are phenytoin; sulfonamides (including vaginal creams and eyedrops); barbiturates; penicillins; allopurinol; and recently nonsteroidal anti-inflammatory drugs, especially phenylbutazone and oxicam derivatives.[1,2,7] The exact pathogenesis of this so-called drug allergy is quite obscure. Presumably, some combination of humoral and/or cellular-mediated immunity other than the classically described types I–IV hypersensitivity reactions is operative. An association of TEN with HLA-B12 has been reported.[6,7] On both clinical and histologic grounds, most dermatologists would classify TEN as being the most severe expression of erythema multiforme–Stevens-Johnson syndrome.

With respect to differential diagnosis, the two other conditions that need to be considered are staphylococcal scalded skin syndrome (SSSS) and toxic shock syndrome (TSS). Although it is much more commonly seen in children, SSSS can occur in adults.[3] Those adults are often immunocompromised and always have a very-high-grade infection (i.e., a visceral abscess or endocarditis) with *Staphylococcus aureus*, phage group II. Although these patients are usually very ill from sepsis, the blistering and skin shedding in SSSS, which are due to a circulating staphylococcal exotoxin, are very superficial, so that most of the epidermis is left in place. The erosions heal within a few days, and fluid loss is minimal. Perioral blisters and erosions are seen, but the oral cavity is spared. The differential diagnosis between TEN and SSSS can be made quickly by a frozen-section examination of either a punch biopsy or simply a piece of the shedding epidermis.[4] The depth of epidermal involvement is easily determined.

TSS (see article *Toxic Shock Syndrome*) usually presents with various systemic symptoms such as vomiting, myalgias, and disorientation, followed quickly by a generalized red macular/urticarial rash with swelling of the palms and soles. Blisters almost never occur,[5] and the only epidermal shedding that takes place is on the palms and soles, and that does not happen until around the tenth day as the illness is resolving. Hypotension is common in the early phase of TSS but is seen only in the later phase of TEN after most of the epidermis is lost.

The management of TEN is somewhat controversial. Obviously, the suspected inciting drug should be stopped immediately. Some authorities believe that high-dose systemic steroids may be helpful if given very early in the course of the disease. However, once the epidermis becomes necrotic, there seems to be little rationale for steroids; indeed, at that stage they would be expected to delay wound healing and increase the risk of infection.[7]

Meticulous nursing and supportive medical care, preferably in a unit experienced in treating extensive burns, are the major factors that will determine whether or not the outcome is favorable.

KEY FEATURES

Toxic epidermal necrolysis (TEN) is almost always caused by a drug, especially phenytoin (dilantin), sulfonamides, penicillins, barbiturates, and allopurinol.

The oral mucosa, esophagus, trachea, and conjunctiva develop severe erosions in TEN.

Staphylococcal scalded skin syndrome (SSSS) is usually a milder disease than TEN, with the epidermal shedding being much more superficial and with minimal mucous membrane involvement.

Toxic shock syndrome (TSS) almost never has blisters.

Systemic steroids *may* help in TEN if given early enough and in high enough doses.

BIBLIOGRAPHY

1. Rasmussen J: T.E.N. Med Clin North Am 64:901, 1980.
   One of the best extensive reviews of the topic.

2. Scully R: Case records of the MGH. N Engl J Med 299:33, 1978.
   Case of trimethoprim-sulfamethoxazole (Bactrim)–induced TEN.

3. Neefe L, Tuazon L, et al: S.S.S.S. in adults. Am J Med Sci 277:99, 1979.
   Excellent extensive review of the topic.

4. Hurwitz R, et al: T.S.S. or T.E.N.? J Am Acad Dermatol 7:246, 1982.
   Discusses clinical and histologic differential diagnoses.

5. Elbaum DJ, et al: Bullae in a patient with T.S.S. J Am Acad Dermatol 10:267, 1984.
   Exceptions to the rule do occur.

6. Revuz J, Penso D, Roujeau J-C, et al: Toxic epidermal necrolysis: Clinical findings and prognosis factors in 87 patients. Arch Dermatol 123:1160, 1987.
7. Guillaume J-C, Roujeau J-C, Revuz J, Penso D, Touraine R: The culprit drugs in 87 cases of toxic epidermal necrolysis (Lyell's syndrome). Arch Dermatol 123:1166, 1987.
   Large clinical series from Créteil, France, summarized in a series of reports and an accompanying editorial. The most common culpable drugs identified were nonsteroidal anti-inflammatory drugs (especially phenylbutazone and oxicam derivatives), sulfonamides (especially trimethoprim/sulfamethoxazole), anticonvulsants (especially barbiturate), allopurinol, and chlormezanone. Overall mortality was 25%, the leading cause being sepsis with Staphylococcus aureus *or* Pseudomonas aeruginosa. *Multivariate analysis showed age, extent of necrolysis, and BUN to be of independent prognostic value. HLA-A, -B, and -DR typing of survivors demonstrated a statistically significant increase in HLA-B12 over normal controls. In an accompanying editorial, the authors stress the need for aggressive supportive care and caution against the use of corticosteroids.*

Heat Illness

James Feldman, M.D.

Acute heat illnesses present a spectrum of disorders from painful muscle cramps to heat stroke, a fulminant multi-system disorder with a significant morbidity and mortality. Patients at all ages are at risk for acute heat illness; this clinical entity may pose a diagnostic challenge in that the cardinal features are nonspecific and may be found in a variety of infectious, toxic-metabolic, endocrine, or structural disorders. Management of the patient with severe heat illness presents a challenge because of the complexity of the neurologic, metabolic, hemodynamic, and hematologic abnormalities. A favorable outcome depends on rapid assessment and treatment.

Heat loss as environmental temperature surpasses 99° F is mediated by evaporation and sweating alone rather than by radiation and convection, the major sources of heat loss at lower temperatures. Efficiency of heat dissipation by sweating is limited by humidity, air temperature, and movement as well as by the ability to sweat. Any alteration in the multiple components that are necessary for normal thermal homeostasis may result in an improper temperature response to heat stress. Some of these considerations include vigorous exertion overwhelming heat dissipation capacity; an impaired sweating mechanism on the basis of congenital or acquired abnormalities (drugs, scleroderma, cystic fibrosis); impaired cardiac output or volume depletion limiting dermal blood flow; failure to remove clothing; or an abnormally large volume to surface area ratio, as in obesity.

The ability to tolerate heat stress may be modified by the process of acclimatization. Features of this process include improved cardiac and peripheral metabolic efficiency and increased sweating capacity initiated at lower temperatures as well as renal and sweat sodium conservation. Increased secretion of aldosterone appears to play a significant role in this process.[1]

Environmental measurements used to quantify thermal stresses include not only absolute temperature but also humidity and air movement. The THI (temperature humidity index), (dry bulb + wet bulb F) × 0.4 + 15, is one such measure. At a THI greater than 65, the risk of heat stroke rises. Most people feel uncomfortable at a THI greater than 80.[4] The WBGT index (70% wet bulb + 20% black globe + 10% dry bulb) is another such measure.[2]

The pathogenesis of heat syndromes does not appear to depend only on the absolute core or environmental temperature. Such variables as duration of thermal exposure, dehydration, and other factors may play significant roles. Core temperatures greater than 42° C have been shown to damage mammalian tissues through direct thermal injury.[1,3] On the other hand, significant core temperature elevations have been observed in marathon runners without apparent adverse effects.[18] Thus, it is difficult to define a temperature that is "too high" for an individual patient.

Heat disorders are classified as heat cramps, heat exhaustion, and heat stroke. The last category may be divided into exertional heat stroke, affecting strenuously exercising or working young patients (miners, athletes, military recruits); and epidemic heat stroke, affecting generally older patients with underlying chronic illnesses in the setting of a sustained heat wave.

Heat cramps are painful skeletal or abdominal muscle cramps that occur in young patients during or following strenuous activities. The patients are usually acclimatized, although heat cramps may occur during the early phase of acclimatization.[1,2] Elderly patients, in general, are unable to undertake the sustained exertion required. Heat cramps are believed to result from excess sodium losses despite water intake; the exact mechanism is not known.[1,5] Body temperature remains normal. Heat cramps are distinguished from exertional rhabdomyolysis by the absence of myoglobinuria or associated features of rhabdomyolysis. Treatment consists of oral or intravenous rehydration with electrolyte-containing solutions. Systemic symptoms should suggest heat exhaustion or the prodromal phase of heat stroke.

Heat exhaustion occurs during periods of exertion in high temperatures or during a heat wave and arises from sodium and water deficits incurred by sweating. Mild CNS symptoms such as irritability, lassitude, weakness, or headache may be noted. Gastrointestinal symptoms of nausea or vomiting may be present. Muscle cramps may occur. Body temperature may be subnormal, normal, or elevated. Sweating is present. Serum sodium concentration may be normal, low, or high, depending on the relative sodium and water deficits. The presence of significant neurologic symptoms such as confusion, delirium, or psychosis suggests the prodromal phase of heat stroke. Treatment consists of removal of the patient to a cooler environment and volume repletion.

Heat stroke, the most serious of heat illnessss, has been defined by the triad of hyperpyrexia (temperature greater than 40.6° C [105° F]), anhidrosis, and significant neurologic dysfunction. Specific components of this triad, such as absence of sweating, are not required (especially in exertional heat stroke).[1,3,9] The limitations of defining an absolute temperature have been pointed out earlier. Among the many disorders that may present with similar features are such infectious diseases as falciparum malaria, meningococcemia, typhus, and Rocky Mountain spotted fever; many forms of encephalitis; such toxic ingestions as salicylates, tricyclic antidepressants, phenothiazines, anticholinergics, or such stimulants as cocaine or amphetamines; withdrawal states such as delirium tremens; endocrine disorders such as thyroid storm or diabetic ketoacidosis (DKA); and such structural abnormalities as midbrain hemorrhage or hypothalamic lesions. Rare mimics that can usually be identified appropriately by the clinical setting include the malignant hyperthermia syndrome following the use of anesthetic agents or muscle relaxants or the neuroleptic malignant syndrome following the administration of phenothiazines, butyrophenones, or thioxanthenes.

Risk factors have been identified for both exertional and epidemic heat stroke.[1,5,14,17] Specific risk factors for classic heat stroke include age greater than 65; minority or lower socioeconomic status; lack of air conditioning; habitation of upper stories of a multilevel dwelling; as well as the use of alcohol, major tranquilizers, drugs with anticholinergic properties, or diuretics. Infants with a history of upper respiratory infection, diarrhea, or neurologic disability may be at increased risk. Environmental conditions usually require a temperature greater than 95° F with more than 48 hours of sustained temperature higher than 90° F and relative humidity of 50–75%.[6] Risk factors for exertional heat stroke have been defined for specific populations such as Marine recruits and joggers.[13]

A variety of signs and symptoms have been observed in patients with heat stroke. Neurologic symptoms include coma, delirium, seizures, decortication and rigidity. Hyperventilation is common, and hemoptysis has been noted; pulmonary edema is considered an unusual presenting feature. Hypotension is a common finding. Gastrointestinal symptoms such as nausea, vomiting, or diarrhea may be noted. It is important to note that prodromal symptoms are not found in a large number of the patients who develop either exertional or epidemic heat stroke.[1,3,8,9,14]

The laboratory abnormalities that are found in both forms of heat stroke have been reviewed; complications such as acute renal failure, rhabdomyolysis, and disseminated intravascular coagulation (DIC) appear more commonly in those with exertional heat stroke.[9] The CSF is usually clear, although xanthochromia and an elevated protein may be found. ECG changes include sinus tachycardia, reversible ST–T wave changes suggesting ischemia, Q–T interval prolongation, and the development of intraventricular conduction abnormalities.[15] Thrombocytopenia and abnormal coagulation studies are common findings; active DIC may occur.[16,20] The serum sodium concentration can be low or high, potassium levels are usually normal or low, and hypoglycemia has been reported. A respiratory alkalosis or a mixed acid-base disturbance is found. Amylase levels are often elevated, although rarely is clinical or pathologic evidence of pancreatitis documented.[1,3,9] Transaminase, creatine kinase, and uric acid levels are usually elevated. The urine sediment may demonstrate granular or pigmented casts with evidence of myoglobinuria; a chronic interstitial nephritis has been reported.[1,3,5] Hemodynamic monitoring reveals either a hyperdynamic or hypodynamic pattern that may be complicated by volume depletion. The peripheral vascular resistance is low, presumably because of vasodilation and increased dermal blood flow. The reduction in cardiac output is due to volume depletion, thermal myocardial injury, or elevated pulmonary vascular resistance.[10–12]

Although such factors as prolonged coma greater than two hours, persistent hypotension, SGOT* greater than 1000, and fever greater than 106° F have been suggested as poor prognostic findings,[1–4,19] recovery has been noted despite profound hyperpyrexia (temperature 116° F) or prolonged coma.[9,20] The significance of a markedly elevated SGOT has not been con-

---

*SGOT = serum glutamate oxaloacetate transaminase.

firmed in several series.[5,8,9] Data regarding outcome must also be viewed in light of the general absence of standardized pre-hospital management even within a collected experience. A serum lactate level greater than 3.3 mmol/L initially was found to predict a poor outcome in classic heat stroke victims.[9]

Optimal management recommendations are difficult to make because of the absence of adequately controlled trials of different cooling methods or therapeutic interventions. Heat stroke should be considered in any patient at risk for either exertional or environmental heat syndrome who exhibits neurologic symptoms or syncope.[1,3] An accurate core temperature with a rectal probe capable of readings greater than 42° C should be obtained. The airway should be appropriately managed with strong consideration for endotracheal intubation because of the complications encountered during the cooling period. Cooling should be immediately initiated while additional historical information is obtained, such as travel history, past medical history, and known toxic ingestion; also, a more detailed physical examination should be performed at this time, with particular attention paid to stigmata of the infectious agents that may mimic heat stroke. Cooling techniques include ice bath immersion, ice packs, or a body cooling unit that utilizes the entire body surface area for cooling.[7] Evaporative techniques cool up to four times more rapidly than an ice water bath.[22] Although core cooling techniques such as cardiopulmonary bypass, peritoneal lavage, nasogastric lavage, or intratracheal cold helium administration have been reported in animal models, the risks or benefits from such core cooling techniques are not yet defined in human studies. Some authors recommend the use of a "lytic" cocktail containing such drugs as chlorpromazine and meperidine to limit shivering during the cooling period. Potent arguments against the use of a phenothiazine for this purpose include the potentiation of hypotension, lowering of the seizure threshold, and impairment of heat dissipation. Israeli military experience has demonstrated that diazepam decreases shivering and prevents seizures when administered during the cooling period.[21] Thiamine and 50% dextrose should be administered to all patients with a significant alteration in mental status. Hypoglycemia has been noted in patients with heat stroke.[23] Mannitol has been suggested for prophylaxis of acute renal tubular necrosis, particularly in exertional heat stroke.[1,3,4] Heparin has been used to treat DIC.[20] There are case reports on the use of dantrolene sodium in heat stroke.[20] It has been suggested that dantrolene be considered when prominent muscular hyperactivity is noted in the setting of heat stroke.[23]

Complications should be anticipated during the cooling period. Seizures may occur and should be managed with standard agents such as diazepam. Volume status may be difficult to assess. Deficits in exertional heat stroke may be moderate, approximately 1200 ml/4 hours.[20] Elderly patients who may have been exposed to a prolonged period of hyperthermia may incur greater fluid deficits, yet are at risk for complications from aggressive fluid resuscitation.[11] Therefore, hypotension not rapidly reversed by cooling and modest volume infusion should be evaluated by central hemodynamic monitoring. If a vasopressor is required, isoproterenol may offer the advantage of avoiding peripheral vasoconstriction with associated impairment of heat dissipation.[10] The core temperature should be rapidly lowered to approximately 102° F. Additional studies such as blood smear for a patient with malaria exposure, lumbar puncture to rule out meningitis, or toxicologic studies may be undertaken when indicated. All laboratory studies should be temperature corrected. The patient should be managed in an intensive care setting with frequent assessment of neurologic, cardiovascular, renal, and coagulation status. Despite aggressive cooling and resuscitation, significant mortality or residual neurologic deficits, including hemiparesis and cognitive or personality changes, may occur.

Both exertional and epidemic heat stroke can be prevented by identifying groups at risk and by modifying work, exercise load, or environmental conditions. A multi-agency working group can allow a community to reduce the incidence of epidemic heat stroke significantly. A cooperative effort can be developed involving media, at-risk groups such as the elderly, local government, and emergency services. A graded plan can be developed that is triggered by estimates of environmental risk. Initial approaches may include public information outlining simple preventive measures (such as avoid the sun, dress coolly, avoid alcohol) as well as recognition and emergency measures for the heat-related disorders. As a heat wave and environmental risk escalate, more aggressive measures can be taken, including the establishment of air conditioned shelters with a means of transportation for elderly and disabled citizens as well as the distribution of air conditioners.

Exertional heat stroke can be prevented by proper education of athletes, coaches, and sports officials. Such practices as avoiding mid-day workouts, encouraging fluid intake, and prohibiting the use of rubber type sweat suits during hot weather can prevent the tragic death of a young athlete. Employers placing workers at occupational risk can prevent heat stroke by education and simple preventive measures such as shortening periods of heavy exertion, encouraging breaks and fluid intake, and providing facilities for cooling. Given the serious cost in lives and long-term disability, prevention is by far the wisest approach to the heat-related disorders.

KEY FEATURES

A. Heat cramps
  1. Benign painful muscle cramps
  2. Affect young patients during or following strenuous activity

      3. Self-limited or responsive to rehydration
- B. Heat exhaustion
  1. Mild systemic symptoms accompanying salt and water losses from sweating
  2. Core temperature subnormal, normal, or elevated
  3. Resolution of symptoms with rehydration and cool environment
- C. Heat stroke
  1. Severe neurologic dysfunction and profound temperature elevation, often with anhidrosis
  2. Exertional heat stroke in young athletes, miners, military recruits
  3. Epidemic heat stroke in extremes of age, underlying chronic illness, congenital or acquired sweat limitations; significant morbidity and mortality
- D. In addition to routine supportive measures, treatment of heat stroke includes the following:
  1. Airway management, 100% oxygen
  2. Establish large-bore IV normal saline
  3. Cardiac monitor
  4. Administer 100 mg thiamine, Chemstrip for glucose, administer 25 gm 50% dextrose
  5. Consider early administration of diazepam during cooling
  6. Initiate rapid cooling to 102° F
  7. Moderate volume resuscitation 1200 ml/4 hr
  8. Manage seizures with standard measures
  9. Nasogastric tube and Foley catheter placement
  10. Central hemodynamic monitoring for hypotension not rapidly corrected by cooling and moderate volume expansion
  11. Isoproterenol if cardiotonic drug required
  12. Consider mannitol administration, particularly in exertional heat stroke
  13. Search for infectious, toxic, or endocrine disorders that mimic heat stroke. Consider CT scan; perform LP and blood cultures
  14. Avoid aspirin and other antipyretics
  15. Temperature-correct laboratory data
  16. ICU surveillance of renal, coagulation, neurologic, and hemodynamic status

REFERENCES

1. Knochel JP: Environmental heat illness—an eclectic review. Arch Intern Med 133:841, 1974.
   A detailed review with excellent discussion of pathophysiology of heat-related syndromes, illustrative case studies, and extensive bibliography.

2. Clowes GH, O'Donnell TF: Heat stroke—current concepts. N Engl J Med 291:564, 1974.
   A concise although limited discussion.

3. Shibolet S, Lancaster MC, Danon Y: Heat stroke: A review. Aviat Space Environ Med 47:280, 1976.
   A complete review of experimental, clinical, and therapeutic aspects of heat stroke.

4. Goldfrank L, Osborn H, Weisman R: Heat stroke—toxicologic emergencies. Hosp Physic 8:24, 1980.
   Case presentation with practical discussion.

5. Stine RJ: Heat illness—collective review. JACEP 8:154, 1979.
6. Wheelher M: Heat stroke in the elderly. Med Clin North Am 60:1288, 1976.
   Emphasizes geriatric physiology and considerations in elderly victims of heat stroke.

7. Khogali M, Weiner JS: Heat stroke: Report on 18 cases. Lancet 2:276, 1980.
   A description of a body cooling unit used on heat stroke victims on the Mecca pilgrimage. Five patients required more than 1 hour to reach 38° C. Two of eighteen patients died.

8. Beller GA, Boyd AE: Heat stroke: A report of 13 consecutive cases without mortality despite severe hyperpyrexia and neurologic dysfunction. Milit Med 140:464, 1975.
   Study of military recruit victims of heat stroke. There was a mean rectal temperature of 107.6° F. Hypotension, coma, and hypokalemia were common findings. Nonstandardized management was used; normal recovery was seen.

9. Hart GR, et al: Epidemic classical heat stroke: Clinical characteristics and course of 28 patients. Medicine 61:189, 1982.
   A detailed study of 28 patients with classic heat stroke from the Parkland Memorial Hospital in Dallas, Texas. Emphasizes differences between exertional and classic heat stroke. Report on a survivor with a temperature of 116° F. Initial lactate level greater than 3.3 mmol/L was a poor prognostic finding.

10. O'Donnell T, Clowes G: The circulatory abnormalities of heat stroke. N Engl J Med 287:734, 1972.
    Indocyanine green dye curves were obtained on military recruits with heat stroke. Identification of hyperdynamic and hypodynamic profiles was made.

11. Sprung C: Hemodynamic alterations of heat stroke in the elderly. Chest 75:362, 1979.
    Demonstrates results similar to data from military recruits. Studied seven elderly victims of New York heat wave. Circulatory failure appeared to result from peripheral pooling or hypovolemia.

12. Malamud N, Haymaker W, Custer RP: Heat stroke—a clinicopathological study of 125 fatal cases. Milit Surg 99:397, 1946.
    Old but detailed pathologic findings in military victims of heat stroke.

13. The American College of Sports Medicine Position Statement on the Prevention of Heat Injuries During Distance Running. Med Sci Sports 7:VII, 1975.
    Detailed guidelines from the ACSM.

14. England AC 3d, et al: Preventing severe heat injury in runners: Suggestions from the 1979 Peachtree Road Race experience. Ann Intern Med 97:196, 1982.
    Emphasizes that prodromal symptoms are infrequently observed in running-induced heat stroke. Fluid intake at this middle distance (10 km) did not influence heat stroke risk.

15. Costrini AM, Pitt HA, Gustafson SB, Uddin DE: Cardiovascular and metabolic manifestations of heat stroke and severe heat exhaustion. Am J Med 66:296, 1979.
16. O'Donnell TF: Acute heat stroke—epidemiologic, biochemical, renal and coagulation studies. JAMA 234:824, 1975.
    Fifteen Marine recruits with heat stroke were analyzed.

17. Kilbourne EM, et al: Risk factors for heatstroke: A case-control study. JAMA 247:3332, 1982.

Results from 1980 heat wave in St. Louis and Kansas City, MO.

18. Pugh LG, Corbett JL, Johnson RH: Rectal temperatures, weight losses and sweat rates in marathon running. J Appl Physiol 23:347, 1957.
19. Kew M, Bersohn I, Seftel H: The diagnostic and prognostic significance of the serum enzyme changes in heatstroke. Trans R Soc Trop Med Hyg 65:325, 1971.
      Review of the findings in South African miners with heatstroke. Standard reference for the significance of SGOT greater than 1000.

20. Perchick JS, Winkelstein A, Shadduck RK: Disseminated intravascular coagulation in heat stroke: Response to heparin therapy. JAMA 23:480, 1975.
      Case report of a 14-year-old athlete with severe heat stroke. Recovery occurred despite prolonged coma. Authors uncertain whether heparin use was beneficial or coincidental to recovery.

21. Stewart, CE, Dwyer B (eds): Preventing the progression of heat injury. Emergency Med Rep 8:121, 1987.
      Concise and up-to-date review with 46 references.

22. Graham BS, Lichenstein MJ, et al: Nonexertional heatstroke. Physiologic management and cooling in 14 patients. Arch Intern Med 146:87, 1986.
23. Olson KR, Benowitz NL: Environmental and drug-induced hyperthermia. Emerg Med Clin 2:459, 1984.
      Excellent summary of pathophysiology and treatment of heat syndromes.

The Ethanol Withdrawal Syndrome

James J. Heffernan, M.D.

Alcoholism may legitimately be considered the United States' third largest health problem, with a cost of $60 billion and an association with 200,000 deaths yearly.[1] Ninety million Americans consume alcoholic beverages in one form or another, and 10 million are considered problem drinkers. Alcohol is a factor in half of the 50,000 annual motor vehicle fatalities, in two of every three homicides, in half of deaths by fire, and in one of three suicides. The direct medical complications of alcohol abuse are many and varied, with effects on central and peripheral nervous systems, heart, muscles, bone marrow, liver, pancreas, gut mucosa, and intermediary metabolism. Alcohol use has been associated with the development of carcinomas of the aerodigestive tract and breast. The fourth leading cause of death in males aged 25–44 in the United States is cirrhosis, overwhelmingly related to alcohol abuse; the three leading causes of death for the same age cohort, accidents, homicide, and suicide, also bear strong associations with alcohol use, as noted previously.[17]

The symptoms of the ethanol withdrawal syndrome vary from mild to life-threatening and most commonly come to the attention of the health care system when a patient with a history of ethanol abuse presents (1) seeking detoxification or (2) seeking treatment for another medical problem, often alcohol related, that has interrupted his or her ability to maintain customary intake. It is likely that the overwhelming majority of minor withdrawal symptoms go unrecognized, undiagnosed, and untreated, because the large number of problem drinkers vary their intake but do not come into contact with the health care system, or do so in a manner in which alcohol abuse is not considered. Fever, altered mental status, hypertension, agitation, and tachycardia are just a few of the symptoms of ethanol withdrawal that may become manifest after hospital admission and/or surgery, the true cause of which often remains unappreciated, despite investigation, unless one has considered the possibility of the withdrawal state.

Although ethanol withdrawal symptoms have been described for millenia and delirium tremens for several centuries, clear characterization of the syndrome dates from the classic descriptions of Victor and Adams in 1953, confirmed by the experimental work, using human volunteers, of Isbell, Fraser, Wikler, and colleagues in 1955.[2-4] The full spectrum of symptoms is wide, ranging through tremulousness, sleep disturbance, nystagmus, hyperreflexia, nausea, vomiting, sweating, tachycardia, fever, agitation, hallucinosis, seizures, and delirium tremens (DTs). Most classification systems have considered seizures and DTs to be *major withdrawal phenomena,* and all others to be *minor withdrawal symptoms.* Some investigators have considered hallucinosis to occupy an intermediate position. Such schemata have arisen from the dose dependence of withdrawal symptoms demonstrated in earlier studies. In the aforementioned work of Isbell and coworkers, all of four experimental subjects who consumed a moderately high daily ethanol intake for 7–34 days experienced weakness, anorexia, diaphoresis, and tremulousness on sudden abstinence. Of the six patients who consumed a greater daily amount for a sustained period of 48–87 days, all experienced the mild symptoms just noted, as well as insomnia, nausea, vomiting, hyperreflexia, diarrhea, hypertension, and fever; moreover five of six patients developed hallucinosis, two of six seizures, and three of six DTs.[3,4] In the earlier clinical review by Victor and Adams of 266 consecutive patients admitted to the Boston City Hospital with obvious complications of alcoholism, 18% developed atypical hallucinatory states, 12% seizures, and 5% DTs. These earlier studies also demonstrated the other hallmarks, besides dose dependence, of ethanol withdrawal, specifically, tolerance, and withdrawal while drinking. Although the nominal fatal blood alcohol level is 400 mg/dl, individuals with a history of sustained heavy consumption may occasionally survive levels in excess of 700 mg/dl without ventilatory support; in the habituated drinker, drunkenness may not be sustained and a rapid progression to major withdrawal phenomena may occur at blood ethanol levels of 250 mg/dl.[17] Point scoring systems have been developed to quantify the ethanol withdrawal syndrome;[13] it is not clear that such systems offer any clear clinical advantages over the traditional system of nomenclature in predicting individual outcomes, but they may enhance comparisons in different clinical trials.

Although it is true that all ethanol withdrawal symptoms may become manifest during continued consumption, especially in the setting of restricted intake and/or supervening medical illness, there is generally a progression in the development of specific withdrawal reactions on cessation of drinking. Sleep disturbances and hallucinosis may be present during intoxication or withdrawal. Nystagmus, nausea, vomiting, tremulousness, anxiety, and a sense of foreboding generally develop within hours of the decay in the blood alcohol level. Evidence of enhanced central sympathetic activity—hyperventilation, tachycardia, hypertension, hyperreflexia, low-grade fever—is generally apparent to some extent within the first 24 hours of cessation of drinking. Withdrawal seizures, when they occur, generally do so within the first 12–48 hours, but they may develop without other identifiable cause up to 5 and possibly up to 9 days after abstention from alcohol.[2,8,12] In up to two thirds of patients, multiple seizures occur, generally in a flurry over a period of several hours. Of those with pure withdrawal seizures, only a small percentage progress to status epilepticus; however, withdrawal from alcohol and other substances was the second most common cause of status epilepticus in a major review from an urban emergency department. A substantial minority of those experiencing withdrawal seizures progress to DTs, some directly in the postictal period but more after a lucid interval.

The majority of those developing DTs do not experience antecedent seizures. The rather broad peak of onset for the development of DTs, 24–96 hours after the last drink, is later than that for withdrawal seizures. This condition is, by definition, an agitated (and tremulous) confusional state accompanied by florid autonomic hyperactivity and perceptual disorders.[4] Tremulousness and hallucinosis in an oriented, responsive patient are not sufficient to make the diagnosis. Delirium tremens is indeed a medical emergency with a substantial mortality and morbidity from metabolic derangements, self-induced trauma, dehydration/volume depletion, cardiopulmonary events, and associated medical conditions.[16] This most serious of ethanol withdrawal phenomena generally lasts 12–48 hours with appropriate treatment. Patients experiencing only minor withdrawal symptoms usually show substantial improvement with appropriate care in 40–50 hours;[1] nonetheless, some minor symptoms, especially anxiety and tremulousness, may persist for weeks.

The mechanisms that result in ethanol tolerance, addiction, and withdrawal are poorly understood. Because ethanol diffuses freely into all aqueous compartments of the body and is miscible with fats, its acute actions are felt to reflect primarily membrane effects in neuronal tissues. It has been postulated that condensation of derivative aldehydes into opiate-mimicking tetrahydroisoquinolines may explain, in part, ethanol's addiction potential. It has also been postulated that ethanol may interfere with formation or release of an as yet unidentified excitatory neurotransmitter with subsequent up-regulation of precursors resulting in tolerance and withdrawal. There is little experimental evidence in humans to support either theory convincingly at this point.[17]

MANAGEMENT

Although ethanol does not appear to act at specific receptors, cross-tolerance has long been noted among ethanol, general anesthetic agents, and a variety of sedative drugs, many of which do appear to exert their effects at specific receptors. Administration of one such agent may abort or reduce the withdrawal reaction from another. This principle has been the mainstay of management in ethanol withdrawal reactions.

A number of well-planned and executed clinical trials have been conducted over the past several decades, comparing numerous pharmacologic agents in the management of various aspects of the ethanol withdrawal syndrome. Cross-tolerance exists among ethanol, paraldehyde, barbiturates, and benzodiazepines, but the weight of evidence to date favors the use of benzodiazepines, for reasons of safety and efficacy.[4-7,11,12,17] Numerous trials have demonstrated the superiority of diazepam or chlordiazepoxide over placebo in alleviating minor withdrawal symptoms and in reducing the incidence of seizures and DTs.[4,5,7,12,19] In another major study, parenteral diazepam resulted in more rapid calming and significantly fewer side effects than did paraldehyde in a group of patients with DTs.[11] The effects of thiamine, hydroxyzine, and chlorpromazine have not been shown to differ from those of placebo, and pooled data suggest that use of phenothiazines enhances the likelihood of seizures.[4,7,17] Although there is a theoretical advantage in the use of benzodiazepines with inactive metabolites and short or intermediate duration of action (e.g., oxazepam, lorazepam) in patients with liver disease, there are no comparisons to date that have demonstrated any clear advantage in efficacy or safety over diazepam or chlordiazepoxide. However, both oxazepam and lorazepam, and a longer acting benzodiazepine, chlorazepate, have been used effectively in the treatment of ethanol withdrawal and are probably comparable in efficacy with the earlier benzodiazepines.[18,19] Because of concern over erratic absorption from intramuscular injection sites, it remains standard practice to administer diazepam and chlordiazepoxide by mouth or intravenously: for the treatment of minor withdrawal symptoms, chlordiazepoxide 25–100 mg PO q4–6h (dosage adjusted to control symptoms), tapering over five days; for DTs, diazepam 5 mg IV q5–15 minutes, in a closely monitored patient, to achieve mild sedation. The patient who has been receiving oral benzodiazepines for minor withdrawal symptoms but who subsequently develops DTs will generally require only small dosages of parenteral diazepam to achieve control of agitation. On the other hand, the patient who presents *de novo* with DTs may have prodigious requirements for parenteral medication to achieve adequate sedation, e.g., >2000 mg diazepam IV over 24 hours.[11] In the patient with minor withdrawal symptoms who is NPO, the use of phenobarbital intramuscularly has been advocated.[17] Lorazepam possesses reliable absorption from intramuscular sites, and it has been used effectively but is not formally approved for treatment of withdrawal states.[18]

As noted previously, there are substantial data to support the contention that early treatment of minor withdrawal symptoms with benzodiazepines reduces the incidence of withdrawal seizures.[4,5,7,12,19] Indeed, benzodiazepines form the mainstay of seizure and DT prophylaxis. One randomized, prospective, placebo-controlled trial demonstrated a further highly significant reduction in seizures by the addition of phenytoin 100 mg PO tid to standard chlordiazepoxide therapy during the withdrawal period in a group of patients with a prior history of seizures.[8] It is not unreasonable to consider supplementing benzodiazepine therapy with phenytoin for a limited period in patients with a prior history of seizures who are experiencing ethanol withdrawal, although this remains controversial. There are no controlled data to address the question of optimal therapy following presentation with a single withdrawal seizure.

Carbamazepine has been advocated as an agent effective for a number of the manifestations of the ethanol withdrawal syndrome on the basis of limited human data.[9] Clonidine has been shown to reduce pulse, blood pressure, and withdrawal score in a small, short-term crossover trial but has not been shown to reduce the risk of DTs and carries its own risk of inducing hypotension.[5,14] It has been reported that atenolol added to standard prn oxazepam accelerated normalization of abnormal vital signs, clinical features, and behavioral features (and reduced oxazepam consumption) in a group of patients experiencing ethanol withdrawal.[13] Unfortunately, the general applicability of this study is questionable because of the exclusion of sicker patients, the lack of data as to the magnitude of the clinical effect, and the fact that no one in the atenolol or placebo groups experienced seizures or DTs, thus making it impossible to assess the potential risk or benefit of atenolol in the subset of patients most likely to experience a fatal or morbid outcome from ethanol withdrawal.

The patient who presents with ethanol withdrawal symptoms also requires scrupulous attention to general medical care. Thiamine, folate, magnesium (calcium), and phosphate deficits; dehydration/volume depletion; acid-base disturbances; infection; unrecognized trauma; hepatic dysfunction; pancreatitis; gastrointestinal hemorrhage; marrow suppression; rhabdomyolysis; ethanol-associated dysrhythmias ("holiday heart")—all must be antic-ipated and treated when present. New onset seizures with focal findings on examination obligate an emergency CT scan of the head.[10] Abnormal mental status or seizures in the setting of fever warrant a lumbar puncture. Close monitoring of the DT patient is mandatory, preferably restrained in the swimmer's position. Although fever is common among patients experiencing the spectrum of ethanol withdrawal symptoms, it is especially common among those with DTs and in up to half of such instances has been associated with pneumonia.[15]

The prognosis for minor ethanol withdrawal symptoms is generally that of comorbid disease, most often also ethanol related—pancreatitis, pneu-mococcal pneumonia, upper gastrointestinal hemorrhage, and so forth. With-drawal seizures generally respond to standard measures and appropriate prophylaxis. Delirium tremens is still associated with a 5–15% mortality rate, traditionally among those with liver disease, pneumonia, high fever, and seizures.[16]

KEY FEATURES

The physiologic basis of ethanol intoxication, tolerance, addiction, and withdrawal remains incompletely understood.

The acute actions of ethanol are felt to reflect membrane effects in neuronal tissues; cross-tolerance has been noted among ethanol, nu-merous general anesthetic agents, paraldehyde, barbiturates, and ben-zodiazepines.

The clinical hallmarks of ethanol addiction and withdrawal are dose dependence, tolerance, and withdrawal while intoxicated.

Withdrawal symptoms are generally classified as minor, interme-diate, and major; the more serious withdrawal reactions generally attend heavier consumption for longer periods:

1. *Minor*: tremulousness, sleep disturbance, nystagmus, nausea/vomiting, diaphoresis, tachycardia, tachypnea/hyperventila-tion, low-grade fever, agitation

2. *Intermediate*: hallucinosis

3. *Major*: seizures, delirium tremens (DTs)

Minor withdrawal symptoms generally are manifested within hours of cessation of ethanol consumption.

Withdrawal seizures generally occur 12–48 hours after cessation of drinking but may present up to a week later; multiple seizures in a brief flurry over several hours are common.

Those who develop DTs usually do so 24–96 hours after the last drink; minor withdrawal symptoms are almost always apparent beforehand, and a substantial minority of those who experience withdrawal seizures will progress to DTs.

All patients who present with the ethanol withdrawal syndrome require attention to potential thiamine, folate, magnesium (calcium), and phosphate deficits; dehydration/volume depletion; and acid/base disturbances.

Infection, trauma, and the specific medical complications of ethanol abuse—hepatic dysfunction, pancreatitis, gastrointestinal hemorrhage, bone marrow suppression, rhabdomyolysis, cardiac effects—must be identified and treated when present.

Minor withdrawal symptoms should be treated with oral benzodiazepines, tapering over 4–5 days; in the patient who is NPO, intramuscular phenobarbital or lorazepam (not formally approved for this indication) is a reasonable alternative. (Concern remains over the predictability of absorption from IM sites of those benzodiazepines approved for use in withdrawal states.)

Oral phenytoin or intramuscular phenobarbital may be considered in those with a prior history of withdrawal-associated seizures; such withdrawal seizure prophylaxis should be maintained only for the duration of withdrawal.

The treatment of choice for a patient with DTs remains intravenous diazepam with close monitoring.

Limited data suggest the possible utility of beta blockers (especially atenolol), clonidine, and carbamazepine for various withdrawal symptoms; however, these agents have not yet been shown to be safe in those progressing to more serious withdrawal states.

The mortality rate of minor withdrawal symptoms is generally that of comorbid disease, usually ethanol related. The mortality rate associated with DTs remains 5–15%, traditionally among those with concurrent liver disease, pneumonia, high fever, and seizures.

REFERENCES

1. West WJ, Maxwell DS, Noble EP, Solomon DH: Alcoholism. Ann Intern Med 100:405, 1984.
   Good discussion of the public health aspects of the problem of alcoholism.

2. Victor M, Adams RD: The effect of alcohol on the nervous system. Res Publ Assoc Res Nerv Ment Dis 32:526, 1953.
   Excellent descriptive review of the clinical features of ethanol intoxication and withdrawal in 266 consecutive patients admitted to the Boston City Hospital with obvious complications of alcoholism. Five per cent of such patients developed DTs, with an attendant mortality rate of 15%. Seizures occurred in 12% and atypical hallucinatory states in 18% of the overall study group.

3. Isbell H, Fraser HF, Wikler A, et al: An experimental study of the etiology of "rum fits" and delirium tremens. Quart J Stud Alcohol 16:1, 1955.
   Representative study in volunteers demonstrating the hallmarks of the ethanol withdrawal syndrome: (1) dose dependence, (2) withdrawal while drinking, and (3) tolerance. Only subjects in the higher consumption group experienced hallucinosis (5/6), seizures (2/6), or DTs (3/6).

4. Thompson WL: Management of alcohol withdrawal syndromes. Arch Intern Med 138:278, 1978.
   Excellent focused review drawing heavily on human studies from the last few decades. Treatment recommendations generally still applicable.

5. Treatment of alcohol withdrawal. Med Lett Drug Ther 28:75, 1986.
   Brief discussion citing limited number of fairly recent references. Advocates benzo-diazepines as mainstay of therapy with possible consideration of the use of adrenergic blocking agents to relieve some symptoms of withdrawal.

6. Sellers EM, Kalant H: Alcohol intoxication and withdrawal. N Engl J Med 294:757, 1976.
   Good discussion of the various pharmacologic agents used to treat the ethanol withdrawal state.

7. Kaim SC, Klett CJ, Rothfeld B: Treatment of the acute alcohol withdrawal state: A comparison of four drugs. Amer J Psychiat 125:12, 1969.
   Randomized prospective trial of chlordiazepoxide, chlorpromazine, hydroxyzine, or thiamine against placebo among 537 hospitalized alcoholics with symptoms of withdrawal. Only 2% of those treated with chlordiazepoxide sustained seizures and/or DTs compared with 10–16% among those in the other treatment and placebo groups.

8. Sampliner R: Diphenylhydantoin control of alcohol withdrawal seizures: Results of a controlled study. JAMA 230:1430, 1974.
   Randomized prospective trial of chlordiazepoxide and diphenylhydantoin (phenytoin) (100 mg PO tid) versus chlordiazepoxide and placebo in 157 patients with prior history of seizures and recent heavy ethanol consumption admitted to a detoxification unit. The diphenylhydantoin-treated group experienced no seizures during the treatment period (and 2 afterward) compared with 11 among those in the placebo-treated group (P <.005).

9. Ballenger JC, Post RM: Carbamazepine in alcohol withdrawal syndromes and schizophrenic psychoses. Psychopharmacol Bull 20:572, 1983.
   The authors cite a number of human and animal studies suggesting a role for carbamazepine in the management of ethanol withdrawal.

10. Feussner JR, Linfors EW, Blessing CL, Starmer CF: Computed tomography in alcohol withdrawal seizures. Ann Intern Med 94:519, 1981.
    Among 151 alcoholic patients with withdrawal seizures, 50% of CT scans were normal, 34% showed generalized atrophy, and 15% demonstrated focal structural lesions. When focal neurologic deficits were present, 30% of CT scans showed focal lesions (18% potentially reversible), compared with 6% (1% potentially reversible) when such deficits were absent (P<.0002).

11. Thompson WL, Johnson AD, Maddrey WL, et al: Diazepam and paraldehyde for treatment of severe delirium tremens. Ann Intern Med 82:175, 1975.
    Randomized, prospective trial in 34 consecutive patients comparing diazepam and paraldehyde in the treatment of DTs. Diazepam resulted in significantly more rapid calming effect. Those with pneumonia, pancreatitis, and/or hepatitis required more medication and a longer period to achieve desired effect. Nine untoward reactions occurred, only among paraldehyde-treated patients (sudden death, apnea, injuries).

12. Sellers EM, Naranjo CA, Harrison M, et al: Diazepam loading: Simplified treatment of alcohol withdrawal. Clin Pharmacol Ther 34:824, 1983.
    Diazepam and supportive care were significantly better than placebo and supportive care in a randomized, prospective trial of 50 patients. Seizures (5/25), hallucinosis (1/25), and dysrhythmia (1/25) occurred only among placebo-treated patients.

13. Kraus ML, Gottlieb LD, Horwitz RI, Anscher M: Randomized clinical trial of atenolol in patients with alcohol withdrawal. N Engl J Med *313*:905, 1985.

    Prospective trial comparing atenolol and oxazepam to placebo and oxazepam in the treatment of ethanol withdrawal. Abnormal vital signs, clinical features, and behavioral features resolved more quickly in the atenolol-treated group. However, 72 patients with severe withdrawal reactions were excluded before randomization; no patient in either treatment arm had a seizure or experienced DTs.

14. Wilkins AJ, Jenkins WJ, Steiner JA: Efficacy of clonidine in treatment of alcohol withdrawal state. Psychopharmacology *81*:78, 1983.

    Clonidine was significantly better than placebo in reducing pulse, blood pressure, and withdrawal sign score in small, short-term, randomized, prospective, crossover trial.

15. Rose HD, Golbert TM, Sanz CJ, et al: Fever during acute alcohol withdrawal. Am J Med Sci *260*:112, 1970.

    Temperature was greater than 101° F in 27% of patients with minor withdrawal symptoms and in 82% of patients with DTs. Among those with DTs, fever was attributed to pneumonia in 50% and dehydration in 25%.

16. Tavel ME, Davidson W, Batterton TD: A critical analysis of mortality associated with delirium tremens. Am J Med Sci *242*:18, 1961.

    Retrospective review of 39 fatalities associated with DTs, representing 11.8% of all cases with DTs over the study period. Liver disease, pneumonia, seizures, and temperature greater than 104° F were more common among fatal cases.

17. Clark WD: Alcohol addiction and withdrawal. *In* Noble J (ed): Textbook of General Medicine and Primary Care. Boston, Little, Brown, 1987, pp 1627–1631.

    Broadly written, practical summary.

18. Hosein IN, de Frietas R, Beaurbrun MH: Intramuscular/oral lorazepam in acute alcohol withdrawal and incipient delirium tremens. Curr Med Res Opin *5*:632, 1978.

19. Haddox VG, Bidder TG, Waldron LE, Derby P: Chlorazepate use may prevent alcohol withdrawal convulsions. West J Med *146*:695, 1987.

Thromboembolic Disease

Arthur H. Eskew, M.D.

BACKGROUND

Deep venous thrombosis and pulmonary embolism are a major cause of morbidity and mortality in inpatient populations. It has been estimated that up to 630,000 pulmonary emboli occur annually in the United States, involving some 500,000 hospital admissions. Autopsy data suggest that pulmonary emboli are directly fatal in some 100,000 cases annually and may be a contributory factor in an additional 100,000. The incidence of resulting pulmonary hypertension and chronic cor pulmonale in the survivors is unknown, but it may be significant in those patients whose thromboembolism remains undiagnosed and untreated.[1]

The incidence of deep venous thrombosis (DVT) is unknown in ambulatory populations, but it is a common clinical entity in hospitalized surgical and selected medical patients. Roughly one third of general surgical patients over the age of 40 will have symptomatic or asymptomatic deep venous thrombosis demonstrable by various diagnostic modalities. Most of these are clinically inapparent thrombi limited to the calf veins. The incidence may approach 50–70% in those undergoing emergency hip surgery; the incidence of pulmonary embolism approaches 20% in these patients, with a 4–7% fatal embolism rate. Most symptomatic deep venous thrombi are located in the thigh, and roughly 50% of patients with DVT have clinically unsuspected embolism suggested by simultaneous ventilation-perfusion (V/Q) lung scanning.[2–4]

The most effective therapy for thromboembolic disease is preventative. For most general medical patients, subcutaneously administered mini-dose heparin (5000 U q12h) employed during periods of prolonged immobility is effective in reducing thrombotic and embolic episodes. This regimen is also effective in most general surgical patients, although combined modalities offer superior efficacy with equal or less risk. Therapy is begun postoperatively as soon as it seems prudent to do so, consideration being given to the type and extent of surgery. The incidence of major bleeding and wound hematoma is generally acceptable except for neurosurgical patients, and calcium heparin may provide less risk than the sodium salt. Therapy is continued for the duration of postoperative immobility.[4]

For patients undergoing hip and knee surgery, both elective and emergency, as well as for patients undergoing open prostatectomy, mini-dose heparin is not protective.[2] Other high-risk categories include the elderly, those with a history of previous thrombosis, and patients with malignancy. In these instances, more aggressive measures are necessary. A number of protocols, employing adjusted-dose subcutaneous heparin, low-dose oral sodium warfarin (coumadin), heparin-dihydroergotamine (DHE) combinations, and pneumatic compression stockings, have been demonstrated to be superior to mini-dose heparin.[2–4] Optimally, anticoagulant therapy should be begun prior to surgery, although fear of untoward hemorrhagic side effects has limited this practice. The heparin-DHE combination has the advantages of relatively short duration of action and every-12-hour dosing, and laboratory monitoring is not required. Oral Coumadin offers the advantages of allowing titration of the degree of anticoagulation and the continuation of therapy for long periods of time if necessary. Mechanical modalities such as graded compression stockings and intermittent pneumatic compression offer efficacy and do not predispose the patient to bleeding.[3] The use of antiplatelet therapy alone in the prevention of thromboembolism is controversial and at present cannot be recommended.[4]

PATHOPHYSIOLOGY AND CLINICAL FEATURES

The pathophysiology of venous thrombosis is accurately described by Virchow's triad of stasis, endothelial injury, and hypercoagulability.[5] From this, the clinical risk factors for thrombosis and subsequent embolism can easily be extrapolated. The inaccuracy of history and physical examination in the diagnosis of venous thromboembolism is well known; the commonly associated signs and symptoms, including pain, swelling, and Homans sign, occur with approximately equal frequency in patients with and without deep venous thrombosis.[6] A palpable, tender, deep venous cord, if present, is helpful but is not a common finding.[6] In the case of pulmonary embolism, the most common signs and symptoms, which include dyspnea, tachypnea, tachycardia, chest pain, apprehension, and fever, are so nonspecific as to have little predictive value in an individual patient, though their presence may be the only indicator to the clinician of the possibility of embolism.[7] Therefore, objective diagnostic testing is always indicated in cases of suspected deep venous thrombosis and/or pulmonary embolism before or shortly after the institution of therapy.

EVALUATION OF SUSPECTED THROMBOEMBOLISM

The initial evaluation of the patient with suspected deep venous thrombosis includes a thorough history and physical examination, focusing on possible alternative diagnoses and on the identification of risk factors for venous thromboembolism. Laboratory studies are selected based on suspected underlying and/or contributory conditions. Coagulation studies and a platelet count are necessary for monitoring subsequent heparin therapy.

Contrast venography remains the diagnostic reference standard for establishing the presence or absence of deep venous thrombosis, but the exact sensitivity and specificity of the procedure are unknown.[6] Venography offers the advantages of being readily available and allowing direct and rapid visualization of both the proximal and the distal deep venous systems. Disadvantages include some degree of invasiveness as well as the risks of contrast reaction and local complications. In addition, contast venography induces phlebitis in a small percentage of patients subjected to the study.[2]

Impedance plethysmography (IPG) represents a sensitive and specific alternative for establishing the diagnosis of proximal deep venous thrombosis.[8] It is, however, insensitive to thrombosis limited to the deep veins of the calf.[2] Furthermore, any entity that obstructs venous return to the thorax from the lower extremity, including pregnancy, pelvic and abdominal tumor, and obesity, may cause a false positive result. Major advantages include its safety, reproducibility, and low cost. Conversely, ^{125}I-labeled fibrinogen scanning is extremely sensitive to actively forming calf-vein thrombosis (albeit somewhat lacking in specificity) but is notably inaccurate in determining the presence or absence of clot in the veins of the thigh.[2,9] Additional disadvantages with this study include a 24–48 hour delay in establishing a diagnosis and the potential for concentration of the ^{125}I isotope by the thyroid. At present, ^{125}I scanning has been most extensively used as a research tool. Its clinical utility remains unclear, although it has been purported that the combined use of IPG and ^{125}I scanning may approach the diagnostic accuracy of venography in patients with clinically suspected DVT.[9] Doppler ultrasound, despite its disadvantage of being somewhat operator dependent in its interpretation, may approach IPG in sensitivity to proximal thrombosis and is clearly superior to IPG in the detection of thrombi in the calf veins.[2,6]

The initial evaluation of the patient with suspected pulmonary embolism must include a thorough history and physical examination, primarily aimed at excluding other entities, such as angina pectoris, spontaneous pneumothorax, or esophageal disorders, that might account for the observed signs and symptoms. A PA and a lateral chest radiograph should always be obtained; they are essential in interpreting subsequent studies and may also indicate an alternative diagnosis, obviating further consideration of thromboembolism. A baseline (room air) arterial blood gas determination is not of much diagnostic use because a normal PaO_2 is compatible with the presence of embolism, but it may be helpful in guiding supplemental oxygen therapy. Electrocardiography may reveal evidence of acute right ventricular strain (S1, Q3, T3), usually seen with massive emoblism.[1] Coagulation studies (aPTT, PT, and platelets) are obtained at baseline to guide subsequent anticoagulation.

Pulmonary angiography is the diagnostic reference standard for establishing the presence or absence of pulmonary embolism. Because of its relatively invasive nature and what is occasionally perceived to be unacceptable risk in performing angiography on critically ill patients with suspected embolism, perfusion lung scanning is usually employed first. Perfusion lung scanning is extremely sensitive to the presence of even small peripheral emboli, so that a normal scan effectively excludes the diagnosis of pulmonary embolism.[10–12] However, one of the various patterns that can be seen on an abnormal perfusion scan is sufficiently specific to confirm the presence of embolism.[10–12] Ventilation scanning improves the diagnostic accuracy of perfusion scanning; the finding of a segmental or greater perfusion defect with ventilation mismatch (high probability scan) has greater than

90% positive predictive value for venous thromboembolism and in most instances obviates the need for further study.[10] The finding of an abnormal but not "high probability" scan is of insufficient predictive value, and further work-up is indicated.[10-12] Either venography of IPG is useful in this setting, since proximal lower extremity thrombophlebitis is the pathophysiologic precursor in most cases of pulmonary embolism and is usually treated in the same manner. Pulmonary angiography can be reserved for those cases in which the V/Q scan is abnormal but not diagnostic and venography or IPG yields normal results.[10]

TREATMENT OF THROMBOEMBOLIC DISEASE

Once it has been established that deep venous thrombosis or pulmonary embolism is present, intravenous heparin is the treatment of choice in most patients. The efficacy of heparin in the treatment of thromboembolic disease was established in the early 1960s when it was shown that heparin reduced both overall mortality in pulmonary embolism and the risk of recurrent embolization.[13] Whether or not heparin is effective in preventing permanent damage to the valves of the deep venous system or in preventing the post-phlebitic syndrome is unknown. Heparin exerts its anticoagulant activity by combining with its circulating cofactor antithrombin III (ATIII) and enhancing its ability to inhibit activated clotting Factors II, IX, X, XI, and XII, involved in the intrinsic and common coagulation pathways.[14] Heparin also has some activity in inhibiting platelet aggregation, and it may have a small amount of intrinsic fibrinolytic activity.[14] Therapy is initiated with an IV bolus of 5000–10,000 U, followed by a continuous intravenous infusion of 1000 ± 500 U/hour, adjusted so as to maintain the aPTT at 1.5–2.0 times the control value.[14] During the initial stages of acute thrombosis, substantially larger amounts of heparin may be required. A mild and inconsequential depression in the platelet count, probably owing to sequestration, is frequently seen following the initiation of heparin therapy.[14] A more profound reduction in the platelet count, probably on an immunologic basis, is associated with paradoxical thrombosis, most commonly of the arterial system. This complication is seen in several per cent of treated patients in some studies. It is recommended that heparin therapy be discontinued if the platelet count[14] falls below 100,000/mm^3. The optimum duration of intravenous heparin therapy is not well established, but traditionally the drug is administered for 7–14 days. The last several days of heparin therapy are used to initiate and stabilize oral Coumadin therapy so as to achieve and maintain a prothrombin time of 1.2–1.5 times control (using rabbit brain thromboplastin).[15] Oral warfarin therapy is continued for a period of 3–6 months, or indefinitely if there has been recurrent thromboembolism or if a significant risk factor for recurrence persists. In the setting of pregnancy or in other instances in which warfarin is contraindicated, adjusted-dose subcutaneous heparin is employed for 3–6 months or until delivery, at which time warfarin is substituted. Those patients who have an absolute contraindication to anticoagulation or who have documented recurrence of pulmonary embolism while adequately anticoagulated should be considered for plication of the inferior vena cava (IVC) or for placement of a filtering device in the IVC.

Thrombolytic Therapy in the Treatment of Thromboembolism

The rationale for the use of thrombolytic agents in the treatment of thromboembolic disease is based upon the theoretical consideration that fibrinolytic therapy will more rapidly normalize the hemodynamic disturbance associated with the thrombus or embolus as compared with conventional heparin therapy. Whether or not thrombolytic therapy prevents venous valvular damage and subsequent venous hypertension, or prevents permanent damage to the pulmonary vascular bed and reduces the incidence of persisting pulmonary hypertension, remains to be conclusively demonstrated. [16,17]

Currently, there are two thrombolytic agents approved by the FDA for use in the treatment of venous thromboembolism. Streptokinase, a protein first isolated from group C streptococci, is itself not an enzyme. Once administered, it forms a 1:1 stoichiometric complex with circulating plasminogen, forming a streptokinase-plasminogen activator complex. This activator complex enzymatically cleaves circulating free plasminogen to form plasmin, the major endogenous fibrinolytic enzyme. Thus a generalized fibrinolytic state is established in the circulation. The second agent, urokinase, itself is a proteolytic enzyme that acts directly to convert circulating plasminogen to plasmin. [18–20]

The administration of thrombolytic therapy necessitates admission of the patient to an ICU. Streptokinase is currently approved for treatment of both deep venous thrombosis and pulmonary embolism. The standard dosage involves a 250,000 U IV volus given over 30 minutes, followed by a continuous IV infusion of 100,000 U/hour. For the treatment of deep venous thrombosis, various experts have advocated a duration of therapy ranging from 12 to 72 or more hours. There is no conclusive evidence that longer periods of therapy provide a therapeutic advantage, and they may result in an increased complication rate. When streptokinase is used in the treatment of pulmonary embolism, a 24-hour infusion is recommended. Allergy is a common occurrence with streptokinase. Approximately 25% of patients will experience a febrile reaction, with the incidence of more serious reactions ranging from

2 to 18% in various studies. For this reason, premedication with corticosteroids and/or antihistamines is commonly employed.[16]

Urokinase is currently approved only for the treatment of pulmonary embolism. It is administered in a 4400 U/kg loading dose over 5 minutes, followed by a 2200 U/kg/hour infusion. It is substantially more expensive than streptokinase, but allergic reactions are rare.[16]

At the completion of the fibrinolytic infusion, the patient is switched to conventional heparin followed by warfarin therapy.

The issue of laboratory monitoring with fibrinolytic therapy is controversial. Prior to therapy, a baseline PT, aPTT, and platelet count should be obtained. A bleeding time is useful in detecting unsuspected pre-existing hemostatic defects. During therapy, the purpose of laboratory monitoring is simply to confirm the establishment of a lytic state. This can be accomplished by demonstrating a prolongation of the aPTT, although many investigators advocate following the thrombin time, the euglobulin lysis time, or the level of fibrin degradation products. Some authors have claimed that it is necessary to depress fibrinogen levels to less than 100 mg% in order to achieve effective thrombolysis, whereas others claim that fibrinogen levels less than 100 mg% are associated with excessive bleeding complications. Generally speaking, no laboratory parameter is felt to correlate with either bleeding risk or the probability of successful therapy.[16,17] Following the cessation of therapy, an aPTT is recommended to establish a baseline for subsequent anticoagulant therapy. Clinical experience has indicated that an inordinate number of bleeding complications occur during the interface between thrombolytic and anticoagulant therapy. For this reason, it is probably advisable to delay anticoagulation until the aPTT has returned to baseline.

One of the factors that has limited the use of thrombolytic agents in the treatment of thromboembolic disease is the difficulty in selecting patients who will benefit from therapy.[17] Absolute contraindications to therapy include active internal bleeding or recent (within 2 months) stroke or other active intracranial disease. Relative major contraindications include recent (within 10 days) major surgery, obstetrical delivery, organ biopsy or previous puncture of noncompressible vessels, recent serious gastrointestinal bleeding, recent serious trauma, and severe hypertension (systolic >200 mmHg or diastolic >110 mmHg). Relative minor contraindications include recent minor trauma (including cardiopulmonary resuscitation), high likelihood of left heart thrombus, bacterial endocarditis, hemostatic defects, pregnancy, age >75 years, and diabetic hemorrhagic retinopathy. Minimizing the complications of therapy involves careful patient selection, sound documentation of a valid indication, limiting venipuncture to the arms with the use of pressure dressings, avoidance of arterial punctures and puncturing uncompressible vessels, and limiting the concomitant use of drugs that may increase the risk of bleeding.[16,17]

The superiority of thrombolytic therapy over heparin in the treatment of deep venous thrombosis has not been conclusively proved. A pooled analysis[21] of the available randomized, controlled studies revealed that streptokinase was 3.7 times more likely than heparin to achieve significant thrombolysis in the deep veins, as judged by venography (p<.0001).[21] However, this result was achieved at a cost of a 2.9-fold increase in the risk of serious hemorrhage (p = .04). This analysis was limited by much variability in the treatment protocols used in the various studies. The results of various nonrandomized studies all support a marked superiority of streptokinase. The results of studies that attempted to address the question indicate that significant thrombolysis documented by phlebography can be expected in from 25 to 65% of patients treated with streptokinase, and in a substantially smaller proportion of those treated with heparin. Significant thrombolysis appears to be more likely if the duration of symptoms is less than 72 hours at the time of presentation. Little information is available regarding long-term effects; however, a few studies have suggested that streptokinase is more effective than heparin in preventing post-phlebitic syndrome. There are no data available that conclusively show that streptokinase preserves venous valvular integrity to a greater extent than heparin.

The use of thrombolytic agents in the treatment of pulmonary embolism has been more adequately studied. In the Urokinase Pulmonary Embolism Trial (UPET)[22] 160 patients were randomized to treatment with either urokinase or heparin. In phase II of the study, the Urokinase-Streptokinase Pulmonary Embolism Trial (USPET),[23] 167 patients were randomized to treatment with 12 or 24 hours of urokinase or to 24 hours of streptokinase. All patients underwent pulmonary angiography to establish the diagnosis and had right heart catheterization for monitoring. It was required that patients had a clinical event that suggested that embolization had taken place within 5 days of enrollment. The effects of therapy were assessed by serial pulmonary angiograms and by following hemodynamic parameters.

The results of the phase I trial indicated that patients treated with urokinase achieved a significantly greater degree of clot lysis than heparin-treated patients when assessed at 24 hours by angiography. This difference was also apparent in those patients who underwent perfusion lung scanning. Similarly, a significant difference between the two groups was seen in pulmonary artery pressures but not in the arterio-venous oxygen difference or in the cardiac index. Analysis of a subgroup of patients with initial cardiac index less than 2.7 suggested a trend toward more marked improvement, but this failed to reach statistical significance. There was also a trend toward greater response in younger patients, those with larger emboli, and patients with underlying cardiorespiratory disorders. After 24 hours, the observed difference between the two groups began to diminish and was unappreciable at 5 days. This lack of difference in the angiographic picture persisted at follow-up at 1 year. There was no difference in mortality between the two groups.

In phase II, no significant difference was found between the treatment groups; however, when a subgroup of patients who met the criteria for massive pulmonary embolism (filling defects in two or more lobar arteries on the initial angiogram) were analyzed, 24 hours of urokinase was significantly better than 24 hours of streptokinase in mean per cent improvement of the perfusion defect on angiogram and in improvement in pulmonary artery pressures. The incidence of recurrence of pulmonary embolism was 19% in the heparin group and 15% in the urokinase group (NS).

The UPET and USPET trials were remarkable for the high incidence of bleeding complications in both study groups, occurring in 45% of the urokinase group and in 27% of the heparin group in phase I. The most common hemorrhagic complications were overt bleeding and unexplained falls in hematocrit. If bleeding occurring at the sites of invasive procedures were to be excluded, the incidence of bleeding complications in the two groups would be identical.

Based on these data, it is suggested that patients who are most likely to benefit from thrombolytic therapy are those with massive or submassive pulmonary embolism who demonstrate marked circulatory compromise, as well as those patients with significant pre-existing cardiopulmonary disorders. There is some evidence to suggest that the use of thrombolytic therapy may preserve the function of the pulmonary microvascular bed,[24] although it is currently unclear who is most likely to benefit in this regard.

Other Therapies

There have been case reports involving the use of tissue plasminogen activator in the treatment of massive pulmonary embolism.[25,26] Systematic studies are needed in order to demonstrate whether or not this relatively clot-specific thrombolytic agent will provide a clear advantage over currently available modalities.

Suction embolectomy has been advocated as an effective alternative therapy in those patients with large central emboli and with significant circulatory compromise. In this procedure, a suction cup–tipped catheter is introduced into the pulmonary artery via the central venous circulation and is used to extract accessible emboli.[27]

Emergency surgical embolectomy is still rarely used in patients with large central emboli and shock; however, the excessively high mortality rate associated with this procedure (50–75%) and the ready availability of less invasive therapies militate against the use of this treatment.

KEY FEATURES

I. Pathophysiology and clinical features
   A. The pathophysiology of venous thromboembolism involves stasis, endothelial injury, and hypercoagulability.
   B. Risk factors thus include bed rest and other causes of immobility, trauma, surgery and malignancy, estrogen use, and nephrotic syndrome, to name a few.
   C. The history and physical examination are unreliable in making the diagnosis of venous thromboembolism; thus, objective diagnostic testing is always indicated.

II. Evaluation
   A. Deep venous thrombosis
      1. A thorough history and physical examination should be performed, with emphasis placed on excluding other disease entities that may explain symptoms and obviate further consideration of DVT.
      2. Laboratory studies are selected to obtain an appropriate data base. Coagulation studies and a platelet count are mandatory for monitoring subsequent anticoagulant therapy.
      3. Venography remains the diagnostic reference standard for the diagnosis of DVT.
      4. Impedance plethysmography (IPG) represents a sensitive and relatively specific alternative for establishing the diagnosis of *proximal* thrombosis. It is insensitive to thrombus limited to the calf.
      5. ^{125}I-labeled fibrinogen scanning is very sensitive to fresh thrombus below the knee, although it lacks specificity. The clinical utility of this study has not been firmly established.
      6. Doppler ultrasound is another useful noninvasive modality, although its sensitivity and specificity are somewhat operator dependent.
   B. Pulmonary embolism
      1. A thorough history and physical examination should be completed, with attention paid to ruling out other disease entities.
      2. A PA and a lateral chest radiograph should always be obtained; they are essential in interpreting subsequent studies and may suggest an alternative diagnosis.
      3. Arterial blood gas analysis is not useful diagnostically but is useful in guiding supplement O_2 therapy.
      4. ECG may reveal evidence of acute right ventricular strain with massive embolism.
      5. Pulmonary angiography is the diagnostic reference standard in pulmonary embolism; its relatively invasive nature makes it the modality of last resort in some patients.
      6. Perfusion lung scanning is relatively noninvasive and is extremely sensitive to the presence of pulmonary embolism. A negative scan virtually rules this out.
      7. Ventilation lung scanning improves the specificity of perfusion scanning. The finding of a segmental or greater perfusion

defect with ventilation mismatch is sufficiently diagnostic to justify treatment.
   8. A positive venogram or IPG is diagnostically useful in suspected pulmonary embolism.
   9. Pulmonary angiography can be reserved for those cases in which the V/Q scan is abnormal but nondiagnostic and the venogram or IPG yields normal results.
III. Treatment of thromboembolism
   A. Anticoagulant therapy
      1. Intravenous heparin is the treatment of choice in most patients with documented thromboembolism.
      2. Therapy with heparin is started with an initial IV bolus of 5000—10,000 U followed by a constant infusion of 1000 ± 500 U/hour, adjusted so as to maintain the aPTT at 1.5–2.0 times the control value.
      3. During the initial stages of acute thrombosis, substantially larger doses may be required.
      4. Profound thrombocytopenia associated with paradoxical arterial thrombosis is an occasional side effect of heparin therapy. Heparin should be discontinued if the platelet count falls below 100,000.
      5. Those patients who have or develop an absolute contraindication to anticoagulation should undergo interruption of the inferior vena cava.
      6. Heparin therapy is tradionally continued for 7–14 days (the optimum duration of therapy is yet to established) and is followed by 3–6 months of oral anticoagulation.
   B. Thrombolytic Therapy
      1. Streptokinase aand urokinase are currently the only two thrombolytics approved for use in thromboembolism. (Urokinase is approved only for treatment of pulmonary embolism.)
      2. Admission to an ICU is necessary.
      3. Patients being considered for therapy should be carefully screened for the presence of contraindications.
      4. Streptokinase is given in an initial 250,000 U IV bolus over 30 minutes, followed by an infusion of 100,000 U/hour.
      5. Urokinase is given in a 4400 U/kg loading dose over 5 minutes, followed by an infusion of 2200 U/kg/hour.
      6. The length of the infusion varies slightly, according to the indication, but is usually continued for 12–24 hours.
      7. Following thrombolytic therapy, conventional anticoagulant therapy is instituted after the aPTT returns to baseline.
      8. No laboratory parameter has been shown to correlate with either bleeding complications or successful thrombolysis.
      9. During therapy, laboratory monitoring should be used to confirm the establishment of a lytic state. The aPTT, TT, fibrinogen, and fibrin degradation products can all be used for this purpose.

698   MISCELLANEOUS DISORDERS

REFERENCES

1. Dalen JE, Alpert JS: Natural history of pulmonary embolism. Prog Cardiovasc Dis 17:259–270, 1975.
    A thorough review of the epidemiology and clinical course of pulmonary embolism. Contains some discussion of late complications.

2. Becker DM: Venous thromboembolism: Epidemiology, diagnosis, prevention. J General Intern Med 1(Nov/Dec): 1986.
    A useful review.

3. Colditz GA, Tuden RL, Oster G: Rates of venous thrombosis after general surgery: Combined results of randomised clinical trials. Lancet 2:143–146, 1986.
    Analysis of pooled studies comparing various methods of prophylactic antithrombotic regimens. Combined modalities were found to be more effective than any single modality. Combined use of gradient compression stockings and intermittent pneumatic compression appeared to achieve the best results.

4. Hull RD, Raskob GE, Hirsch J: Prophylaxis of venous thromboembolism—an overview. Chest 89(5):375S–383S, 1986.
    A review of prophylactic antithrombotic measures.

5. Hirsch J, Hull RD, Raskob GE: Epidemiology and pathogenesis of venous thrombosis. J Am Coll Cardiol 8:104B–113B, 1986.
6. Hirsch J, et al: Clinical features and diagnosis of venous thrombosis. J Am Coll Cardiol 8:114B–127B, 1986.
    A practical discussion of the identification of and the approach to patients with suspected thrombophlebitis.

7. Bell WR, Simon TL, et al: The clinical features of submassive and massive pulmonary emboli. Am J Med 62:355–360, 1977.
    A review of the common signs and symptoms of pulmonary embolism that emphasizes the nonspecificity of the presentation and the need for objective diagnostic testing.

8. Hull R, Hirsch J, et al: Diagnostic efficacy of impedance plethysmography for clinically suspected deep venous thrombosis: A randomized trial. Ann Intern Med 102:21–26, 1985.
9. Hull R, Hirsch J, et al: Replacement of venography in suspected venous thrombosis by impedance plethysmography and 125I fibrinogen scanning; a less invasive approach. Ann Intern Med 94:12–15, 1981.
    A prospective study of 322 patients in whom the combination of IPG and 125I-labeled fibrinogen scanning was compared with venogram. The results yielded a sensitivity of 90%, a specificity of 95%, and both positive and negative predictive values of 93% for IPG plus 125I scan as compared with venogram. These results were valid only if care was taken to exclude patients with conditions known to produce false positive results on either IPG or 125I scan.

10. Hirsch J, et al: Diagnosis of pulmonary embolism. JACC 8:128B–138B, 1986.
    A thorough review of the clinical features and diagnostic work-up of pulmonary embolism. The authors review their own previously published prospective data exploring the utility of ventilation-perfusion scanning as compared with other commonly employed modalities.

11. Hull RD, Hirsch J, et al: Pulmonary angiography, ventilation scanning and venography for clinically suspected pulmonary embolism with abnormal perfusion lung scan. Ann Intern Med 98:891–899, 1983.
    The first report of a randomized, prospective series of patients referred with a di-

agnosis of suspected pulmonary embolism. An attempt was made to obtain V/Q scan, pulmonary angiography, and venography on all patients enrolled. It was found that ventilation scanning increased the probability of detecting pulmonary embolism in patients with large perfusion defects and ventilation mismatch, but V/Q match was not helpful in ruling out pulmonary enbolism. The predictive value of small perfusion defects with mismatch was insufficient. It was concluded that pulmonary angiography in concert with venography was necessary in most patients.

12. Hull RD, Hirsch J, et al: Diagnostic value of ventilation-perfusion lung scanning in patients with suspected pulmonary embolism. Chest 88(6):819–828, 1985.

    The entire series of patients, including those previously published (see reference 20). A negative perfusion lung scan effectively rules out the diagnosis of pulmonary embolism, whereas only the finding of segmental or greater perfusion defects with ventilation mismatch was adequately predictive to allow a diagnosis to be made. Pulmonary angiography could not be performed in some patients, particularly those who were deemed too ill to undergo the procedure. The results of this study may not be applicable to this subset; however, the results indicate that the practice of using a low-probability V/Q scan to rule out pulmonary embolism is incorrect. Venography and IPG were found to be useful adjuncts in the work-up of suspected pulmonary embolism. The following table summarizes these findings:

Frequency of Pulmonary Embolism Associated with the Individual Ventilation-Perfusion Scan Patterns

Ventilation-Perfusion Scan Pattern	Frequency of Pulmonary Embolism
One or more segmental or greater defects	
Mismatch	51 of 59 (86%)
Match	10 of 28 (36%)
One or more subsegmental defects	
Mismatch	16 of 40 (40%)
Match	6 of 24 (25%)
Intermediate	5 of 24 (21%)

13. Barritt DW, Jordan SC: Anticoagulant drugs in the treatment of pulmonary embolism: A controlled trial. Lancet 1:1309–1312, 1960.

    An early study that demonstrated the clear reduction in mortality associated with the use of anticoagulation in the treatment of pulmonary embolism.

14. Wessler S, Gitel S: Pharmacology of heparin and warfarin. Am J Coll Cardiol 8:10B–20B, 1986.

    A thorough and useful review of the mechanisms, indications, administration, monitoring, and side effects of heparin and warfarin.

15. Hyers TM, Hull MB, Weg JG: Antithrombotic therapy for venous thromboembolic disease. Chest 89(2):27S–35S, 1986.

    A review of anticoagulant therapy, both prophylactic and therapeutic.

16. Marder VJ: The use of thrombolytic agents: Choice of patients, drug administration and laboratory monitoring. Ann Intern Med 90:802–808, 1979.

    A review of the clinical issues associated with the use of thrombolytic therapy in the treatment of thromboembolism, with emphasis on contraindications.

17. Thrombolytic therapy in thrombosis: A National Institutes of Health consensus development conference. Ann Intern Med 93:141–144, 1980.

18. Verstraete M, Collen D: Pharmacology of thrombolytic drugs. J Am Coll Cardiol 8:33B–40B, 1986.
19. Verstraete M, Collen D: Thrombolytic therapy in the eighties. Blood 67(6):1529–1541, 1986.
    References 17–19 represent comprehensive reviews of thrombolytic therapy.

20. Hessel LW, Kluft C: Advances in clinical fibrinolysis. Clin Hematol 15(2):443–463, 1986.
21. Goldhaber SZ, Buring JE, et al: Pooled analyses of randomized trials of streptokinase and heparin in phlebographically documented acute deep venous thrombosis. Am J Med 76:393–397, 1984.
    Analysis of pooled selected randomized controlled studies comparing streptokinase to heparin in the treatment of DVT. The relative risk of thrombolysis was 3.7 with streptokinase, while the relative risk of serious bleeding was 2.9. The authors discuss the shorcomings of their analysis.

22. Urokinase Pulmonary Embolism Trial Study Group: Urokinase pulmonary embolism trial (phase I results): A cooperative study. JAMA 214(12):2163–2172, 1970.
23. Urokinase Pulmonary Embolism Trial Study Group: Urokinase pulmonary embolism trial (phase II results): A cooperative study. JAMA 229(12):1606–1613, 1974.
24. Sharma GVRK, et al: Effect of thrombolytic therapy on pulmonary capillary blood volume in patients with pulmonary embolism. N Engl J Med 303(15):842–845, 1980.
    An analysis of pulmonary capillary volume and diffusing capacity in a subgroup of patients of 40 patients from the urokinase pulmonary embolism trial, of whom 21 received thrombolytic therapy and 19 received heparin alone. Pulmonary capillary volume was abnormally low in the heparin group, both at two weeks and one year, as compared with the thrombolytic group, which had normal values at both points. In addition, there were significant differences in the diffusing capacity: at two weeks 69% vs. 85%, and at one year 72% vs. 93% of predicted values for heparin and thrombolytics, respectively. It was postulated that thrombolytic therapy might exert this effect by either clearing small peripheral emboli more effectively or by more effectively dealing with peripheral thrombi and thus preventing recurrent embolic events. It is suggested by the authors that this might have important implications for patients with preexisting cardiopulmonary disease, which deserves further study (see also references 22 and 23).

25. Bounameaux H, et al: Thombolytic treatment with recombinant tissue-type plasminogen activator in a patient with massive pulmonary embolism. Ann Intern Med 103(1):64–65, 1985.
26. Goldhaber SZ, Markis JE, et al: Acute pulmonary embolism treated with tissue plasminogen activator. Lancet 2:886–889, 1986.
27. Greenfield LJ, Zocco JJ: Intraluminal management of acute massive pulmonary embolism. J Thorac Cardiovasc Surg 77:402–410, 1979.

Index

Note: Page numbers in *italics* indicate illustrations; those
followed by t indicate tables.

701

Pain *(Continued)*
  elbow, 591–593
  foot, 593
  hand and forearm, 593
  headache, 443–445. See also *Headache.*
  in cancer, management of, 280–284
  in pelvic inflammatory disease, 353, 354
  in peptic ulcer disease, 181
  in sickle cell anemia, 236–238, 237t
  in spinal cord compression, 514
  in synovitis vs. soft tissue rheumatism, 590
  low back, acute, 596–599
  lower extremity, 593
  neuropathic, in cancer, 283
  physiology of, 281
  shoulder, 591–592
  transcutaneous electrical nerve stimulation for, 281, 284
Palindromic rheumatism, 586
Pancreatic abscess, in acute pancreatitis, 218
Pancreatic enzyme replacement, for chronic pancreatitis, 223
Pancreatic phlegmon, in acute pancreatitis, 218
Pancreatic pseudocyst, in acute pancreatitis, 218, 219
Pancreatitis, acute, 216–220
  alcoholic, acute, 217
    chronic, 221, 222
  chronic, 221–224
  gallstone, 217
    treatment of, 219–220
  idiopathic, 217
PaO$_2$, in acute respiratory failure, 550, 551
  in adult respiratory distress syndrome, 530–531
  in asthma, 546
Papilledema, and increased intracranial pressure, 446, 456
Para-aminosalicylic acid, for tuberculosis, 579, 581
  toxicity of, 581
Paradoxical thrombosis, in anticoagulation therapy, 691
Paraldehyde, and metabolic acidosis, 375
Paralysis, and spinal cord compression, 514–515
  differential diagnosis of, 486–487
  pharmacologic, for tetanus, 296, 297
Paralytic ileus, chemotherapy-induced, 231
Parapneumonic pleural effusion, 564–566
Parathyroid hormone, deficiency of, and hypocalcemia, 139–141
Paroxysmal atrial tachycardia, 71, 73, 76–77
Paroxysms, hypertensive, in pheochromocytoma, 175, 176

Partial thromboplastin time, prolonged, 261–265
Pathologic fractures, pain management for, 283
PEEP. See *Positive end-expiratory pressure.*
Pelvic inflammatory disease, 353–356
Penicillin, anaphylactic reaction to, 606–608
  for aspiration pneumonia, 541–542
  for brain abscess, 319
  for endocarditis, 307–308
  for meningitis/encephalitis, 313–314
  for pelvic inflammatory disease, 355t
  for septic arthritis, 620, 622
  for spontaneous bacterial peritonitis, 289
  for tetanus, 296
Pentamidine, for *P. carinii* pneumonia, in AIDS, 365–366, 366t
Peptic ulcer disease, 181–184, 188
Percutaneous nephrolithotomy, 413
Percutaneous pleural biopsy, 564
Perfusion lung scanning, for pulmonary embolism, 690
Pericardial effusion, and cardiac tamponade, 82
  and pericarditis, 81–82
  causes of, 81
  diagnosis of, 82, 83
  pericardiocentesis for, 84, 85
Pericardial friction rub, 82
  in myocardial infarction, 7
Pericardial tamponade. See *Cardiac tamponade.*
Pericardiocentesis, 84, 85
Pericarditis, acute, 81–86
  clinical presentation of, 82
  diagnosis of, 83–84
  pathophysiology of, 81–82
  physical examination in, 82–83
  treatment of, 84–85
  viral, vs. myocardial infarction, 7
  vs. myocardial infarction, 82, 83
Pericardium, anatomy of, 81
Peridiverticulitis, 209
Perilymphatic fisutla, and vertigo, 475, 479
Periodontal disease, and aspiration pneumonia, 537, 538
Peripheral neuropathy, and isoniazid, 580
Peripheral vestibular dysfunction, vs. transient ischemic attacks, 425
Peritoneal dialysis, complications of, 418
  in acute renal failure, 388–389
  in chronic renal failure, 418, 418t
  in salicylate poisoning, 646
Peritoneal lavage, in acute pancreatitis, 219
Peritonitis, spontaneous bacterial, 287–291
Peroneal nerve compression, 593

Perphenazine, as chemotherapy antiemetic, 230
Phalen's maneuver, 593
Phenobarbitol, for ethanol withdrawal syndrome, 683, 685
Phenothiazines, toxicity of, 230
Phenoxybenzamine, for pheochromocytoma, 176
Phentolamine, for malignant hypertension, 118
  for pheochromocytoma, 176
Phenylephrine, for acute sinusitis, 344
  for shock, 106
Phenytoin, blood level of, isoniazid and, for tuberculosis, 580
  for ethanol withdrawal syndrome, 683
Pheochromocytoma, 175–178
Phlebitis, vs. Baker's cyst, 602
Phlebotomy, for chronic obstructive pulmonary disease, 553
  for pulmonary edema, 44
Phosphasoda, for hypophosphatemia, 145
Phosphates, intravenous, for hypercalcemia, 138, 139
Phosphodiesterase inhibitors, for propranolol overdose, 651
  toxicity of, 654–656
Phosphorus, deficiency of, 143–146
Physostigmine, for tricyclic antidepressant overdosage, 626
Pituitary, disorders of, 121–131
  and antidiuretic hormone secretion, 123–130
    key features of, 130–131
    vascular aspects of, 121–123
  postpartum necrosis of, 122–123, 130
  transsphenoidal microsurgery of, for Cushing's syndrome, 172
Pituitary apoplexy, 121–122, 130
  coma in, 494
Pituitary Cushing's syndrome, 168. See also Cushing's syndrome.
Plasma, fresh frozen. See Transfusion.
Plasmapheresis, for hyperviscosity syndrome, 269
  in Guillain-Barré syndrome, 488
  in myasthenia gravis, 469, 470
Plasmodium falciparum, 357–361
Platelet(s), decreased, in heparin therapy, 691
  in thrombocytopenia, 254–259
Platelet transfusion, and purpura, 257
  in disseminated intravascular coagulation, 250
  in thrombocytopenia, 257–258
Platelet washout, in blood transfusion, 277

Plethysmography, impedance, in thromboembolic disease, 689–691
Pleura, anatomy of, 561
Pleural biopsy, percutaneous, 564
Pleural calcification, 568
Pleural disease, 561–570
  and empyema, 564–565
  biopsy in, 564
  pathology of, 561–563
  types of, 564–570
Pleural effusion, biochemical composition of, 563
  cellular content of, 562–563
  chylous, 566
  culture of, 563
  exudative, 562
  parapneumonic, 564–566
  pseudochylous, 566
  transudative, 562
  tuberculous, 563, 575–576
    vs. malignant, 563
Pleural metastasis, 563, 568, 570
Pleural tuberculosis, 575–576
Pneumococcal sepsis, in sickle cell anemia, 237t, 239
Pneumocystis carinii pneumonia, in AIDS, 363, 365, 366t, 367
Pneumonia, 320–325
  aspiration, 321, 333. See also Aspiration syndromes.
  atypical, 321
  and Legionnaires' disease, 328
  in AIDS, 363, 365, 366t
  Legionnaires', 327–331
  necrotizing, 538–539
  pleural effusion in, 564–566
Pneumothorax, 566–567, 569
Poisoning, acetaminophen, 629–631
  and acute confusional states, 501t
  antifreeze, 632–635
  beta blocker, 649–652
  carbon monoxide, 571–573
  cocaine, 657–661
  ethylene glycol, 632–635
  from chemical fumes, 571–572, 573t
  isopropyl alcohol, 632–635
  methanol, 632–635
  propranolol, 649–652
  salicylate, 642–647
  theophylline, 654–656
  tricyclic antidepressant, 625–627, 628t
Poliomyelitis, vs. Guillain-Barré syndrome, 486–487
Polyarticular arthritis, acute, 585–588
  chronic, 588

DATE DUE

MAY 1 0 1992			
APR 1 2 1992			
GAYLORD			PRINTED IN U.S.A.